Children's Speech Sound Disorders

Children's Speech Sound Disorders

THIRD EDITION

Caroline Bowen, AM PhD CPSP
Speech-Language Pathologist
Senior Honorary Research Fellow in Linguistics, Macquarie University,
Sydney, Australia
Honorary Research Fellow, School of Health Sciences, Speech-Language Pathology,
University of KwaZulu-Natal, Durban, South Africa
Adjunct Fellow, Graduate School of Health, University of Technology, Sydney, Australia

WILEY Blackwell

Registered Offices
John Wiley & Sons, Inc., 111 River Street, Hoboken, NJ 07030, USA
John Wiley & Sons Ltd, The Atrium, Southern Gate, Chichester, West Sussex, PO19 8SQ, UK

For details of our global editorial offices, customer services, and more information about Wiley products visit us at www.wiley.com.

Wiley also publishes its books in a variety of electronic formats and by print-on-demand. Some content that appears in standard print versions of this book may not be available in other formats.

Library of Congress Cataloging-in-Publication Data

Names: Bowen, Caroline, editor.
Title: Children's speech sound disorders, 3rd edition / Dr. Caroline Bowen.
Description: Third edition. | Hoboken, NJ : John Wiley & Sons, 2023. | Includes bibliographical references and index.
Identifiers: LCCN 2023017899 | ISBN 9781119743118 (paperback) | ISBN 9781119743163 (epub) | ISBN 9781119743149 (adobe pdf)
Subjects: LCSH: Speech disorders in children.
Classification: LCC RJ496.S7 B69 2023 | DDC 618.92/855--dc23/eng/20230428
LC record available at https://lccn.loc.gov/2023017899

Cover Image: © Gary Radler Photography
Cover Design: Wiley

Set in 9.5/12pt TimesLTStd Integra Software Services Pvt. Ltd, Pondicherry, India

Dedication

To my 2020–2023 officemate and sunrise barista, Don; my four Wiley Managing Editors: Louise Barnetson, Jenny Seward, Anne Hunt, and Vallikkannu Narayanan; my Content Refinement Specialist Purushothaman Govindhasamy, and my contributors. I'm thankful to have been stuck at home with him; to have been gently encouraged by them; and to have journeyed to inspiring places of the mind with the great 58.

Contents

Acknowledgement of Country

I acknowledge the diverse people of the Dharug Nation upon whose ancestral lands this book was conceived and written. I pay respect to their Elders past, present and emerging, recognising them as the traditional custodians of knowledge for this place. I understand that the health, social, and emotional well-being of Aboriginal and Torres Strait Islander peoples are grounded in the deep and continuing connection to culture, country, waters, language, and community, and I am sorry that sovereignty was never ceded.

Contributors

Kristen Allison, PhD
Assistant Professor
Department of Communication Sciences & Disorders
Bouvé College of Health Sciences
Northeastern University
Boston, MA
USA

Areej Asad, PhD
Speech Language Therapist and Postdoctoral
    Research Fellow
Section of Audiology
School of Population Health
Faculty of Medical and Health Sciences
The University of Auckland
Auckland
New Zealand

Elise Baker, PhD
Conjoint Associate Professor Allied Health School
    of Health Sciences, Western Sydney University
    Southwestern Sydney Local Health District
    Campbelltown, NSW Australia

Martin J. Ball, PhD
Honorary Professor of Linguistics
School of Languages, Literatures, Linguistics and
    Media
Bangor University
Bangor
Wales

Barbara May Bernhardt, PhD
Professor Emerita
School of Audiology and Speech Sciences
University of British Columbia
Vancouver, BC
Canada

Daniel Bérubé, PhD
Assistant Professor of Speech-Language
    Pathology
Faculté des sciences de la santé
Université d'Ottawa
Ottawa, ON
Canada

James Robert Bitter, EdD
Professor
Department of Counseling and Human Services
East Tennessee State University
Box 70701
Johnson City, TN
USA

Kenneth M. Bleile, PhD
Professor
Department of Communication Sciences and
    Disorders
University of Northern Iowa
Cedar Falls, IA
USA

Nicole Caballero, MS
Speech-Language Pathologist
Department of Communication Sciences and
    Disorders
Syracuse University
Syracuse, NY
USA

Joanne Cleland, PhD
Reader in Speech and Language Therapy
University of Strathclyde
Glasgow
Scotland

Kathryn Crowe, PhD
Adjunct Research Fellow
Charles Sturt University
Bathurst, NSW
Australia
Postdoctoral Researcher
University of Iceland / Háskóli Íslands
Reykjavík
Iceland

Barbara Dodd, PhD
Honorary Professorial Fellow
Department Audiology and Speech Pathology
The University of Melbourne
Melbourne, VIC
Australia

Liz Fairgray, MSc
Speech-Language Therapist and Auditory Verbal
    Therapist
Listening and Language Clinic
Discipline of Speech Science
School of Psychology
Faculty of Science
The University of Auckland
Auckland
New Zealand

Peter Flipsen Jr., PhD
Professor of Speech Pathology
School of Communication Sciences and Disorders
Pacific University
Forest Grove, OR
USA

Silke Fricke, PhD
Senior Lecturer
Health Sciences School, Division of Human
    Communication Sciences
The University of Sheffield
Sheffield
UK

Karen Froud, PhD
Associate Professor of Neuroscience & Education
Director, Neurocognition of Language Laboratory
Department of Biobehavioral Sciences
Teachers College
Columbia University
New York, NY
USA

Brian A. Goldstein, PhD
Chief Academic Officer
Executive Dean, College of Rehabilitative
    Sciences
University of St. Augustine for Health Sciences
San Marcos, CA
USA

Barbara W. Hodson, PhD
Professor Emeritus
Communication Sciences and Disorders
Wichita State University
Wichita, KS
USA

David Ingram, PhD
Professor in Speech and Hearing
Department of Speech and Hearing Science
Arizona State University
Tempe, AZ
USA

Deborah G. H. James, PhD
Associate Professor
Course Chair and Head of Speech Pathology
College of Health and Biomedicine
Victoria University
Melbourne, VIC
Australia

Victoria Joffe, DPhil
Dean, School of Health and Social Care
Professor, Speech and Language Therapy
School of Health and Social Care
The University of Essex
UK

Breanna I. Krueger, PhD
Assistant Professor
Division of Communication Disorders
University of Wyoming, WY
USA

Gregory L. Lof, PhD
Professor Emeritus
Department of Communication Sciences and
    Disorders
School of Health and Rehabilitation Sciences
MGH Institute of Health Professions
Boston, MA
USA

Lesley C. Magnus, PhD
Professor
Department of Communication Disorders
Memorial Hall 104K
Minot State University
500 University Ave W
Minot, ND
USA

Glenda Mason, PhD
Lecturer
School of Audiology and Speech Sciences
University of British Columbia
Vancouver, BC
Canada

Patricia McCabe, PhD
Professor of Speech Pathology
Discipline of Speech Pathology
Sydney School of Health Sciences
The University of Sydney
Sydney, NSW
Australia

Rebecca J. McCauley, PhD
Professor
Department of Speech and Hearing Science
The Ohio State University
Columbus, OH
USA

Karen Leigh McComas, EdD
Professor of Communication Disorders
Executive Director Center for Teaching and
    Learning
Marshall University
Huntington, WV
USA

Sharynne McLeod, PhD
Professor of Speech and Language Acquisition
Charles Sturt University
Bathurst, NSW
Australia

Brigid C. McNeill, PhD
Professor
University of Canterbury
Christchurch
New Zealand

Adele Miccio, PhD (1959–2009)
Professor of Communication Sciences and
    Disorders and Applied Linguistics
Co-Director of the Center for Language Science
Pennsylvania State University
University Park, PA
USA

Nicole Müller, DPhil
Professor Speech & Hearing Sciences
University College Cork
Cork
Ireland

Benjamin Munson
Professor and Chair
Department of Speech-Language-
    Hearing Sciences
University of Minnesota
Minneapolis, MN
USA

Roslyn Neilson, PhD
Speech-Language Pathologist
Language, Speech and Literacy Services
Jamberoo, NSW
Australia

Megan Overby, PhD
Associate Professor (retired)
Department of Speech-Language Pathology
Duquesne University
Pittsburgh, PA
USA

Michelle Pascoe, PhD
Associate Professor
Division of Communication Sciences and
    Disorders
University of Cape Town
South Africa

Lindsay Pennington, PhD
Reader in Communication Disorders
Population Health Sciences Institute
Faculty of Medical Sciences
Newcastle University
UK

Karen E. Pollock, PhD
Professor
Department of Communication Sciences and
    Disorders
University of Alberta
Edmonton, AB
Canada

Raul F. Prezas, PhD
Professor
Department of Speech-Language Pathology
Dr. Pallavi Patel College of Health Care Sciences
Health Professions Division
Nova Southeastern University
Davie, FL
USA

Suzanne C. Purdy, PhD
Professor and Head
School of Psychology
Faculty of Science
The University of Auckland
Auckland
New Zealand

Melissa Randazzo, PhD
Assistant Professor
Department of Communication Sciences &
    Disorders
Adelphi University
Garden City, New York, NY
USA

Dennis M. Ruscello, PhD
Professor Emeritus
Department of Communication Sciences and Disorders
West Virginia University
Morgantown, WV
USA

Susan Rvachew, PhD
Associate Dean and Director
School of Communication Sciences and Disorders
Faculty of Medicine and Health Sciences
McGill University
Montréal, QC
Canada

Blanca Schäfer, PhD
Speech and Language Therapist
Frankfurt
Germany

James M. Scobbie, PhD
Professor of Speech Sciences
Queen Margaret University
Edinburgh
Scotland

Amy E. Skinder-Meredith, PhD
Clinical Professor
Department of Speech and Hearing Sciences
Washington State University
Spokane, WA
USA

Ruth Stoeckel, PhD
Clinical Speech-Language Pathologist
Mayo Clinic (retired)
Rochester, MN
USA

Carol Stoel-Gammon, PhD
Professor Emerita
Department of Speech and Hearing Sciences
University of Washington
Seattle, WA
USA

Edythe A. Strand, PhD
Emeritus Professor of Speech Pathology: Mayo
    College of Medicine
Emeritus Consultant, Department of Neurology:
Mayo Clinic
Rochester, MN
USA

Holly Teagle, AuD
Associate Professor
Section of Audiology
School of Population Health
Faculty of Medical and Health Sciences
The University of Auckland
Auckland
New Zealand

Donna Thomas, PhD
Lecturer
Discipline of Speech Pathology, Faculty of
    Medicine and Health
The University of Sydney
Sydney, NSW
Australia

Alayo Tripp, PhD
Postdoctoral Researcher
Department of Speech-Language-Hearing Sciences
University of Minnesota
Minneapolis, MN
USA

Rebecca Waring, PhD
Lecturer in Speech Pathology Department of
    Audiology & Speech Pathology University of
    Melbourne, VIC
Australia

A. Lynn Williams, PhD
Associate Dean and Professor
Department of Audiology and Speech-Language
    Pathology
College of Clinical and Rehabilitative Health
    Sciences
East Tennessee State University
Johnson City, TN
USA

Pamela Williams, PhD
Honorary lecturer
University College London Hospitals NHS
    Foundation Trust
Royal National ENT Hospital Administrative Base
London
UK

Krisztina Zajdó, PhD
Associate Professor
Department of Special Education/Speech-
    Language Pathology
Széchenyi István University/University of Győr
Győr
Hungary

Part I
A Practical Update

Introduction to Part I

The first two editions of *Children's Speech Sound Disorders* appeared six years apart (Bowen 2009; 2015a) and a further eight-to-nine years of robust research enquiry and publications have amassed to inform the third edition. Once again, the aim of this 2024 work is to provide an accessible, theoretically sound, evidence driven textbook on child speech for a wide readership. Most readers will be academics, clinical educators, clinicians, and undergraduate, graduate, and doctoral students in speech–language pathology/speech and language therapy (SLP/SLT), with a smattering of family members of children with speech sound disorders (SSD). They will be located where English is spoken as a first or additional language; and where SLP/SLT services are delivered in English—in-person and via telepractice—in expat networks and communities, international schools, and other multilingual settings.

New in This Edition

19 New Authors

The new authors here, some writing in conjunction with previous contributors—shown in parentheses—are: Kristen Allison, Daniel Bérubé and Glenda Mason (with Barbara May Bernhardt), Kathryn Crowe (with Sharynne McLeod), Breanna Krueger, Lindsay Pennington, Raul F. Prezas and Lesley C. Magnus (with Barbara W. Hodson), Melissa Randazzo (with Karen Froud), Brigid McNeill, Blanca Schäfer and Silke Fricke, Holly Teagle (with Areej Asad, Liz Fairgray and Suzanne C. Purdy), James Scobbie and Joanne Cleland, Donna Thomas and Nicole F. Caballero (with Pam Williams), Alayo Tripp (with Benjamin Munson), and Rebecca Waring (with Barbara Dodd).

Children's Speech Sound Disorders, Third Edition. Caroline Bowen.
© 2023 John Wiley & Sons Ltd. Published 2023 by John Wiley & Sons Ltd.

23 New Topics

The new topics are: Application of constraint-based nonlinear phonology across languages (Barbara May Bernhardt, Daniel Bérubé and Glenda Mason, A45); Applying crosslinguistic research evidence to debunk unhelpful myths about speech acquisition (Krisztina Zajdó, A43); Clinical decision-making as a dynamic process (Ruth Stoeckel, A25); Crosslinguistic knowledge about children's speech acquisition (Sharynne McLeod and Katherine Crowe, A42); Ethical issues in evidence based clinical decision-making (Suze Leitão, A1); Executive function in speech sound disorder (Rebecca Waring and Barbara Dodd, A6); Facilitating phonological awareness development in children with speech sound disorders (Brigid McNeill, A22); Implementing interventions with optimal fidelity (Elise Baker, A26); Improving speech intelligibility in developmental dysarthria (Lindsay Pennington, A30); Lifelong speech and psychological consequences of Childhood Apraxia of Speech (Patricia McCabe, A34); Measuring speech intelligibility in children with motor speech disorders (Kristen Allison, A29); Phonemic placement and shaping in targeting fricatives and affricates (Kenneth Bleile, A36); Prompts that help children when picture naming (Deb James, A11); Putting teachers and SLPs/SLTs on the same page: Phonemic awareness and responding to students' errors (Roslyn Neilson, A49); Selecting treatment words for a complexity approach to phonological intervention (Breanna Krueger, A35); Social factors in phonological acquisition: Sociophonetics and social identification (Benjamin Munson and Alayo Tripp, A40); Speech perception and production in children with hearing loss: Assessment and management (Areej Asad, Liz Fairgray, Holly Teagle and Suzanne Purdy, A12); Syllable Repetition Test for differential diagnosis (Susan Rvachew, A9); Towards the development of speech assessments, normative data and interventions for children acquiring the languages of Southern Africa (Michelle Pascoe, A39); Telepractice in SSD: Application for assessment, treatment, training, and clinical education (Pam Williams, Donna Thomas and Nicole Caballero, A46); Visual biofeedback (VBF): Practical options for articulatory feedback in the speech clinic (Joanne Cleland and James Scobbie, A47); and, Why is /ɹ/ such a challenge for SLPs/SLTs? (Peter Flipsen Jr., A37).

The Structure of This Text

Maintaining an E^3BP focus (Dollaghan, 2007), this book is in two parts. Part I concerns theoretical and empirical developments since the previous edition, and leading earlier work in the classification, diagnosis and management of children affected by Speech Sound Disorder (SSD). Against this scientific backdrop, the emphasis in Part II is on the practicalities of day-to-day assessment and treatment of children for their SSD and associated issues.

The Author

I composed about two-thirds of the book, including the questions put to the 58 contributors who wrote the other third. I write from the perspective of a semiretired Australian speech-language pathologist with an international outlook, 42 years of clinical experience, a modest research output, close familiarity with our refereed literature and a commitment to both strong theory and ethical evidence-based practice or E^3BP (Dollaghan, 2007; Hoffman et al., 2017; Leitão, A1).

As a professional, committed to, but only moderately successful in maintaining work–life balance, I am mindful of the time limitations, competing priorities, and other barriers that make it hard for clinicians to access research literature relating to child speech as regularly as they would wish; to synthesize and integrate what they have read; and apply that knowledge in their work, with good fidelity (Baker, A26). These restrictions mean that clinically applicable information tends to remain in academe, often, but not inevitably refusing to cross the theory–therapy and research–practice gaps (see Froud & Randazzo, A51 for an optimistic view of this). Speaking clinician-to-clinician, clinician-to-researcher, and researcher-to-clinician, this edition sets out once again with the aspirational goal of making critical theory-to-evidence-to-practice connections plain.

It has been my privilege, since 2005, to present invited Continuing Professional Development (CPD) events on children's speech in Australia, Canada, Denmark, Éire, England, Hong Kong, Iceland, India, Indonesia, Malaysia, New Zealand, Northern Ireland, Norway, Pakistan, the Philippines, Portugal, Scotland, Singapore, South Africa, Turkey, the United Arab Emirates, and the US. All travel plans stopped abruptly in March 2020 when intended visits to, Kuwait, Kuala Lumpur and Penang in Malaysia, Mexico, New Zealand, Pakistan, Singapore, Vietnam, and Western Australia rescheduled more than once and then postponed indefinitely or cancelled due to the COVID-19 pandemic.

The Contributors and Their Contributions

Meanwhile, the 58 contributors to this book—distributed across 11 countries: Australia, Canada, Éire, England, Hungary, Iceland, New Zealand, Northern Ireland, Scotland, South Africa, and the US—also experienced the hard-hitting consequences of the pandemic (Kearns et al., 2021) as they wrote. Many of them are mentioned above, and the others—all previous contributors and familiar names in our field—are:

> *James Robert Bitter, Karen Golding-Kushner, Brian Goldstein, Victoria Joffe, Gregory L. Lof, Rebecca J. McCauley, Karen Leigh McComas, Adele W. Miccio (d), Nicole Müller and Martin J. Ball, Megan Overby, Karen E. Pollock, Dennis M. Ruscello, Amy E. Skinder-Meredith, Carol Stoel-Gammon, and Edythe A. Strand.*

The Contributors: My Questions and Their Answers

The uniqueness of this text lies not only in the trying circumstances the authors weathered, but also in the relevance to clinical practice of their 51 expert essays, each about 2000 words in length. The authors are nationally and internationally respected academicians, clinicians, and researchers, representing the fields of audiology, clinical phonetics (Ball, 2021) and clinical phonology, (Ball, 2016; Ball et al., 2010; Grunwell, 1987): other branches of linguistics; family therapy (Bitter, 2021) and the history and development of SLP/SLT clinical and research practice (Armstrong et al., 2017; Duchan & Felsenfeld, 2021; Stansfield, 2020). Some are widely published, and their names are prominent in our field; others are early-career researchers and rising stars.

Their pertinent, reader-friendly essays numbered A1–to—A51 are responses to a question or questions numbered Q1–to—Q51 about major areas of their work and how they relate to theoretically sound, evidence based SLP/SLT practice. The questions are not entirely my own. Most are built on queries and discussion in social media. e.g., to my Twitter handle @speechwoman and to www.facebook.com/groups/E3BPforSSD, and in CPD, ProD, or 'training' events and conference talks. Note that while my Twitter identity remains, I can be found in social media at https://lingo.lol/web/@CarolineBowen which is SLP/SLT related, and https://nerdculture.de/@speechwoman which is more eclectic.

The first two essays are here in the introduction to Part I, with two SLPs focusing on the fundamentals of best practice. Responding to Q1, in A1, Suze Leitão considers the ethical issues that arise in the process of evidence based clinical decision-making. Then, in A2, Sharynne McLeod writes about the advantages of using the World Health Organization (2021) *International Classification of Functioning, Disability and Health—Children and Youth* (ICF-CY) in our work, and honouring the ethical principles embedded in the *Universal Declaration of Human Rights* (UDHR: https://www.un.org/en/about-us/universal-declaration-of-human-rights in our engagement with clients, colleagues, and the community. A related essay, A3, is in Chapter 1 where Nicole Müller and Martin Ball explain the use, impact, and importance of linguistic sciences to SLP/SLT education, scholarship, and accountable clinical practice as the 'theoretical backbone' of the work we do.

The contributors' task was complex. It is a big thing, even for an expert, to capture central aspects of a major body of work in a few approachable and well-considered paragraphs, and all the authors delivered skilfully. Their straight answers provide quick, readable, and sufficiently detailed information for busy colleagues. The references they cite provide helpful leads to journal articles linked with

Digital Object Identifiers (DOIs), books, and other readings for those seeking more information.

URLs, DOIs, and Link Shorteners

The technical names for a clickable electronic **link** that allows internet users to 'go' from one place on the internet to another are **hyperlink** and **Uniform Resource Locator** (URL). Two handy types of URL are the DOI® (**Digital Object Identifier**) and the PMID (**PubMed Reference Number**). The style guide used in writing this book was the 7th edition of the *Publication Manual of the American Psychological Association*: American Psychological Association (2020) which advises using the DOI System (International DOI® Foundation [IDF], 2019). A DOI is a unique alphanumeric string, used to identify content and provide a persistent link to its internet location. DOIs are found in database records and the reference lists of published works. A DOI assigned to an article increases its visibility and accessibility. Rather than expressing a DOI as an unlinked number (e.g., doi:10.1000/123123) the current APA format presents DOIs as direct URLs such as the fictional https://doi.org/10.123123 where '10.123456' refers to the DOI number. This: https://doi.org/10.1136/bmj.1.4852.8 is a real DOI that links to the openly accessible 1954 article by Morley, Court and Miller that introduced the term developmental dysarthria (Morley et al., 1954). By including DOIs in this work, readers of digital editions can click through to research evidence of interest.

Unduly long DOIs may be shortened using the IDF's **link shortener**: https://shortdoi.org Because a work can only have one link and one shortened link, the software will create a short DOI for a DOI that has never had one or retrieve the short DOI of one that has.

URLs are allotted to selected content that is available online (e.g., links to pdfs), but which have no DOIs. Note that some resources may have both.

Pseudonyms

The book is peppered with illustrative examples of real children with SSD, used with their parents' permission and where possible with the children's permission too. Except for Aaliyah, Gerri, Luke, Madison, and Shaun (who said, '*I want them to know it's me*'), the children and their family members, SLPs/SLTs and teachers have pseudonyms and details have been anonymized where necessary. Many of the children chose their aliases, but slight persuasion was needed to reduce doubling-up of names from children's media: e.g., Belle (Beauty and the Beast), Elsa of Arendelle (Frozen), Harry (Potter), Jack Sparrow (Pirates of the Caribbean), and Moana Walaliki (Moana).

Evidence and Evidence-based Practice (EBP)

In discussions of Evidence-Based Practice (e.g., Ash et al., 2020; Greenwell & Walsh, 2021; Higginbotham & Satchidanand, 2019) connections between clients and practitioners, good science, academic curiosity, and clinical thinking are in constant focus. Reflecting on the multidimensional nature of EBP, I put Q1 to Suze Leitão.

Dr. Suze Leitão, a Life-Member of Speech Pathology Australia (SPA), has a long-standing clinical and research interest in children with speech, language, and literacy difficulties. She is an Associate Professor teaching into the speech pathology course in the Curtin School of Allied Health in Western Australia and holds a position as the Director of Graduate Research. She was the national Chair of the SPA Ethics Board from 2010 to 2019. Her current program of research is around investigating disorders of speech, language, and literacy, developing the evidence base for assessments and interventions, and supporting the mental health of children and adolescents with Developmental Language Disorder (DLD) and Dyslexia. In recent years, her teaching in the areas of ethics and professional issues and clinical decision making has caused her to reflect on the mix of art and science involved in clinical decision-making.

Q1.   Suze Leitão: Ethics, Evidence, and Intervention for Clients with SSD

Ethical issues arise for clinicians when assessing, treating, and discharging clients with speech sound disorders as we endeavour to draw on the evidence base. These include relegating treatment to non-SLPs, taking (or not taking) fidelity and practicability into account when selecting an intervention and intervention targets, waiting lists, cherry-picking intervention techniques, incorporating non-EBP methods into clients' programs, and talking to clients openly about Evidence-Based Practice (EBP). Evidence is more than research. Although critical consumption of research is foundational to ethical and evidence-based practice, we need to consider the other fundamental contributors of client factors, clinician factors and workplace factors. How do clinicians navigate this increasingly complicated world while operating within an ethical and professional framework?

A1.   Suze Leitão: Ethical Issues in Evidence Based Clinical Decision-making

Evidence-based clinical decision-making sounds like an easy and ethical framework to apply to guide our professional practice with clients with speech sound disorders. Well, yes…and no.

While there is no doubt that evidence-based practice (EBP) is our professional and ethical responsibility—and it is indeed a very useful 'guide'—we are often confronted with situations for which there is no easy 'answer'.

We can of course turn to the research literature to help us tackle tricky issues around selecting assessment protocols and treatment approaches, schedules, dosage, and targets that are theoretically informed and supported by well-designed treatment studies. But even here, when we do find clear guidelines, we need to consider the other contributions to EBP—in other words, client perspectives and values, clinician perspectives and expertise, as well as workplace contexts. The original notion of an evidence-based triangle with the three elements of research evidence, client values and preferences and clinical expertise, has, in many ways, grown as we now consider 4 perspectives as described by Hoffman et al. (2017), all of which drive our clinical reasoning in an integrated fashion, as shown in Figure A1.1.

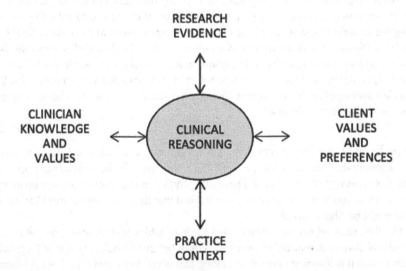

Figure A1.1 Evidence Based Practice as described by Hoffman et al., 2017 / Elsevier.

Now decision-making can start to get tricky as we walk the tightrope between maintaining fidelity to a researched treatment approach (the research evidence) with its implementation in the real-world lives of our clients, their families, and our workplaces (taking account of client values and preferences, clinician knowledge and values, as well as the practice context).

Let's say you have a child on your caseload with Childhood Apraxia of Speech (CAS) who is considered suitable for Rapid Syllable Transition treatment (ReST). You read and critique a key article and, following the evidence, you plan to deliver ReST 4 times per week in blocks of 12–15 sessions followed by a break of 6–8 weeks (Murray et al., 2015). However, this frequency of delivery carries a significant cost and time load for this family to attend a clinic that often. There is evidence that a minimum of twice a week is efficacious, but you know that overall, therapy is more effective with a greater treatment intensity (Namasivayam et al., 2015). A family's availability (and finances) may however preclude you from implementing any therapy at the recommended dosage—so how does this then impact on your confidence in the approach? How sure can you be of achieving the results as outlined in the research base? How do you reconcile the EBP evidence and real-world implementation? Perhaps you could consider supplementing your delivery with that of a non SLP/SLP—maybe a teaching assistant or family member. This now brings issues of fidelity into play—what is the evidence if the treatment is delivered by a non-speech pathologist? If you provide training, how can you be sure that the treatment is being delivered as intended? How do you allocate time to monitor and check delivery? These examples illustrate the complexity of implementing EBP and drawing on the research, whatever treatment you are considering—ReST or any other. These examples are also a reminder that the other aspects of EBP are also key to success!

Client perspectives also bring a range of ethical considerations to our practice. What about the time when a family contacts you asking you to try out a treatment that they have heard about from a friend or on the internet? They have heard this will bring about the outcome they want for their child and are determined to give it a go. They ask you to have a look at 'XYZ Therapy' and send you the details of their searches. Your heart sinks as you click on the link in their email and are immediately directed to a shiny website offering a free 'screening' and a pop-up assistant who wants to schedule you a consultation. You search in vain for the research tab. You find something called 'research' and click on to find…a page of testimonials. After ten minutes you stop searching and ask yourself—well what about the underlying theory—why would this treatment work? In the words of Heather Clark (2003):

> 'At least two strategies are available to clinicians selecting management techniques for specific individuals: The approach that is advocated by evidence-based practice is to refer to research reports describing the benefits of a particular treatment. The question asked in this case is, "Is this treatment beneficial?" In the absence of adequately documented clinical efficacy, clinicians may select treatments based on theoretical soundness. The question asked in this case is, "Should this treatment be beneficial?" This second method of treatment selection has potential for success if the clinician has a clear understanding of both the nature of the targeted impairment and the therapeutic mechanism of the selected treatment technique.'

Clark, 2003, p. 1

So, is there evidence of 'theoretical soundness'? No, no luck there either. It is hard to reconcile the broad-brush description of this 'amazing therapy' ('XYZ Therapy' will fix most things apparently), with any theory or mechanism of change that you have ever studied in your career. So, you begin to consider why this family wants you to try this approach—what is it that they are looking for? Why do they think this treatment might be 'the' answer?

At times like this, drawing on your professional Code of Ethics and reflecting on values and beliefs can be a useful tool. As Jess Berentson-Shaw reminds us in her 2018 book *A Matter of Fact: Talking Truth in a Post-truth World*, it is listening rather than talking that is our most useful tool in understanding and connecting with people to communicate about research. Taking a narrative approach, involving listening to and exploring, the stories of our families and clients focuses us on the individual context, and is consistent with an emphasis on the ethical principle of autonomy in clinical decision making (Kenny et al., 2010). Again, this reminds us that implementing EBP is not simply a matter of 'applying' the research.

Turning to clinician factors—a speech pathologist may lack experience in a particular area of practice such as Childhood Apraxia of Speech, or a specific condition associated with a SSD, and may choose to post on a social media platform, such as a clinician Facebook group, asking for input. How much information is enough to request advice? How much is too much? The description of a client and their context at times can verge on revealing a client's, family's or maybe even another clinician's identity, raising potential breaches of confidentiality. Has the questioner sought consent? Are the Facebook responses moderated? How does the questioner critically evaluate the advice?

And, finally, what about the workplace context? COVID-19 certainly pushed the skill set of many clinicians a long way with the rapid uptake of telehealth in all its forms, but it has also opened a whole new raft of workplaces and, hence, ethical considerations relating to the notion of practice context. An SLP/SLT offering services via telehealth may now find themselves in competition with local clinicians from across state, and even national borders. Now we need to learn about and reflect on what might be local rules and ethical guidelines, and how these might apply differently across the borders.

Consider advertising for example. The rules around advertising in Australia for speech pathologists are quite clear.

> *'The speech pathologist will ensure the content of all advertising they own, operate or control:*
>
> - *Is accurate*
> - *Is based on evidence*
> - *Does not misrepresent the profession or the profession's scope of practice*
> - *Does not use client information and images in advertising without careful consideration*
> - *Does not solicit or encourage unnecessary or indiscriminate use of services through the use of inducements such as gifts, discounts or prizes*
> - *Denotes approved membership and professional qualification information only'*
>
> Speech Pathology Australia, 2021

The Board of Directors of Speech Pathology Australia (SPA) supports the profession's code of ethics in relation to advertising, and SPA reminds clinicians of their professional responsibility. While membership of SPA is not compulsory in Australia, most clinicians are members and, accordingly, must not describe themselves using terms such as 'expert' or 'specialist'. In contrast, while the guidelines regarding accuracy in advertising in the UK are similar (see below), these terms, and the NHS terms 'highly specialist SLT' and 'highly specialist speech and language team', can be used.

> *Advertisements must not be misleading, false, unfair or exaggerated. In particular, you should not claim your personal skills, equipment or facilities are better than anyone else's, unless you can prove this is true. https://hcpcdefencebarristers.co.uk/health-care-professions-council-code-practice*

Testimonials are also not allowed in SPA members' advertisements or on professional websites. But what about other countries? Is this acceptable or even common? Practitioners offering services to families of children with SSDs need to investigate local rules and regulations and consider the impact of delivering their services in this way.

The evidence base for our profession is growing and it is our professional and ethical responsibility to draw on it to support our clinical decision-making. But herein lies the art—we must also take care not to lose sight of the client as an individual, their views, and their autonomy.

I recommend that SLPs/SLTs carefully consider the evidence they find and interpret it within the wider context that includes client-, family-, clinician-, agency- and service-related factors and frameworks. Reflect on, and learn from, those messy real-life clinical contexts that we work in. The outcomes of our decisions may not be what we expect, and this may, or may not, be a bad thing. What is important though, is that we learn from them and continue to develop our clinical decision-making skills whether we are student, novice, or experienced.

To reiterate, our clinical decision-making may well involve a mix of scientific objective facts and artistic subjective interpretations, it should draw on all perspectives, in other words, considerations beyond the research literature. That is the real world of decision-making. However, every decision we make will be framed by our own personal and professional moral and ethical codes and life experience and must be consistent with that.

Children with Speech Sound Disorders

Children with speech sound disorders can have any combination of difficulties with perception, articulation/motor production, and/or phonological representation of speech segments (consonants and vowels), phonotactics (syllable and word shapes), and prosody (lexical and grammatical tones, rhythm, stress, and intonation) that may impact speech intelligibility and acceptability.

International Expert Panel on Multilingual Children's Speech, 2012, p. 1.

Children with SSD have gaps and simplifications in their speech sound systems that *can* make what they say difficult to understand. While the speech of some of them is usually, or even always fully intelligible to familiar and unfamiliar listeners, others can be unclear, hard to understand, or unintelligible. Yet, most poorly intelligible, and unintelligible children persist in trying to communicate effectively, despite limitations in their speech sound repertoires, syllable structure and stress pattern inventories, and their odd pronunciation. Some 70 percent of the world's languages include tones: pitch changes that distinguish words or convey grammatical inflections. Children with SSD who are acquiring a tonal language—Bantu, Cantonese, Mandarin, Norwegian, Punjabi, Thai, or Vietnamese, for example—may also have missing or incorrect tones.

Children with SSD may, in an unconscious bid to accommodate their difficulties, use phonological patterns (Hodson, 1982) or phonological processes (Grunwell, 1975; Ingram, 1974, 1989), that should not occur in the utterances of otherwise typically developing children of their ages (Hustad et al., 2020, 2021; Mahr et al., 2021). For example, English-learning children of 4 or 5, with protracted speech development, may persist in saying *doe* for *go*, *tight* for *kite*, or *save* for *shave*. Sometimes they appear to leave a gap, and the listener hears, for example, *roe* for *rope*, *off* for *cough*, *toss* for *Thomas*, *knees* for *sneeze*, or *bend* for *spend*; and sometimes they almost seem to play consonant pick 'n' mix with productions like *beats* for *speech*, and *Getty* for *Jesse*. They can have poor stimulability, persistent phonological patterns/processes in the form of systemic and substitution errors, syllable structure or phonotactic errors, consonant distortions, vowel deviations (Pollock, A20), and atypical prosody including atypical syllable and word stress, and timing.

Any or all these troublesome speech difficulties can occur singly. For example, Aaliyah 12;2 (years; months) had a mild articulation disorder involving [v] replacing /ð/ and [vz] replacing /ðz/. These substitutions were immediately noticeable in her social and linguistic milieu, drawing continual criticism, occasional mimicry, and teasing by family, teachers, and peers. Aaliyah said words like *them these those brother weather* and *breathing* correctly but pronounced word-final /ð/ as [v] e.g., *clove* for *clothe*. Where /ðz/ occurred in plurals (as in *booths cloths mouths* and *paths*) and present progressive verbs (as in *breathes soothes* and *loathes*) she would produce /vs/ (e.g., *loaves* for *loathes*). Using clinical judgement (Records et al., 1994), her SLT classified her speech difficulty as 'mild' on initial presentation, but soon realized that for Aaliyah it loomed large.

Table i.1 SSD severity scale based on percentages of consonants correct (PCCs) drawn from conversational speech samples (Adapted from Shriberg & Kwiatkowski, 1982).

Descriptor	PCC
Mild SSD to normal speech	>85%
Mild to moderate SSD	65–85%
Moderate to severe SSD	50–65%
Severe SSD	<50%

Mild, Moderate and Severe SSD

In one of two contributions, Flipsen Jr., A7 describes measuring the severity of involvement in SSD as 'a continuing puzzle'. An early and useful attempt to solve the puzzle by quantifying severity objectively, with severity interval descriptors, came from Shriberg and Kwiatkowski (1982, p. 265). Their four-interval scale, based on percentage of consonants correct (PCC) data, is displayed in Table i.1.

The four descriptors refer to speech sound disorder in general and they, and the percentages of consonants correct are applicable to children aged 4;1 through 8;6. For example, the term 'mild to moderate SSD' may be applied to describe the *conversational speech* of a child aged 4;1–8;6 with a PCC of 65–85%, noting that clinical judgement (Diepeveen et al., 2020; Records et al., 1994) is used by the SLP/SLT where the percentages overlap. It would be misuse of the descriptors to say that same child had a 'mild to moderate articulation disorder', or 'mild to moderate phonological disorder' or 'mild to moderate childhood apraxia of speech'. Also, because the scale was developed using conversational speech samples the descriptors may not be applied to PCCs derived from single word naming tests.

Co-occurrence

SSDs can, and often do, occur in children and young people in combination with

- each other (e.g., persistent phonological patterns *and* articulation errors)
- other communication disorders (e.g., SSD *and* a fluency disorder)

- biomedical conditions that *usually* impact speech (e.g., cleft lip and palate)
- disorders that *may* impact speech (e.g., foetal alcohol spectrum disorder: FASD)
- conditions that *may* affect speech (e.g., phenylketonuria: PKU)
- syndromes that *may* affect speech (e.g., velo-cardio-facial syndrome: VCFS)
- teratogens that *may* affect speech (e.g., alcohol, recreational drugs, and nicotine)
- disorders, conditions, and syndromes that are not known to affect speech or language specifically or communicative function in general

The SSD Umbrella

Children's speech sound disorders can encompass a mix of anatomic (e.g., cleft lip and palate), sensory (e.g., hearing impairment), motoric (e.g., childhood apraxia of speech), perceptual (e.g., compromised auditory discrimination), phonetic (articulatory), or phonemic (linguistic) difficulties.

The SSD Umbrella displayed in Figure i.1. (Bowen, 2015b), and the variation of it in Figure 3.1, is dubbed 'simplified' because it is an extremely pared back account of the underlying bases for SSD, especially when compared with the thorough Speech Disorders Classification System (SDCS) (Shriberg et al., 2019) discussed in Chapter 2.

The umbrella was designed to aid explanations for parents of their child's SSD, particularly where they had cooccurring speech difficulties (e.g., CAS and phonological disorder). The umbrella's five (metaphoric) 'levels' of speech function—**anatomic or sensory, motoric, perceptual, phonetic**, and **phonemic**—work in concert, and are inseparable in real life, so the word 'levels' is in quotation marks. Besides interacting with each other, they work in conjunction with a developing child's cognitive, psycholinguistic and neuromotor functions in the context of their personal characteristics (e.g., personality, temperament, resilience, intellectual level, and emotional growth) and their communicative milieu, particularly their family context.

In Figure i.1, 'Children's Speech Sound Disorders' is the overarching umbrella term for the range of speech difficulties children can experience. Hanging

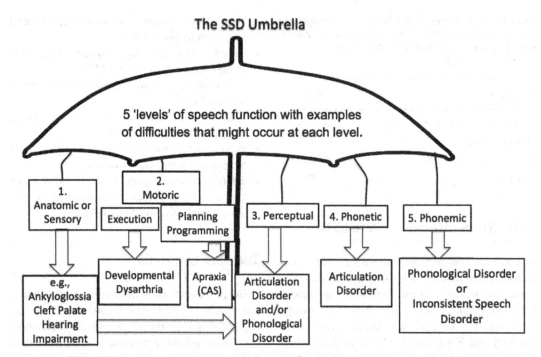

Figure i.1 The SSD Umbrella (Caroline Bowen / https://www.speech-language-therapy.com/index. php?option=com_content&view=article&id=190): A simplified classification system for the five underlying 'levels' of speech form and function, and the speech sound disorders that may arise when difficulties affect one or more of the five, in any combination. Reflecting the inconsistent nature of terminology related to SSD, Developmental Dysarthria is also called Childhood Dysarthria, and Articulation Disorder and Phonological Disorder are also called Articulation Impairment and Phonological Impairment.

from it are the five levels of speech function (1. anatomic or sensory, 2. motoric, 3. perceptual, 4. phonetic, and 5. phonemic) that may be compromised or impaired, accounting, at least in part, for the related speech disorder.

McLeod & Baker (2017, p. 39) also provide a simple conceptualization of children's speech with two umbrella terms: *speech sound disorders* (SSD) and a separate category, *speech difference* which does not come into the SSD realm, but rather encompasses dialectal difference, and differences attributable to multilingual acquisition, sociolinguistic factors (Munson & Tripp, A40), etc. In their schema, **SSD** has two categories suspended from it: first, **Phonology**, subdivided into *Phonological impairment*, and *Inconsistent speech disorder*; and second, **Motor speech**, subdivided into *Articulation impairment*, *Childhood apraxia of speech (CAS)*, and *Childhood dysarthria*.

Form and Function: Articulation and Phonology

SSDs that affect the **phonetic form**, also called **phonetic realisations** or **surface forms**, of speech sounds (the **phones**) are typically classified as **articulation disorders** and are usually associated with no known cause, or some combination of anatomic, sensory, motoric, and perceptual difficulties. SSDs affecting the **phonemic function** (or **linguistic function**) of speech sounds (the **phonemes**) in a language are usually classified as **phonological disorders** (American Speech-Language-Hearing Association Practice Portal, n.d. a).

The **function** of phonemes is to communicate or 'make meaning' (Grunwell, 1985a; Stoel-Gammon & Dunn, 1985). They do so by signalling meaningful contrasts between words, called phonemic contrasts. The following words exemplify phonemic contrasts in the word-initial position: *buy chai dye fie guy hi lie my nigh pie rye shy sigh thy tie vie why*. Next is a list containing phonemic contrasts in the word-final position: *beach bead beef beak beam bean beep bees beat*, and this one: *ban bane bean Ben bin bun bone boon* contains vowel and diphthong contrasts, generally referred to as vowel contrasts.

Minimal Pairs Involving Minimal Meaningful Contrasts

One Feature Difference If you take any two words from the lists where the vowel remains the same and the consonants differ by only one feature—in **place** of articulation, or in **manner** of articulation, or in **voice**—you will have a **minimal pair** that forms a **minimal meaningful contrast**. For example, *tie* and *dye* differ only in terms of voice and so do *pie* and *buy*. The /t/ in *tie* and /p/ in *pie* are voiceless and the /d/ in *dye* and /b/ in *buy* are voiced, so minimal pairs *tie-die* and *pie-buy* both form **minimal oppositions**. Likewise, any two words that contain the same consonants but different vowels, like *bin* and *Ben* where the short vowels differ, *bean* and *boon* where the long vowels differ, *bane* and *bone* where the diphthongs differ, or combinations like *bin-bone* (short vowel vs. diphthong), *bean-bone* (long vowel vs. diphthong) also form minimal pairs that are minimally opposed.

Minimal Pairs in Which the Contrast Is Not Minimal

More Than One Feature Difference Words pairs from the lists like *buy* and *sigh* that differ by more than one feature are still considered to be minimal pairs forming minimal meaningful contrasts because they differ by only one sound (i.e., one phone) when they are spoken, *and* they are represented by a single phoneme. The /b/ in *buy* is a voiced labial stop and the /s/ in *sigh* is a voiceless alveolar fricative, so the minimal pair involves three feature differences: a **voicing contrast** (voiced vs. voiceless), a **place of articulation contrast** (labial vs. alveolar), and a

manner of articulation contrast (stop vs. fricative), noting that 'stops' or stop consonants are also referred to as 'plosives' and that both terms are correct. Similarly, words from the lists that differ by two features, like *shy* and *tie*, are also minimal pairs (minimal meaningful contrasts), differing in place and manner, but sharing the voicing feature because both initial sounds are voiceless. So, *buy* vs. *sigh* and *shy* vs. *tie* do not comprise minimal *oppositions*, because they differ by more than one feature.

Types of Speech Sound Disorder

Below the five levels of speech function in Figure i.1 are types of SSD associated with each level: **developmental dysarthria, childhood apraxia of speech, articulation disorder**, and **phonological disorder**, as follows.

1. **SSDs with an Anatomic (Structural) and/or Sensory Basis**.

    The examples given for these two types of difficulty are ankyloglossia (tongue-tie) which seldom impacts speech (Salt et al., 2020; Wang et al., 2021), and cleft palate and hearing impairment which generally do. Wang and colleagues concluded that there was no clear connection between ankyloglossia and speech disorders, pointing to the need for more widely accepted uniform grading systems and well-designed clinical studies. The first two examples, ankyloglossia and cleft palate, are 'structural' involving body structure and the third is 'sensory', relating to the auditory sense (hearing) and it concerns body function (see McLeod, A2 for explanations of body structure and function within the World Health Organization, 2007, ICF-CY Framework). Anatomic differences and sensory impairment can affect the phonetic form *and* the phonological function of speech sounds, giving rise to articulation and/or phonological disorders.

2. **SSDs with a Motoric Basis**.

    Motoric or 'motor speech' disorders (typically abbreviated as MSD) are subdivided into **motor execution** and **motor planning/motor programming** difficulties, which, you guessed it, can cooccur. The motor execution category includes the dysarthrias found in children and young people, referred to collectively as developmental dysarthria (Pennington, A30) or childhood dysarthria. They are **spastic** dysarthria, **flaccid** dysarthria, **ataxic** dysarthria, **hyperkinetic** dysarthria, and **mixed** dysarthria. An additional type, **hypokinetic** dysarthria, is mainly seen in Parkinson's disease in adults. The dysarthrias in children and young people have many different causes, including cerebral palsy, neonatal stroke, and traumatic brain injury (TBI). In affected individuals, the speech mechanism, including the muscles of respiration, may be paralysed, weak or poorly co-ordinated. The dysarthrias can affect all motor speech processes—breathing, phonation, articulation, resonance, and prosody. Meanwhile, Childhood Apraxia of Speech (CAS) 'is a developmental, neurological SSD that affects motor planning and/or programming' (ASHA, 2007; and see, n.d. b; Murray et al., 2021).

3. SSDs with a Perceptual Basis.

Difficulties with speech perception may be implicated in both articulation disorder and phonological disorder. Charles Van Riper (b 1905 d 1994) a pioneer in intervention for articulation disorders, had just retired when David Ingram's *Phonological Disability in Children* was published, inspiring the so-called phonological revolution. Two years before he died, the third edition of Van Riper's co-authored introduction to general American phonetics, first published in 1954, was reissued (C. G. Van Riper & Smith, 1992). In it, the word 'phonology' appeared once, in passing (p. 1); 'phoneme' was defined as 'a sound family' (p. 8) and more helpfully 'a family of allophones meaningfully different from any other sounds' (p. 9), and throughout its 243 pages both phonemes and phones are rendered in phonetic square brackets (e.g., [s]) with not a virgule ('slashes' like the pair here: /s/) to be found.

But let's not get waylaid by presentism (Burke, 2020; Hunt, 2002). Presentism is the tendency to interpret the past in presentist terms, or attitudes towards the past that are governed by present-day attitudes, information, experiences, and values (Meyerowitz, 2020). Although Van Riper's publications suggest that he was loosely acquainted with the prevailing clinical phonology buzz (see, C. Van Riper & Erickson, 1996, pp. 208, 230–236), he was ahead of his time in stressing the importance of speech perception in intervention.

'Van Riper therapy': an auditory-phonetic or sensory-motor intervention for articulation disorder (Van Riper, 1939) is known in clinical circles as **traditional articulation therapy**. It invariably began with 'ear training' as foundational for what would follow. The client was taught to identify or hear the 'standard sound' (the desired target, e.g., /k/), then to discriminate the standard sound from their error (e.g., [t] replacing /k/) by scanning and comparing. Next, they performed auditory stimulation activities such as auditory sequencing, before moving on to production drill and the client's first experience of attempting to say their new sound in increasingly complex syllable, word, phrase and connected speech contexts (Van Riper, 1978, p. 179).

Abundant evidence from research teams in Canada, New Zealand and the USA quelled lurking thoughts that SLPs/SLTs may have harboured that Van Riper was somewhat passé on the speech perception topic. Confirmation that a large section of the SSD population has more difficulty with speech perception than their peers with age-typical speech came from Munson et al., 2005, 2006, Sutherland & Gillon, 2007; and a robust body of work by Rvachew and colleagues, including intervention studies: Rvachew, 1994, Rvachew et al., 1999, 2003, 2004.

In a client with SSD, it is possible that one or more errors are due to the child's inability to perceive the difference between his or her misproduction and the target correctly produced, but this difficulty may not be readily apparent via clinical observations and requires appropriate testing (Rvachew, A18).

4. SSDs with a Phonetic Basis.

As noted above, SSDs affecting the **phonetic form** of vowel and consonant **phones** are usually classified as articulation disorders and considered to be associated with some combination of 'functional' (cause unknown), anatomic, sensory, motoric, and auditory-perceptual difficulties. It is important to know that alongside fluency and voice disorders, articulation disorders comprise a sub-category of **speech disorders**. An individual with an articulation disorder has difficulty producing (articulating) the phones in the language(s) they speak.

5. SSDs with a Phonemic Basis.

Finally, SSDs affecting the **function** of speech sounds (as phonemes that contrast to 'make meaning') are typically classified as **phonological disorders**. Also importantly, phonological disorders are a sub-category of **language disorders**, just as **phonology**—in company with morphology, syntax, semantics, and pragmatics—is a component of language (see, Figure i.2).

Phonology

Ingram (1989) considered that phonology, as a discipline within linguistics, embraced the threefold study of **phonemes**, **mapping rules**, and **phones**, summarized below and then displayed in Figure i.3.

The nature of the underlying representations of speech sounds—how these linguistic units are stored in the mind—these are

ABSTRACT CONCEPTS OF SOUNDS, CALLED PHONEMES

Phonemes are the smallest linguistic units that, in combination with other phonemes, signal meaning differences between words. When transcribed individually and in words and longer utterances, phonemes appear in virgules e.g., /d/ /ɹ/ /i/ /m/ /z/.

———

Phonological rules or processes—these are

RULES THAT MAP BETWEEN PHONEMES AND PHONES, CALLED MAPPING RULES

Map (-ping, -ped) is a term used to characterize a feature of model construction in scientific enquiry. It is applied to several areas in linguistics and phonetics.

Mapping refers to the correspondence between the elements defined in a model of a situation, and the elements recognized in the situation itself (Crystal, 1991).

———

The nature of the phonetic representations—how sounds are articulated—these are

SPOKEN, CONCRETE SURFACE FORMS, CALLED PHONES

Listeners *hear* phones (not phonemes). When transcribed individually, and in words, and longer utterances, phones appear in square brackets e.g., [d] [ɹ] [i] [m] [z]; [dɹimz]; [ɪn jɔ dɹimz]

———

Figure i.2 Venn diagram illustrating relationships between diagnostic terms. Developmental language Disorder (DLD) and Speech Sound Disorder SSD are nested within the broader Speech, Language and Communication Needs (SLCN) category (Bishop et al., 2017). Impaired phonology (Phonological Disorder) resides in the Language Disorder/DLD subcategory. Used by permission of D. V. M. Bishop.

UNDERLYING REPRESENTATIONS: ABSTRACT CONCEPT OF THE SOUNDS   IN THE MIND

PHONEME   PHONEME   PHONEME   PHONEME   PHONEME

/d/   /ɹ/   /i/   /m/   /z/

MAPPING RULES THAT COMMUNICATE BETWEEN UNDERLYING REPRESENTATIONS AND SURFACE FORMS

SURFACE FORMS / PHONETIC REALIZATIONS THAT THE LISTENER HEARS   SPOKEN

PHONE   PHONE   PHONE   PHONE   PHONE

[d]   [ɹ]   [i]   [m]   [z]

UNDERLYING REPRESENTATIONS: ABSTRACT CONCEPT OF THE WORD(S)   IN THE MIND

PHONEMIC REPRESENTATION OF 'IN YOUR DREAMS'

/ɪn jɔ ˈdɹimz/

MAPPING RULES THAT COMMUNICATE BETWEEN UNDERLYING REPRESENTATIONS AND SURFACE FORMS

CONCRETE SURFACE FORMS / PHONETIC REALIZATIONS OF WORD(S)   SPOKEN

PHONETIC REALIZATION OF 'IN YOUR DREAMS' THAT THE LISTENER HEARS

[ɪn jɔ ˈdɹimz]

Figure i.3 Underlying representation, mapping rules and surface forms for 'dreams' and 'in your dreams' in a non-rhotic variety of English.

Serendipity

Considering Figure i.3, and Ingram's (1989) conceptualization of the three-way study of phonology as incorporating **phonemes** ↔ and **mapping rules** and ↔ **phones**, knowing how phonemes may be represented in a child's mind relies on serendipity and *listening*! Such chance revelations are easily missed. Fortuitous glimpses of two boys' probable underlying representations for /l/ serve as examples: they are Luke 2;9 (years; months) with typically developing speech, and Farez 4;3 with a phonological disorder.

Picture Luke, who called himself 'Yukie' ['juki] at the time, walking on the beach, one hand in mine, and the other clasping a newly purchased ice-cream. His satisfied expression is obvious to a friendly stranger who says smilingly, 'You're a lucky boy!' I feel his grip tighten, look down at his cross little face, as he grumbles, 'Yukie *aren't* a yucky boy'. Might /'juki/ and /'jʌki/ have been his underlying representations for 'Lukie' and 'lucky'? Probably. Were all instances of prevocalic /l/ stored in his mind as /j/? Impossible to say. Impossible to test.

Farez is drawing a picture for his SLP, and a pencil rolls onto the floor and out of view beneath a large toy truck. He searches unsuccessfully.

Farez: I lost the yellow.
[ˌaɪ ˈwɒst və ˈjɛˌwoʊ]
SLP: You [wɒst] it?
Farez: You said it wrong.
[ˈju ˌsɛdɪt ˈwoŋ]
Farez: I can't say lost like you say lost.
[ˈaɪ kant seɪ ˈwɒst waɪk ˈju seɪ ˈwɒst]
Farez: Oh look; look there, it's under the truck!
[oʊ ˈwʊk | ˈwʊk ˌvɛə | ɪts ˈʌnˌdə və ˈtɹʌk]
SLP: It is! It's **THERE…THERE**, under **THE** truck.

Farez (exasperated, and aware of being corrected on yet another sound): *Yes.*
[ˈjɛs]

Did Farez have /l/ as his underlying representation for the surface form [l]? Perhaps. He was aware of his error production in *lost* and identified the error when the SLP produced *lost* as [wɒst]. Figure i.4 shows three possible phonemic representations for his utterance: one matching the adult target, the next matching his production, and the last one showing some variability, with *lost* reflecting the target and *yellow* (a notoriously difficult word for young children to pronounce) corresponding with his production.

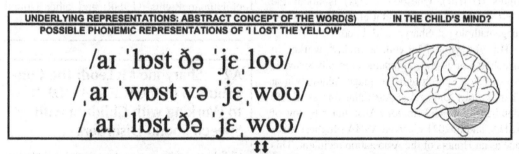

UNDERLYING REPRESENTATIONS: ABSTRACT CONCEPT OF THE WORD(S) IN THE CHILD'S MIND?
POSSIBLE PHONEMIC REPRESENTATIONS OF 'I LOST THE YELLOW'

/aɪ ˈlɒst ðə ˈjɛˌloʊ/
/ˌaɪ ˈwɒst və ˈjɛˌwoʊ/
/ˌaɪ ˈlɒst ðə ˈjɛˌwoʊ/

⇅

MAPPING RULES THAT COMMUNICATE BETWEEN UNDERLYING REPRESENTATIONS AND SURFACE FORMS

⇅

CONCRETE SURFACE FORMS / PHONETIC REALIZATIONS OF WORD(S) SPOKEN BY THE CHILD
PHONETIC REALIZATION OF 'I LOST THE YELLOW' THAT THE LISTENER HEARS

[ˌaɪ ˈwɒst və ˈjɛˌwoʊ]

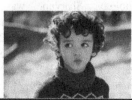

Figure i.4 Three possible underlying (phonemic) representations for Farez's phonetic realization of 'I lost the yellow' as [ˌaɪ ˈwɒst və ˈjɛˌwoʊ]. (David Sanchez / Pixabay).

As well as making the communication process arduous and sometimes frustrating for children like Farez, their poor speech clarity places additional demands on their communicative partners: parents, siblings, and others close to them. Often, these important individuals must apply extra effort, listening super-attentively to decipher what the speech-impaired children are saying, regularly finding themselves in the roles of advocate, apologist, codebreaker, go-between, and personal interpreter.

World Health Organization and the United Nations

Whether they are monolingual or multilingual, have an isolated SSD or have an SSD as one of several issues, their lives will be affected in the areas of Body Function, Body Structure, Activity and Participation, Environmental Factors and Personal Factors. These are the headings itemized in the World Health Organization's ICF-CY: the children and youth version of the *International Classification of Functioning, Disability and Health* (WHO, 2021). They, in common with everyone—with or without a disability—have rights, put forth in the United Nations' Universal Declaration of Human Rights (UDHR). Question 2 (Q2) is about the ICF-CY and the UDHR, and it goes to speech–language pathologist, Sharynne McLeod.

Dr. Sharynne McLeod, a tireless worker in speech research and communication advocacy, is Professor of Speech and Language Acquisition at Charles Sturt University, Australia. She is a Life Member of Speech Pathology Australia, a Fellow of ASHA, and in 2021 received ASHA's highest accolade as an Honors of the Association recipient. This award is reserved for whose contributions have been of such excellence that they have enhanced or altered the course of the professions of SLP and/or Audiology. Sharynne was named Australia's Research Field Leader in Audiology, Speech and Language Pathology in 2018, 2019 and 2020 Best in the World in 2019 based on the 'quality, volume and impact' of research. More recently, in 2022 she was elected as a Fellow of the Academy of the Social Sciences in Australia. She has co-authored 11 books and over 200 journal articles and chapters focusing on speech acquisition, speech sound disorders, and

multilingualism. Her web presence (https://www.csu.edu.au/research/multilingual-speech), Multilingual Children' Speech, has free resources in over 60 languages. She was editor-in-chief of the International Journal of Speech-Language Pathology (2005–2013) and edited a special issue on Communication Rights which she presented at the United Nations in 2019. Prof McLeod provided expertise into the World Health Organization's children and youth version of the International Classification of Functioning, Disability and Health as well as the Rehabilitation Competency Framework.

Q2.   Sharynne Mcleod: The ICF and Communication Rights

What are the benefits of using the ICF for the client, their families, people associated with the client such as SLPs/SLTs and teachers, and the wider community? What do you see as the major advantages for the client when the physical, mental, social, and environmental aspects of his or her condition or disorder are carefully considered and acknowledged, and how does all of this relate to communication rights as outlined in the Universal Declaration of Human Rights (UDHR) and other United Nations conventions?

A2.   Sharynne McLeod: The Contribution of the ICF and UDHR to Working with Children with Speech Sound Disorders

Children with speech sound disorders bring more than their ears and mouths to a conversation. Each of the children we interact with brings a unique combination of factors such as relationships with family, friends, teachers, and acquaintances; aspects of their lives that are important to them; their personality, capacity to learn and so forth. As SLPs/SLTs we often take these factors into consideration, but rarely do so in an explicit fashion (Blake & McLeod, 2018; McLeod, 2004). Instead, our reports and clinic files predominantly contain information about children's speech output such as their ability to produce consonants and vowels correctly.

For over four decades the World Health Organization has been developing an extensive classification system to be used throughout the world to support the health and wellness of all people. This started with the *International Classification of Impairment, Disabilities and Handicaps* (ICIDH) (WHO, 1980), *International Classification of Functioning, Disability and Health* (WHO, 2001), the *International Classification of Functioning, Disability and Health—Children and Youth* (ICF-CY) (WHO, 2007). The ICF sits within the World Health Organization's family of classifications, which also includes:

- International Statistical Classification of Diseases and Related Health Problems (ICD)
- International Classification of Health Interventions (ICHI)

The five components of the ICF (listed below) have direct relevance to children with speech sound disorders (McLeod, 2006; McLeod & McCormack, 2007). A description of the history and application of the ICF-CY to children's communication is contained in McLeod and Threats (2008).

1. ICF: Body Structure

Structures of the ear, nose, mouth, larynx, pharynx, and respiration are routinely screened by SLPs/SLTs to determine their potential contribution to speech sound disorders. For most children with speech sound disorders, Body Structure is not considered to be a causal factor (Shriberg et al., 1986). In some cases, such as when children have a craniofacial anomaly (e.g., cleft lip and palate), impairment in Body Structure can impact on children's ability to speak intelligibly and may also impact on their Activity and Participation in society (Cronin et al., 2020).

2. ICF: Body Function

Articulation, voice, fluency, hearing, respiration, intellectual and specific mental functions such as temperament and personality functions are classified amongst Body Functions in the ICF-CY. SLPs/SLTs working with children with speech sound disorders routinely consider these aspects in their assessment and intervention practices. Most of the SLP/SLT assessment, analysis, and intervention tools for children with speech sound disorders fall under the category of Body Function (McLeod & Threats, 2008). Thus, although not specifically stated in the ICF-CY, Body Function can include measures such as the percentage of consonants correct, the occurrence of cluster reduction and the inventory of consonants phones (McLeod, Harrison et al., 2013).

3. ICF: Activities and Participation

Learning and applying knowledge; general tasks and demands; communication; interpersonal interactions and relationships; major life areas such as education; and community, social and civic life are all included in the ICF-CY as categories of Activities and Participation. There are a few tools specifically designed to consider children's Activities and Participation including: *Focus on the Outcomes of Communication Under Six* (FOCUS©) (Thomas-Stonell et al., 2010), *Intelligibility in Context Scale* (ICS) (McLeod, 2020; McLeod et al., 2012) and the *Speech Participation and Activity Assessment of Children* (SPAA-C) (McLeod, 2004). When we as SLPs/SLTs set goals for children with speech sound disorders, it is important that we acknowledge and include these broader aspects of their lives. Thus, communicating intelligibly on the sporting field and in the playground are relevant goals for SLPs/SLTs working in this framework. It is also helpful if we consider the possible mismatch between capacity and performance in these life areas. As children grow older, the impact of speech sound disorders on individuals' Activities and Participation may include an impact on social, educational, occupational, behavioural outcomes (McCormack et al., 2011; McCabe, A34) as well as on quality of life for these individuals and their families (for a review see, McCormack et al., 2009).

4. ICF: Environmental Factors

Products and technology; support and relationships; attitudes; services, systems and policies are all included as Environmental Factors in ICF-CY. Each of these areas can act as facilitators and/or barriers to children with speech sound disorders. In most children's lives, perhaps the most prominent Environmental Factor is their family. As SLPs/SLTs we need to be aware of facilitating involvement of parents and siblings in assessment and intervention (McLeod, Daniel et al., 2013; Watts Pappas et al., 2016). Another relevant Environmental Factor is the attitudes of family, friends, acquaintances, people in authority (such as teachers), health professionals, and society (Overby et al., 2007). The attitudes people hold towards children with speech sound disorders can either be facilitative or a barrier in these children's lives. Consequently, there may be times when our intervention goals need to be directed towards others, rather than the children with speech sound disorders. For example, McCormack et al. (2010) found that preschool children were concerned that adults had difficulties understanding them so recommended that intervention could focus both on children's 'speech problem' as well as the adults' 'listening problem'. Finally, Environmental Factors include the policies and services that are available for children with speech sound disorders. In some nations such as the USA and UK, legislation ensures that children with speech sound disorder are provided with relevant services, and these act as an environmental facilitator. In other nations, such as Australia, SLP/SLT services are not legislated (McLeod et al., 2010), and access to services may be difficult due to long waiting lists (McGill et al., 2020) acting as an environmental barrier.

5. ICF: Personal Factors

Age, gender, race, other health conditions, coping styles, overall behaviour pattern and character style are all included in the ICF as relevant personal factors. Unlike the other components of the ICF, detailed and coded descriptions of Personal Factors are not included in the manual. However, it is helpful if SLPs/SLTs explore relevant personal factors for each child they engage with.

More than the Sum of Its Parts

To summarize, the ICF is far more than these five discreet components. The interaction between each of these components is essential for realizing the goal of health and wellness. The advantage of engaging with this comprehensive classification system is that it enables holistic consideration of children with speech sound disorder to envisage and facilitate fuller participation in society (cf., Cronin et al., 2020). Advocacy for increased access to specialized services and updated legislation and policies are recommended to support children's ability to communicate.

6. Communication Rights

The right to communicate includes 'the right to freedom of opinion and expression' that has been articulated in Article 19 of the Universal Declaration of Human Rights (UDHR, United Nations, 1948), Articles 12 and 13 of the Convention on the Rights of the Child (United Nations, 1989) and Article 21 of the Convention on the Rights of Persons with Disabilities (United Nations, 2006). Article 19 continues by saying 'this right includes freedom to hold opinions without interference and to seek, receive and impart information and ideas through any media and regardless of frontiers' (United Nations, 1948). If people have a communication disability (speech, language, and communication needs), they may have limitations to the attainment of other human rights, including self-determination, education, work, and other freedoms (McCormack et al., 2018; McLeod, 2018). The Universal Declaration of Communication Rights International Communication Project, 2014 (Mulcair et al., 2018) has been signed by over 10,000 SLPs/SLTs and others and states:

We recognise that the ability to communicate is a basic human right.

We recognise that everyone has the potential to communicate.

By putting our names to this declaration, we give our support to the millions of people around the world who have communication disorders that prevent them from experiencing fulfilling lives and participating equally and fully in their communities.

> *We believe that people with communication disabilities should have access to the support they need to realise their full potential.*
>
> (Mulcair et al., 2018)

In 2019, members of the International Communication Project went to the United Nations in New York to promote communication rights and the 70th anniversary of the Universal Declaration of Human Rights (International Communication Project, 2019), and present the special issue of the *International Journal of Speech-Language Pathology* dedicated to communication rights (McLeod, 2018).

People with communication disabilities (including children with speech sound disorders) often require support to realize their communication rights (McLeod, 2018; Roulstone & McLeod, 2011). Creativity is required to enable children with speech sound disorders to realize their right to 'seek, receive and impart information and ideas' and SLPs/SLTs are encouraged to consider 'any media' and new 'frontiers' (United Nations, 1948). Our Speech-Language-Multilingualism team (and others) have undertaken a number of studies where we have listened to children with speech sound disorders by invited them to draw themselves talking to someone, colour faces with different emotions to indicate how they feel about issues, answer questions from the SPAA-C (McLeod, 2004), and allowed us to join them in their daily routines while also talking with their siblings, friends, family and other important adults (e.g., McCormack et al., 2010; McLeod, Harrison et al., 2013). Children have been able to articulate their frustrations, concerns, solutions, and dreams, empowering us to advocate for children's participation in decision-making (Lundy, 2007). By aligning service delivery and advocacy with international classifications (e.g., ICF) and conventions (e.g., UDHR) SLPs/SLTs can work together to change the lives of people across the world.

Summing Up

The topics covered briefly so far in the introduction to Part 1 represent some of the components that are integral to best practice and include:

- The importance of **ethical** Evidence-Based Practice (aka EBP/E^{3}BP/E^{4}BP) as a professional responsibility and code of conduct, with due regard for the research literature, theoretical rigour, treatment fidelity as far as it is possible, and the role of critical and clinical thinking—taking a holistic view of individual clients in their unique communicative milieu.
- The significance of the World Health Organization's ICF-CY: a dynamic classification system that allows **just** and **fair** (holistic and equitable) consideration of children with SSD that is directed to the goal of their health, wellness, and meaningful participation, as effective communicators, in civil society.
- The relevance of the connection between the Universal Declaration of Human Rights (UDHR)—which espouses fundamental entitlements and freedoms for all—and other universal Declarations and Conventions on one hand, and on the other, our **values** and roles as SLPs/SLTs and our relationships with and responsibilities to clients, their families, colleagues, and the wider community.
- The meanings of a small selection terms, with their abbreviation and acronyms. relative to children's speech that are in constant use in SLP/SLT professional practice, necessitating an agreed understanding by SLPs/SLTs.

Attention now turns, in Chapter 1, to what we know as SLPs/SLTs; the knowledgebase we draw upon, and that shapes our thinking, conduct, and practice, as students, clinicians, researchers, academics, and administrators.

References

American Psychological Association. (2020). *Publication manual of the American Psychological*

Association 2020: The official guide to APA style (7th ed.).

Armstrong, L., Stansfield, J., & Bloch, S. (2017). Content analysis of the professional journal of the Royal College of Speech and Language Therapists, III: 1966–2015—into the 21st century. *International Journal of Language & Communication Disorders*, *52*(6), 681–688. https://doi.org/10.1111/1460-6984.12313

Ash, A. C., Christopulos, T. T., & Redmond, S. M. (2020). "Tell me about your child": A grounded theory study of mothers' understanding of language disorder. *American Journal of Speech-Language Pathology*, *29*(2), 819–840. https://doi.org/10.1044/2020_AJSLP-19-00064

ASHA (2007). Childhood apraxia of speech: Technical report. http://www.asha.org/policy/TR2007-00278

ASHA (n.d.a) *Speech Sound Disorders: Articulation and Phonology*. (Practice Portal). https://www.asha.org/Practice-Portal/Clinical-Topics/Articulation-and-Phonology

ASHA (n.d.b). *Childhood Apraxia of Speech* (Practice Portal). www.asha.org/Practice-Portal/Clinical-Topics/Childhood-Apraxia-of-Speech

Ball, M. J. (2016). *Principles of clinical phonology. Theoretical Approaches*. Psychology Press.

Ball, M. J. (Ed.). (2021). *Manual of clinical phonetics*. Routledge.

Ball, M. J., Müller, N., & Rutter, B. (2010). *Phonology for communication disorders*. Psychology Press.

Berentson-Shaw, J. (2018). *A matter of fact: Talking truth in a post-truth world* (Vol. 67). Bridget Williams Books.

Bishop, D. V. M., Snowling, M. J., Thompson, P. A., Greenhalgh, T., & Consortium, T. C. A. T. A. L. I. S. E. (2017). Phase 2 of CATALISE: A multinational and multidisciplinary Delphi consensus study of problems with language development: Terminology. *Journal of Child Psychology & Psychiatry*. https://doi.org/10.1111/jcpp.12721

Bitter, J. R. (2021). *Theory and practice of family therapy and counseling* (3rd ed.). American Counseling Association.

Blake, H. L., & McLeod, S. (2018). The international classification of functioning, disability and health: Considering individuals from a perspective of health and wellness. *Perspectives of the ASHA Special Interest Groups*, *3*(17), 69–77. https://doi.org/10.1044/persp3.SIG17.69

Bowen, C. (2009). *Children's speech sound disorders* (1st ed.). Wiley-Blackwell.

Bowen, C. (2015a). *Children's speech sound disorders* (2nd ed.). Wiley-Blackwell. https://doi.org/10.1002/9781119180418

Bowen, C. (2015b). *The SSD umbrella*. Five Levels of Speech Function with Examples of Difficulties that Might Occur at Each Level. Author. https://www.speech-language-therapy.com

Burke, M. B. (2020). Liberated presentism. *The Review of Metaphysics*, *73*(3), 569–603. https://philpapers.org/rec/BURLP-2

Clark, H. M. (2003). Neuromuscular treatments for speech and swallowing. *American Journal of Speech-Language Pathology*, *12*(4), 400–415. https://doi.org/10.1044/1058-0360(2003/086)

Cronin, A., McLeod, S., & Verdon, S. (2020). Applying the ICF-CY to specialist speech-language pathologists' practice with toddlers with cleft palate speech. *The Cleft Palate-Craniofacial Journal*, *57*(9), 1105–1116. https://doi.org/10.1177/1055665620918799

Crystal, D. (1991). *A dictionary of linguistics & phonetics*. Basil Blackwell.

Diepeveen, S. J. H., Haaften, L. V., Terband, H., Swart, B. J. M. D., & Maassen, B. (2020). Clinical Reasoning for Speech Sound Disorders: Diagnosis and Intervention in Speech-Language Pathologists' Daily Practice. *American Journal of Speech-Language Pathology*, *29*(3), 1529–1549. https://doi.org/10.1044/2020_AJSLP-19-00040

Dollaghan, C. A. (2007). *The handbook for evidence-based practice in communication disorders*. Paul H. Brookes Publishing Co.

Duchan, J. F., & Felsenfeld, S. (2021). Professional issues: A view from history. In M. W. Hudson & M. DeRuiter, *Professional issues in speech-language pathology and audiology* (5th ed., pp. 57–80). Plural Publishing.

Greenwell, T., & Walsh, B. (2021). Evidence-based practice in speech-language pathology: Where are we now? *American Journal of Speech-Language Pathology*, *30*(1), 186–198. https://doi.org/10.1044/2020_AJSLP-20-00194

Grunwell, P. (1975). The phonological analysis of articulation disorders. *British Journal of Disorders of Communication*, *10*(1), 31–42. https://doi.org/10.3109/13682827509011272

Grunwell, P. (1985a). *Phonological assessment of child speech (PACS)*. NFER–Nelson.

Grunwell, P. (1987). *Clinical phonology* (2nd ed.). Williams & Wilkins.

Higginbotham, J., & Satchidanand, A. (2019). *Triangle to diamond: Recognizing and using data* to inform our evidence-based practice, ASHA Journals Academy. ASHA. https://academy.pubs.asha.org/2019/04/from-triangle-to-diamond-recognizing-and-using-data-to-inform-our-evidence-based-practice

Hodson, B. (1982). Remediation of speech patterns associated with low levels of phonological performance. In M. Crary (Ed.), *Phonological intervention, concepts, and procedures* (pp. 97–115). College-Hill Press Inc.

Hoffman, T., Bennett, S., & Del Mar, C. (2017). *Evidence-based practice across the health professions* (3rd ed.). Elsevier.

Hunt, L. (2002, May). *Against presentism*. American Historical Society News Magazine: Perspectives on History. American Historical Association. https://www.historians.org/publications-and-directories/perspectives-on-history/may-2002/against-presentism

Hustad, K. C., Mahr, T. J., Natzke, P., & Rathouz, P. J. (2020). Development of speech intelligibility between 30 and 47 months in typically developing children: A cross-sectional study of growth. *Journal of Speech, Language and Hearing Research, 6*(63), 1675–1687. https://doi.org/10.1044/2020_JSLHR-20-00008

Hustad, K. C., Mahr, T. J., Natzke, P., & Rathouz, P. J. (2021). Speech development between 30 and 119 months in typical children I: Intelligibility growth curves. *Journal of Speech, Language and Hearing Research, 64*(10), 3707–3719. https://doi.org/10.1044/2021_JSLHR-21-00142

Ingram, D. (1974). Phonological rules in young children. *Journal of Child Language, 1*(1), 49–64. https://doi.org/10.1017/S0305000900000076

Ingram, D. (1989). *Phonological disability in children* (2nd ed.). Whurr Publishers.

International Communication Project (2019). *International communication project holds event at UN*. https://internationalcommunicationproject.com/2019/05/international-communication-project-event-united-nations

International DOI Foundation (2019). DOI® Handbook. https://www.doi.org/hb.html

International Expert Panel on Multilingual Children's Speech (2012). *Multilingual children with speech sound disorders: Position paper*. Research Institute for Professional Practice, Learning and Education (RIPPLE), Charles Sturt University. http://www.csu.edu.au/research/multilingual-speech/position-paper

Kearns, A., Gallagher, A., & Cronin, J. (2021). Quality in the time of chaos: Reflections from teaching, learning and practice. *Perspectives of the ASHA Special Interest Groups, 6*(5), 1310–1314. https://doi.org/10.1044/2021_PERSP-21-00095

Kenny, B., Lincoln, M., & Balandin, S. (2010). Experienced speech-language pathologists' responses to ethical dilemmas: An integrated approach to ethical reasoning. *American Journal of Speech-Language Pathology, 19*(2), 121–134. https://doi.org/10.1044/1058-0360(2009/08-0007)

Lundy, L. (2007). 'Voice' is not enough: Conceptualising article 12 of the United Nations convention on the rights of the child. *British Education Research Journal, 33*(6), 927–942. https://doi.org/10.1080/01411920701657033

Mahr, T. J., Soriano, J. U., Rathouz, P. J., & Hustad, K. C. (2021). Speech development between 30 and 119 months in typical children II: Articulation rate growth curves. *Journal of Speech, Language and Hearing Research, 64*(11), 4057–4070. https://doi.org/10.1044/2021_JSLHR-21-00206

McCormack, J., Baker, E., & Crowe, K. (2018). The human right to communicate and our need to listen: Learning from people with a history of childhood communication disorder. *International Journal of Speech-Language Pathology, 20*(1), 142–151. https://doi.org/10.1080/17549507.2018.1397747

McCormack, J., Harrison, L. J., McLeod, S., & McAllister, L. (2011). A nationally representative study of the association between communication impairment at 4-5 years and children's life activities at 7–9 years. *Journal of Speech, Language and Hearing Research, 54*(5), 1328–1348. https://doi.org/10.1044/1092-4388(2011/10-0155)

McCormack, J., McLeod, S., McAllister, L., & Harrison, L. J. (2009). A systematic review of the association between childhood speech impairment and participation across the lifespan. *International Journal of Speech-Language Pathology, 11*(2), 155–170. https://doi.org/10.1080/17549500802676859

McCormack, J., McLeod, S., McAllister, L., & Harrison, L. J. (2010). My speech problem, your listening problem, and my frustration: The experience of living with childhood speech impairment. *Language, Speech, and Hearing Services in Schools, 41*(4), 379–392. https://doi.org/10.1044/0161-1461(2009/08-0129)

McGill, N., Crowe, K., & McLeod, S. (2020). "Many wasted months": Stakeholders' perspectives about waiting for speech-language pathology services. *International Journal of Speech-Language Pathology, 22*(3), 313–326. https://doi.org/10.1080/17549507.2020.1747541

McLeod, S. (2004). Speech pathologists' application of the ICF to children with speech impairment. *International Journal of Speech-Language Pathology, 6*(1), 75–81. https://doi.org/10.1080/14417040410001669516

McLeod, S. (2006). The holistic view of a child with unintelligible speech: Insights from the ICF and ICF-CY. *International Journal of Speech-Language Pathology, 8*(3), 293–315. https://doi.org/10.1080/14417040600824944

McLeod, S. (2018). Communication rights: Fundamental human rights for all. *International Journal of Speech-Language Pathology, 20*(1), 3–11. https://doi.org/10.1080/17549507.2018.1428687

McLeod, S. (2020). Intelligibility in context scale: Cross-linguistic use, validity, and reliability. *Speech, Language and Hearing, 23*(1), 9–16. https://doi.org/10.1080/2050571X.2020.1718837

McLeod, S., & Baker, E. (2017). *Children's speech: An evidence-based approach to assessment and intervention* (pp. 39). Pearson.

McLeod, S., Daniel, G., & Barr, J. (2013). "When he's around his brothers ... he's not so quiet": The private and public worlds of school-aged children with speech sound disorder. *Journal of Communication Disorders, 46*(1), 70–83. https://doi.org/10.1016/j.jcomdis.2012.08.006

McLeod, S., Harrison, L. J., McAllister, L., & McCormack, J. (2013). Speech sound disorders in a community study of preschool children. *American Journal of Speech-Language Pathology, 22*(3), 503–522. https://doi.org/10.1044/1058-0360(2012/11-0123)

McLeod, S., Harrison, L. J., & McCormack, J. (2012). Intelligibility in context scale: Validity and reliability of a subjective rating measure. *Journal of Speech, Language, and Hearing Research, 55*(2), 648–656. https://doi.org/10.1044/1092-4388(2011/10-0130)

McLeod, S., & McCormack, J. (2007). Application of the ICF and ICF-children and youth in children with speech impairment. *Seminars in Speech and Language, 28*(4), 254–264. https://doi.org/10.1055/s-2007-986522

McLeod, S., Press, F., & Phelan, C. (2010). The (in)visibility of children with communication impairment in Australian health, education, and disability legislation and policies. *Asia Pacific Journal of Speech, Language, and Hearing, 13*(1), 67–75. https://doi.org/10.1179/136132810805335173

McLeod, S., & Threats, T. T. (2008). The ICF-CY and children with communication disabilities. *International Journal of Speech-Language Pathology, 10*(1–2), 92–109. https://doi.org/10.1080/17549500701834690

Meyerowitz, J. (2020). 180 Op-Eds: Or how to make the present historical. *Journal of American History, 107*(2), 323–335. https://doi.org/10.1093/jahist/jaaa335

Morley, M. E., Court, D., & Miller, H. (1954). Developmental dysarthria. *British Medical Journal, 2*(1), 8–10. 4852. https://doi.org/10.1136/bmj.1.4852.8

Mulcair, G., Pietranton, A. A., & Williams, C. (2018). The international communication project: Raising global awareness of communication as a human right. *International Journal of Speech-Language Pathology, 20*(1), 34–38. https://doi.org/10.1080/17549507.2018.1422023

Munson, B., Baylis, A., Krause, M., & Yim, D.-S. (2006). Representation and access in phonological impairment. *Paper presented at the 10th Conference on Laboratory Phonology*, Paris, France, June 30-July 2. De Gruyter. https://doi.org/10.1515/9783110224917.4.381

Munson, B., Edwards, J., & Beckman, M. E. (2005). Relationships between nonword repetition accuracy and other measures of linguistic development in children with phonological disorders. *Journal of Speech, Language, and Hearing Research, 48*(1), 61–78. https://doi.org/10.1044/1092-4388(2005/006)

Murray, E., Iuzzini-Seigel, J., Maas, E., Terband, H., & Ballard, K. (2021). Differential diagnosis of childhood apraxia of speech compared to other speech sound disorders: A systematic review. *American Journal of Speech-Language Pathology, 30*(1), 279–300. https://doi.org/10.1044/2020_AJSLP-20-00063

Murray, E., McCabe, P., Heard, R., & Ballard, K. J. (2015). Differential diagnosis of children with suspected childhood apraxia of speech. *Journal of Speech, Language and Hearing Research, 58*(1), 43-60. https://doi.org/10.1044/2014_JSLHR-S-12-0358

Namasivayam, A. K., Pukonen, M., Goshulak, D., Hard, J., Rudzicz, F., & Lieshout, P. (2015). Treatment intensity and childhood apraxia of speech. *International Journal of Language & Communication Disorders, 50*(4), 529-546. https://doi.org/10.1111/1460-6984.12154

Overby, M., Carrell, T., & Bernthal, J. (2007). Teachers' perceptions of students with speech sound disorders: A quantitative and qualitative analysis. *Language, Speech, and Hearing Services in Schools, 38*(4), 327–341. https://doi.org/10.1044/0161-1461(2007/035)

Records, N., Jordan, L., & Tomlin, B. J. (1994). Clinical judgement: A familiar concept, but a poorly understood process. *NSSLHA Journal*, *21*(November), 74–81. https://doi.org/10.1044/nsshla_21_74

Roulstone, S., & McLeod, S. (Eds.). (2011). *Listening to children and young people with speech, language, and communication needs*. J&R Press.

Rvachew, S. (1994). Speech perception training can facilitate sound production learning. *Journal of Speech and Hearing Research*, *37*(2), 347–357. https://doi.org/10.1044/jshr.3702.347

Rvachew, S., Nowak, M., & Cloutier, G. (2004). Effect of phonemic perception training on the speech production and phonological awareness skills of children with expressive phonological delay. *American Journal of Speech-Language Pathology*, *13*(3), 250–263. https://doi.org/10.1044/1058-0360(2004/026)

Rvachew, S., Ohberg, A., Grawburg, M., & Heyding, J. (2003). Phonological awareness and phonemic perception in 4-year-old children with delayed expressive phonology skills. *American Journal of Speech-Language Pathology*, *12*(4), 463–471. https://doi.org/10.1044/1058-0360(2003/092)

Rvachew, S., Rafaat, S., & Martin, M. (1999). Stimulability, speech perception and the treatment of phonological disorders. *American Journal of Speech-Language Pathology*, *8*(1), 33–43. https://doi.org/10.1044/1058-0360.0801.33

Salt, H., Claessen, M., Johnston, T., & Smart, S. (2020, July). Speech production in young children with tongue-tie. *International Journal of Pediatric Otorhinolaryngology*, *134*, 110035. https://doi.org/10.1016/j.ijporl.2020.110035

Shriberg, L. D., & Kwiatkowski, J. (1982). Phonological disorders III: A procedure for assessing severity of involvement. *Journal of Speech and Hearing Disorders*, *47*(3), 256–270. https://doi.org/10.1044/jshd.4703.256

Shriberg, L. D., Kwiatkowski, J., Best, S., Hengst, J., & Terselic-Weber, B. (1986). Characteristics of children with phonologic disorders of unknown origin. *Journal of Speech and Hearing Disorders*, *51*(2), 140–161. https://doi.org/10.1044/jshd.5102.140

Shriberg, L. D., Kwiatkowski, J., & Mabie, H. L. (2019). Estimates of the prevalence of motor speech disorders in children with idiopathic speech delay. *Clinical Linguistics & Phonetics*, *33*(8), 679–706. https://doi.org/10.1080/02699206.2019.1595731

Speech Pathology Australia (2021, March). Code of Ethics—Advertising. https://www.speechpathology australia.org.au/SPAweb/About_Us/SPA_Documents/Advertising/Advertising.aspx [Accessible to SPA Members]

Stansfield, J. (2020). Giving voice: An oral history of speech and language therapy. *International Journal of Language & Communication Disorders*, *55*(3), 320-331. https://doi.org/10.1111/1460-6984.12520

Stoel-Gammon, C., & Dunn, C. (1985). *Normal and disordered phonology in children*. University Park Press.

Sutherland, D., & Gillon, G. T. (2007). The development of phonological representations and phonological awareness in children with speech impairment. *International Journal of Language and Communication Disorders*, *14*(2), 229–250. https://doi.org/10.1080/13682820600806672

Thomas-Stonell, N., Oddson, B., Robertson, B., & Rosenbaum, P. (2010). Development of the FOCUS© (Focus on the Outcomes of Communication Under Six): A communication outcome measure for preschool children. *Developmental Medicine and Child Neurology*, *52*(1), 47–53. https://doi.org/10.1111/j.1469-8749.2009.03410.x

United Nations (1948). *Universal declaration of human rights*. http://www.un.org/en/universal-declaration-human-rights

United Nations (1989). *Convention on the rights of the child*. https://www.unicef.org/crc

United Nations (2006). *Convention on the rights of persons with disabilities*. https://www.un.org/development/desa/disabilities/convention-on-the-rights-of-persons-with-disabilities.html

Van Riper, C. (1939). *Speech correction: Principles and methods*. Prentice-Hall.

Van Riper, C. (1978). *Speech correction: Principles and methods* (6th ed.). Prentice-Hall.

Van Riper, C., & Erickson, R. L. (1996). *Speech correction: Principles and methods* (9th ed.). Pearson.

Van Riper, C. G., & Smith, D. E. (1992). *An introduction to general American phonetics* (3rd ed.). Harper Collins Publishers.

Wang, J., Yang, X., Hao, S., & Wang, Y. (2021). The effect of ankyloglossia and tongue- tie division on speech articulation: A systematic review. *International Journal of Paediatric Dentistry*, *32*(2), 144–156. https://doi.org/10.1111/ipd.12802

Watts Pappas, N., McAllister, L., & McLeod, S. (2016). Parental beliefs and experiences regarding involvement in intervention for their child with speech sound disorder. *Child Language*

Teaching and Therapy, 32(2), 223–239. https://doi.org/10.1177/0265659015615925

World Health Organization. (1980). *ICIDH: International classification of impairment, disabilities, and handicaps.* World Health Organization.

World Health Organization. (2001). *ICF: International classification of functioning, disability and health.* World Health Organization.

World Health Organization (WHO Workgroup for development of version of ICF for Children & Youth). (2007). *International classification of functioning, disability, and health - Version for children and youth: ICF-CY.* World Health Organization.

Chapter 1
The Evolution of Current Practices

Conceptual frameworks are easy to ignore. Like the air we breathe, their presence is everywhere once they are looked for. Yet, they are often taken for granted, under-estimated and under-examined. One way to reveal the influence of frameworks today is to study their use in unfamiliar contexts. For example, an examination of past practices of speech therapists raises questions about what practitioners did then as well as how and why they did it. Such an investigation creates the distance needed for clinicians to apprehend aspects of their own practice that are ordinarily taken for granted.

Duchan, 2006a, p. 736

Historians are uncommon in SLP/SLT circles, so we are fortunate to have the handful of people who have documented the profession's development, notably: Linda Armstrong, Judith Felsen Duchan, Margaret Eldridge, and Jois Stansfield who is dual qualified as an SLT and as a historian (Stansfield, 2022). Some oral historians have focused on specific topics within SLP/SLT, for example, Denyse Rockey (1980) concentrated on stuttering, and Alison McDougall (2006) explored the development of Speech Pathology in Australia. Other detailed professional association histories have been compiled: Robertson et al. (1995), and Stansfield (2020a, 2020b), on the RCSLT; Malloy (2021) on the NZSTA; and Leahy et al. (2021) on the growth of SLT and the IASLT in the Republic of Ireland. Linda Armstrong and Jois Stansfield contribute amply to the University of Strathclyde's Archives and Special Collections which houses the RCSLT's historical papers; see https://guides.lib.strath.ac.uk/archives/slt

Duchan (2001 to date) believes too little work has been done on the evolution of current practices. She observes that most histories of the origins of speech pathology in the United States consider organisational matters and place the profession's genesis in about 1925, when people interested in speech disorders and speech correction established professional associations. This institutional emphasis is observed in the chronologies by Margaret Eldridge, recording the development of speech therapy in Australia (Eldridge, 1965) and worldwide (Eldridge, 1968a, 1968b). By contrast, Duchan (2001 to date) has produced and maintains a lively web-based history, augmented by journal articles (e.g., Duchan, 2002, 2006b, 2010; Duchan & Hewett, 2023) and book chapters, (e.g., Duchan, 2009; Duchan & Felsenfeld, 2021). Duchan's contribution is broad in scope and distinctive because it includes systematic records of the science and ideas underlying practice.

Aside from brief biographies in textbooks, auto-biographical statements are unusual in SLP/SLT. But remarkably, McDougall (2006) and Stansfield (2020a) took fresh approaches by using an oral history methodology to explore the life stories of early members of the profession in Australia and in the UK, respectively. McDougall's account included interviews, conducted in 2002 by oral historian Jo Wills, tracing the history of the profession in Australia from 1929 to 2004. Stansfield interviewed 19 women who qualified in Britain between 1945 and 1968, to provide unique insights into challenges and changes in the UK profession as reported by post-WW2 practitioners.

Much of the memoir by Leahy et al. (2021) is based on the experiences of the class of 1969 at Trinity College Dublin. It contains reminiscences of the roles of carbon paper, typewriters, a Black & Decker Language Master that proclaimed that 'Dougal had lots of work to do at his party', temperamental photocopiers that unreliably spat out expensive photocopies, contact paper—the laminator's sticky antecedent—and bespoke therapy materials conceived, designed, and executed by resourceful SLTs.

Resources were largely of the DIY variety—literally cut and paste! They were the pen and paper days—you drew a picture and labelled it and that's what it became for the child in your clinic (it didn't have to resemble the actual object much!)

Leahy et al., p. 12

Given few specialised therapy materials in the early days, the quality and scope of resources was dependant on the ingenuity, talents, and creative ability of each individual SLT. As with assessments, any clinical equipment was supplemented with everyday objects, toys, colouring pencils, and copybooks. The earliest cohorts of students were offered optional drawing classes as part of their curriculum.

Leahy et al., p. 30

An innovative historical standout is Armstrong et al.'s (2017) history of speech and language therapy traced through 50 years' professional publications in the RCSLT's *International Journal of Language & Communication Disorders* (IJLCD) and its predecessors. Their study provides an in-depth content analysis of the IJLCD from 1966 to 2015, illuminating shifts in clinical and research priorities, and the increased complexities of the profession's practice.

Unlike the rich histories cited above, the timeline in Table 1.1 provides just a glimpse of the notable SLP/SLT and linguistics influences on contemporary child speech practice, from the 1930s to the 2020s, set against key professional association milestones. Striving to dodge the trap of presentism (Meyerowitz, 2020) which is what historians call the practice of evaluating past events, and people's attitudes, values, and motivations by present-day criteria, in the subsequent sections, connections are made between our histories of practice and practice today.

Early Conceptualisations of 'Normal' and 'Deviant' Speech

The book *Speech Pathology: A Dynamic Neurological Treatment of Normal Speech and Speech Deviations* (Travis, 1931) was written by an SLP professor whose passion was stuttering. It contained just one paragraph on articulation therapy and an appendix containing a list of initial–medial–final-sound production practice words and was warmly welcomed by reviewers (e.g., Buswell, 1932). His next book, *The Handbook of Speech Pathology* (Travis, 1957), or 'the Travis Handbook', as it was affectionately called, also offered a tiny contribution to articulation assessment and therapy. Nonetheless, it was highly regarded as a standard text, providing outlines of the neurophysiological bases and clinical subtypes of fluency, articulation and voice disorders, and aphasia.

Uninfluenced by linguistics theory of the day – the Linguistic Society of America was founded in 1924 – Travis presented a view of disorders that had the speech sound (phone) as the basic unit of

Table 1.1 Timeline 1924—2025: Milestones in the history of SLP/SLT management for children's speech sound disorders set against selected key developments in the MRA signatories' professional associations

1924	IALP formed	International Association of Logopedics and Phoniatrics
1924	LSA founded	Linguistic Society of America
1925	AASC formed	American Academy of Speech Correction
1926	An early use of the term speech therapy	Winifred Kingdon Ward appointed Director of Speech Therapy, West End Hospital for Nervous Diseases (London)
1927	ASSDS formed	American Society for the Study of Disorders of Speech
1931	Lee Edward Travis	*Speech Pathology: A Dynamic Neurological Treatment of Normal Speech and Speech Deviations* (Book)
1933	Ruth Lewis, Toronto's first qualified Speech Therapist	Lewis was a Canadian psychologist interested in children's speech problems who studied Speech Therapy in England
1934	Irene Poole	Produced a schedule for 'normal' articulatory proficiency
1934	ASSDS became ASCA	American Speech Correction Association
1934	Irene Poole	Created a developmental schedule for 'normal' articulation.
1934	ATSD (Remedial) formed	Association of Teachers of Speech and Drama (UK)
1935	BSST formed	British Society for Speech Therapists
1937	Robert West	*The Rehabilitation of Speech* (Book)
1937	Samuel T. Orton	*Reading, Writing and Speech Problems in Children* (Book)
1938	Stinchfield and Young	Developed a motor-kinesthetic therapy for speech defects
1939	Charles Van Riper	Proposed a social theory of speech acquisition
1940	Grant Fairbanks	Wrote a voice/articulation drill book with minimal pairs
1940	Theory–Therapy Gap and Research–Practice Gap	It was becoming evident that the principles of practice were often at odds with theory and research
1941	Roman Jakobson	Developed a linguistics theory of phonological universals
1943	Berry & Eisenson	Mildred Berry and Jon Eisenson linked a linguistic-mentalist acquisition theory with articulatory-motor therapy
1939–45	World War II Veterans needed SLP/SLT services	Education, neurology, physiology, psychology, and psychiatry (but not linguistics) informed SLP/SLT practice
1945	ATST and BSST merged	College of Speech Therapists (CST) founded in the UK
1946	NZSTA formed	New Zealand Speech Therapy Association
1947	ASCA became ASHA	American Speech and Hearing Association
1948	Kurt Goldstein	Discussed symbol formation, heralding 'Psycholinguistics'
1949	ACST inaugurated	Australian College of Speech Therapists (ACST)
1954	ACST incorporated	ACST was incorporated. Its name changed in 1975 and 1996
1957	Lee Edward Travis	*The Handbook of Speech Pathology* (Book)
1965	NZSTA was incorporated	NZSTA (Inc) became an incorporated society
1952	Helmer R. Myklebust	Used the same term symbol formation
1957	Charles Osgood	Talked about mediation/psycho-linguistic processing
1957	Mildred Templin	*Certain Language Skills in Children* (Book)
1959	CST defined 'dyslalia'	Dyslalia included in CST *Terminology for Speech Pathology*
1959	Margaret Hall Powers	Powers defined functional articulation disorder
1964	CSHA formed	Canadian Speech and Hearing Association
1965	NZSTA incorporated	New Zealand Speech Therapy Association Inc
1966	Catherine Easton Renfrew	Wrote about 'the persistence of the open syllable' in JSHR
1968	*The Sound Pattern of English* (SPE) published	Linguists, Noam Chomsky, and Morris Halle elaborated generative phonology and distinctive features theory (Book)

(Continued)

Table 1.1 (*Continued*)

1968	Jon Eisenson	Discussed symbol formation
1968	Charles Ferguson	Developed contrastive (phonological) analysis
1969–92	CST accreditation in Ireland	CST (later RCSLT) accredited ST education in Ireland
1970s	American behaviourism	3-position testing and traditional 'artic' therapy dominated
1971	IAST	The Irish Association of Speech Therapists (IAST) founded|
1972	Muriel Morley	Saw no neuromotor basis for functional articulation disorder
1972	Catherine Easton Renfrew	Published *Speech Disorders in Children*
1973	David Stampe	Explicated natural phonology and phonological processes
1975	Pamela Grunwell	Showed the relevance to SLP/SLT of clinical linguistics
1975	AASH	Australian Association of Speech and Hearing
1976	David Ingram seminal book	*Phonological Disability in Children* evoked a paradigm shift
1978	ASHA's name changed	American Speech-Language-Hearing Association
1979	Frederick Weiner	*Phonological Process Analysis*
1979	David Stampe	Expounded natural phonology and phonological processes
1980	Barbara Hodson	*The Assessment of Phonological Processes*
1980	Shriberg & Kwiatkowski	*Natural Process Analysis*
1981	Frederick Weiner	Presented an account of conventional minimal pairs therapy
1981	David Ingram	*Procedures for the Phonological Analysis of Child Speech*
1982	Stephen E. Blache	Applied distinctive features theory to child speech practice
1983	Hodson & Paden's impactful (especially in the United States) book	*Targeting Intelligible Speech* by Barbara Williams Hodson and Elaine Pagel Paden about cycles/patterns intervention
1984	Dana Monahan	Published (perhaps the first) assessment/therapy package/kit
1985b	Pamela Grunwell	*Phonological Assessment of Child Speech*: PACS
1985	Marc Fey	Published the formative 'Inextricable constructs' article
1985	Carol Stoel-Gammon and Carla Dunn	Published the scholarly and accessible (to clinicians) *Normal and Disordered Phonology in Children*
1985	CASHA renamed CASLPA	Canadian Association of Speech-Language Pathologists and Audiologists
1986	Dean and Howell	Published on linguistic awareness, heralding *Metaphon*
1986	Elbert and Gierut	*Handbook of Clinical Phonology* (Book)
1988	CPLOL	The Comité Permanent de Liason des Orthophonists-Logopèdes de l'UE (CPLOL) formed
1989	Lancaster and Pope	Developed and described auditory input therapy for under 3s
1990	Dean, Howell, Hill, Waters	Published the *Metaphon Resource Pack* (Intervention kit)
1992	Marc Fey	Headed up a challenging LSHSS clinical forum
1993	Lawrence Shriberg	Published the early, middle, and late 8 acquired consonants
1993	IAST became IASLT	IAST added 'language' to its title
1995	RCSLT Royal patronage	The Royal College of Speech and Language Therapists
1996	AASH became SPA	Speech Pathology Australia
1997	Ball and Kent	*The New Phonologies* for clinicians and linguists (Book)
1997	Joy Stackhouse and Bill Wells	Published the first volume of an influential series on the psycholinguistic framework (Books)

Table 1.1 (*Continued*)

1998–9	B. May Bernhardt and Joseph Stemberger	Developed clinical applications of non-liner phonology, including assessment and intervention resources
2001	WHO—children and youth classification	International Classification of Functioning, Disability and Health ICF-CY
2004	MRA between ASHA, RCSLT, SAC, and SPA	The International Mutual Recognition Agreement (of credentials) between four associations was inaugurated
2008	IASLT and NZSTA	Ireland and New Zealand became MRA signatories
2012	International Expert Panel on Multilingual Children's Speech (IEPMCS)	IEPMCS, led by Sharynne McLeod, published the *Multilingual Children with Speech Sound Disorders: Position Paper*
2014	CASLPA renamed SAC	Speech-Language and Audiology Canada
2014	IASLT and CORU	Registration of the SLT profession with CORU established
2018	McLeod & Crowe	Published updated the 'norms' for articulatory acquisition
2019	Telehealth/Telepractice	Telepractice burgeoned due to, the COVID-19 pandemic
2020	Online conferences/meetings	Upsurge in hybrid and online conferences due to COVID
2021	Williams, McLeod & McCauley published	*Interventions for Speech Sound Disorders in Children, 2nd edition* (Book)
2021	CPLOL became ESLA	European Speech and Language Therapy Association
2024	IALP's Centenary	International Association of Logopedics and Phoniatrics
2025	ASHA's Centenary	American Speech-Language-Hearing Association

speech. There was a hopeful sign that more was to come when Wellman et al. (1931) reported on the development of 'speech sounds' in young children. Publications by other American SLPs followed, with such revealing titles as: *The Rehabilitation of Speech* (West et al., 1937), *Reading, Writing and Speech Problems in Children* (Orton, 1937), and *Children with Delayed or Defective Speech: Motor-Kinesthetic Factors in Their Training* (Stinchfield & Young, 1938). Robert West wrote the first section of West et al. (1937) covering articulation difficulties due to 'oral deformities' and hearing impairment. Speech remediation suggestions in the book's second half included muscle relaxation, non-speech oral motor exercises: NS-OME (Lof, A24), phonetic placement strategies (Bleile, A36), and drill.

Another flurry of influential 'child speech' publications between 1939 and 1943 started with *Speech Correction: Principles and Methods* (Van Riper, 1939). This monumental work endured for nine editions (C. Van Riper & Erickson, 1996) a feat only matched by Bernthal et al. (2022) in their *Speech Sound Disorders in Children: Articulation & Phonological Disorders*. The SLP/SLT community was deeply saddened when its first author, John E. Bernthal died on July 25, 2021. A steadfast ally of countless practitioners and researchers in child

speech worldwide, Dr. Bernthal was a contributor to the first two editions of this book and the third co-author—since their sixth edition—Peter Flipsen Jr., has contributed to all three. Back to Van Riper.

Van Riper's Legacy

Charles Van Riper (1905–1994), who had a doctorate in clinical psychology and no formal SLP qualification, emphasised the significance of social context on the day-to-day experience of speech-impaired individuals, with portents of the ICF-CY (McLeod, A2). His social perspective is revealed in his famous definition:

> *Speech is defective when it deviates so far from the speech of other people in the group that it calls attention to itself, interferes with communication, or causes its possessor to be maladjusted to his environment.*
>
> Van Riper, 1939, p. 51

Van Riper's cultural sensitivity and matchless insight into what he called the 'penalties' of communication impairment may have stemmed from his intrapersonal and interpersonal experiences of stuttering. Discussing what people with communication 'differences' might make of their social situations, and what they might perceive others to read into their symptoms, he wrote – long before person first language was a thing – '*The difference in itself was not so important as its interpretation by the speech defective's associates*' (p. 66). He reflected sourly on the likely reactions of the said associates, writing: '*Personality is not merely individuality but evaluated individuality*' (p. 67). So intensely important was the social level for him that he recommend trainee speech correctionists undertake assignments, such as lisping for a day, to develop empathy for individuals with speech difficulties and a sensitivity to their emotional landscapes. The social aspect was present in his intervention advice, too, when he suggested that correctionists should work with *teachers and parents* in pursuing therapy goals.

The original phonetically oriented approaches to articulation disorders were described by Gutzmann (1895) and Kussmaul (1885) in Europe, Ward (1923) in the UK, and in the United States, Mosher (1929), Nemoy and Davis (1937), Scripture and Jackson (1919), and West et al. (1937). These authors progressively modified and elaborated earlier methodologies, but the text that is usually credited with popularizing their phonetic, sound-by-sound techniques is Van Riper's *Speech Correction*, published in 1939.

Paradoxically, although Van Riper espoused a sincerely held social view of speech impairment and disability, his speech intervention approach—classically referred to as 'Traditional Articulation Therapy' or, slightly tongue-in-cheek, 'Van Riper Therapy'—was not communication focused. Like his predecessors, he combined disparate elements in an atomistic array of peripheral procedures, including stimulus–response routines; sensory training (called auditory stimulation) comprising auditory discrimination, 'ear training' and auditory sequencing; and production drill. These became part of an auditory–phonetic (or sensory–motor) therapy that is still implemented.

In the same productive period, practical manuals, books of exercises, source books, and workbooks for speech correctionists appeared, replete with word and sentence lists for production practice, listening lists, rhymes, and stories alongside therapy tips, advice, ideas, techniques, and activities for use in speech lessons (e.g., Fairbanks, 1940; Nemoy & Davis, 1937; Twitmeyer & Nathanson, 1932).

Among the techniques that Van Riper did *not* incorporate into intervention, but which were gaining in popularity, were motorkinesthetic (or motokinesthetic) tactile manoeuvres. In keeping with his grumpy reputation (John E. Bernthal 1997, personal correspondence) Van Riper (1939, pp. 198–201) describes them with heavy sarcasm.

We have previously mentioned the Motokinesthetic Method invented by Edna Hill Young as one of the approaches used in teaching a child with delayed speech to talk. It has also been used in the elimination of misarticulations. Essentially, this method is based upon intensive stimulation; however, the stimulation is not confined to sound alone but to tactile and kinesthetic sensations as well. The therapist, by manipulation and stroking and pressing the child's face and body as she utters the stimulus syllable, helps him recognize the place of articulation, the direction of movements, the amount of air pressure, and so on. Watching an expert motokinesthetic therapist at work on a lisper is like attending a show put on by a magician. The case lies on a table with the therapist bending over him. First, she presses on his abdomen to initiate breathing as she strongly makes the s sound; then to produce a syllable from the patient, her fingers fly swiftly to close his jaws, spread the lips, and tap a front tooth, thereby signaling a narrow groove of the tongue or the focus of the airstream. Then her magical fingers squeeze together to draw out the sibilant hiss as a continuant.

One therapist, when working with a child, used to 'draw out' the s, wind it around the child's head three times then insert it into her ear, thus insuring that it would be prolonged enough to be felt. Each sound has its own unique set of deft manipulations, and considerable skill is required to administer motokinesthetic therapy effectively.

Viewed by the cold eye of the modern speech scientist, many of the motokinesthetic cues seem inappropriate; and a therapist would need sixty fingers and thirty arms to provide sufficient cues to take care of the necessary integration and coarticulation. Moreover, much of our research has indicated that standard sounds are produced in different ways by different people, and that their positioning vary widely with differing phonetic contexts. We suspect that much of the effectiveness of this method is due to its powerful suggestion (the laying on of hands), to its accompanying auditory stimulation, or to the novelty to the situation, which may free the case to try new articulatory patterns. We have used it successfully with some very refractory cases, but we always have felt a bit uncomfortable when doing so, as though we were the Magical Monarch of Mo in the Land of Hocus Pocus.

Disparities between Theory, Therapy and Practice

The release of *The Defective in Speech* (Berry & Eisenson, 1942, and see, Berry & Eisenson, 1956) provided an alternative interpretation of what might improve children's speech production. They guided a swing away from Van Riper's auditory perceptual training, refocusing on auditory memory span and the motor execution component of speech output, in treatment that saw the therapist administering general bodily relaxation procedures and speech musculature exercises. Today, these are generally referred to synonymously as non-speech oral motor exercises (NS-OME), oral motor therapy, oral motor treatment, or oromotor exercises (the more prominent UK term, sometimes called oromotor work). Apparently ignoring the social context of and consequences for the client of his or her communication impairment, Berry and Eisenson wrote about the mechanism of first-language learning for the first time in the speech pathology literature. They embraced the associative—imitative model (Allport, 1924) from psychology theory, conceptualising speech in linguistic–mentalist terms. But again, these insights were not reflected in their intervention suggestions. Like Van Riper's, their therapy belied any appreciation of language, and they proceeded from bottom up, starting with tongue, lip, and jaw exercises, with stimulation of individual phones, and using phonetic placement techniques and repetitive motor drill.

In her analysis of these inconsistencies, Duchan (2001 to date) highlights the genesis of

'a familiar trait in our professional development, the theory–therapy gap', also commenting that 'a second identifiable gap was between research findings and therapy practices', pointing to an evident interdisciplinary gap that saw speech pathologists failing to take much advantage of the developmental psychology research that flourished from the 1920s to the 1950s—a reminder of historian Peter Burke. 'Knowledges' makes me flinch slightly, but following Foucault, Burke sees knowledge or knowledge traditions as plural. He wrote:

> *It takes a polymath to 'mind the gap' and draw attention to the knowledges that may otherwise disappear into the spaces between disciplines, as they are currently defined and organized.*
>
> Burke, 2012

Dyslalia, Functional Articulation Disorder, and 'Patterns'

SLP/SLT was still a young profession when speech sound disorders in children were called 'dyslalia' or 'functional articulation disorders.' In its *Terminology for Speech Pathology*, the College of Speech Therapists (1959) defined dyslalia as: '*Defects of articulation, or slow development of articulatory* **patterns**, *including: substitutions, distortions, omissions and transpositions of the sounds of speech.*' Contemporaneously in the United States, Powers (1959, p. 711) defined it, with a different name, using the word 'functional' in its medical pathology connotation 'of currently unknown origin' or 'involving functions rather than a physiological or structural cause'. If Powers entertained the idea of introducing the acronym 'SODA' (for [S] substitution, [O] omission, [D] distortion, and [A] addition) she did not mention it. What she *said* was,

> *...the term functional articulation disorder encompasses a wide variety of deviate speech* **patterns**. *These can be described in terms of four possible types of acoustic deviations in the individual speech sounds: omissions, substitutions, distortions, and additions. An individual may show one or any combination of these deviations.*

How interesting it is to find that as early as 1959 SLTs in Britain and SLPs in the United States had an agreed definition and terminology and included the notion of speech *patterns* when they described speech development and disorders. Nonetheless, it is noted that they did so without considering speech sounds' organisation and representation, cognitively. The 'phoneme', and abstract theoretical constructs like it, were the domain of clinical linguistics, and it would not be until 20 years or more after the formulation of the British and American definitions that the beginnings of practical 'assessment connections' and 'therapy connections' (Grunwell, 1975; Ingram, 1976) would be forged between phonological theory and SLP/SLT practice.

In the UK and Australia, the name 'dyslalia' remained in vogue until the 1960s when the preferred US term, 'functional articulation disorder', gained currency. The preoccupation of therapists, in the 1960s through to the mid-1970s, with individual sounds in the so-called 'three positions' (i.e., the initial, medial, and final positions of sounds in words, e.g., for /f/ in *phone*, *sofa*, and *laugh* respectively), still constituted a strictly phonetic, sound-by-sound approach to the problem, somehow isolating the linguistic function of speech from the mechanics or motoric aspects of speech. It is enlightening to return to Grunwell's 1975 critique of contemporary practice and her proposal for a more linguistically principled approach to assessment and remediation than those that evolved from practice in the 1930s.

Functional articulation disorders were graded (subjectively) in severity as mild, moderate, or severe. In the severe category were the children with 'multiple dyslalia' or 'multiple misarticulations' whose speech was generally unintelligible to people outside of their immediate families. It was readily acknowledged that children with severe functional articulation disorders could usually imitate or quickly be taught how to produce most speech sounds (Morley, 1972). In other words, the supposed motor execution problem or 'articulation' disorder appeared to reside in the children's difficulty in employing speech sounds for word production, which they *could* produce in isolation. Intervention concentrated on the mechanical aspects of establishing the production of individual phonemes, one at a time, context by context.

By defining the problem in articulatory terms and focussing in therapy on accurate production, SLPs/SLTs failed to consider something that they already knew—that speech serves as the spoken medium of language in a system of contrasts and combinations that signal meaning–differences. That is, while children acquire the pronunciation patterns of a language and learn the correspondences between articulatory *movements* and sounds, they also discover relationships between *meanings* and sounds.

Linguistic Theory and Sound Patterns

In the 1940s and beyond, linguistics theory blossomed in the hands of Jakobson (1941/1968), who studied child language, aphasia, and phonological universals; Velten (1943), who investigated in the growth of phonemic and lexical patterns in infants; and Leopold (1947), who explored sound learning in the first two years of life. These linguistics developments eventually proved highly relevant to practice, but, in and around the World War II period, the profession tended towards neurology, physiology, psychology, and psychiatry for elucidation, and not linguistics or education. By the 1950s, however, the literature revealed that scholars knew something more was going on in speech besides auditory, visual, and tactile perception and motor execution of sounds. The idea of an inner process or underlying representation as a clinical construct was imminent. Eisenson (1968) talked about symbol formation; Goldstein (1948) and Myklebust (1952) alluded to inner language; and Osgood (1957) used two terms: mediation and psycholinguistic processing.

The linguistic linkage that enticed speech-language clinicians to consider speech disorders in terms of sound systems or patterns came when generative linguists Chomsky and Halle (1968), expounded distinctive features theory in *The Sound Patterns of English*, a book so influential in linguistic circles that it is commonly referred to as SPE (see, Zsiga, 2020, pp. 53–86 for details). Contemporaneously, Ferguson (1968) looked at contrastive speech analysis and phonological development (see also, Ferguson, 1978; C. Ferguson & Farwell, 1975; Ferguson et al., 1973). Stampe (1973, 1979) forged another link, but this time in natural phonology, leading most saliently for SLP/SLT to Ingram's innovative work (Ingram, 1974, 1976) uniquely dedicated to the understanding of disordered speech, and to Grunwell (1975, 1981) who was similarly motivated.

Clinical Phonology

The application of phonological theory to child speech practice has a chequered history. From her 2020 vantage point, Stansfield in the UK recalls:

> *Many older SLTs speak of being trained mainly to work with 'articulation' difficulties, and it was not until the late 1960s that linguistics raised its head in the speech therapy world, with pragmatics coming later still. On my own course, we had only one hour a week of linguistics for three terms. My 'finals' case book from 1972 described 13 'patients' in detail (present-day students take note, 13!). There is little evidence anywhere in the case book that this linguistic theory was put into practice, although language tests were reported ... as was working with people to increase language, and articulation, voice, and fluency skills.*
>
> Stansfield, 2020a

In the 1970s, linguists and SLPs/SLTs were talking to each other about language in general and clinical phonology particularly. Finally, what SLPs/SLTs had perceived as multiple individual errors were seen as sound class problems, involving multiple members of those classes.

Two phonologists, Pamela Grunwell, and David Ingram were on a mission to help SLPs/SLTs apply phonological principles (see Chapter 4) to treating children with 'phonological disability'; and many clinicians, myself included, devoured everything they wrote! Clinical phonology, according to Grunwell (1987), a British linguist working in the UK, was the clinical application of linguistics at the phonological level. Ingram (1989a), an American working at the University of British Columbia at the time, said phonology embraced the study of: (1) the nature of the underlying representations of speech sounds (how they are stored in the mind); (2) the nature of the phonetic representations (how the sounds are articulated); and (3) phonological rules or processes (the

mapping rules that connect the two) as shown in Figures i3 and i4. In the United States, Elbert and Gierut (1986) and Stoel-Gammon and Dunn (1985) provided further theoretically principled guidance in books about assessment and intervention.

The most radical aspect of the new principles was the concept of changing phonological patterns by stimulating children's underlying systems for phoneme use. Sections of the clinical community were apprehensive. Would the theoretical paradigm shift bring big changes to familiar therapy approaches, goals, procedures, and activities? Mark Fey mitigated these uncertainties in a reassuring article, in which he wrote:

> .... *adopting a phonological approach to dealing with speech sound disorders does not necessitate the rejection of the well-established principles underlying traditional approaches to articulation disorders. To the contrary, articulation must be recognized as a critical aspect of speech sound development under any theory. Consequently, phonological principles should be viewed as adding new dimensions and new perspectives to an old problem, not simply as refuting established principles. These new principles have resulted in the development of several procedures that differ in many respects from old procedures yet are highly similar in others.*
>
> Fey, 1985, p. 255

In their response to Q3., Nicole Müller and Martin Ball, both linguists, explore the development of the application of linguistic sciences to speech SLP/SLT practice.

Dr. Nicole Müller received a master's degree from the University of Bonn, Germany, and a doctorate from the University of Oxford, England. She has taught at the University of Central England, Birmingham, at Cardiff University, Wales, the University of Louisiana at Lafayette, Linköping University, Sweden, and is now the Professor of Speech and Hearing Sciences at University College Cork, Ireland. Her research combines interests in clinical linguistics, dementia, and bilingualism, with occasional forays into phonetics, speech disorders, and aphasia. She co-edits the book series *Communication Disorders across Languages*.

Dr. Martin J. Ball is Honorary Professor of Linguistics at Bangor University in Wales. He is co-editor of the *Journal of Monolingual and Bilingual Speech* (Equinox), and the book series *Communication Disorders Across Languages* (Multilingual Matters). His main research interests include sociolinguistics, clinical phonetics and phonology, and the linguistics of Welsh. Among his recent books are *Phonetics for Speech Pathology 3rd edition*, with colleagues (Ball et al., 2021)) and *Manual of Clinical Phonetics* (edited, Ball, 2021). Professor Ball is an honorary Fellow of the Royal College of Speech and Language Therapists, and a Fellow of the Learned Society of Wales.

Q3.   Nicole Müller and Martin J. Ball: Application of Linguistic Sciences

Crystal (2001) defined clinical linguistics, which originated in the 1970s, as 'the application of the linguistic sciences to the study of language disability in all its forms'. It has become an independent discipline, with its own scholarly association and a peer-reviewed journal, as well as being a core curriculum subject in the education of SLPs/SLTs. On one hand, it informs SLP/SLT assessment, target selection, and intervention practices, and on the other, it provides a tool for the critical evaluation of competing linguistic theories and methodologies. In the process, each discipline impacts the other. How did these two-way influences evolve, and what, in your estimation, are the contributions of clinical linguistics to SLP/SLT practice and vice versa? Since the previous editions of this book, there has been an increase in therapists working with children with speech sound disorders in the predominantly English-speaking, industrialized world. More recently, there has been a striking and necessary rise in telepractice (Williams, Thomas, & Caballero, A46.). Have these changes brought with them new roles and research directions for clinical linguists?

A3.   Nicole Müller and Martin J. Ball: Clinical Linguistics (and Phonetics)

Students of speech-language pathology/therapy (SLP/SLT) at times find it difficult to understand why we burden them with the study of linguistic (and phonetic) theory. To clinical linguists and phoneticians, the motivation is obvious: To us, doing SLP/SLT without a thorough grounding in linguistic and phonetics is like doing engineering without physics: One (physics, or linguistics/phonetics) provides a conceptual basis, and indeed a language and analytical tools, to be able to talk about and do the practical work associated with the other.

The term clinical linguistics gained currency in SLP/SLT and linguistics in the wake of David Crystal's publication of a book with that title in 1981. Crystal defined clinical linguistics as the 'application of linguistic science to the study of communication ability, as encountered in clinical situations' (Crystal, 1981, p. 1) and expanded on this definition later: '[C]linical linguistics is the application of the theories, methods, and findings of linguistics (including phonetics) to the study of those situations where language handicaps are diagnosed and treated' (Crystal, 1984, p. 31). In other words, clinical linguistics provides the theoretical backbone to develop tools for use in SLP/SLT. Other linguists have used a wider definition and include, under the umbrella term clinical linguistics, research that uses data gathered from participants with a variety of language disorders to test hypotheses and models formed based on typical language, or more often, based on native speaker intuition and introspection of how language works (see for example, Ball & Kent, 1987; Müller & Ball, 2013, for further discussion).

Like other scientists and philosophers, linguists construct categories and build models that aid them in thinking about phenomena they encounter in the real world. In other words, they build theories to understand the world we live in. The theories and interpretive categories we use to analyse language produced by people with a variety of language disorders, to develop assessment and diagnostic procedures, and to better understand the defining characteristics of language disorders are imports into the clinical domain: There are no linguistic theories applied to disordered language that don't start out as theories of typical language. Most modern linguistic frameworks, including phonological theories, have been applied in the clinical context. Some aspiring or practising clinicians may, on reading this, think, 'but I'm not interested in all this theorizing. I want to know which tools to use in practice.' We need to keep in mind, though, that we can't think without theorizing, and categorizing: Thinking, talking about, and striving to understand any phenomenon necessarily involves building models and theories. The labels and categories that SLPs/SLTs use to analyse the characteristics of disordered language (or speech) rest on a set of assumptions about the nature of the phenomena analysed, and these assumptions can differ dramatically between different theories of language. Further, when we use categories and labels provided by linguistic theories, we also need to ask ourselves whether we use them as descriptive and analytical devices only, or whether we assume that the categories we use represent psychological or mental realities.

Generative Theory

There is a sizeable body of work that applies Chomskyan generative linguistics, in its various versions, to the study of impaired language, including phonology. Some key assumptions in generative theory are that language is a modular cognitive system that is independent of other cognitive systems, and that it is a complex of mental representation with a grammar at its core. Modular systems have distinct, clearly separable components (e.g., lexicon, phonology, morphology, and syntax in language). From such a perspective, language impairments are viewed as selective deficits within the mental grammar of a speaker (see for example, Clahsen, 2008; Schulz & Friedmann, 2011). The aim of the linguist working within a Chomskyan generative model is to build a generative account of mental

categories and operations. Language use, in the generative tradition of clinical linguistics, is of interest only insofar as it can give insight into the mental representations that give rise to it. This means that for the generative linguist, it is not an object of investigation in and of itself.

Usage-Based Approaches

In contrast, usage-based approaches to language theorize that grammar emerges from general cognitive abilities, and that language learning uses the same cognitive abilities as other types of learning, for instance, the ability to make inferences, categorization, memory, and motoric abilities (see, M. Barlow & Kemmer, 2000, for an overview of usage-based models; Vogel Sosa & Bybee, 2008, on cognitive phonology; Martínez-Ferreiro et al., 2020 for a recent review of usage-based and functional approaches in aphasia). A usage-based approach to language learning gives a crucial role to language use in a continuous process of modifying and building a child's language, which in turn is seen as a dynamic, emergent system. This is very different from considering the role of input as that of a mere trigger for the setting of a finite number of pre-determined parameters in a child's internal grammar (as in the principles and parameters account of generative linguistics).

Implications For SLP/SLT Practice

Why do such differences matter in clinical practice? And why does it matter whether we consider models as aids to our thinking, or as representing mental or psychological reality? Let us consider a concept all SLPs/SLTs have learned about at some point, namely the phoneme. It is typically defined as the smallest unit of sound in any one language that can bring about a change in meaning between words (which gives us the clinically useful notion of the minimal pair or minimal group). Phonemes represent contrastivity in spoken language. If we treat phonemes as entities that have a reality as mental representations in the Chomskyan generative tradition, then we will most likely conceptualize them as made up of distinctive features, and think of language use, or input, as a trigger for the setting of feature specifications. From this theoretical perspective, it should be immaterial whether an SLP/SLT targets phonemic contrasts in intervention using many different examples of minimal pairs or only a few, since any one minimal pair could serve as a sufficient representation of a target contrast. On the other hand, we can use the term phoneme as a descriptive summary: certain minimal differences between otherwise similar sequences of articulator configurations result in output that represents different meanings. Thus, the syllables /dɪp/ and /tɪp/ illustrate that fortis and lenis plosives in English represent different phonemes. The term phoneme summarizes a complex of cognitive as well as physical processes that link the meanings of words with sound production, hearing, and perception. In other words, the symbols /t/ and /d/ are a very economical way of representing that a fortis versus a lenis alveolar plosive, in an otherwise identical syllable structure, is 'different enough' in English to represent different words with distinct meanings. We can further note that this difference is expressed in word-initial position typically by an aspirated voiceless plosive [tʰ] versus a partially devoiced plosive [d̥], and to these latter categories we typically refer as allophones of their respective phonemes. This way of thinking, in our view, aligns well with usage-based theories of language: From this perspective, phonology is considered as an emergent property of vocabulary learning. In terms of intervention, it would therefore make the most sense to use many different exemplars in input and output to facilitate the emergence of the target contrast.

Communication in Real Life

SLPs/SLTs need linguistics (including phonetics) because linguistic frameworks provide tools to discover patterns in the language (and speech) produced by adults and children with language, speech (or other) impairments, which in turn can contribute to understanding communication successes and breakdowns and inform intervention. We believe that is it most useful to take models as aids to thinking, and a further important

assumption that we make about a clinically useful linguistics is that it should be data driven; in other words, the starting point should always be language used in context. This means, in turn, that we need to contextualize theoretical notions by reference to communication in real life: To return to our earlier example, we represent the English phonemes /t/ and /d/ by IPA symbols for static articulatory configurations. However, speech is about movement, coordination, precision, and timing, and about context, and goal setting and intervention must take this into consideration.

A large proportion of clinical linguistic research is, still, on monolingual English speakers. Increasing linguistic diversity in majority English-speaking countries, and the reality of working with multilingual clients represent a significant opportunity for clinical linguists. There are well-established traditions of multilingualism research in sociolinguistics and speech and language development that can inform work in the clinical realm investigating the nature of multilingual language systems, language use (code-switching, for instance), and indeed language and speech norms, which in some multilingual context can be very fluid (see for example, McLeod & Goldstein, 2012, on speech sound disorders; Babatsouli et al., 2017, on language acquisition; Müller et al., 2019, on bilingualism) in the context of rapid language change; (see Pascoe, A39. on the development of speech assessments, normative data, and interventions for children acquiring the languages of Southern Africa).

There is also a well-established linguistic tradition of analysing language use in interaction, for instance, within Systemic Functional Linguistics (see for example, Hersh et al., 2018). The analytical categories used in this tradition, for instance, speech function and exchange structures, will lend themselves to analysing remote therapeutic interaction via telehealth platforms. Remote service delivery and communication with clients have become the norm rather than the exception for many students and clinicians in the wake of the COVID-19 pandemic, and while face-to-face work will remain crucial for many clients, we can confidently predict that telehealth will remain an important mode of communication in SLP/SLT, and thus it represents an important analytic focus for clinical linguists.

Articulation Development

In work whose impact was far-reaching, Irene Poole, a speech teacher at the University Elementary School in Ann Arbor, Michigan, who was pursuing a doctorate, produced a developmental schedule for phonetic development (Poole, 1934). This was consistent with the prevailing, and persisting, view that intervention for speech impairment should be based on typical developmental expectations of 'articulatory proficiency'. Other accounts of phonetic mastery criteria have followed, up to the time of writing. They include (Arlt & Goodban, 1976; Kilminster & Laird, 1978; Prather et al., 1975; Sander, 1972; Smit et al., 1990; Templin, 1957); and, through to more up-to-date, peer-reviewed accounts of acquisition by Crowe and McLeod (2020), McLeod (2022, pp. 57–108), and McLeod and Crowe (2018).

A study of phonetic age-norms by Kilminster and Laird (1978) involved single-word citation naming by children aged 3;0–8;6 (years;months) in Queensland, Australia, with the aim of determining the ages, in years and months, by which 75% of children had mastered 24 English phones. Most developmental profiles of phonetic acquisition are similarly structured, but Shriberg (1993) took a fresh approach when he produced a clinically useful breakdown of the 'early-8', 'middle-8' and 'late-8' acquired sounds, based on monosyllabic words in conversational speech samples: reflecting the approximate *order* of acquisition rather than

approximate *ages* of acquisition. The norms provided by Kilminster and Laird, and Shriberg's early-, middle- and late-8 are contrasted in Table 1.2, together with a more recent study (McLeod & Crowe, 2018).

It is common for SLPs/SLTs to show parents a consonant acquisition chart in explaining their child's speech development progress. When this relates, for example, to a five-year-old who is essentially on-track with just /dʒ, tʃ, ʃ and ʒ/ missing or erred this can be helpful and potentially reassuring for the parent in the sense of the difficulty being mild or moderate, with not much delay in development. The clinician might then show them the McLeod and Crowe (2018) order of acquisition, explaining reassuringly that the child '*has all her four- to five-year-old sounds except /dʒ/ and /tʃ/ and all her five- to seven-year-old sounds except, /ʃ/ and /ʒ/*'. On the other hand, if the child is a 12-year-old with an intellectual impairment and a limited phonetic inventory, it is somehow less dispiriting for parents if the therapist focuses on *order* rather than *age* of acquisition, by saying something like, '*she's conquered all 13 of the early sounds and /v/ from the middle sounds, so she's over halfway there, with 10 sounds to go*'.

McLeod and Crowe's 'new norms', especially for /ɹ/, flagged a potential impact on service eligibility and funding for students within US schools (Storkel, 2019) triggering a social media kerfuffle (Harold, 2018; updated 2019, 2020), among US

Table 1.2 Developmental schedules for phonetic development of English-speaking children in Australia (1978), the United States (1993), and internationally (2018)

Age of acquisition Kilminster & Laird, 1978[a] Australian children	Order of acquisition Shriberg, 1993[b] United States children	Order of acquisition* McLeod & Crowe, 2018[c] English-speaking children
3;0 p b t d k g m ŋ w j h	Early 8	Early 2;0–3;11
3;6 f	m n j b w d p h	p, b, m, d, n, h, t, k, g, w, ŋ, f, j
4;0 l ʃ tʃ		
4;6 s z dʒ	Middle 8	Middle 4;0–4;11
5;0 ɹ	t ŋ k g v tʃ dʒ	l, dʒ, tʃ, s, v, ʃ, z
6;0 v		
8;0 ð	Late 8	Late 5;0–6;11
8;6 θ	ʃ ʒ l ɹ s z ð θ	ɹ, ʒ, ð, θ

*McLeod & Crowe list consonants in age of acquisition order, from youngest to oldest.
[a]Data source: single-word citation naming of picture stimuli.
[b]Data source: monosyllabic words in conversational speech samples.
[c]Data source: single words; 90–100% acquisition criteria averaged across eight studies.

SLPs. Many were applying the Smit et al. (1990) norm of 8;0–8;11 for /ɹ/ far later than McLeod and Crowe's (A42) 5;0–5;11.

Regarding /r/ and /ɹ/, in phonetics /r/ is the voiced alveolar trill that is present, for example, in Scottish English and Spanish. The R-sound we hear from most English speakers is the voiced, alveolar (or postalveolar) approximant /ɹ/. In the SLP/SLT literature, particularly in older US publications, /ɹ/ and [ɹ] are (incorrectly) rendered as /r/ and [r]. Speakers of rhotic varieties of English pronounce the 'R' as /ɹ/ in words like *red* [ɹɛd] and *barrow* ['bæɹoʊ], and as the rhotic vowels /ɝ/ or /ɚ/ in words such as *butterfly* ['bʌtɚˈflaɪ], *dollar* ['dɑlɚ], *cracker* ['kɹækɚ], *first* [fɝst], *turning* ['tɝnɪŋ], terse [tɝs] and *church* [tʃɝtʃ]. Most people in the United States speak a rhotic variety of English, so the 'R-norms' for that language group cover /ɹ/ and the rhotic vowels /ɝ/ and /ɚ/. For more on American phonetics, refer to Shriberg et al. (2018) and see Flipsen Jr. A37 on treating R-errors.

Entertaining the *possibility* that consonant acquisition data drawn from children in the United States might differ from English-speaking children's speech data from elsewhere due to differences between word position, transcription, and analysis conventions, Crowe and McLeod (2020) reviewed age of acquisition information specifically intended to guide SLPs working with US children acquiring English. Their study, which included English consonant acquisition data from close to 19,000 children living in the United States (see Table 1.3), echoed their 2018 cross-linguistic findings. It is pleasing that Crowe and McLeod (2020), McLeod and Crowe (2018), and Storkel (2019) are openly accessible; 'pleasing' because,

> *These data inform SLPs' clinical decision making and consideration of eligibility for services to support best practice to enhance children's communicative competence.*
>
> Crowe & McLeod, 2020, p. 2167

Clinically relevant normative data began emerging in the 1970s when practice was heavily influenced by the medical model and American behaviourism; 'SODA' articulation analysis of errors of (S) substitution, (O) omission, (D) distortion and (A) addition; and 'Traditional Articulation Therapy'

Table 1.3 Developmental schedule for phonetic development of English-speaking children in the United States (2020)

Order of acquisition*
Crowe & McLeod, 2020[a]
United States children
Early 2;0–3;11
b, n, m, p, h, w, d, g, k, f, t, ŋ, j (all stops, nasals, and glides)
Middle 4;0–4;11
v, ʤ, s, ʧ, l, ʃ, z
Late 5;0–6;11
ɹ, ð, ʒ, θ

*Consonants are listed in order of age of acquisition from youngest to oldest.
[a]Data source: single words; 90% acquisition criteria across 15 studies of typical speech

(Van Riper, 1978; C. Van Riper & Erickson, 1996). Van Riper Therapy, or at least close variations of it, continued, and continues to be widely implemented.

> *Any contemporary view of treatment needs to stress what is new. Thus, non- contemporary roots might cause clinicians to not take traditional motor approaches seriously. In addition, after so much emphasis has been placed on analyzing our clients' phonemic systems, clinicians wonder whether a traditional phonetic approach should still be used. It should be; there is definitely a place for these methods in our contemporary understanding of speech sound disorders and their remediation. These procedures are certainly used as a part of many phonological treatment procedures. … there might be a time in the course of every treatment, for articulation or phonological disorders, when these principles could be used briefly to obtain a specific sound.*
>
> Bauman-Waengler, 2020, p. 271

When Brumbaugh and Smit (2013) surveyed 2,084 US clinicians working with 3–6-year-olds, they mustered 489 usable responses. Of the 489, 49% *often* or *always* used traditional intervention with children with SSD, and 33% *sometimes* did. These findings were like those of Joffe and Pring (2008) in the UK; Pascoe et al. (2010) in South

Africa; McLeod and Baker (2014) in Australia; Oliveira et al. (2015) in Portugal; Hegarty et al. (2018) in the UK; Hegarty et al. (2020) in Northern Ireland; and L. M. Furlong et al. (2021) in Victoria, Australia.

Traditional Articulation Therapy and Eclectic Practice

Eclectic or hybrid approaches (Lancaster et al., 2010; Joffe, A23; McLeod & Baker, 2014) may see SLPs/SLTs:

- Mismatching assessment and intervention processes, e.g., using a 3-position articulation test to determine treatment targets for a phonological intervention such as Multiple Oppositions Intervention (Williams, A19).
- Mingling interventions, e.g., administering a mix of *Metaphon* (E. C. Dean et al., 1995) and Core Vocabulary Therapy (Dodd, 2005).
- Combining *components* of different approaches that are associated with reasonable levels of evidence when administered as part of a 'package', according to an empirically validated protocol. Such amalgamations might include delivering aspects of the Nuffield Dyspraxia Programme (Williams A33) with aspects of Language-Based Intervention for Speech and Language Disorders (Tyler, 2002).
- Cherry-picking screening, assessment, and intervention processes that they 'like', or that the client will at least tolerate, or at best enjoy, to devise their preferred blend of assessment and intervention approaches, procedures, and activities.

As Wren et al. (2018, p. 417) sniped, *clinicians tend to favour the use of just two or three named approaches, often combined into one eclectic package, presumably with the expectation that one of the elements within the package will target the child's specific needs.*

L. M. Furlong et al. (2021) described their exploration, via guided interviews, of the *intervention processes* that 11 Australian SLPs working in the state of Victoria used to treat children with SSDs, defining *intervention processes* as

...the series of therapeutic actions and steps directed toward remediation of an SSD. These therapeutic actions and steps broadly relate to target selection, selection of a therapy approach, and the structural and procedural aspects of therapy sessions.

L. M. Furlong et al., 2021, p. 3

They found that SLPs frequently worked eclectically, employing a mixture of four intervention procedures: minimal pair activities, traditional articulation approaches, auditory discrimination, and *Cued Articulation* (Passy, 2010).

Cued Speech was developed by R. Orin Cornett (b. 1913 d. 2002) in 1966 as a visual system of communication used with and among deaf or hard-of-hearing people. By contrast, *Cued Articulation* is a system of logical hand cues, and colour-coded letters (e.g., green for /s/ and /z/, pink for /f/ and /v/, purple for / tʃ/ and /dʒ/). It was first published in 1986, to aid in teaching children to say 26 consonants and 23 vowels. It remains popular among SLPs in Queensland, and in Victoria where SLP Jane Passy devised it while working with children with severe speech and language problems. Teachers trained in the technique applied it in literacy classes. Passy also ran training courses for teachers in the UK where Joffe and Pring (2008) found that 30.6% of the British SLTs they surveyed used *Cued Articulation* for speech intervention often/always; 26% sometimes; and 42% rarely/never. Helen Botham continues Passy's work, focusing on literacy, particularly phonological awareness (PA) and improving teacher knowledge of the links between PA and reading. (Botham, 2020). An innovation was a *Cued Articulation App* for iPad and Android tablets (Passy et al., 2014).

L. M. Furlong et al. (2021) further found that SLPs based their choices of initial therapy targets on typical order of acquisition criteria, or child or family preferences as to 'what to work on', prioritising clients' needs in choosing therapy targets, and in their choices of therapy approaches.

The eclecticism story recurs internationally. For example, Joffe and Pring (2008) surveyed UK SLTs, and reported that they combined three 'therapies': auditory discrimination, meaningful minimal contrast, and phonological awareness that addressed different levels of input and output processing (see Schäfer & Fricke A21). Also in the UK, Lancaster et al. (2010) combined perceptual processing (e.g., phonological awareness), and production tasks. Pascoe et al. (2010) in culturally and linguistically diverse (CALD) Western Cape, South Africa found that their 28 survey participants used a wide variety of therapies, eclectically with few adhering to a single approach to treating SSD. They deemed this appropriate in their local context, given their CALD demographic and the frequent need for clinicians to improvise (e.g., by administering informal assessments only). They ranked the therapies participants implemented, in most to least popular order as: 1. Auditory discrimination, 2. Phonological awareness (Gillon, 2000), 3. Parent-based programs, 4. Articulation work/motor-skills training (Van Riper & Emerick, 1984), 5. Core vocabulary (Dodd, 2005), 6. Meaningful minimal-contrast pairs (Weiner, 1981a, 1981b), 7. Cued articulation (Passy, 1990) and 8. Whole language approach (Hoffman et al., 1990), followed by seven that were less popular.

In Portugal, Oliveira et al. (2015) built on Lousada et al. (2013) and found that therapists combined phonological awareness, auditory discrimination, and meaningful minimal contrast therapy. They commented that *'The great majority of SLTs combined several approaches in their intervention. There was also a high percentage of SLTs that used articulation-based approaches, namely articulation work (31%) in cases of phonologically based disorders.'* (p. 182).

In Britain, Hegarty et al. (2018) revealed a similar but more arresting example of 'articulation work' as the fourth most popular approach for phonological impairment, which they called 'phonological SSD' in their survey, reflecting its cognitive-linguistic basis. They conducted a UK-wide survey of 166 therapists' management of children with phonological impairment, which included inconsistent speech disorder (Dodd, 2005). Disappointingly, they found that close to half of their respondents *'always or often used traditional articulation therapy to remediate phonological impairment, even though this approach has been found to be less effective for this difficulty'* (p. 995). The SLTs used speech discrimination (79.5%), conventional minimal pairs (77.3%), phonological awareness therapy (75.6%), and traditional articulation therapy (48.4%).

Following Hegarty et al. (2018), Hegarty et al. (2020) concluded, from focus groups and interviews

with SLTs in Northern Ireland, that *'There is a research-practice gap in which SLPs' current practices are driven by organisational factors, their own preferences and child-specific factors.'* Their participants suggested that the development of time-saving, evidence-based tools might help address this gap.

In their 2021 article, Furlong et al. considered eclecticism problematic, because

1. Implementation fidelity (Baker A26.) for both content and dose of the various therapy elements is difficult to replicate and measure; and
2. the therapies often used within eclectic frameworks may only be supported by evidence for their isolated use, not in combination with other therapies.

Revolution?

Did the hackneyed term 'paradigm shift' (Kuhn, 1962) exaggerate what happened? *Was* there a phonological revolution? *Did* the new principles change practice? Certainly, there were changes in the way some SLPs/SLTs understood phonological *theory* and chose *assessments* (e.g., Grunwell, 1975, 1985a; Hodson, 1980; Hodson & Paden, 1981; Ingram, 1981; Shriberg & Kwiatkowski, 1980; Weiner, 1979), but did the *intervention* work of Elbert, Dunn, Gierut, Grunwell, Hodson, Ingram, Paden, Stoel-Gammon, and others alter what happened in therapy? The answer probably must be, 'not much'.

Indeed, Barbara Williams Hodson, co-developer with Elaine Pagel Paden of patterns/cycles therapy (Hodson & Paden 1983, Hodson & Paden, 1991), bemoaned SLPs' devotion to sound-by-sound therapy in 2004. Interviewed by Thinking Publications (2004), for their website, she said, *'The one thing I wish most is that SLPs would work on patterns when serving an unintelligible child, rather than to focus on teaching isolated sounds to a criterion'*. Apparently, little had changed by 2013, when Brumbaugh and Smit reported that 33% of their American respondents frequently used the cycles phonological patterns approach and suggested that *'SLPs who treated preschoolers were using hybrid interventions, influenced primarily by traditional intervention, but also by minimal pairs and cycles approaches'* (p. 316).

Where the questions in this book are directed to more than one author, thumbnail biographies appear before their Q&A in the order in which they appear on the piece. The only exception is Q5/A5, where Dr. Hodson's bio appears first, as a courtesy and to reflect her high standing within the profession.

Dr. Barbara Williams Hodson is a Professor Emerita at Wichita State University. Dr. Hodson has published two phonology tests (one in Spanish), a computer software program, and three books, which include *Evaluating and Enhancing Children's Phonological Systems: Research and Theory to Practice*, research articles in scholarly national and international journals, and numerous textbook chapters. She has delivered clinical phonology presentations nationally and internationally. Her major professional goal has been to develop more effective assessment and remediation procedures for children with highly unintelligible speech. Dr. Hodson has been recognized by peers with, among other tributes, the American Speech-Language-Hearing Foundation's Frank R. Kleffner Lifetime Clinical Career Award (2004), the Wichita State University's (WSU) Excellence in Research Award (2008), and the highest award of the profession in the United States, ASHA Honors (2009). Dr. Hodson established the Barbara Williams Hodson Scholarship in Communication Sciences and Disorders in 2012 to recognize and reward outstanding researchers in the WSU College of Health Professions.

Dr. Raul F. Prezas is an Associate Professor in the Department of Speech and Hearing Sciences at Lamar University in Texas. He has over 15 years' of clinical experience in university, public school, and home health settings; particularly working with culturally and linguistically diverse populations. His interests include speech disorders, phonological development, bilingual/multicultural assessment, and treatment, working with children with highly unintelligible

speech, and phonological treatment models and outcomes. In addition to publications in several journals, including the *American Journal of Speech-Language Pathology*, he has written several book chapters and articles related to his interest areas. He served on the International Expert Panel on Multilingual Children's Speech, which included efforts to establish international screening tools and guidelines for speech sound assessment and treatment in various populations. He is a member of ASHA's Continuing Education Board. Dr. Prezas has been invited to present his research and share his experiences at numerous workshops, webinars, and conventions throughout the United States and its unincorporated territory Puerto Rico; and Canada, Chile, England, Scotland, and Wales.

Dr. Lesley C. Magnus is a Professor in the Department of Communication Sciences and Disorders at Minot State University in North Dakota. She has worked in the field for more than 35 years as a clinician, teacher, and mentor. After 10 years of clinical work in Paediatric SLP, Dr. Magnus returned to Wichita State University to complete her Doctor of Philosophy in Communication Disorders and Sciences under Dr. Barbara Hodson. Magnus' professional interests and work lie in the areas of phonology, speech sound disorders, working with children with highly unintelligible speech, cleft lip and palate, and early language disorders in children. Dr. Magnus has co-authored book chapters and articles related to her interest areas. Dr. Magnus is a certified S-LP(C) and SLP in Canada and the United States, respectively. In addition, she is past president of the Saskatchewan Association of Speech Language Pathologists and Audiologists. At her university, Dr. Magnus won The Most Dedicated Advisor in 2015 and the Academic Advisor of the year in 2021. She presents locally, nationally, and internationally on the topics of Phonological Intervention.

Q5.   Raul Prezas, Lesley Magnus, and Barbara Hodson: A Phonological Patterns Focus

Professor Hodson, a clinical phonology pioneer and household name in SLP/SLT circles, has pursued at least three long-standing clinical interests. First, helping children with difficult-to-understand speech to achieve intelligibility. Second, the initial and ongoing expansion of the Cycles Phonological Pattern Approach (CPPA) and within that, the role of metaphonology. And third, implementation of CPPA with multilingual populations.

In previous editions of this book, she discussed some possible reasons why many clinicians in the United States still focus on mastering phonemes one-at-a-time until a pre-specified criterion is reached, even when working with children who have highly unintelligible speech. For the third edition, I put the following questions to Dr. Hodson and her co-authors, Drs Prezas and Magnus.

Does the apparent resistance to working 'phonologically' and focusing on speech patterns persist, and if so, why might that be? Do SLPs/SLTs have other concerns about CPPA's implementation? What is 'metaphonology' and why is it integral to CPPA? What recommendations are there for applying CPPA when working with bilingual children at the severe end of the phonological disorder scale, including Spanish-speaking children and others with culturally and linguistically diverse (CALD) backgrounds?

A5.   Raul Prezas, Lesley Magnus, and Barbara Williams Hodson: The Cycles Phonological Pattern Approach: Expediting Intelligibility

In our experience, there is an increasing body of clinicians who understand that children with highly unintelligible speech require intervention that goes beyond the traditional phoneme-oriented approach. Social media has been helpful in conveying this message and clinical researchers (e.g., Dr. Kelly Farquharson Bevens on Instagram @classlab_fsu) and clinicians (e.g., Amy Graham, also on Instagram @grahamspeechtherapy) and others, use social media platforms to impress on their followers that a *phonological* intervention is essential for many children. While clinicians are now more inclined to focus on phonological patterns there remains a need for further clarification of the 'what', 'when', and 'how' of specific treatment targets to use. Furthermore, graduate students' and practitioners' effectiveness as interventionists is heightened when they are imbued with the principle that target selection for this highly unintelligible population involves a careful, individualized process of balancing complex sounds (within the child's Zone of Proximal Development; Vygotsky, 1962) and earlier developing sounds in a theoretically sound framework.

Expediting intelligibility in highly unintelligible children remains a central undertaking for SLP/SLT practitioners. Drawing on our experience of delivering CPPA workshops in the United States, the UK, and New Zealand, we perceive that choosing appropriate targets, and not clinicians' resistance to a phonological approach, is now the main concern. Unfortunately, many recently qualified US SLPs still report that while they learned about various phonological interventions as graduate students, they are not taught either in classes or in clinics *how* to provide pattern-oriented treatment. Accordingly, they are often astounded in our workshops at the gains in clients' intelligibility with one hour per week of patterns-oriented intervention over 24 months, or fewer.

The CPPA

The *Cycles Phonological Pattern Approach: CPPA* (Hodson, 2010; Prezas et al., 2021) is based on several decades of clinical practice and research and is designed specifically for children 2;5 to 14;0 with highly unintelligible speech (in the severe to profound range, with a score of 101–150 or >151 respectively on the 2004 *Hodson Assessment of Phonological Patterns-3* (HAPP-3)). The HAPP-3 is a pattern-oriented assessment that helps to identify major phonological error patterns requiring intervention. It employs object and picture stimuli to collect a 50-single-word sample. Major error patterns are classified as omissions of sound segments, major substitutions, major assimilations, syllable-structure/context-related changes, voicing alternations, and other deviations/distortions.

CPPA offers a model with clear target pattern guidelines that eliminate guesswork in determining which patterns to target and when. Initiated in 1975 in an experimental clinic for young children, aged 3;6 to 8;10 with highly unintelligible speech, CPPA was a response to the observation that some children required years of intervention to 'master' all the sounds and word structures (see Hodson & Paden, 1991). Clearly, an alternative approach was needed and, in the mid 1970s, Grunwell (1975) and Ingram (1976) helped practitioners and researchers see beyond individual phonemes. When broad patterns were targeted via CPPA, children's intelligibility gains were enhanced, and progress occurred more rapidly than was typical with a sound-by-sound approach.

Practical guidance for clinicians has arisen from CPPA's implementation over the years. First, for example, singleton /s/ and even /f/ are often mistakenly targeted initially with highly unintelligible clients who 'stop' fricatives (e.g., replacing /s/ and /f/ with [t]). When such children attempt to produce word initial /s/, they may produce /s/ accurately, but then insert /t/, so that *sun* becomes *stun*. Once children have been taught to delete /t/ and can say *sun*, words with /s/+stop clusters are produced with /s/ singletons (e.g., *stun* becomes *sun*). Therefore, it was hypothesised that targeting /s/ clusters before /s/ singletons might be more expedient for this client population. Moreover, as children start incorporating /s/ clusters into conversational speech, their intelligibility improves (e.g., Gordon-Brannan et al., 1992).

Second, children with highly unintelligible speech need practice with all their error types. Targeting phonological patterns in cycles, in time periods varying from 5 to 16 hours depending on each child's needs, was explored at the first experimental phonology clinic (Hodson & Paden, 1991) and adjusted frequently to establish appropriate frequency and duration of treatment cycles.

Typically, a consonant phoneme or two-element consonant cluster (e.g., /st/) is targeted for 1 hour per week, in one 60-minute session, two 30-minute sessions, or three 20-minute sessions, with each pattern usually targeted from 2 to 5 hours in aggregate per cycle. This timeframe is increased to 120 minutes per target for children with cognitive delays (Berman, 2001). Thus, targets for the CPPA are Phonological Patterns (e.g., syllables or 'syllableness'; final consonants). Training individual phones in particular word positions (e.g., initial /b/) may be done as an intermediary step but not as a goal.

Some SLPs/SLTs may consider CPPA and think, 'wait a minute, why am I targeting /b/, I thought this was a patterns approach?' By way of explanation, it can be beneficial to introduce a placeholder sound, that a child can produce well, for certain phonological patterns (e.g., initial consonants; final consonants). Therefore, in this case, /b/ is targeted as a 'placeholder' for word-initial consonants. This provides them with accurate kinaesthetic feedback for the sound, correctly produced in a real word and in a position of the word where an error pattern is occurring. This in turn provides them with a kinaesthetic image, where the term 'kinaesthetic image' refers to the brain's perception of relative movements and positions of body parts (see the servomechanism explanation by Fairbanks, 1954). To introduce a placeholder for /b/ you might choose 'buy' (if the child says it correctly) and do activities around 'buy' in the session. Placeholder sounds often, but not necessarily, involve the early developing /p, b, m, or w/ (noting that /w/ does not occur in same languages).

Theoretical and Underlying Concepts of CPPA

The CPPA is based on developmental phonology theories, cognitive psychology principles, and ongoing clinical phonology research. It is aligned most closely with two theories: Gestural Phonology (Browman & Goldstein, 1986, pp. 219–252; Prezas et al., 2021) and Dynamic Systems (De Bot et al., 2007; Rvachew & Bernhardt, 2010). It is based on eight underlying concepts, listed in Table A5.1 (Hodson, 2010; Hodson & Paden, 1991).

It is important to note that articulatory difficulty is increased gradually throughout the CPPA so that the child is optimally challenged but successful in producing target words from the outset. Most children between the ages of 3;0 and 5;0 with initial intelligibility below 20% have become essentially intelligible within 3 to 4 cycles (i.e., approximately 30 to 40 contact hours) and simultaneously demonstrated significantly improved phonological systems (e.g., Gordon-Brannan et al., 1992).

CPPA addresses a combination of earlier developing sounds and complex patterns and aligns with Vygotsky's Zone of Proximal Development (ZPD; Vygotsky, 1962). Following ZPD, later developing sounds (e.g., liquids) and sound combinations (clusters) are combined with earlier developing sounds

Table A5.1 Underlying concepts

1	Children with 'normal' hearing typically acquire the adult sound system primarily by *listening*.
2	Phonological acquisition is a *gradual* process.
3	*Phonetic environment* in words can facilitate or inhibit correct sound productions.
4	Children associate *auditory* and *kinaesthetic* sensations that enable later *self-monitoring*.
5	Children *generalise* new speech production skills to other targets
6	An optimal *'match'* facilitates learning.
7	Children learn best when they are *actively involved/engaged* in phonological remediation.
8	Enhancing child's *metaphonological* skills enhances the child's speech and early literacy skills.

Source: Adapted from Hodson (2010)

(Prezas et al., 2021). This creates a balance between more stimulable patterns and complex and later developing targets at an optimal moment within a child's ZPD.

Non-stimulable sounds should be addressed to *make* them stimulable, but not targeted for production practice until the child produces them correctly, noting that stimulable sounds and patterns show greater generalization than those that are non-stimulable (Rudolf & Wendt, 2014).

Targeting Phonological Patterns

Typically, a phoneme (e.g., a stop such as final /k/), cluster (e.g., an initial /s/ cluster), or syllable structure (e.g., final consonants) is targeted for 1 hour per week. At least two exemplars (e.g., initial /sp/ and /st/) of the current target are presented before moving to another sound class (e.g., velars, liquids), cluster (e.g., final /st/), or syllable structure (e.g., weak, or unstressed syllables) within the cycle.

Most target patterns are recycled one or more times with gradually increased articulatory difficulty in each successive cycle. Table A5.2 provides information about the typical CPPA session structure.

Ongoing clinical research has seen phonological patterns classified as *Primary* (those targeted first and recycled as needed until they began emerging in conversational speech) and *Secondary* (see Figure A5.1).

Stimulability, Amplification, and Imagery

It is critical that the child be *stimulable* for their targets, and this may require tactile cues and amplification at first. Once stimulable, the child begins to develop an accurate kinaesthetic image. Continued use of amplification aids in this process. We use a small portable battery-operated amplifier and child-sized headphones and have elicited sounds with the amplifier that had remained non-stimulable when other methods were employed. Sounds that are initially non-stimulable (e.g., /k/) are worked on ('facilitated') for a few minutes each session and are targeted when the child achieves stimulability. If non-stimulable sounds are targeted, repeated incorrect production can be counterproductive because they reinforce the inaccurate kinaesthetic image (Prezas et al., 2021).

Metaphonology as an Integral Component of CPPA

Learning to read and spell an alphabetic language requires children to understand that sounds in spoken words can be represented by letters on a page (Hodson, 2010). This is called sound-symbol association or phoneme-grapheme correspondence and is an aspect of metaphonological awareness. It is critical for literacy acquisition because it underpins children's ability to make phoneme-grapheme connections rather than attempting to memorize whole words. Children who can make such connections are primed to use these strategies in reading, written expression, and spelling.

Table A5.2 Typical Clinical Session Structure

1	**Review**	Child produces practice words (depicted on large index cards) from the previous treatment session.
2	**Listening Activity**	Clinician reads approximately 20 words using slight amplification (this takes 30 seconds). Child then says new production-practice words for the day while still wearing amplifier headset.
3	**Experiential-play motivational production-practice activities**	Child says practice word by naming picture or object with correct production of the target pattern for the session before 'taking a turn'. Clinician provides assists (e.g., modelling, tactile cue) as needed so that the child achieves 100% 'correctness' for the target pattern in the practice words.
4	**Metaphonological Activity**	Incorporation of a metaphonological activity: (e.g., rhyming, syllable segmentation).
5	**Probing**	Probing by clinician to determine optimal target (e.g., singleton phoneme, consonant cluster) for next session's target pattern.
6	**Listening Activity**	Second reading of week's listening list with slight amplification (by parent if possible).
7	**Home Program**	Parents/caregivers are given the following from this day's session to practice with their child for 2 minutes every day. (a) week's listening list to read to their child, (b) week's production-practice word (picture) cards for child to name, (c) metaphonological activity (e.g., folder with 4-line rhyme, syllable segmentation)

Children with highly unintelligible speech are predisposed to concomitant deficits in metaphonological awareness and literacy (Prezas et al., 2021). The Critical Age Hypothesis (Bishop & Adams, 1990) tells us that children must be intelligible by the age of 5;6, especially if they also have semantic and syntactic difficulties, or their literacy acquisition may be compromised (Zajdó, A43).

School-age children with moderate to severe phonological impairment, with scores of 50–100 and 101–150 respectively on the HAPP-3, perform poorly on metaphonological tasks (Hodson, 2010). Clinical research findings support the use of metaphonological awareness activities with children who are highly unintelligible (Gillon, 2017, p. 139).

Metaphonological awareness tasks, integrated with phonological intervention, may help children's literacy and aspects of speech (e.g., by working on final consonants *after* focusing on rimes in rhyming activities; Hodson, 2010).

Metaphonological awareness tasks include explicitly identifying graphemes and phonemes, and riming tasks such as nursery rhymes or songs with repetition, syllable segmentation, and alliteration tasks for preschoolers. School-age children can continue these tasks, adding final phoneme identity, blending of syllables and/or phonemes, segmentation of syllables and/or phonemes, and manipulation of phonemes.

CPPA and Multilingual Children with Severe SSD

The CPPA can be adapted to meet the needs of multilingual children with highly unintelligible speech. The eight underlying concepts of CPPA displayed in Table A5.1 are universal and a framework for a Spanish-English CPPA is available (see, Prezas et al., 2021). The primary recommended targets of CPPA align with most languages (e.g., shared versus unshared sounds; see, Kester, 2014). Sounds shared across languages should be targeted first, followed by unshared sounds. Careful selection of targets for multilingual children, taking dialect and language of intervention into account, is needed to preserve the unique linguistic characteristics of CLD children (Prezas et al., 2021). By targeting shared sounds first, clinicians who do not speak the child's L1 (e.g., Spanish) can feel more confident about targeting sounds in the child's L2 (e.g., English) as targeting a shared sound in one language may generalize to the other (Paradis, 2001).

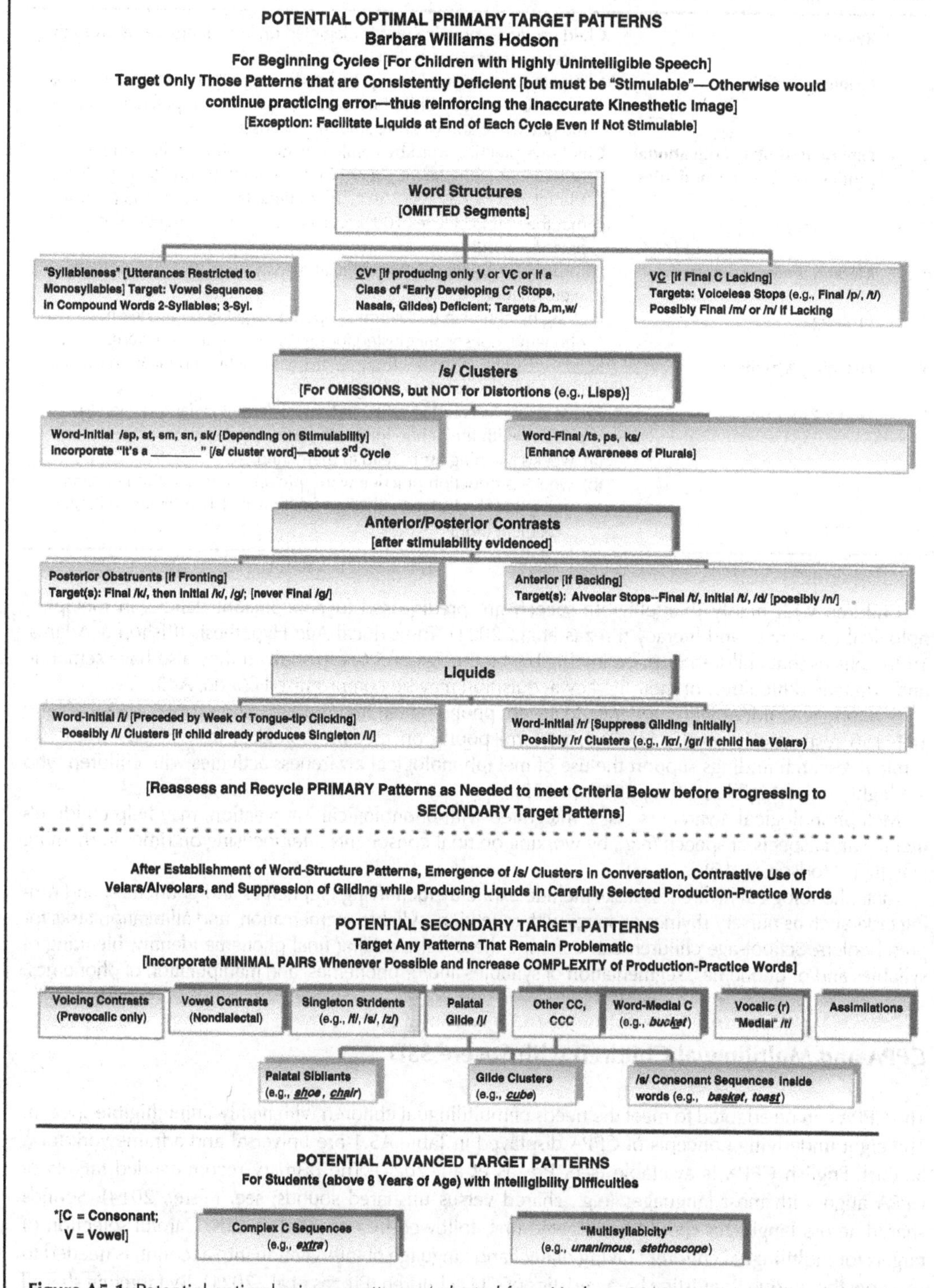

POTENTIAL OPTIMAL PRIMARY TARGET PATTERNS
Barbara Williams Hodson
For Beginning Cycles [For Children with Highly Unintelligible Speech]
Target Only Those Patterns that are Consistently Deficient [but must be "Stimulable"—Otherwise would
continue practicing error—thus reinforcing the Inaccurate Kinesthetic Image]
[Exception: Facilitate Liquids at End of Each Cycle Even if Not Stimulable]

Word Structures
[OMITTED Segments]

"Syllableness" [Utterances Restricted to Monosyllables] Target: Vowel Sequences in Compound Words 2-Syllables; 3-Syl.

CV* [If producing only V or VC or if a Class of "Early Developing C" (Stops, Nasals, Glides) Deficient; Targets /b,m,w/

VC [If Final C Lacking] Targets: Voiceless Stops (e.g., Final /p/, /t/) Possibly Final /m/ or /n/ if Lacking

/s/ Clusters
[For OMISSIONS, but NOT for Distortions (e.g., Lisps)]

Word-Initial /sp, st, sm, sn, sk/ [Depending on Stimulability] Incorporate "It's a _____" [/s/ cluster word]—about 3rd Cycle

Word-Final /ts, ps, ks/ [Enhance Awareness of Plurals]

Anterior/Posterior Contrasts
[after stimulability evidenced]

Posterior Obstruents [If Fronting] Target(s): Final /k/, then initial /k/, /g/; [never Final /g/]

Anterior [If Backing] Target(s): Alveolar Stops--Final /t/, initial /t/, /d/ [possibly /n/]

Liquids

Word-Initial /l/ [Preceded by Week of Tongue-tip Clicking] Possibly /l/ Clusters [if child already produces Singleton /l/]

Word-Initial /r/ [Suppress Gliding Initially] Possibly /r/ Clusters (e.g., /kr/, /gr/ if child has Velars)

[Reassess and Recycle PRIMARY Patterns as Needed to meet Criteria Below before Progressing to SECONDARY Target Patterns]

After Establishment of Word-Structure Patterns, Emergence of /s/ Clusters in Conversation, Contrastive Use of Velars/Alveolars, and Suppression of Gliding while Producing Liquids in Carefully Selected Production-Practice Words

POTENTIAL SECONDARY TARGET PATTERNS
Target Any Patterns That Remain Problematic
[Incorporate MINIMAL PAIRS Whenever Possible and Increase COMPLEXITY of Production-Practice Words]

| Voicing Contrasts (Prevocalic only) | Vowel Contrasts (Nondialectal) | Singleton Stridents (e.g., /f/, /s/, /z/) | Palatal Glide /j/ | Other CC, CCC | Word-Medial C (e.g., bucket) | Vocalic (r) "Medial" /r/ | Assimilations |

Palatal Sibilants (e.g., shoe, chair)

Glide Clusters (e.g., cube)

/s/ Consonant Sequences inside words (e.g., basket, toast)

POTENTIAL ADVANCED TARGET PATTERNS
For Students (above 8 Years of Age) with Intelligibility Difficulties

*[C = Consonant; V = Vowel]

Complex C Sequences (e.g., extra)

"Multisyllabicity" (e.g., unanimous, stethoscope)

Figure A5.1 Potential optimal primary patterns. (adapted from Hodson, 2010).

Implementing a Bilingual CPPA

The implementation of a bilingual CPPA requires exploration of sounds shared between languages initially, following the CPPA framework in English (see, Figure A5.1).

Begin with shared sounds and then move to unshared sounds in English, assuming English is the child's L2 and SLPs'/SLTs' L1. Note that anterior/posterior contrasts should be targeted with multilinguals before /s/ clusters if there are no /s/ clusters in the L1 (e.g., in Japanese). Many languages have multisyllabic words. Thus, the CPPA concept of 'syllableness' can be targeted in therapy. The term 'syllableness' was coined by Hodson and means the production of the correct number of syllables in multisyllabic words, with the emphasis on including the correct number of syllables and not the phonemic errors (Hodson, 2010).

Singleton Consonants and Anterior/Posterior Contrasts

Many languages have shared phonemes that are phonemes used in *CPPA*. These include: /p/ /b/ /m/ /w/ /t/ /d/ /k/ /g/. Many other languages share these phonemes, or almost do with slight variations in place and/or manner of articulation. Those that correspond fully with the CPPA consonant inventory include most varieties of English, French, Japanese, Tagalog, Bengali (Barman, 2009), and Welsh (S. Munro et al., 2005). Spanish almost corresponds except for /t/ which is dentalised (Prezas et al., 2021) as it is in Vietnamese. In German, /w/ only occurs in loan words. There is no /w/ in Russian either, and /t/ and /d/ are dentalised (Kester, 2014). In the Mahji dialect of Punjabi there is no /w/, and stops may be aspirated (Chohan & García, 2019). Urdu has no /w/, /t/ and /d/ are dentalised and, in some cases, stops are aspirated (Ranjha, 2014). There are slight variations with /t/ and /d/ in Polish (Schwartz, 2019). Singleton consonants can be addressed in the initial position primarily and, in some cases, final position depending on the language. Anterior and posterior contrasts can also be addressed with the languages listed above.

Clusters with /s/, Liquid /l/, Trilled /r/, and Retroflex/Tapped /ɾ/

Clusters and sequences involving /s/ occur in the following languages among others: Welsh has /sb/, /sd/, /sg/ (S. M. Munro et al., 2007), and so does Polish (Schwartz et al., 2019). French and Russian have initial /s/ clusters and so does German with initial /sp/ and /st/ as well as final /st/ (Kester, 2014). The /sm/ occurs in Urdu (Ranjha, 2014). Spanish has /s/ sequences (Prezas et al., 2021).

Liquid /l/ is also shared in other languages (with allophonic variations occurring in some languages). These languages include Spanish, Vietnamese, German, French, Tagalog, Russian (palatal /l/), Polish (lingual dental), Bengali, Urdu, and Welsh. Trilled /r/ and retroflex/tapped /ɾ/ (where noted) occur in Spanish (includes retroflex), Punjabi (includes retroflex), Tagalog (includes retroflex), Bengali, Urdu, and Japanese.

Other Considerations for Multilingual Children

The language abilities of multilingual children (e.g., language strengths and weaknesses) should be monitored in therapy and considered when making clinical decisions about targets for therapy. Communicate with multilingual parents and other family and community members where relevant, speak the language of kindness, honour their names, and encourage families to continue to speak to their children in their home, more dominant language (Goldstein, A41.; Palafox, 2019). Monolingual English-speaking SLPs/SLTs should be familiar with best practices for bilingual assessment and intervention, including what to target in therapy. Work closely with interpreters and colleagues to provide appropriate services and always exert your good-faith effort to meet the needs of multilingual and culturally and linguistically diverse children.

Models of Phonological Acquisition

It is axiomatic in the literature to say that, because so little is known about normal phonological development, a cohesive linguistic theory of phonological disorders has yet to be formulated. Ingram (1989a) examined various bids in the field of linguistics to construct a phonological theory that covered normal *and* disordered phonological acquisition, indicating that the most likely sources of elucidation of *normal* acquisition might be universalist/structuralist theory (Jakobson, 1941/1968), natural phonology theory (Stampe, 1969), or the Stanford cognitive model (Macken & Ferguson, 1983). Of them, only Stampe's was directly tied to a phonological theory.

Behaviourist Model

The behaviourist model dominated linguistics from the 1950s to the early 1970s. It applied a psychological theory of learning to explain how children came to distinguish and produce the sound system of the ambient language. Its adherents included Mowrer (1952, 1960), Murai (1963), and Olmstead (1971). They recognised the role of contingent reinforcement in gradually 'shaping' a child's babbling into meaningful adult forms through classical conditioning. A key aspect of the model was the emphasis on continuity between babbling and early speech. Behaviourists believed that the infant associated the vocalisations of the mother (usually) with primary reinforcements, such as food and nurture, with the vocalisations assuming secondary reinforcement status.

Eventually, the infant's vocalisations became secondary reinforcers (providing self-reinforcement) due to their similarity to adult models. From this point, the caregiver could refine the sound repertoire of the infant through selective reinforcement. The behaviourist framework did not presuppose, or show any interest in, an innate order of speech sound acquisition. The sounds acquired depended on the reinforcement obtained from the linguistic environment.

Structuralist Model

The structuralist model (Jakobson, 1941/1968), stemmed from structuralist linguistic theory, and it proposed *discontinuity* between babbling and speech. In addition, the structuralists postulated an innate, universal order of acquisition, with distinctive features emerging hierarchically and predictably. Jakobson regarded babbling as a random activity virtually unrelated to the development of the sound system. Evidence of regularities in prelinguistic vocal patterns (C. A. Ferguson & Macken, 1980; Oller et al., 1976) has, however, weakened this position. As well, mid-1970s research challenged Jakobson's hypothesis of a sequence of phonemic oppositions as the basis for the earliest stages of phonological development. Kiparsky and Menn (1977) demonstrated that the child's word count is too small to provide objective evidence of the distinctive features 'unfolding' in the way proposed by Jakobson. Really, the developmental order of phonemic oppositions has proved difficult to ascertain, because analysis must take account of the adult targets attempted as well as the child's phonetic repertoire. To complicate matters, children seem to selectively *avoid* saying words containing certain consonants that are difficult for them to produce (C. Ferguson & Farwell, 1975; Schwartz & Leonard, 1982). Evidence of lexical avoidance (or 'lexical selection') lent weight to the theory that, in the first-fifty-words-stage, children target whole words (Ingram, 1989a, pp. 17–22). The phonetic variability readily observed in children in the 9- to 18-month-age range may also provide evidence against a universal order of phoneme acquisition. Irrespective of such shortcomings, Jakobson's views exerted a strong, enduring influence on linguist thought. Ingram (1989a p. 162) counted the structuralist model as one of the 'most likely candidates' for a theory of normal phonological acquisition. He talks about this in A4 and addresses the topic of whole word measures of correct speech production in A11 in the following chapter.

Dr. David Ingram received his PhD from Stanford University in 1970, where he studied language universals under Professor Joseph

Greenberg and phonological acquisition in children under Professor Charles Ferguson. His interest in language disorders was developed during two subsequent years as a Research Associate at the Scottish Rite Institute for Childhood Aphasia. He was a professor at the University of British Columbia from 1972 to 1998 and a professor at Arizona State University where he retired in 2018. His research is on language acquisition in typically developing children and children with language and phonological disorders. The focus is on both English-speaking children and children acquiring other languages. The language areas of primary interest to him are phonological, morphological, and syntactic acquisition. He has published over 100 articles and is particularly known for his seminal work, *Phonological Disability in Children* (Ingram, 1976, 1989a), and his comprehensive textbook, *First Language Acquisition* (Ingram, 1989a).

Q4. David Ingram: Theory and Speech Sound Disorders

Do you continue to regard the structuralist model as a front runner in the formulation of a theory of normal acquisition (Ingram, 1989a) and what are the other contenders? How do you see a theory of acquisition informing the development of theories of disorder and intervention, and now can clinicians use this information?

A4. David Ingram: The Role of Theory In SSD

The effort to determine a theoretical account of children's SSD has a long history of moving from simpler to more complex explanations. Originally, SLP/SLT began with little if any theory, treating speech sound errors as errors with individual sounds, and subsequent treatments based on the intuitively reasonable assumption that improvement would result from drill and repetition. These early efforts were supported by subsequent acceptance in many circles of behaviourism, a movement clearly described in the present book.

With what appeared to me to be the demise of behaviourism (Chomsky, 1959), a new era of linguistic explanations emerged, with the result over time being a daunting range of possible theoretical accounts (cf. summaries in Ball & Kent, 1997). In the 1970s, the field of SLP/SLT was sympathetic to these efforts, and the proposals have constituted sections of most textbooks since (e.g., Bauman-Waengler, 2020; Stoel-Gammon & Dunn, 1985; Williams et al., 2021). At least two potential problems arose with these efforts at theoretical explanation. For one, phonological theories became more and more complex and abstract, and de facto harder to assimilate and make clinically relevant. Second, no clear theoretical approach won out, in the sense of demonstrating it is, without argument, the best and clinically most relevant account. The positive from all this is the impression that a range of intervention approaches 'work' (with some debate whether one or another might be even more effective). This results from: (1) that many theories have shown success, and (2) that children with a range of speech sound problems respond to different approaches. This leads the authors to the intuitively reasonable conclusion that specific theories, and their subsequent treatment approaches, may work better for some disorders than others.

Like behaviourism, however, this intuitively reasonable assumption is problematic. It can be challenged on both the side of treatment and the side of theory. It is certainly good news that a range of treatment approaches work, and good news that SLPs/SLTs know them. There is the implication that a reasonable arsenal of treatment approaches is sufficient to treat SSD. A range of available treatment approaches, however, is no guarantee of future success without some theoretical grounding. There is no foundation for the prediction that what worked with one child will work with another child, just because the two children appear to be similar based on some assessment. Nor does it make sense simply to run a child through the approaches until one 'clicks'. We need to understand the disorders better than that, and a better understanding can only come from some theoretical approach.

Let's say I am a practicing SLP/SLT with excellent skills in two quite different treatment approaches. On the one hand, I am very experienced in using a cycles approach (in a group setting) with target selection based on using developmentally appropriate sounds. At the same time, I am also well informed in using a maximal contrast approach, involving intense one-on-one intervention with target sounds well beyond the child's current developmental level. I evaluate two children: Barbara and Judy. I conclude from my clinical intuitions that Barbara will benefit from a cycles model, whereas Judy will be best served with maximal oppositions intervention.

At one level, this is evidence-based practice. When I meet with Barbara's parents, I will discuss the cycles approach and refer to Hodson (2004, 2015) and other references as needed. When meeting with Judy's parents, however, my justification will be through discussing work by Gierut (2001) and Morrisette (2021) and the references therein. I will move past the idea that 'one theory fits all'. I also have an additional option. If one or neither child responds to my treatment choices, I can just switch them to the other approach. Or, if I get to attend a national convention in the interim, I can bring home a new approach I might learn at a workshop there. I also don't need to worry much about theories throughout the whole process.

Is what I have just described 'best' practice? I don't know. I am inclined, however, not to give up seeking a single theoretical basis for these decisions. In Ingram and Ingram (2001), we discuss a situation like the one above. We offer the hypothesis that there may be two subgroups of children with SSD: one with poor whole-word skills and one with good whole-word skills. The former group will be children with poor intel-

ligibility, who are having difficulties matching their speech sounds to the target models. The latter group, on the other hand, are matching the target words relatively well (over 50% of the segments) but are possibly delayed in terms of their speech. We go on to suggest that the former children are candidates for a developmental approach, such as the one described for Barbara. The latter children, however, with good matching skills, may respond well to the maximal contrast approach as mentioned for Judy. Importantly, these decisions follow a single theory, a theory that incorporates whole-word abilities into our account of how children acquire their phonological systems. Within this theory, it makes more sense to select the treatments as mentioned, and less sense to do it the opposite way.

Here is another example. In Ingram (1989a), I contrast two theories of language acquisition: a maturational approach and a constructionist (Piagetian) approach. These theories make very different claims about how language is acquired. It is known that certain syntactic constructions are acquired late, for example, more complex forms of passive sentences. A maturational account would say that this is because the grammatical principles needed to form passive sentences do not mature until later, say age 6. A constructionist approach would predict that these sentences could be acquired earlier through the right combination of exposure to them and internal developments of the child's language acquisition. Can these theories co-exist?

We know that children acquire certain English sounds late, such as the dental fricatives, /θ/ and /ð/. Let us say I assess two four-year-old children both of whom are struggling in the production of fricatives and are being considered for intervention. I reach the following conclusions. One child, Dan, strikes me as very constructionist in his learning, whereas the other child, Tom, appears maturational. My recommendations are as follows. Dan will start an intervention program where we will use auditory bombardment (or what Hodson, 2015 called focused auditory input) to stimulate his acquisition of the dental fricatives. We will work on a selective vocabulary with these sounds, which in turn may lead to internal gains in his language knowledge. Tom, however, cannot learn to articulate these sounds yet because his speech development needs to mature. No amount of intervention will help Tom, who will be left alone to acquire these sounds at age six when his maturation is complete. This choice of intervention does not make sense to me. It would be based on what I see as a misunderstanding that somehow theories can co-exist.

Here is one further example. Let us consider a theory of phonological acquisition that proposes children use phonological processes to simplify speech. This theory has many processes, including Fronting (which changes k to t, e.g., 'key' is [ti]), and Backing (which changes t to k, e.g., 'tea' is [ki]). Another theory, NeoJakobson Theory, says that children's productions reflect their underlying distinctive features. This theory allows Fronting, but not Backing, as a natural process. On Thursday, I assess two children: one who shows Fronting (David) and one who is doing Backing (Caroline). My conclusions are that David is using the phonological process theory to acquire his speech sounds, whereas Caroline is using the NeoJakobson theory. The problem with the phonological process theory (as stated) is that it makes up any process it needs and is therefore too powerful. By explaining everything, it explains nothing. The more restricted theory is to be preferred. How then, can the NeoJakobson Theory account for our data? The theory states that children's first feature distinction is between a labial consonant and a non-labial consonant. The first non-labial consonant can either be a [t] or a [k]. Most children will opt for the [t], a more common sound in early productions, and this choice is the predicted, or unmarked, sound. Some children, however, may select to produce [k] instead, since it still has the same underlying value of the [t], that is, both being non-labial. This becomes, therefore, the less common, or more marked, choice. It is

not always easy to evaluate theories and decide that one is more explanatory than the other, but the bottom line is that such evaluations are the way theories are assessed, not by saying they all happily coexist.

If I am to stand by and defend the simplistic view that one theory fits all, then I should provide some suggestions on what this theory might look like. In Ingram (1997), I outline the basic properties of such a theory. The first point to make is that our theory for SSD has, in the short term, different goals from phonological theory. The latter has as its goal the characterization of the phonological systems of the thousands of languages that exist in the world. Our goal is to have a theoretical account of the phonological systems of children's first words, often fewer than a thousand in number. This goal does not require the extent of theorisation or formalism needed in linguistic theory. As suggested in Ingram (1997), it is possible to isolate the shared assumptions of phonological theory in general to form the basis of our theory of SSD. Here are some of those shared characteristics: the acquisition of an early lexicon involves the acquisition of phonological representations; these early representations, like adult representations, consist of phonological features; the early representations of children are underspecified, that is, they do not contain the full range of features of those for adult speakers; children first acquire a subset of the features underlying all languages; my research leads me to suggest these early features are consonantal, sonorant, labial, dorsal, continuant, voice; the child's productions are speech sounds that have one or more of these features; the first syllables are constructed from a small set, that is, CV, CVC, VC, CVCV, CVCVC; children's productions attempt to match the adult models, in typical development around 70%.

So yes, I support a structuralist approach as asked. I'll finish with one of my favourite quotes: 'Theory without practice is speculation, practice without theory is dangerous'.[1]

[1] Source lost in time.

Biological Model

Locke (1983a; 1983b, 1993c) stressed universality in his proposal of a biological model of phonological development. However, Locke emphasised *biological* constraints rather than linguistic ones. Rejecting Jakobson's idea of discontinuity between babbling and speech, Locke postulated relatively rigid maturational control over the capabilities of the speech production mechanism. For Locke, phonology began before 12 months of age with the pragmatic stage when certain babbled utterances gained communicative intent. At the same time, the phonetic repertoire was essentially 'universal', constrained by the anatomical characteristics of the vocal tract. During the 'cognitive stage' that followed, the biological constraints persisted while the child learned to store and retrieve relatively stable forms of phonemes learned from adult language models. At 18 months, in the 'systemic stage', biologically determined babbling production patterns gave way to more adult-like speech. These speech attempts reflected phonologically the target language. Patterns found *only* in adult speech were acquired and patterns not contained in it were 'lost'.

Natural Phonology Model

Meanwhile, Stampe (1969) proposed his natural phonology model of phonological acquisition. He posited that children come innately equipped with a universal repertoire of phonological processes: stopping, fronting, cluster reduction, and so on. These processes were 'mental operations' that change or delete phonological units, reflecting the natural limitations and capacities of speech production and perception. In Stampe's view, natural processes amounted to articulatory restrictions, which came into play *like* reflexes. Note that this is a simile and does not imply reflexes in the physiological 'knee jerk' sense. The effect of these 'reflexes' was to prevent accurate production of sound differences. This occurred despite the sounds being perceived correctly auditorily and stored as 'correct' adult phonemic contrasts in the linguistic mechanism in the brain. The processes operated to constrain and restrict the speech mechanism *per se*. Stampe held

that these universal, innate simplifications of speech output involved children's cognitive, perceptual, and production domains. He believed that the processes simplified speaking in three possible ways. Given a potential phonological contrast, a process favoured the member of the opposition that was the:

1. least complex to produce,
2. least complex to perceive; or,
3. least complex to produce and perceive.

For instance, given the choice of saying /d/ or /ð/, the assumption was that /d/ was easier, because, in typical development, it was acquired earlier (see Table 1.2); for example, *this* (/ðɪs/) is often realised by young children as [dɪs] (an example of Stopping).

The child's developmental task was to suppress the natural phonological processes to achieve full productive control of the phonemes of the ambient language. Stampe also believed that, from the onset of meaningful speech, children possessed a fully developed, adult-like, phonological perceptual system. Thus, while they exhibited natural processes in output, they already had an underlying representation (a mental image or internal knowledge of the lexical items) of the appropriate adult target form (so 'this' would be /ðɪs/ underlyingly and [dɪs] on the surface). Stampe relied heavily on a deterministic explanation of phonological change. He maintained that children 'used' processes for the phonological act of simplifying pronunciation.

The progression to adult-like productions (for instance, the use of consonant clusters) represented mastery of increased constraints (upon output phonology). This development occurred through the suppression of natural processes and consequent revision of the universal system. Change occurred through a passive mechanism of suppression as part of maturation. Stampe did not consider cognitive constraints related to the pragmatics of communication, or of the active learning of a language-specific phonology through problem solving, as in the cognitive model. Possibly the most contentious aspect of Stampe's interpretation of Natural Phonology was his (unsupported) claim that the processes were psychologically real, with Neil Smith (Smith, 1973, 1978) concluding that there was no psychological reality to the child's system because there was no evidence for the 'reflex mechanism' proposed by Stampe in applying, or rather 'using', phonological processes.

Prosodic Model

The prosodic model of Waterson (1971, 1981) introduced another novel theoretical construct. It involved a perceptual schema in which '*a child perceives only certain of the features of the adult utterance and reproduces only those he is able to cope with*' (Waterson, 1971, p. 181) in the early stages of word production. Waterson (1971), Braine (1974), Macken (1980), and Maxwell (1984) asserted that, in infants, both perception and production are incomplete at first. Both developed and changed before they could become adult like. Unlike the more generally applied phonological process-based (segmental) descriptions, Waterson's schema provided a gestalt of child production rather than a segment-by-segment comparison with the adult target. Waterson's approach is useful in describing the word productions of toddlers and may explain those that are not obvious reductions of adult forms.

Cognitive/Stanford Model

The Stanford or cognitive model of phonological development (Ferguson, 1968; Kiparsky & Menn, 1977; Macken & Ferguson, 1983), and Menn's (1976) 'interactionist discovery model', construed the child as *Little Linguist*, a captivating idea that dates back at least as far as Comenius (1659). Comenius insisted that, for a child, language learning was never an end but rather a means of finding out about the world and forming new concepts and associations. In problem-solving mode, the child met successions of challenges and mastered them, thereby gradually acquiring the adult sound system.

Because the child was involved actively and 'cognitively' in the construction of his or her phonology, the term cognitive model was used. Phonological development was an individual, gradual, and creative process (Ferguson, 1978). The Stanford team proposed that the strategies engaged in the active construction of phonology were individual for each child and influenced by internal factors: the characteristics and predispositions of the child, and external factors: the characteristics of the environment. The external factors might include the child's ordinal position in the family, family size, child-rearing practices, and interactional style of the adults close to the child.

Levels of Representation

Both David Stampe and Neil Smith recognised only two levels of representation. Stampe saw phonological processes as mapping from the underlying representation to the surface phonetic representation, whereas Smith (1973) saw realisation rules assuming this function. Stampe and Smith insisted that the child's phonological rules or processes were innate or learned extremely early. Then, Ingram (1974) coined the term 'organisational level' to connote a third, intervening component, related to, but distinct from, the child's perceptual representation of the adult word. A similar three-level arrangement, implicit in Jakobson's distinctive features theory, was central to cognitive or Stanford theory.

Smith rejected the hypothesis that each child has a unique system and assumed full, accurate perception and storage of adult speech targets. He proposed a set of ordered and universal phonological tendencies and realisation rules. Realisation rules were physical expressions of abstract linguistic units. Any underlying form had a corresponding realisation in substance. In this instance, phonemes were 'realised' or manifested in 'phonic substance' as phones (whereby meanings were transmitted). Smith's understanding was that the processes acted as a filter between the correctly stored adult word and the set of sounds produced by the child. Again, the problem arose of the child being perceived as passively allowing the realisation rules to 'apply' in reflecting the adult word.

Theories of Development, Disorder, and Intervention

The theoretical assumptions upon which any speech-intervention approach is based are derived first from a **theory development**, or how children *normally* learn the speech sound system through a combination of maturation and learning. Exploring this idea, Stoel-Gammon and Dunn (1985) posited four basic interacting components necessary for the formulation of a model of phonological development:

1. An auditory–perceptual component, encompassing the ability to attend to and perceive linguistic input.
2. A cognitive component, encompassing the ability to recognise, store and retrieve input and to compare input with output.
3. A phonological component, encompassing the ability to use sounds contrastively and to match the phonological distinctions of the adult language.
4. A neuromotor component, encompassing the ability to plan and execute the articulatory movements underlying speech.

From the practitioner's beliefs and assumptions about *normal* development comes a theory of *abnormal* phonological development: that is, a **theory of disorders** that explains why some children do not acquire their phonology along typical lines. Then, from the theories of normal and abnormal acquisition, and their formalisms, a **theory of intervention** can evolve. A theory of intervention (or **theory of therapy**) depends on how the individual clinician understands, interprets, incorporates, adapts, and modifies knowledge of normal and abnormal acquisition, and what theoretical assumptions are made in the process. Michie and Abraham (2004) suggested that intervening *without* a theory of therapy could lead to '*reinventing the wheel rather than re-applying it*'. They explained that, if we can isolate which parts of a treatment are doing the work (the 'active ingredients') of facilitating desired goals, it is possible to 'finetune' therapy to maximise effective components and reduce components that do not exert much effect on outcomes.

A theory of intervention, or how best to improve the speech of a child with SSD beyond the progress expected with age must logically rely on *assessment procedures* that are congruent with the SLP's/SLT's theories of development, disorders, and intervention (Fey, 1992a, 1992b; Ingram, A4). In this connection, Table 1.1 shows increasing availability of speech assessments based around Natural Phonology

and emphasising phonological process analysis. These included Weiner (1979), Hodson (1980), Shriberg and Kwiatkowski (1980), Ingram (1981), and L. Khan and Lewis (1983); L. M. L. Khan & Lewis (2002); Grunwell (1985b), and E. Dean et al. (1990). Phonological process analysis introduced the concept of an abstract level of knowledge. This was revolutionary in its time and was the phonological version of syntactic deep structure.

The first intervention inspired by Natural Phonology appeared in the literature when Frederick Weiner had a novel idea. Calling it 'the method of meaningful contrast' (Weiner, 1981a), he described what is sometimes called the 'conventional' (J. A. Barlow & Gierut, 2002) minimal pair approach. In rapid succession, Blache (1982) presented a systematic approach to minimal pairs and distinctive feature training; Hodson and Paden (1983) wrote the first edition of *Targeting Intelligible Speech*, describing their 'patterns' approach, popularly called 'cycles therapy', and rebadged by Hodson as the *Cycles Phonological Pattern Approach: CPPA* (Prezas et al., A5); Monahan (1984, 1986) devised a therapy kit called *Remediation of Common Phonological Processes*; and Elbert and Gierut (1986) wrote the *Handbook of Clinical Phonology*. While these achievements occurred in the United States, Grunwell (1983, 1985b) provided intervention guidance; Dean and Howell (1986) wrote an inspiring article about the metalinguistic aspect of therapy with portents of the (now out of print) *Metaphon Resource Pack* (E. Dean et al., 1990); and Lancaster and Pope (1989) developed a practical manual, *Working with Children's Phonology*, focusing on an auditory input therapy (a naturalistic recast approach) approach for very young children and older children with cognitive challenges. Still in the UK, the first in a book series (Stackhouse & Wells, 1997) on assessment and intervention within a psycholinguistic framework appeared (Schäfer & Fricke, A6).

A clinical forum on phonological assessment and treatment, edited by Marc Fey, was published in 1992 in ASHA's *Language, Speech, and Hearing Services in Schools*. Other forums followed in 2001, 2002, 2004, and 2006, but this one, with articles by Edwards (1992), Elbert (1992), Fey (1985, 1992a, 1992b), Hodson (1992), Hoffman (1992), Kamhi

(1992) and Schwartz (1992), remains extraordinarily helpful as an introduction.

Fey (1992b) captured the clear distinction between intervention approaches, intervention procedures, and intervention activities when he described and applied a structural plan for analysing the form of language interventions, such as phonological therapies. This hierarchical plan (displayed in Table 1.4) was adapted from Fey (1986) by Bowen (1996) and discussed in Bowen and Cupples (1999a) and Bowen (2010)

For clinicians, one good reason for *knowing*, or *deducing* the theoretical underpinnings of the interventions in their repertoire is that it helps in

choosing which to use, or how to combine them, or aspects of them, according to client needs. On *'deduction'* Duchan (personal correspondence 2008) wrote, '*I feel that we can look at any intervention and deduce its theoretical underpinnings or at least the assumptions it is based on, even if the clinician cannot articulate them. For example, drill relies on an assumption, or theory that learning is like exercise, the more you practice saying a sound or word, the better you "know" or can say it next time*'.

Fey's useful 1986 hierarchy covered the steps in modifying and adapting theoretical principles into a practicable intervention. It shows the progression

Table 1.4 Fey's (1986) theory-to-intervention hierarchy applied to clinical phonology

1. PHONOLOGICAL THEORY
**THE CLINICIAN'S OWN
THEORY OF DEVELOPMENT,
THEORY OF DISORDERS, and
THEORY OF INTERVENTION**
that are CONGRUENT WITH each other, and CONGRUENT WITH:

↑↓
2. PHONOLOGICAL ASSESSMENT APPROACHES
↑↓
CONGRUENT WITH
3. PHONOLOGICAL INTERVENTION APPROACHES
**INCORPORATING GOAL SELECTION AND GOAL ATTACK VIA
3 LEVELS OF INTERVENTION GOALS**

LEVEL 1: BASIC INTERVENTION GOALS
**(1) To facilitate cognitive reorganisation of the child's phonological system, and phonologically oriented processing strategies;
(2) to improve the child's intelligibility.**

LEVEL 2: INTERMEDIATE INTERVENTION GOALS
**To target *groups* of sounds related by an organising principle
(e.g., phonological processes / patterns / rules; or phoneme collapses)**

LEVEL 3: SPECIFIC INTERVENTION GOALS
To target a sound, sounds or structure, using vertical strategies, e.g., working on it until a criterion is reached, then moving to a new goal; or horizontal strategies, e.g., targeting several sounds within a process, and/or targeting more than one process simultaneously, and/or targeting syllable structures, metrical stress, etc. simultaneously with another target; or cyclical strategies, e.g., addressing several goals cyclically, focusing on only one goal per treatment session.
↓
4. INTERVENTION PROCEDURES
e.g., stimulability training, or phonetic production
↓
5. INTERVENTION ACTIVITIES
Contexts and events, such as games and tasks

Source: Available from: www.speech-language-therapy.com/images/14.png.

from (1) a given **phonological theory** (e.g., Natural Phonology) to (2) a **phonological analysis** that is congruent with the theory of development (e.g., Independent and Relational Analyses) to (3) the **phonological therapy approach** under consideration (e.g., Conventional Minimal Pairs Therapy), informed by (1) and (2). It then allows description of three levels of intervention goals—basic goals, intermediate goals, and specific goals—with goal-selection and goal-attack as critical components. From these arise (4) the intervention procedures of choice within the selected therapy model or a coherent combination of models and (5) intervention activities that are both consistent with the preceding four levels and suitable for a particular client.

The 'other' clinical forums, so useful to clinicians, referred to above include those edited by Barlow (2001, 2002); Helm-Estabrooks et al. (2002); Williams (2002a, 2002b); Bernhardt (2004); McLeod (2006). Clinical forums dealing with discrete approaches are also available to guide the clinician. For example, one on *Metaphon* (E. C. Dean et al., 1995) and one on *Parents and Children Together: PACT* (Bowen & Cupples, 1999a, 1999b). More recently we have seen an outstanding 2022 forum: Innovations in Treatments for Children with Speech Sound Disorders which begins with Farquharson and Tambyraja (2022).

Table 1.1 takes us on a century-long excursion from the formation of the International Association of Logopedics and Phoniatrics in 1924 to ASHA's centenary in 2025, via the Travis articulation paragraph in 1931, the impact of phonology in the 1970s, the ICF-CY view of speech impairment post 2001, and the rise and rise of telepractice from the early 2020s. The influence of clinical linguistics on child speech *theory* and its increasing presence in textbooks, journal articles, and university curricula are unmissable. But a commensurate manifestation of linguistics in everyday clinical practice is harder to detect.

Theory and Practice Now, and in the Future

Is linguistic theory exhausted as a source of ideas and insights about the prevention, assessment, and treatment of SSD, like behavioural psychology that ran out of puff in the 1970s? Will new progress come via information-processing models like the psycholinguistic model of speech processing and production (Schäfer & Fricke, A6; Stackhouse & Wells, 1997, 2001); or advances in neurophysiological processing of phonological information (Gerwin et al., 2021); or studies of the neurophysiological underpinnings of linguistic processing and representation (Froud & Randazzo, A51); or cognitive psychology investigations of key domain-general cognitive processes (e.g., Waring & Dodd, A7)? Will big new insights come from biology, particularly developmental neurology, and genetics? Or, is progress largely dependent on research and funding and the economics of clinical service provision? What would happen if every child with an SSD had enough affordable, accessible intervention in the care of clinicians with manageable caseload numbers?

These tantalising questions notwithstanding, we clinicians should be well acquainted with certain linguistic principles because they can help us devise evidence-based therapies that are conducive to treatment efficacy (Ingram, A4; Müller & Ball, A5).

Terminology

A Dictionary of Terms Dealing with Disorders of Speech was published in 1929 and its second revision was in 1946. Commenting on the review process, a Nomenclature Committee member declared:

> ...*speech rehabilitation has remained in a state of suspended, pre-scientific adolescence' and that 'it is impossible to talk about a problem, much less develop a theory, without a specialized, orderly nomenclature.*
>
> Wise, 1946, p. 327

Fast forward six decades, through a motherlode of publications—and conversations in classrooms, clinics, and research labs—expounding similar views, to find McNeilly et al. (2007) who told IALP world conference delegates that:

> ...*terminology in communication sciences and disorders 'presents a significant barrier to the profession's advancement in research, clinical effectiveness, public image, and political profile;*

adding influencing attitudes and understanding about something as fundamental and closely tied to one's professional identity as terminology is no small task.

More recently, Diepeveen et al. (2020) amplified the message:

Our findings show that there is no consensus on terminology of the different SSDs and that there are a lot of idiosyncrasies in the diagnostic labels that are used. This makes it difficult to communicate among SLPs, let alone communicate well with other disciplines and parents.

Terminology, nomenclature, and taxonomies (Baker et al., 2018) form an integral and discordant feature of our history and identities as SLPs/SLTs. Seemingly forever, individuals, panels, and committees have worked to streamline the terminology for voice, speech, language, fluency, and literacy, attempting to make it more 'international' and consistent across jurisdictions. The result is the profession's increased awareness that our terminology is unwieldy, and that change is desirable. Implementing change, however, is disappointingly slow and difficult, often with inconclusive outcomes. Conceding that there is a (terminological) elephant-in-the-room the tenor of our history, with the diligent work of our founders, was forward-thinking, optimistic, compassionate, and constructive. Against the historical background, Chapter 2 focuses on children's speech covering current classification, description, and assessment of SSD, and inevitably, terminology.

References

Allport, G. (1924). *Social psychology*. Houghton-Mifflin Co.

Arlt, P. B., & Goodban, M. T. (1976). A comparative study of articulation acquisition as based on a study of 240 normals, aged three to six. *Language, Speech, and Hearing Services in Schools*, 7(3), 173–180. https://doi.org/10.1044/0161-1461.0703.173

Armstrong, L., Stansfield, J., & Bloch, S. (2017). Content analysis of the professional journal of the Royal College of Speech and Language Therapists, III: 1966–2015—into the 21st century. *International Journal of Language & Communication Disorders*, 52(6), 681–688. https://doi.org/10.1111/1460-6984.12313

Babatsouli, E., Ingram, D., & Müller, N. (Eds.). (2017). *Crosslinguistic encounters in language acquisition. Typical and atypical development*. Multilingual Matters.

Baker, E., Williams, A., McLeod, S., & McCauley, R. (2018). Elements of phonological interventions for children with speech sound disorders: The development of a taxonomy. *American Journal of Speech-Language Pathology*, 27(3), 906–935. https://doi.org/10.1044/2018_AJSLP-17-0127

Ball, M. J. (Ed.). (2021). *Manual of clinical phonetics*. Routledge.

Ball, M. J., & Kent, R. D. (1987). Editorial. *Clinical Linguistics & Phonetics*, 1(1), 1–5. https://doi.org/10.1080/02699208708985000

Ball, M. J., & Kent, R. D. (Eds.). (1997). *The new phonologies: Developments in clinical linguistics*. Singular.

Ball, M. J., Rahilly, J., Lowry, O., Bessell, N., & Lee, A. (2000). *Phonetics for speech pathology* (3rd ed.). Equinox.

Barlow, J. A. (2001). Recent advances in phonological theory and treatment. *Language, Speech, and Hearing Services in Schools*, 32(4), 225–298. https://doi.org/10.1044/0161-1461(2001/020)

Barlow, J. A. (2002). Recent advances in phonological theory and treatment, part II. *Language, Speech, and Hearing Services in Schools*, 33(1), 4–8. https://doi.org/10.1044/0161-1461(2002/001)

Barlow, J. A., & Gierut, J. A. (2002). Minimal pair approaches to phonological remediation. *Seminars in Speech and Language*, 2(1), 57–68. https://doi.org/10.1055/s-2002-24969

Barlow, M., & Kemmer, S. (Eds.). (2000). *Usage-based models of language*. CSLI Publications.

Barman, B. (2009). A contrastive analysis of English and Bangla phonemics. *The Dhaka University Journal of Linguistics*, 2(4), 19–42. https://doi.org/10.3329/dujl.v2i4.6898

Bauman-Waengler, J. (2020). *Articulatory and phonological impairments: A Clinical focus* (6th ed.). Pearson Education, Inc.

Berman, S. (2001). Speech intelligibility and the down syndrome child. *Poster session presented at the annual convention of the American Speech-Language-Hearing Association*, New Orleans, LA. ASHA.

Bernhardt, B. (2004). Maximizing success in phonological intervention. *Child Language Teaching and Therapy*, 20(3), 195–198. https://doi.org/10.1191%2F0265659004ct271ed

Bernthal, J. E., Bankson, N. W., & Flipsen, P., Jr. (2022). *Speech sound disorders. Articulation and phonological disorder in children* (9th ed.). Paul H. Brookes Publishing.

Berry, M. D., & Eisenson, J. (1942). *The defective in speech*. Appleton-Century-Crofts.

Berry, M. D., & Eisenson, J. (1956). *Speech disorders: Principals and practices of therapy*. Appleton Century Crofts.

Bishop, D. V. M., & Adams, C. (1990). A prospective study of the relationship between specific language impairment, phonological disorders, and reading retardation. *Journal of Child Psychology and Psychiatry*, 31(7), 1027–1050. https://doi.org/10.1111/j.1469-7610.1990.tb00844.x

Blache, S. E. (1982). Minimal word pairs and distinctive feature training. In M. Crary (Ed.), *Phonological intervention: Concepts and procedures*. College-Hill Press Inc.

Botham, H. (2020). Cued articulation video and app course. Sounds for Literacy. https://www.soundsforliteracy.com.au/Video-App.html

Bowen, C. (1996). Evaluation of a phonological therapy with treated and untreated groups of young children. *Unpublished doctoral dissertation*. Macquarie University. http://hdl.handle.net/1959.14/304812

Bowen, C. (2010). Parents and children together (PACT) intervention for children with speech sound disorders. In A. L. Williams, S. McLeod, & R. J. McCauley (Eds.), *Interventions for speech sound disorders in children* (pp. 407–426). Paul H. Brookes Publishing Co.

Bowen, C., & Cupples, L. (1999a). Parents and children together (PACT): A collaborative approach to phonological therapy. *International Journal of Language & Communication Disorders*, 34(1), 35–55. https://doi.org/10.1080/136828299247603

Bowen, C., & Cupples, L. (1999b). A phonological therapy in depth: A reply to commentaries. *International Journal of Language & Communication Disorders*, 34(1), 65–83. https://doi.org/10.1080/136828299247649

Braine, M. D. S. (1974). On what might constitute a learnable phonology. *Language*, 50(2), 270–299. https://doi.org/10.2307/412438

Browman, C. P., & Goldstein, L. M. (1986). Towards an articulatory phonology. *Phonology Yearbook*, 3, 219–252. https://doi.org/10.1017/S0952675700000658

Brumbaugh, K. M., & Smit, A. B. (2013). Treating children ages 3–6 who have speech sound disorder: A survey. *Language Speech, and Hearing Services*

in Schools, 44(3), 306–319. https://doi.org/10.1044/0161-1461(2013/12-0029)

Burke, P. (2012). *A social history of knowledge II: From the encyclopédie to Wikipedia* (Vol. 2). Polity Press.

Buswell, G. T. (1932). Speech pathology: A dynamic neurological treatment of normal speech and speech deviations by Lee Edward Travis. *The Elementary School Journal*, 32(10), 793–794. https://doi.org/10.1086/456817

Chohan, M. N., & García, M. I. (2019). Phonemic comparison of English and Punjabi. *International Journal of English Linguistics*, 9(4), 347–357. https://doi.org/10.5539/ijel.v9n4p347

Chomsky, N. (1959). A review of B. F. Skinner's verbal behavior. *Language*, 35(1), 26–58. https://doi.org/10.4159/harvard.9780674594623.c6

Chomsky, N., & Halle, M. (1968). *The sound pattern of English*. Harper and Row.

Clahsen, H. (2008). Chomskyan syntactic theory and language disorders. In M. J. Ball, M. R. Perkins, N. Müller, & S. Howard (Eds.), *The handbook of clinical linguistics* (pp. 165–183). Blackwell.

College of Speech Therapists. (1959). *Terminology for speech pathology*.

Comenius, J. A. (1659). *Orbis sensualium pictus*. (Facsimile of first English edition of 1659). Sydney University Press.

Crowe, K., & McLeod, S. (2020). Children's English consonant acquisition in the United States: A review. *American Journal of Speech-Language Pathology*, 29(4), 2155–2169. https://doi.org/10.1044/2020_AJSLP-19-00168

Crystal, D. (1981). *Clinical linguistics*. Springer.

Crystal, D. (1984). *Linguistic encounters with language handicap*. Blackwell.

Crystal, D. (2001). Clinical linguistics. In M. Aronoff & J. Rees-Miller (Eds.), *The handbook of linguistics* (pp. 673–682). Blackwell.

De Bot, K., Lowie, W., & Verspoor, M. (2007). A dynamic systems theory approach to second language acquisition. *Bilingualism: Language and Cognition*, 10(1), 7–21. https://doi.org/10.1017/S1366728906002732

Dean, E., & Howell, J. (1986). Developing linguistic awareness: A theoretically based approach to phonological disorders. *British Journal of Disorders of Communication*, 21(2), 223–238. https://doi.org/10.3109/13682828609012279

Dean, E., Howell, J., Hill, A., & Waters, D. (1990). *Metaphon resource pack*. NFER Nelson.

Dean, E. C., Howell, J., Waters, D., & Reid, J. (1995). Metaphon: A metalinguistic approach to the treatment of phonological disorder in children. *Clinical Linguistics & Phonetics*, 9(1), 1–19. https://doi.org/10.3109/02699209508985318

Diepeveen, S. J. H., Haaften, L. V., Terband, H., Swart, B. J. M. D., & Maassen, B. (2020). Clinical reasoning for speech sound disorders: Diagnosis and intervention in speech-language pathologists' daily practice. *American Journal of Speech-Language Pathology*, 29(3), 1529–1549. https://doi.org/10.1044/2020_AJSLP-19-00040

Dodd, B. (2005). *Differential diagnosis and treatment of children with speech disorder* (2nd ed.). Whurr.

Duchan, J. F. (2001 to date). *A history of speech-language pathology*. http://www.acsu.buffalo.edu/~duchan/new_history/overview.html

Duchan, J. F. (2002). What do you know about your profession's history? *The ASHA Leader*, 7(23). https://doi.org/10.1044/leader.FTR.07232002.4

Duchan, J. F. (2006a). How conceptual frameworks influence clinical practice: Evidence from the writings of John Thelwall, a 19th-century speech therapist. *International Journal of Language and Communication Disorders*, 41(6), 735–744. https://doi.org/10.1080/13682820600570773

Duchan, J. F. (2006b). The phonetic notation system of Melville Bell and its role in the history of phonetics. *Canadian Journal of Speech Language Pathology and Audiology*, 30(1), 14–17. https://cjslpa.ca/files/2006_JSLPA_Vol_30/No_01_1-80/Duchan_JSLPA_2006.pdf

Duchan, J. F. (2009). The conceptual underpinnings of John Thelwall's elocutionary practices. In S. Poole (Ed.), *John Thelwall: Radical romantic and acquitted felon* (pp. 139–145). Pickering & Chatto.

Duchan, J. F. (2010). The early years of language, speech, and hearing services in U.S. schools. *Language, Speech, and Hearing Services in Schools*, 41(2), 152–160. https://doi.org/10.1044/0161-1461(2009/08-0102)

Duchan, J. F., & Felsenfeld, S. (2021). Professional issues: A view from history. In M. W. Hudson & M. DeRuiter, *Professional issues in speech-language pathology and audiology* (5th ed., pp. 57–80). Plural Publishing.

Duchan, J. F., & Hewitt, L. E. (2023). How the charter members of ASHA responded to the social and political circumstances of their time. *American Journal of Speech-Language Pathology*, 32(3), 1037–1049.

Edwards, M. L. (1992). In support of phonological processes. *Language, Speech, and Hearing Services in Schools*, 23(3), 233–240. https://doi.org/10.1044/0161-1461.2303.233

Eisenson, J. (1968). Developmental aphasia: A speculative view with therapeutic implications. *Journal of Speech and Hearing Disorders*, 33(1), 3–13. https://doi.org/10.1044/jshd.3301.03

Elbert, M. (1992). Consideration of error types: A response to Fey's 'Articulation and phonology: Inextricable constructs in speech pathology'. *Language, Speech, and Hearing Services in Schools*, 23(3), 241–246. https://doi.org/10.1044/0161-1461.2303.241

Elbert, M., & Gierut, J. (1986). *Handbook of clinical phonology: Approaches to assessment and treatment*. College-Hill Press.

Eldridge, M. (1965). *A history of the Australian college of speech therapists*. Melbourne University Press.

Eldridge, M. (1968a). *A history of the treatment of speech disorders*. E. & S. Livingstone.

Eldridge, M. (1968b). *A history of the treatment of speech disorders*. F.W. Cheshire.

Fairbanks, G. (1940). *Voice and articulation drillbook*. Harper.

Fairbanks, G. (1954). Systematic research in experimental phonetics: A theory of the speech mechanism as a servosystem. *Journal of Speech and Hearing Disorders*, 19(2), 133–139. https://doi.org/10.1044/jshd.1902.133

Ferguson, C., & Farwell, C. (1975). Words and sounds in early language acquisition. *Language*, 51(2), 419–439.

Ferguson, C. A. (1968). Contrastive analysis and language development. *Monograph Series on Language and Linguistics*, 21, 101–112. Georgetown University.

Ferguson, C. A. (1978). Learning to pronounce: The earliest stages of phonological development in the child. In F. D. Minifie & L. L. Lloyd (Eds.), *Communicative and cognitive abilities - early behavioural assessment* (pp. 273–297). University Park Press.

Ferguson, C. A., & Macken, M. (1980). Phonological development in children: Play and cognition. *Papers and Reports on Child Language Development*, 18, 138–177.

Ferguson, C. A., Peizer, D. B., & Weeks, T. A. (1973). Model-and-replica phonological grammar of a child's first words. *Lingua*, 31(1), 35–65.

Fey, M. E. (1985). Clinical forum: Phonological assessment and treatment. Articulation and phonology: Inextricable constructs in speech pathology. *Language, Speech, and Hearing Services in Schools*, 23(3), 225–232. https://doi.org/10.1044/0161-1461.2303.225

Fey, M. E. (1986). *Language intervention with young children*. College-Hill Press.

Fey, M. E. (1992a). Phonological assessment and treatment. Articulation and phonology. *Language, Speech, and Hearing Services in Schools*, 23(3), 224. https://doi.org/10.1044/0161-1461.2303.224

Fey, M. E. (1992b). Phonological assessment and treatment. Articulation and phonology: An addendum. *Language, Speech, and Hearing in Schools*, 23(3), 277–282. https://doi.org/10.1044/0161-1461.2303.277

Furlong, L. M., Morris, M. E., Serry, T. A., & Erickson, S. (2021). Treating childhood speech sound disorders: Current approaches to management by Australian speech-language pathologists. *Language, Speech, and Hearing in Schools*, 52(2), 581–596. https://doi.org/10.1044/2020_LSHSS-20-00092

Gerwin, K. L., Brosseau-Lapré, F., & Weber, C. (2021). Event-related potentials elicited by phonetic errors differentiate children with speech sound disorder and typically developing peers. *Journal of Speech, Language and Hearing Research*, 64(12), 4614–4630. https://doi.org/10.1044/2021_JSLHR-21-00203

Gierut, J. (2001). Complexity in phonological treatment: Clinical factors. *Language, Speech, and Hearing in Schools*, 32(4), 229–241. https://doi.org/10.1044/0161-1461(2001/021)

Gillon, G. T. (2000). The efficacy of phonological awareness intervention for children with spoken language impairment. *Language, Speech and Hearing Services in Schools*, 31(2), 126–141. https://doi.org/10.1044/0161-1461.3102.126

Gillon, G. T. (2017). *Phonological awareness: From research to practice* (2nd ed.). Guilford Press.

Goldstein, K. (1948). *Language and language disturbances*. Grune and Stratton.

Gordon-Brannan, M., Hodson, B., & Wynne, M. (1992). Remediating unintelligible utterances of a child with a mild hearing loss. *American Journal of Speech-Language Pathology*, 1(4), 28–38. https://doi.org/10.1044/1058-0360.0104.28

Grunwell, P. (1975). The phonological analysis of articulation disorders. *British Journal of Disorders of Communication*, 10(1), 31–42. https://doi.org/10.3109/13682827509011272

Grunwell, P. (1981). *The nature of phonological disability in children*. Academic Press.

Grunwell, P. (1983). Phonological development in phonological disability. *Topics in Language Disorders*, 3(2), 62–76. http://dx.doi.org/10.1097/00011363-198303000-00010

Grunwell, P. (1985a). Developing phonological skills. *Child Language Teaching and Therapy*, 1(1), 65–72. https://doi.org/10.1177%2F026565908500100108

Grunwell, P. (1985b). *Phonological assessment of child speech (PACS)*. NFER-Nelson.

Grunwell, P. (1987). *Clinical phonology* (2nd ed.). Williams & Wilkins.

Gutzmann, A. (1895). *Die Gesundheitspfl.ege der Sprache*. F. Hirt.

Harold, M. P. (2018 December; Updated 2019, August 2020). That one time a journal article on speech sounds broke the SLP internet [Blog post]. https://www.theinformedslp.com/how-to/that-one-time-a-journal-article-on-speech-sound-norms-broke-the-slp-internet

Hegarty, N., Titterington, J., McLeod, S., & Taggart, L. (2018). Intervention for children with phonological impairment: Knowledge, practices, and intervention intensity in the UK. *International Journal of Language & Communication Disorders*, 53(5), 995–1006. https://doi.org/10.1111/1460-6984.12416

Hegarty, N., Titterington, J., & Taggart, L. (2020). A qualitative exploration of speech-language pathologists' intervention and intensity provision for children with phonological impairment. *International Journal of Speech-Language Pathology*, 23(2), 213–224. https://doi.org/10.1080/17549507.2020.1769728

Helm-Estabrooks, N., Bernstein Ratner, N., & Velleman, S. (2002). Updates in phonological intervention. *Seminars in Speech and Language*, 23(1), 1–82. https://doi.org/10.1055/s-002-1630

Hersh, D., Wood, P., & Armstrong, E. (2018). Informal aphasia assessment, interaction and the development of the therapeutic relationship in the early period after stroke. *Aphasiology*, 32(8), 876–901. https://doi.org/10.1080/02687038.2017.1381878

Hodson, B. (1980). *The Assessment of Phonological Processes*. Interstate.

Hodson, B. (1992). Clinical forum: Phonological assessment and treatment. Applied phonology: Constructs, contributions, and issues. *Language, Speech, and Hearing Services in Schools*, 23(3), 247–253. https://doi.org/10.1044/0161-1461.2303.247

Hodson, B. (2010). *Evaluating and enhancing children's phonological systems: Research and theory to practice.* Phonocomp.

Hodson, B., & Paden, E. (1991). *Targeting intelligible speech: A phonological approach to remediation* (2nd ed.). Pro-Ed.

Hodson, B. W. (2004). *Hodson assessment of phonological patterns (HAPP- 3)* (3rd ed.). Pro-ed.

Hodson, B. W. (2015). Cycles phonological patterns approach. In C. Bowen, *Children's speech sound disorders* (2nd ed., pp. 36–40). Wiley-Blackwell.

Hodson, B. W., & Paden, E. P. (1981). Phonological processes which characterize unintelligible and unintelligible speech in early childhood. *Journal of Speech and Hearing Disorders*, 46(4), 369–373. https://doi.org/10.1044/jshd.4604.369

Hodson, B. W., & Paden, E. P. (1983). *Targeting intelligible speech: A phonological approach to remediation.* College-Hill Press.

Hoffman, P., Norris, J., & Monjure, J. (1990). Comparison of process targeting and whole language treatments for phonologically delayed preschool children. *Language, Speech and Hearing Services in Schools*, 21(2), 102–109. https://doi.org/10.1044/0161-1461.2102.102

Hoffman, P. R. (1992). Synergistic development of phonetic skill. *Language, Speech, and Hearing Services in Schools*, 23(3), 254–260. https://doi.org/10.1044/0161-1461.2303.254

Ingram, D. (1974). Phonological rules in young children. *Journal of Child Language*, 1(1), 49–64. https://doi.org/10.1017/S0305000900000076

Ingram, D. (1976). *Phonological disability in children.* Edward Arnold.

Ingram, D. (1981). *Procedures for the phonological analysis of children's language.* University Park Press.

Ingram, D. (1989a). *First language acquisition: Method, description, and explanation.* Cambridge University Press.

Ingram, D. (1997). Generative phonology. In M. J. Ball & R. D. Kent (Eds.), *The new phonologies: Developments in clinical linguistics* (pp. 7–33). Singular Publishing Group Inc.

Ingram, D., & Ingram, K. (2001). A whole word approach to phonological intervention. *Language, Speech, and Hearing Services in Schools*, 32(4), 271–283. https://doi.org/10.1044/0161-1461(2001/024)

Jakobson, R. (1941/1968). *Child language, aphasia, and phonological universals.* Mouton.

Joffe, V., & Pring, V. (2008). Children with phonological problems: A survey of clinical practice. *International Journal of Language & Communication Disorders*, 43(2), 154–164. https://doi.org/10.1080/13682820701660259

Kamhi, A. G. (1992). The need for a broad-based model of phonological disorders. *Language, Speech, and Hearing Services in Schools*, 23(3), 261–268. https://doi.org/10.1044/0161-1461.2303.261

Kester, E. S. (2014). *Difference or disorder? Understanding speech and language patterns in culturally and linguistically diverse students.* Bilinguistics.

Khan, L., & Lewis, N. (1983). *Khan–Lewis phonological analysis.* American Guidance Service.

Khan, L. M. L., & Lewis, N. P. (2002). *Khan–Lewis. Phonological analysis* (2nd ed.). American Guidance Service.

Kilminster, M. G. E., & Laird, E. M. (1978). Articulation development in children aged three to nine years. *Australian Journal of Human Communication Disorders*, 6(1), 23–30. https://doi.org/10.3109/asl2.1978.6.issue-1.04

Kiparsky, P., & Menn, L. (1977). On the acquisition of phonology. In J. Macnamara (Ed.), *Language learning and thought.* Academic Press.

Kuhn, T. S. (1962). *The structure of scientific revolutions.* The University of Chicago Press.

Kussmaul, A. (1885). Die Storungen der Sprache. In H. V. Ziemsson (Ed.), *Handbuch der Speciellen Pathologie und Therapie: Volume 12* (pp. 1–299). F. C. W. Vogel.

Lancaster, G., Keusch, S., Levin, A., Pring, T., & Martin, S. (2010). Treating children with phonological problems: Does an eclectic approach to therapy work? *International Journal of Language & Communication Disorders*, 45(2), 174–181. https://doi.org/10.3109/13682820902818888

Lancaster, G., & Pope, L. (1989). *Working with children's phonology.* Winslow Press.

Leahy, M. M., Thornton, J., Creevey, M., Keane, N., & Rogers, P. (2021). *Speech & language therapy in Ireland: The early years & beyond.* Authors. Irish Association of Speech & Language Therapists.

Leopold, W. F. (1947). Speech development of a bilingual child. In *Sound learning in the first two years.* Studies in Humanities (Vol. 2). Northwestern University Press.

Locke, J. L. (1983a). Clinical phonology: The explanation and treatment of speech sound disorders. *Journal of Speech and Hearing Disorders*, 48(4), 339–341. https://doi.org/10.1044/jshd.4804.339

Locke, J. L. (1983b). *Phonological acquisition and change*. Academic.

Locke, J. L. (1993c). *The child's path to spoken language*. Harvard University.

Lousada, M., Jesus, L. M. T., Capelas, S., Margçá, A, C., Simões, D., Valente, A., Hall, A., & Joffe, V. L. (2013). Phonological and articulation treatment approaches in Portuguese children with speech and language impairments: A randomized controlled intervention study. *International Journal of Language and Communication Disorders*, 48(2), 172–187. https://doi.org/10.1111/j.1460-6984.2012.00191.x

Macken, M. A. (1980). The child's lexical representations: The 'puzzle - puddle - pickle' evidence. *Journal of Linguistics*, 16, 1–17. https://doi.org/10.1017/S0022226700006307

Macken, M. A., & Ferguson, C. A. (1983). Cognitive aspects of phonological development: Model, evidence, and issues. In K. E. Nelson (Ed.), *Children's language, 4*. Lawrence Erlbaum.

Malloy, S. (2021). Commemorating 75 years of advocacy and member service. *Communication Matters*, 44, 12–17. https://www.readkong.com/page/communication-commemorating-75-years-of-advocacy-and-9499168

Martínez-Ferreiro, S., Bastiaanse, R., & Boye, K. (2020). Functional and usage-based approaches to aphasia: The grammatical-lexical distinction and the role of frequency. *Aphasiology*, 34(8), 927–942. https://doi.org/10.1080/02687038.2019.1615335

Maxwell, E. M. (1984). On determining underlying representations of children: A critique of the current theories. In M. Elbert, D. A. Dinnsen, & G. Weismer (Eds.), *Phonological theory and the misarticulating child*. ASHA. *Asha Monographs. 22.*

McDougall, A. (2006). Speech pathology and its professional association in Australia. *Australian Communication Quarterly*, 8(2), 51–59.

McLeod, S. (2006). An holistic view of a child with unintelligible speech: Insights from the ICF and ICF-CY. *International Journal of Speech-Language Pathology*, 8(3), 293–315. https://doi.org/10.1080/14417040600824944

McLeod, S. (2022). Speech sound acquisition. In J. E. Bernthal, N. W. Bankson, & P. Flipsen Jr. (2022), *Speech sound disorders. Articulation and phonological disorder in children* (9th ed.). Paul H. Brookes Publishing.

McLeod, S., & Baker, E. (2014). Speech-language pathologists' practices regarding assessment, analysis, target selection, intervention, and service delivery for children with speech sound disorders. *Clinical Linguistics & Phonetics*, 28(7–8), 508–531. https://doi.org/10.3109/02699206.2014.926994

McLeod, S., & Crowe, K. (2018). Children's consonant acquisition in 27 languages: A cross-linguistic review. *American Journal of Speech-Language Pathology*, 27(4), 1546–1571. https://doi.org/10.1044/2018_AJSLP-17-0100

McLeod, S., & Goldstein, B. (Eds.). (2012). *Multilingual aspects of speech sound disorders in children*. Multilingual Matters.

McNeilly, L., Fotheringham, S., & Walsh, R. (2007). Future directions in terminology. Symposium: Terminology in communication sciences and disorders: A new approach. Copenhagen: *27th World Congress of the International Association of Logopedics and Phoniatrics*. IALP.

Menn, L. (1976). Evidence for an interactionist discovery theory of child phonology. *Papers and reports on language development*, 12, 169–177. Stanford: Stanford University.

Meyerowitz, J. (2020). 180 Op-Eds: Or how to make the present historical. *Journal of American History*, 107(2), 323–335. https://doi.org/10.1093/jahist/jaaa335

Michie, S., & Abraham, C. (2004). Identifying techniques that promote health behaviour change: Evidence-based or evidence-inspired? *Psychology and Health*, 19(1), 29–49. https://doi.org/10.1080/0887044031000141199

Monahan, D. (1984). *Remediation of common phonological processes*. CC Publications.

Monahan, D. (1986). Remediation of common phonological processes. Four case studies. *Language Speech and Hearing Services in Schools*, 17(3), 187–198. https://doi.org/10.1044/0161-1461.1703.199

Morley, M. (1972). *The development and disorders of speech in children* (3rd ed.). Churchill Livingstone.

Morrisette, M. L. (2021). Complexity approach. In A. L. Williams, S. McLeod, & R. J. McCauley (Eds.), *Interventions for speech sound disorders in children* (2nd ed., pp. 91–110). Paul H. Brookes Publishing Co.

Mosher, J. (1929). *The production of correct speech sounds*. Expression.

Mowrer, O. (1952). Speech development in the young child: The autism theory of speech development and some clinical applications. *Journal of Speech and Hearing Disorders*, 17(3), 263–268. https://doi.org/10.1044/jshd.1703.263

Mowrer, O. (1960). *Learning theory and symbolic processes*. John Wiley and Sons.

Müller, N., & Ball, M. J. (2013). *Research methods in clinical linguistics and phonetics.* Wiley-Blackwell.

Müller, N., Muckley, S.-A., & Antonijevic, S. (2019). Where phonology meets morphology in the context of rapid language change and universal bilingualism: Irish initial mutations in development. *Clinical Linguistics and Phonetics,* 33(1–2), 3–19. https://doi.org/10.1080/02699206.2018.1542742

Munro, S., Ball, M. J., Müller, N., Duckworth, M., & Lyddy, F. (2005). Phonological acquisition in Welsh-English bilingual children. *Journal of Multilingual Communication Disorders,* 3(1), 24–49. https://doi.org/10.1080/14769670410001683467

Munro, S. M., Ball, M. J., & Müller, N. (2007). Welsh speech acquisition. In S. McLeod (Ed.), *The international guide to speech acquisition* (pp. 592–607).

Murai, J. (1963). The sounds of infants, their phonemicization and symbolization. *Studia Phonologica,* 3, 18–34. http://hdl.handle.net/2433/52620

Myklebust, H. (1952). Aphasia in childhood. *Journal Exceptional Children,* 19, 9–14.

Nemoy, E., & Davis, S. (1937). *The correction of defective consonant sounds.* Expression Company.

Oliveira, C., Lousada, M., & Jesus, L. M. T. (2015). The clinical practice of speech and language therapists with children with phonologically based speech sound disorders. *Child Language Teaching and Therapy,* 31(2), 173–194. https://doi.org/10.1177/0265659014550420

Oller, D. K., Wieman, L. A., Doyle, W. J., & Ross, C. (1976). Infant babbling and speech. *Journal of Child Language,* 3(1), 1–11. https://doi.org/10.1017/S0305000900001276

Olmstead, D. (1971). *Out of the mouths of babes.* Mouton.

Orton, S. T. (1937). *Reading, writing and speech problems in children: A presentation of certain types of disorders in the development of the language faculty.* W. W. Norton.

Osgood, C. (1957). *A behavioristic analysis of perception and language as cognitive phenomena, contemporary approaches to cognition.* Harvard University Press.

Palafox, P. L. (2019). *The heartbeat of speech-language pathology: Changing the world one session at a time.* Bilinguistics.

Paradis, J. (2001). Do bilingual two-year-olds have separate phonological systems? *International Journal of Bilingualism,* 5(1), 19–38. https://doi.org/10.1177%2F13670069010050010201

Pascoe, M., Maphalala, Z., Ebrahim, A., Hime, D., Mdladla, B., Mohamed, N., & Skinner, M. (2010). Children with speech difficulties: An exploratory survey of clinical practice in the Western Cape. *South African Journal of Communication Disorders,* 57(1), 66–75. https://doi.org/10.4102/sajcd.v57i1.51

Passy, J. (1990). *Cued articulation.* ACER Press.

Passy, J. (2010). *Cued articulation: Consonants and vowels.* ACER Press.

Passy, J., Botham, J., & Botham, H. (2014). *Cued articulation app.* ACER Press.

Poole, I. (1934). Genetic development of articulation of consonant sounds in speech. *Elementary English Review,* 11(6), 159–161. http://www.jstor.org/stable/41381777

Powers, M. H. (1959). Functional disorders of articulation. In L. E. Travis (Ed.), *Handbook of speech pathology and audiology.* Peter Owen.

Prather, E. M., Hedrick, D. L., & Kern, C. A. (1975). Articulation development in children aged two to four years. *Journal of Speech and Hearing Disorders,* 40(2), 179–191. https://doi.org/10.1044/jshd.4002.179

Prezas, R. F., Magnus, L., & Hodson, B. W. (2021). The cycles phonological remediation approach. In A. L. Williams, S. McLeod, & R. J. McCauley (Eds.), *Interventions for speech sound disorders in children* (pp. 251–278). Brookes Publishing Co.

Ranjha, M. I. (2014). Stability of consonant clusters in Urdu. *ELF Annual Research Journal,* 16, 137–156.

Renfrew, C. E. (1972). *Speech disorders in children.* Pergamon Press.

Robertson, S., Kersner, M., & Davis, S. (1995). *From the college of speech therapists to the Royal College of Speech and Language Therapists: A history of the college 1945-1995.* RCSLT.

Rockey, D. (1980). *Speech disorder in nineteenth century Britain: The history of stuttering.* Croom Helm.

Rudolph, J. M., & Wendt, O. (2014). The efficacy of the cycles approach: a multiple baseline design. *Journal of Communication Disorders,* 47, 1–16. https://doi.org/10.1016/j.jcomdis.2013.12.003

Rvachew, S. & Bernhardt, M. (2010). Clinical implications of the dynamic systems approach to phonological development. *American Journal of Speech-Language Pathology,* 19(1), 34–50. https://doi.org/10.1044/1058-0360(2009/08-0047)

Sander, E. K. (1972). When are speech sounds learned? *Journal of Speech and Hearing Disorders*, 37(1), 55–63. https://doi.org/10.1044/jshd.3701.55

Schulz, P., & Friedmann, N. (2011). Specific language impairment (SLI) across languages: Properties and possible loci. *Lingua*, 121(3), 333–338. https://doi.org/10.1016/j.lingua.2010.10.002

Schwartz, G. (2019). When is a cluster really a cluster? *Paper presented at the Approaches to Phonetics and Phonology conference*, Lublin, 21–23 June 2019. Narodowe Centrum Nauki.

Schwartz, R. G. (1992). Advances in phonological theory as a clinical framework. *Language, Speech, and Hearing Services in Schools*, 23(2), 269–276. https://doi.org/10.1044/0161-1461.2303.269

Schwartz, R. G., & Leonard, L. (1982). Do children pick and choose? *Journal of Child Language*, 9(2), 319–336. https://doi.org/10.1017/S0305000900004748

Scripture, M., & Jackson, E. (1919). *A manual of exercises for the correction of speech disorders*. Davis.

Shriberg, L. D. (1993). Four new speech and prosody-voice measures for genetics research and other studies in developmental phonological disorders. *Journal of Speech and Hearing Research*, 36(1), 105–140. https://doi.org/10.1044/jshr.3601.105

Shriberg, L. D., Kent, R. D., McAllister, T., & Preston, J. L. (2018). *Clinical phonetics* (5th ed.). Pearson.

Shriberg, L. D., & Kwiatkowski, J. (1980). *Natural process analysis*. Academic Press.

Smit, A. B., Hand, L., Freilinger, J. J., Bernthal, J. E., & Bird, A. (1990). The Iowa articulation norms project and its Nebraska replication. *Journal of Speech and Hearing Disorders*, 55(4), 779–798. https://doi.org/10.1044/jshd.5504.779

Smith, N. V. (1973). *The acquisition of phonology: A case study*. Cambridge University Press.

Smith, N. V. (1978). Lexical representation and the acquisition of phonology. *Paper given as a forum lecture*, Linguistic Institute, Linguistic Society of America.

Stackhouse, J., & Wells, B. (1997). *Children's speech and literacy difficulties I: A psycholinguistic framework*. Whurr Publishers.

Stackhouse, J., & Wells, B. (2001). *Children's speech and literacy difficulties II: Identification and intervention*. Whurr Publishers.

Stampe, D. (1969). The acquisition of phonetic representation. *Papers from the 5th regional meeting of the Chicago Linguistic Society*. 443–454. Chicago Linguistic Society.

Stampe, D. (1973). *A dissertation on natural phonology. Unpublished doctoral dissertation*, University of Chicago.

Stampe, D. (1979). *A dissertation on natural phonology*. Academic Press.

Stansfield, J. (2020a). Giving voice: An oral history of speech and language therapy. *International Journal of Language & Communication Disorders*, 55(3), 320-331. RCSLT. https://doi.org/10.1111/1460-6984.12520

Stansfield, J. (2020b). 75 years of speech and language therapy. Royal College of Speech and Language Therapists. https://www.rcslt.org/about-us/history

Stansfield, J. (2022). Talking points: Oral histories of Australian and British speech-language pathologists who qualified in the three decades after 1945. *International Journal of Speech-Language Pathology*, 24(6), 573–584. https://doi.org/10.1080/17549507.2022.2032345

Stinchfield, S., & Young, E. H. (1938). *Children with delayed or defective speech: Motor-kinesthetic factors in their training*. Stanford University Press.

Stoel-Gammon, C., & Dunn, C. (1985). *Normal and disordered phonology in children*. University Park Press.

Storkel, H. L. (2019). Using developmental norms for speech sounds as a means of determining treatment eligibility in schools. *Perspectives of the ASHA Special Interest Groups*, 4(1), 67–75. https://doi.org/10.1044/2018_PERS-SIG1-2018-0014

Templin, M. C. (1957). *Certain language skills in children: Their development and interrelationships* (NED-New ed., Vol. 26). University of Minnesota Press. http://www.jstor.org/stable/10.5749/j.ctttv2st

Thinking Publications. (2004). Barbara Hodson: Phonological intervention guru. Thinking Big News, 22(December).

Travis, L. E. (1931). *Speech pathology: A dynamic neurological treatment of normal speech and speech deviations*. D. Appleton and Company.

Travis, L. E. (1957). *Handbook of speech pathology*. Appleton-Century-Crofts.

Twitmeyer, E. B., & Nathanson, Y. S. (1932). *Correction of defective speech*. Blakiston's Son and Co.

Tyler, A. A. (2002). Language-based intervention for phonological disorders. *Seminars in Speech and Language*, 23(1), 69–82. https://doi.org/10.1055/s-2002-23511

Van Riper, C. (1939). *Speech correction: Principles and methods*. Prentice-Hall.

Van Riper, C. (1978). *Speech correction: Principles and methods* (6th ed.). Prentice-Hall.

Van Riper, C., & Erickson, R. L. (1996). *Speech correction: Principles and methods* (9th ed.). Pearson.

Van Riper, C., & Emerick, L. (1984). *Speech correction: An introduction to speech pathology and audiology* (7th ed.). Prentice-Hall.

Velten, H. (1943). The growth of phonemic and lexical patterns in infant language. *Language*, 19(4), 281–292. https://doi.org/10.2307/409932

Vogel Sosa, A., & Bybee, J. L. (2008). A cognitive approach to clinical phonology. In M. J. Ball, M. R. Perkins, N. Müller, & S. Howard (Eds.), *The handbook of clinical linguistics* (pp. 480–490). Blackwell.

Vygotsky, L. S. (1962). *Thought and language*. MIT Press.

Ward, I. (1923). *Defects of speech*. E. P. Dutton.

Waterson, N. (1971). Child phonology: A prosodic view. *Journal of Linguistics*, 7(2), 170–221. https://doi.org/10.1017/S0022226700002917

Waterson, N. (1981). A tentative development model of phonological representation. In T. Myers, J. Laver, & J. Anderson (Eds.), *The cognitive representation of speech*.

Weiner, F. (1979). *Phonological process analysis*. University Park Press.

Weiner, F. (1981a). Treatment of phonological disability using the method of meaningful contrast: Two case studies. *Journal of Speech and Hearing Disorders*, 46(1), 97–103. https://doi.org/10.1044/jshd.4601.97

Weiner, F. (1981b). Systematic sound preference as a characteristic of phonological disability. *Journal of Speech and Hearing Disorders*, 46(3), 281–286. https://doi.org/10.1044/jshd.4603.281

Wellman, B. L., Case, I. M., Mengert, I. G., & Bradbury, D. E. (1931). Speech sounds of young children. *University of Iowa Studies in Child Welfare*, 5(2). The Iowa Child Welfare Research Station: University of Iowa.

West, R., Kennedy, L., & Carr, A. (1937). *The rehabilitation of speech*. Harper and Brothers.

Williams, A. L. (2002a). Prologue: Perspectives in the phonological assessment of child speech. *American Journal of Speech-Language Pathology*, 11(3), 211–212. https://doi.org/10.1044/1058-0360(2002/020)

Williams, A. L. (2002b). Epilogue: Perspectives in the phonological assessment of child speech. *American Journal of Speech-Language Pathology*, 11(3), 259–263. https://doi.org/10.1044/1058-0360%282002%2F020%29

Williams, A. L., McLeod, S., & McCauley, R. J. (2021). *Interventions for speech sound disorders in children* (2nd ed.). Paul H. Brookes Publishing Co.

Wise, H. S. (1946). A revised classification of disorders of speech. *Journal of Speech Disorders*, 11(4), 327–334. https://doi.org/10.1044/jshd.1104.327

Wren, Y., Harding, S., Goldbart, J., & Roulstone, S. (2018). A systematic review and classification of interventions for speech-sound disorder in preschool children. *International Journal of Language & Communication Disorders*, 53(5), 446–467. https://doi.org/10.1111/1460-6984.12371

Zsiga, E. C. (2020). *The phonology / phonetics interface*. Edinburgh University Press.

Chapter 2
Terms, Classification, and Assessment

As the learning of technical terms is difficult at best, writers should not coin unnecessary terms. The Nomenclature Committee is often able to suggest a well-established term which has meaning identical with that of a newly proposed term.

Robbins et al., 1947

Terminology in Speech Sound Disorders

The burdensome terminology (and the temptation *was* there to head this section *TERMS!*) for classifying, describing, and documenting speech development and disorders, groans with acronyms, abbreviations, and synonyms. Mostly, they come from anatomy, education, genetics, linguistics, medicine, psychology, physiology, and sociology. There are also terms that SLPs/SLTs consider their own, or cheerfully own jointly with audiologists, educators, medical practitioners, linguists, psychologists, and others who may or may not have coined them in the first place. Among those we either 'own' or 'share' are the abbreviations CAS, DDK, DTTC,

DVD, NS-OME, OME, E^3BP, PCC, PVM; the acronyms CASANA, DEAP, DEMMS, ReST, and SODA; the terms *consonant harmony*, *phoneme collapse*, *production practice*, *probe word*, *speech banana* (thank you, audiology) *syllable tree* (and you, linguistics), and *relational analysis*; and the words: *fronting*, *metaphonology*, *modelling* (coined by psychologist Albert Bandura), *phonotactics*, *recasting*, *sociophonetics*, and *stimulability*.

As Robbins et al. (1947) admonished, a plethora of synonyms confuse matters, particularly for families of children with SSD and SLP/SLT students. For example, *approximant* and *semivowel*; *assimilation processes* and *harmony processes*; *cluster simplification* and *cluster reduction*; *plosive* and *stop*; *phonetic variation* and *allophonic variation*; *phonological disorder* and *phonological impairment*; *protowords, vocables, phonetically consistent forms*, and *quasi-words*; *systemic process* and *substitution process*; *variegated babbling* and *non-reduplicated babbling*; *velum* and *soft palate*; *vocal cords* and *vocal folds*; *weak syllable deletion* and *unstressed syllable deletion*.

Then there are near synonyms (e.g., *Childhood Apraxia of Speech* and *Developmental Verbal Dyspraxia*) and vernacular names (e.g., *blend* for *consonant cluster*; *glue ear* for *otitis media with effusion*; *tongue-tie* for *ankyloglossia*); homonyms (e.g., *rime* and *rhyme*). Some regularly used abbreviations have multiple meanings (e.g., OME can stand for *otitis media with effusion*, *oral motor exercises* and *oral musculature examination* (see Box 2.1); PA can stand for *phonological awareness* and *phonemic awareness*); and certain words and terms that mean different things are easily confused (e.g., *minimal pair* and *minimal opposition*; *phonological process* and *phonological processing*; and *phonological awareness* and *phonemic awareness*).

Potentially Confusing Nomenclature

When we engage professionally with practitioners and researchers in SLP/SLT, and those in other disciplines, we find that the *same* words are often used to denote *different* concepts and phenomena. Consider how 'language', 'phoneme', and other 'phon words' are understood by teachers, whose definitions may differ from usual SLP/SLT definitions, sometimes leading to miscommunications (Patchell & Hand, 1993; Scarborough & Brady, 2002). Misunderstandings can also result from SLPs'/SLTs' and teachers' use of dissimilar but *similar-sounding* terms such as 'phonological processes' and 'phonological processing'. Differing use of the terms: language, phoneme, phonological processes, phonological processing, phonological disorder/phonological impairment, and several associated terms, are outlined below.

Language

In SLP/SLT, human language is considered partly innate, but also partly learned, as infants, children, and young people interact with other people and the environment. Sometimes referred to as the symbolisation of thought, it is a learned code, or system of rules – incorporating from a very young age, the developing use of appropriate pragmatics in communicative situations. Applying the code enables us to communicate ideas and express wants and needs. Reading, writing, gesturing, and speaking are all forms of language. Self-described 'language nerd' Kenn Apel said that his definition of language

aligned well with the ASHA (1983) definition, except that he would add orthography to the list of language areas (Apel, 2014).

> *Language is a dynamic system that is part of and influenced by the biological, social, cultural, cognitive, and affective domains and contexts of daily life; it is rule-governed and involves the integrated use of all areas of language, including phonology, morphology, syntax, semantics, and pragmatics; it is expressed in a number of modes, including spoken, text, and sign.*
>
> ASHA, 1983

For SLPs/SLTs, language has two main divisions: receptive language – understanding what is said, written or signed; and expressive language – speaking, writing, or signing. By contrast, Patchell and Hand (1993) explain that for teachers, "'*language' tends to refer to schoolwork that involves reading, writing, literature, and advanced discussion skills such as debating, expressing logical reasoning, and so on*".

Phoneme

In Linguistics and SLP/SLT, phonemes are the smallest linguistic units that, in combination with other phonemes, signal meaning differences – or phonemic contrasts – between words (Müller & Ball, A3).

Minimal Pairs

In the meaningful-word-sequence *bin*, *chin*, *din*, *fin*, *gin*, *kin*, *Lynn*, *pin*, *sin*, *shin*, *thin*, *tin*, and *win*, each word sounds different, and each has a different meaning (or two meanings for *gin*, which is a machine or a beverage). These meanings are signalled because the words start with different (initial or onset) phonemes: /b/, /tʃ/, /d/, /f/, /dʒ/, /k/, /l/, /p/, /s/, /ʃ/, /θ/, /t/, and /w/, so that any two of the words listed form a **minimal pair**. 'Minimal', because just one sound changes. Similarly, the meaningful (real) words *bat*, *beat*, *bet*, *bite*, *bit*, *boat*, *boot*, *bought* form various minimal pairs (e.g., *bed-bud*), because each has a different vowel or diphthong. Again, the real words *pack*, *pad*, *Pam*, *pan*, *pat*, *patch* form minimal pairs (e.g., *pack-pat*) because each word has a different final sound.

Minimal Pairs and Minimal Oppositions

All the possible contrastive pairs in the sequence *thin-shin, win-fin, Lynn-bin, gin-kin,* etc., listed above are minimal pairs, but they do not all form a **minimal opposition**. A minimal opposition is present when there is just one feature difference, in place, voice, or manner (PVM) between minimal-pair words. The pairs *bin-din, pin-tin,* and *tin-kin* form minimal oppositions because only **place** of articulation changes (bilabial /b/ and /p/ versus alveolar /d/ and /t/; and alveolar /t/ versus velar /k/) while voice and manner remain the same. The pairs *bin-pin, din-tin,* and *chin-gin* also exemplify minimal oppositions because the difference between them is in **voice** only, and place and manner remain constant. The pairs *tin-sin* and *din-Lynn* are minimal oppositions because the change is in **manner** only (stop versus fricative for *tin-sin* and stop versus lateral approximant for *din-Lynn*) and voice and place remain the same.

Minimal Pairs and Maximal Oppositions

A **maximal opposition** is present when the two words comprising a minimal pair differ by all three features: place, voice, and manner. This occurs in *shin-bin* where the voiceless, postalveolar fricative /ʃ/ contrasts with the voiced, bilabial stop /b/; in *gin-thin* in which the voiced, postalveolar affricate /dʒ/ contrasts with the voiceless, dental fricative /θ/; and in *win-fin* where the voiced, bilabial glide /w/ contrasts with the voiceless, labiodental fricative /f/.

Vowel Minimal Pairs

Minimal pairs are also formed when consonants in a word pair are unchanged and the vowel changes. For instance, *bin-Ben, din-done, fin-fan, gin-John,* or *win-one*; or when a diphthong replaces a diphthong (e.g., *bay-bow,* and *buy-boy*) or a diphthong replaces a vowel (e.g., *bin-bone, chin-chain, fin-phone,* or *pin-pine,* and *tin-tone*).

Rhotic and Non-rhotic Varieties of English

In *non-rhotic* varieties of English, pairs such as *cola-colour, drama-dreamer, lava-liver, panda-gander, soda-cider,* and *scuba-scooter* form minimal pairs because they all end with a neutral vowel or schwa, for example, /koʊlə-kʌlə/, dɹamə-dɹimə/. They do not form minimal pairs in *rhotic* varieties of English, such as the dialects of Ireland, Southwest England, and most of Canada and the United States, because the word-final 'R' is pronounced, for example, [koʊlə-kʌlɝ], and [dɹamə-dɹimɝ].

Near Minimal Pairs

Similar effects are seen in varieties of English that include /bj, kj, dj, fj, hj, mj, nj, pj, sj, and tj/ versus those that do not, in words like *beauty, cue, dew, few, hue, mew, new, pew, sue,* and *tune*. For example, for those who say /bj/ *beauty-booty* [bjuti-buti] is a **near minimal pair**, but for those who do not say /bj/, *beauty-booty* [buti-buti] are homonyms (words that sound the same). A near minimal pair is formed when the structure of the syllable changes with the addition or removal of a phoneme. They come into play when SLPs/SLTs work on structural errors such as **initial consonant deletion (ICD)** (e.g., *eel-seal, eat-feet, old-cold,* and *E-sea*); **final consonant deletion (FCD)** (e.g., *go-goat, bow-boat, doe-dome, hoe-hose, row-road, no-nose,* and *toe-toad*); and cluster reduction (e.g., *nip-snip, nap-snap, no-snow, nail-snail,* and *knees-sneeze,* and *deck-desk, wick-whisk, duck-dusk,* and *tuck-tusk*).

Place-Voice-Manner (PVM) CHART

A simple **Place-Voice-Manner (PVM) Chart** for the language in question is helpful in sorting out the number of feature differences contained in a minimal pair. The PVM Chart in Figure 2.1 is for English and charts for several other languages are available at www.speech-language-therapy.com in the CPD Resources area. The languages include Danish, Icelandic, Indonesian, Irish, Malaysian, Norwegian, European Portuguese, and Turkish. There is also a Place-Aspiration-Manner (PAM) Chart for Cantonese.

PVM Chart: English			PLACE							
			LABIAL		CORONAL				DORSAL	
MANNER		VOICING	Bilabial	Labiodental	Dental	Alveolar	Postalveolar	Palatal	Velar	Glottal
Stop		Voiceless	p			t			k	ʔ
Stop		Voiced	b			d			g	
Fricative		Voiceless		f	θ	s	ʃ			h
Fricative		Voiced		v	ð	z	ʒ			
Affricate		Voiceless					tʃ			
Affricate		Voiced					dʒ			
Nasal		Voiced	m			n			ŋ	
LIQUID	Lateral	Voiced				l				
LIQUID	Rhotic	Voiced					ɹ			
Glide		Voiced	w					j	w	

(OBSTRUENTS: Stop, Fricative, Affricate rows; SONORANTS: Nasal, Liquid, Glide rows)

Figure 2.1 Place-Voice-Manner (PVM) chart for PVM analysis Obstruent: A consonant formed by obstructing outward airflow, causing increased air pressure in the vocal tract. **Sonorant:** A vowel or a consonant produced without turbulent airflow in the vocal tract. A sound is sonorant if it can be voiced continuously at the same pitch. **/w/:** /w/ has two places of articulation (points of narrowest constriction of the vocal tract): bilabial and velar.

A PVM Chart contains every *consonant* phoneme of one language. This is different from the Consonant Chart (2020) provided by the International Phonetic Association (IPA) in its 'Full Chart'. The IPA Full Chart shows *consonant* and *vowel* phonemes of all the world's languages, 'other symbols', diacritics, suprasegmentals, and tones and word accents.

Full Chart

https://www.internationalphoneticassociation.org/IPAcharts/IPA_chart_orig/pdfs/IPA_Kiel_2020_full.pdf

ExtIPA

https://www.internationalphoneticassociation.org/sites/default/files/extIPA_2016.pdf

The IPA (2020) Full Chart is on the back flyleaf of this book alongside the extIPA symbols for disordered speech transcription which are inside the back cover. Both are offered free by the IPA under a Creative Commons Attribution-Sharealike 3.0 Unported License.

Phonemes and Phones

When listening to speech, a listener *hears* or *perceives* phonetic representations of the phonemes, in words. These audible representations are called the surface forms, or phones. In English, they include the consonants [p], [b], [t], [d], [k], [g], [m], [n], [ŋ], [h], [f], [v], [s], [z], [ʃ], [ʒ], [θ], [ð], [tʃ], [dʒ], [ɹ], [l], [j], and [w], and the vowels (for 'vowels', read 'vowels, diphthongs and triphthongs'): [æ], [u], [ɪə], [æʊə], etc., with allophonic variation, also known as phonetic variation. Similarly, what a speaker *says* are phones (also known as phonetic representations or surface forms): ([b], [ʧ], [d], etc., or [ə], [oʊ], etc. In vowel meaningful minimal word-pairs like *open-ocean*, *cry-crow*, and *phone-fun*, either the vowel in the onset (the first sound) or the vowel in the coda (the rest of the word) changes, making their meanings distinct, or 'distinctive'.

Conventionally, in *phonetic* transcription, speech sounds (phones), or the way someone produces a sound, word, or words in real life, are enclosed in square brackets ('[]'). In *phonemic* transcription of the abstract, underlying concepts of speech sounds (the phonemes) the values are signified in virgules (forward slashes: '//'). It is important to know that, as an abstraction, a phoneme incorporates the range of variations, called allophones, that represent how a sound is produced in varying contexts.

Abstract Concepts, or 'Abstractions'

Student SLPs/SLTs are taught in Linguistics classes at university that technically, a phoneme is not a speech sound but rather, an abstract concept a sound, or an *abstraction*, which Scarborough and Brady (2002, p. 304) explained in their useful article, is *the speaker's internalized representation of a single speech sound*. In practice, speech-language clinicians are apt to use terminology loosely, and talk about children practising *saying* phonemes, and clinicians *modelling* (*saying*) phonemes for children to imitate, when what is really going on is saying, or modelling phones.

Calling phonemes abstractions might make them seem difficult to conceptualise, until we remember that we talk and think in abstractions all the time. For example, the word grass conjures an image of grass, or our abstract concept of grass 'in the mind'. But grass is variable: it comes as carefully manicured lawns; vigorous and perennial prairie grass; fast-growing lemon grass ready to add to East Asian broths, soups, and curries; tall, wind-waving pampas grass; and beautiful poa tussock grass, the densely tufted, yearlong green, hardy perennial that grows to 120 cm high throughout Australia. Even bamboo and sugarcane are grasses. 'Grass' is used in vernacular contexts too: a grass is an informer or traitor, and grass is a street name for cannabis. Yet, if someone mentions grass, we immediately draw on a mental abstraction for grass, whatever that might be.

The abstraction will sometimes be conditioned by context. 'Tabby rolled in the fake grass on the balcony' may conjure orderly, evergreen synthetic spears that sometimes demand housework rather than gardening, while 'That grass will be a snake haven if it's not cut' and 'They peddled grass on the streets' evoke different abstractions.

Allophonic Variation (Phonetic Variation)

Like grass, phonemes are variable. These variations are called allophones. Allophones represent any one of two or more speech sounds (phones, phonetic realisations, or surface forms) that are considered variants of the same phoneme. The allophone produced in a word is conditioned by the context. 'Context' can refer to the language, crosslinguistic or dialectal context (e.g., a variety of Arabic compared to a variety of English), and/or the phonetic context, or where the sound occurs in a word or longer utterance, and how it relates to the other sounds.

Language Context

When working with multilingual children with speech sound disorders, it is important to gather information about the phonologies of the languages a child speaks. Consider /n/ cross-linguistically, in Arabic and English for example. In Arabic, /n/ and /ŋ/ are (non-contrastive) allophones of /n/, while in English, /n/ and /ŋ/ are distinctive (contrastive) phonemes (e.g., *pin-ping*). Subtleties such as this mean that SLPs/SLTs must ascertain the system of contrastive phones in a client's Language(s) Other Than English (LOTE) as a component of routine assessment of multilingual children with SSD (McLeod et al., 2017), particularly if we are counted among the vast majority of monolingual English-speaking SLPs/SLTs.

Phonetic Context

An example of phonetic context impacting the production of allophones can be found in the variations that occur in alveolars. Alveolar consonants in

English become 'dental' or are 'dentalised' before [θ] and /ð/, making /t̪/, /n̪/, /d̪/, /s̪/, /z̪/, and /l̪/ allophones of /t/ /n/, /d/, /s/, /z/, and /l/ respectively. Sometimes, our own dentalised production is obvious to us. For instance, compare the alveolar placement for /n/ in *ten*, /d/ in *bread*, and /l/ in *hell*, and notice how the place of articulation for [n], [d], and [l] moves towards the front teeth, becoming dental or interdental, in *tenth*, *breadth*, and *health*. In broad (phonemic) transcription, *month*, *width*, and *health* are transcribed: /mʌnθ/, /wɪdθ/, and /hɛlθ/. In narrow or fine (phonetic) transcription the dental diacritic is below /n/, /d/, and /l/, and they become [n̪], [d̪], and [l̪], and the words are transcribed [mʌn̪θ], [wɪd̪θ], and [hɛl̪θ]. Likewise, in narrow transcription *wet them*, *dice those*, and *freeze these* become ['wɛt̪ˌðəm], ['daɪs̪ˈðoʊz], and ['fɹiz̪ðiz] with the dental diacritic under the coarticulated /t/, /s/, and /z/.

Coarticulation

In conversational speech, *wet them*, *dice those*, and *freeze these*, the final consonant of the first word and the first consonant of the second word are coarticulated. Each of these two-word combinations may sound almost like one two-syllable word unless the speaker is endeavouring to separate the words, applying strong word-stress to both words, as they might aid comprehensibility for a listener in poor listening conditions, or when using speech-to-text transcription software. If, rather than saying ['wɛt̪ˌðəm] with the articulatory movements for /t/ and /ð/ overlapping, a speaker said, distinctly, ['wɛt 'ðɛm] or ['wɛtʰ 'ðɛm] (with excessive aspiration of /t/ indicated by the [ʰ] diacritic), perhaps adding a little extra tongue protrusion to [ð] and changing the vowel in *them* from neutral [ə] to [ɛ], coarticulation would not occur and it is unlikely that the [t] in *wet* would be dentalised.

Assimilation: Consonant Harmony; Vowel Harmony

Coarticulation results in the phonological process (phonological pattern) of assimilation. Assimilation is a normal adaptive articulatory adjustment in which consonants or vowels become more like, or even the same as, a neighbouring phone. Sometimes the articulatory change affects place (P), or manner (M), or voicing (V) only, but assimilations can involve two parameters (e.g., M and V), or all three (P, M, and V). Assimilation can occur within a word (e.g., [mʌn̪θ]) or across word boundaries, between words (e.g., wɛt̪ˌðəm), both of which are examples of dentalisation or dental assimilation. Because two segments become more alike, or 'harmonise' with each other, assimilation processes are also called harmony processes. Harmony processes can involve either or both consonant harmony and vowel harmony. Assimilation or harmony occurs constantly in the world's languages as a natural consequence of normal articulation or coarticulation. It is not confined to young children's developing phonologies.

Phonological Processes

Linguists and SLPs/SLTs understand the synonymous terms 'phonological processes' and 'phonological patterns' to refer to a set of descriptions (not explanations) of the predictable, simplified productions typically found in young children's speech when they are learning to talk, and that persist beyond typical age-expectations in children with SSD.

Four of many phonological processes, or 'processes' are **fronting**, e.g., where a child says *doe* for *go*, *tight* for *kite*, *save* for *shave*; **final consonant deletion**, e.g., in which a child pronounces *rope* as *roe*, *teach* as *tea*, and *rice* as *rye*; **cluster reduction**, e.g., where *knees* replaces *sneeze*, *bend* replaces *spend*, and *moat* replaces *most*; and **stopping of fricatives**, e.g., *pig* or *big* for *fig*, *pate* or *bate* for *face* (where two fricatives are 'stopped' in the same word), and *deep* for *sheep*. These and other commonly observed patterns appear in Table 2.1 with their approximate ages of elimination in years;months they were determined by Grunwell in 1987. Most SLPs/SLPs reserve the terms phonological processes and phonological patterns for such simplified productions, and do not use them in any other sense.

Table 2.1 Phonological processes / phonological patterns commonly observed in typical speech acquisition, with approximate ages of elimination in years;months.

Phonological Process / Phonological Pattern	Adult (target) form vs child's realisation		DESCRIPTION
	ADULT /phonemic/ transcription	CHILD [phonetic] transcription	
Context sensitive voicing 3;0	PIG /pɪɡ/ KISS /kɪs/	[bɪɡ] [ɡɪs]	A voiceless sound is replaced by a voiced sound. In these examples, /p/ is replaced by [b], and /k/ is replaced by [ɡ]. Other examples might include /t/ being replaced by [d], or /f/ being replaced by [v].
Word-final devoicing 3;0	RED /ɹɛd/ BAG /bæɡ/	[ɹɛt] [bæk]	A final voiced consonant in a word is replaced by a voiceless consonant. Here, /d/ has been replaced by /t/, and /ɡ/ has been replaced by [k].
Final consonant deletion 3;3	HIM /hɪm/ ROUGH /rʌf/	[hɪ] [ɹʌ]	The final consonant in the word is omitted. In these examples, /m/ is omitted (or deleted) from 'him' and /f/ is omitted from 'rough'.
Velar fronting 3;9	KISS /kɪs/ GIVE /ɡɪv/ WING /wɪŋ/	[tɪs] [dɪv] [wɪn]	A velar stop or nasal is replaced by an alveolar stop or nasal respectively. Here, /k/ in 'kiss' is replaced by [t], /ɡ/ in 'give' is replaced by [d] and /ŋ/ in 'wing' is replaced by [n].
Palatal fronting 3;9	SHIP /ʃɪp/ TAJ /taʒ/	[sɪp] [taz]	The palato-alveolar fricatives /ʃ/ and /ʒ/ are replaced by alveolar fricatives [s] and [z].
Consonant harmony / Consonant assimilation 4;0	TAKE /teɪk/ DOG /dɒɡ/ GOT /ɡɒt/	[keɪk] [ɡɒɡ] [ɡɒk]	Pronunciation of the whole word is influenced by the presence of a particular sound in the word. Here, /k/ in 'take' causes the /t/ to be replaced [k]; the /ɡ/ in 'dog' causes /d/ to be replaced by [ɡ]; and the /ɡ/ in 'got' causes the /t/ to be replaced by [k].
Weak syllable deletion 4;0	AGO /əɡoʊ/ CARAVAN / ˈkæɹə,væn/	[ɡoʊ] [ˈkæ,væn]	Words of two syllables or more exhibit syllable stress. Here, the unstressed syllables /ə/ and /ɹə/ in 'ago' and 'caravan' respectively have been deleted.
Cluster reduction 4;0	BLUE: blu ANT: ænt	[bu] [æt]	Consonant clusters occur when two or three consonants occur in a sequence in a word. In cluster reduction part of the cluster is omitted. Here, /l/ has been deleted from 'blue' and /n/ from 'ant'.
Gliding of liquids 5;0	REAL /ɹiəl/ LEG /lɛɡ/	[wiəl] [jɛɡ]	The liquid consonants /l/ and /ɹ/ are replaced by the glides /w/ or /j/. In these examples, /ɹ/ in 'real' is replaced by [w], and /l/ in 'leg' is replaced by [j].
Stopping /f/ /s/ 3;0 /v/ /z/ 3;6 /ʃ/ /tʃ/ /dʒ/ 4;6 /θ/ /ð/ 5;0	FUN /fʌn/ VAN /væn/ CHIN /tʃɪn/ JET /dʒɛt/ SIP /sɪp/ ZIP /zɪp/ SHOE /ʃu/ THIN /θɪn/ THAT /ðæt/	[pʌn] [bæn] [tɪn] [dɛt] [tɪp] [dɪp] [tu] [tɪn] [dæt]	A fricative consonant or an affricate consonant is replaced by a stop (plosive). Here, /f/ in 'fun' is replaced by [p]; / /v/ in 'van' is replaced by [b]; /tʃ/ in 'chin' is replaced by [t]; /dʒ/ in 'jet' is replaced by [d]; /s/ in 'sip' is replaced by [t]; /z/ in 'zip' is replaced by [d]; /ʃ/ in 'shoe' is replaced by [t]; /θ/ in 'thin' is replaced by [t]; and /ð/ in 'that' is replaced by [d]. Sometimes a voiceless fricative or affricate is stopped *and* voiced, so that 'fun', 'chin', 'sip', 'shoe' and 'thin' become [bʌn], [dɪn], [dɪp], [du], and [dɪn] respectively.

Phonological Processing

Teachers and cognitive and educational psychologists, and indeed *some* SLPs/SLTs, sometimes use the term 'phonological processes' when discussing 'phonological processing', as in the second sentence from Scarborough and Brady (2002, p. 318):

> ***Phonological processing:*** *The formation, retention, and/or use of phonological codes or speech while performing some cognitive or linguistic task or operation such as speaking, listening, remembering, learning, naming, thinking, reading, or writing.* ***Phonological processes*** *do not require conscious awareness; they can be, and often are, carried out without our attending to them...Even though phonological processing (as defined above) is a mental operation that cannot be directly measured, and even though it plays a role in virtually every kind of task that is used in contemporary research on language and reading, researchers often refer to some tasks and measures, but not others, as indices of phonological processing. Although it is not always stated explicitly, the term tends to be used for tasks that are hypothesized to require relatively more phonological processing than other tasks in a battery, and/or for those in which phonological processing is thought to be so crucial that individual differences in performance largely reflect variability in this component of the overall task. There is not yet full agreement, however, as to which measures meet these criteria.*

Clearly, the terms *phonological processes* in SLP/SLT and Linguistics and *phonological processing* in psycholinguistic theory, cognitive and educational psychology, and in literacy teaching and research, have dissimilar definitions. For speech-language professionals, *phonological processes* (or *phonological patterns*) are speech simplifications, whereas *phonological processing* is crucial in executing numerous cognitive or linguistic tasks. But, because the terms sound similar, they are easily confused. So, if we as SLPs/SLTs use terms like *phonological process, language,* or *phoneme* in discussion or written reports, we must clarify for the listener or reader what *we* mean *and* acknowledge where indicated that they may have equally valid, but different definitions for them.

Speech Sound Disorders and Phonological Disorder

Overarching Headings

In this book the term **speech sound disorders** (SSD) is used as an umbrella heading for the various types of speech impairments in children. By contrast, while she has used SSD in various publications (e.g., Rvachew & Brosseau-Lapré, 2018) Rvachew has preferred **developmental phonological disorders** (DPD) as an overarching term over the years. Grunwell used DPD and many variations of it (e.g., Grunwell, 1989); as did Shriberg (1993) prior to switching to SSD (Shriberg, 2010). I used DPD in my doctoral thesis (Bowen, 1996) and in Bowen (1998), but as a subtype of speech disorder and not as an umbrella heading. Ruscello (1993, 2008) and Shelton (1993) favoured '**sound system disorder**' as the umbrella term. My colleagues at the University of KwaZulu-Natal in Durban, South Africa, cleverly added one key word to this cover term, to create '**speech sound system disorders**' (SSSD) making its meaning clearer, and sounding less like something is wrong with your hi-fi.

Phonological Disorder/Impairment, and Developmental Phonological Disorder

The synonymous and interchangeable terms phonological disorder and phonological impairment refer to a cognitive-linguistic difficulty in learning the phonological system of a language. Phonological disorder is characterised by persistent speech error patterns (or phonological processes) that are characteristic (normal) in typically developing young children's speech. As mentioned above, alternative names have included 'developmental phonological disorder' (e.g., Bowen, 1998; Grunwell, 1989; Rvachew & Brosseau-Lapré, 2018; Shriberg, 1993) as well as 'phonological disability' (e.g., Grunwell, 1983; Ingram, 1976; Weiner, 1981a, 1981b), 'phonological speech disorder' (Gillon, 1998), 'protracted phonological development' (Bernhardt et al., 2015), 'functional phonological disorder' (Gierut, 1998), and uniquely, 'phonological development disorder' (ICD10-CM Diagnosis Code F80.0, 2022).

Misuse of Terms

There is a regrettable tendency among SLPs/SLTs to 'improve on' the term phonological disorder, replacing it with: 'phonological *processing* disorder', 'phonological *process* disorder', or 'phonological *processes* disorder'. These misnomers have crept into our professional discussion, documentation, and reports, and it would be good if they crept right back out again. None of the three terms is an acceptable synonym for 'phonological disorder', 'phonological impairment', or 'developmental phonological disorder'.

Classification of Speech Sound Disorders

In their critical review of classification systems for SSD, Waring and Knight (2013, p. 25) concluded that:

'There is a need for a universally agreed-upon classification system that is useful to clinicians and researchers. The resulting classification system needs to be robust, reliable, and valid. A universal classification system would allow for improved tailoring of treatments to subgroups of SSD which may, in turn, lead to improved treatment efficacy'.

There is a striking but unsurprising influence of the medical model in SLP/SLT. Nowhere is it more evident than in the symptomatologic and aetiologic frameworks used in SSD classification, particularly when they employ terms from the field of human genetics, hence the definitions of genetics terms in Table 2.2.

Table 2.2 Glossary of key genetic terms.

Aetiology (US Etiology)	The study of causes or origins.
Alleles	Humans carry two sets of chromosomes, one from each parent. Equivalent genes in the two sets might be different, for example, because of single nucleotide polymorphisms. An allele is one of the two (or more) forms of a particular gene.
DNA (Deoxyribonucleic acid)	The molecule that encodes genetic information and is capable of self-replication and synthesis of *RNA*. DNA consists of two long chains of nucleotides twisted into a double helix and joined by hydrogen bonds between the complementary 'bases' adenine and thymine or cytosine and guanine. The sequence of nucleotides determines individual *Hereditary* characteristics.
Distal cause	See Proximal cause/Distal cause below.
Endophenotype	Any hereditary characteristic that is normally associated with some condition but is not a direct symptom of that condition. An endophenotype may be neurophysiological, biochemical, cognitive, endocrinological, neuroanatomical, or neuropsychological (including self-report data) in nature.
Environment	All circumstances surrounding an organism or group of organisms, especially: (a) The combination of external physical conditions that affect and influence the growth, development, and survival of organisms. (b) The complex of social and cultural conditions affecting the nature of an individual or community.
Gene	A *hereditary* unit consisting of a sequence of *DNA* that occupies a specific location on a chromosome and determines a particular characteristic in an organism.
Gene expression	The process by which a gene's coded information is converted into the structures present and operating in the cell.
Genome	The complete DNA sequence of an organism.
Genotype	The genotype is the genetic makeup, rather than the physical appearance (*Phenotype*), of an organism or group of organisms. It involves the combination of *Alleles* located on *Homologous Chromosomes* determining a specific characteristic or trait.
Hereditary	(a) Transmitted or capable of being transmitted genetically from parent to offspring. (b) Appearing in or characteristic of successive generations. (c) Of or relating to heredity or inheritance.

Table 2.2 (*Continued*)

Homologous chromosomes	A pair of chromosomes containing the same linear gene sequences each derived from one parent.
Incidence	The number of new cases of a disorder or disease during a given time interval, usually per annum, expressed as *Incidence Proportion (Risk)* or as *Incidence Rate*.
Incidence proportion	The number of new cases divided by the size of the population at risk. For example, if a stable population contains 1000 pre-schoolers and 2 develop a condition over two years of observation, the incidence proportion is 2 cases per 1000 pre-schoolers.
Incidence rate	The number of new cases per unit of person-time at risk. Using the previous example, the incidence rate is 1 case per 1000 person-years, because the incidence proportion (2 per 1000) is divided by the number of years (2). Using person-time rather than just time covers circumstances in which participants exit studies prior to completion.
Inheritance	(a) The process of genetic transmission of characteristics from parents to offspring. (b) A characteristic so inherited. (c) The sum of characteristics genetically transmitted from parents to offspring.
Locus	Locus (pl. loci): The position on a chromosome of a gene or other chromosome marker; also, the DNA at that position. The use of locus is sometimes restricted to mean regions of DNA that are expressed. See *Gene Expression*.
Monogenic disorder	A disorder caused by a mutant allele of a single gene.
Oligogenic disorder	A phenotypic trait produced by two or more genes working together.
Phenotype	The phenotype comprises the observable physical or biochemical characteristics (*Phenotypic Traits*) of an organism, as determined by both genetic makeup (*Genotype*) and environmental influences. It is the expression of a specific trait, such as stature or blood type, based on genetic and environmental influences. (See also *Endophenotype*)
Polygenic disorder	Genetic disorder resulting from the combined action of alleles of more than one gene (e.g., heart disease, diabetes, and some cancers). Although such disorders are inherited, they depend on the simultaneous presence of several alleles; thus, the hereditary patterns usually are more complex than those of single-gene disorders.
Prevalence	The total number (or percentage) of cases of a disease or condition in a population at one time.
Proximal cause Distal cause	Proximal causes are deficiencies within a system that directly bring about impaired performance, while distal causes are the causative factors that produced the deficiencies. The proximal and distal causes interact with environmental inputs over time. Such interactions explain commonalities and individual variation in the developmental path of the SSD that is observed in children with the same subtype. In SSD, the proximal cause is the underlying speech process that *explains* the nature of the speech errors a child produces. 'Proximal' implies 'downstream' or near to the child, or within the child, e.g., difficulties with input processing; difficulties with phonological processing; difficulties with output processing. The distal cause is the *origin* of the impairment in the underlying speech process. Distal implies far from the child (upstream), e.g., family history (heritability) of SSD or reading difficulties; or otitis media with effusion.
RNA (Ribonucleic acid)	A polymeric constituent of all living cells and many viruses, comprising a long, usually single-stranded chain of alternating phosphate and ribose units with the bases adenine, guanine, cytosine, and uracil bonded to the ribose. The structure and base sequence of RNA are determinants of protein synthesis and *Transmission* of genetic information.
Symptom	A symptom is a sign or an indication of disorder or disease, especially when experienced by an individual as a change from normal function, sensation, or appearance. Symptomatic classifications of SSDs are based on speech characteristics or 'symptoms' such as limited phonetic repertoire, or persistence of normal phonological patterns.
Transmission	Genetic transmission is the transfer of genetic information from genes to another generation or from one location in a cell to another location in a cell.

Readers delving into the range of classificatory systems, models, and frameworks quickly discover

- Trichotomous diagnostic distinctions between *articulation disorder*, *phonological disorder*, and *motor speech disorder* (see Figures i.1 and 3.1).
- A dichotomous distinction between (1) *phonological approaches* to intervention for phonological disorder and inconsistent speech disorder and (2) *motor speech approaches* to intervention for articulation disorder, childhood apraxia of speech, and childhood dysarthria (see Figure i.2 and McLeod & Baker, 2017, pp. 38–39).
- A two-way differentiation between speech sound disorders' effects on the form or the function of speech sounds within a specified language system. In that conceptualisation *SSDs affecting the form of speech sounds* are called articulation disorders and are associated with structural (e.g., cleft palate) and motor-based (e.g., apraxia) difficulties, whereas *SSDs affecting the function of speech sounds* within a language system 'are traditionally referred to as phonological disorders and are associated with difficulties in the generation and use of phonemes, phoneme rules, and patterns within the context of spoken language' (Bauman-Waengler, 2020, p. 8).
- A bipartite split between functional and organic SSDs.
  - *Functional speech sound disorders* are often said to have no known cause, or to be *speech sound disorders of unknown origin*. On the functional or idiopathic side are articulation and phonological disorders.
  - *Organic speech sound disorders*, which may be *developmental* or acquired, have known causes. On the organic side are motor/neurological SSDs affecting execution or planning (e.g., cerebral palsy); SSDs due to orofacial anomalies (e.g., cleft palate), surgery, or trauma; sensory/perceptual SSDs due to hearing impairment (e.g., children fitted with hearing aids or cochlear implants); SSD associated with intellectual/cognitive impairment (e.g., Down syndrome); and SSD due to genetic causes including genetic syndromes (e.g., Down syndrome again, Fragile X syndrome, and Velo-Cardio-Facial syndrome). This classification is detailed in the ASHA Practice Portal (American Speech-Language-Hearing Association, n.d.).

ICF-CY, the Psycholinguistic Framework, SDCS, and DDCS

Four prominent classification systems for SSD are:

1. The *International Classification of Functioning, Disability and Health (ICF-CY)* (World Health Organization, 2007): a biopsychosocial framework for all children (including those with SSD).
2. The *Psycholinguistic Framework* (Stackhouse & Wells, 1997a), a processing-based framework for explaining the difficulties of children with SSD.
3. The *Speech Disorders Classification System (SDCS)* (Shriberg, 1980, 1993) comprising an etiological framework for children with SSD.
4. The *Differential Diagnostic Classification System; DDCS* (Dodd, 2005; Leahy & Dodd, 1987), which is a descriptive-linguistic framework for children with SSD that points the way to specific treatment approaches.

Like the Bowen (2015a), Bauman-Waengler (2020), and ASHA (n.d.) approaches 2, 3, and 4 mentioned earlier, The Psycholinguistic Framework, the SDCS, and the DDCS, are based on a medical model (Laing, 1971) with or without components of a social model which takes account of personal factors (e.g., personality, resilience, and preferences) and environmental contexts (e.g., home: family and family structure; school: teachers, peers; and the wider society) that influence a child's life. On the other hand, the first one listed, the ICF-CY (WHO, 2007) is grounded in a systematic biopsychosocial model (Engel, 1977) incorporating organic, psychological, and social factors and their intricate interrelationships.

The dominant model of disease today is biomedical, and it leaves no room within its framework for the social, psychological, or behavioral dimensions of illness. A biopsychosocial model is proposed that provides a blueprint for research, a framework for teaching, and a design for action in the real world of health care.
Engel, 1977, p. 135

In a medical model, impairment is construed as a problem that is situated within the child and the process for practitioners is to address the impairment by removing or reducing its impact. The clinician will evaluate the complaint (the account of the problem provided by the patient, caregiver, or professional), take a history, make a physical examination, administer additional tests where required, consider causes and symptoms, diagnose the complaint, advise treatment or no treatment, convey short-term and long-term prognoses of the consequences of the diagnostic entity with and without treatment, and treat (intervene), if necessary, if that is what the patient (or child's family) wants.

*The **medical model** has served us well. A deep understanding of what is going on in communication, especially when there are communication breakdowns, involves synthesizing what is going on at the biological, psychological, and social levels. Such as synthesis is offered by the causal logic of the medical model. But before we become complacent in thinking that we now have it exactly right, we need to consider the challenges of other models to the well-worn medical approach. One alternative framework to consider when carrying out clinical practice is the **participation model**. It does not allow for an easy combining of levels. Rather, the model may work best if you put what you know about someone's physical and psychological profiles on a back burner. Rather, the focus when interacting with someone ... is to find out how that person is living her life. Your primary interest in the first meeting is not on her diagnosis, or her symptoms, or her psychological test results, but on what she sees as her main worries and hopes.*
Duchan, 2001

1. INTERNATIONAL CLASSIFICATION OF FUNCTIONING, DISABILITY, AND HEALTH (ICF-CY)

The ICF-CY (World Health Organization, 2021) is explained by Sharynne McLeod in A2. It provides a valuable way of conceptualising SSD and thinking deeply about it in terms of body structure (anatomy) and the function and mechanisms (physiology) so strongly aligned with the medical model, and the impact of a speech (or any) impairment, or the absence of impairment, on a child's activities and participation in society, environmental barriers and facilitators, and individual personal factors such as age, gender, race, family structure and sociocultural context, language(s), education, history, and present circumstances.

2. PSYCHOLINGUISTIC FRAMEWORK

The Psycholinguistic Framework (Stackhouse & Wells, 1997a, 1997b) constitutes a broad-based methodology for *profiling*, as opposed to explicitly analysing or 'diagnosing', speech and literacy difficulties in children (Schäfer & Fricke, A21). The aim of profiling does not include determining whether the child has, for example, some combination of articulation disorder, phonological disorder, CAS, or dyslexia. The assessor, who may be a speech-language professional, teacher, or other educational staffer (e.g., a teaching assistant: TA, or Special Educational Needs Coordinator: SENCO) works from a psycholinguistic perspective to produce an individualised profile of the child's strengths and difficulties around input processing, representation, and output processing.

The Framework does not dictate which test measures should be used to generate the profile; neither does it lead to a specified intervention approach. So, SLPs/SLTs can utilise familiar assessment tools and intervention methodologies from their toolkit. For example, they might create independent and relational analyses whose data are drawn from formal measures such as the Diagnostic Evaluation of Articulation and Phonology: DEAP (Dodd, Hua et al., 2002) or the GFTA-3 (Goldman & Fristoe, 2015), HAPP-3 (Hodson, 2004), and/or informal measures (e.g., Limbrick et al., 2013).

3. SPEECH DISORDERS CLASSIFICATION SYSTEM: SDCS

In their timely research, Shriberg, Kwiatkowski et al. (2019) had two major goals. First, they wanted to get initial estimates of the prevalence of each of the four types of motor speech disorders (MSD) in children with idiopathic Speech Delay (SD), and second, they aimed to use these findings to estimate the population-based prevalence of each of the four disorders. By attaining these goals, they could reveal the finishing touches to the Disorders Classification System (SDCS) which entered its fifth decade of careful development in 2021, having begun with Shriberg, 1980; and see Shriberg, 1993; Shriberg et al., 2010. They also presented an update of their behavioural phenotype matrix, the Speech Disorders Classification System Summary (SDCSS).

Shriberg, Kwiatkowski et al. (2019) reported summary assessment, demographic, cognitive-language, and speech information for 415 participants enlisted for studies of idiopathic SD in the USA over several decades, and estimated the prevalence of MSD in idiopathic SD. These estimates, and the updated behavioural phenotype matrix, with the customary abbreviations for the phenotypes, are displayed in Figure 2.2 with the kind permission of Dr. Shriberg. The DOI link in the figure title will take readers to an openly accessible online version of the matrix.

Their 2019 findings showed that there is a substantial prevalence of MSD in children with idiopathic SD, and this caused them to doubt the accuracy of three descriptors frequently applied to CAS – *rare*, *severe*, and *persistent* – in ASHA's 2007 Technical Report, and generally in the MSD literature. Sizing up their results alongside the 2007 document, they concluded that CAS: is a more prevalent MSD, or less rare than once believed; may present as a mild, moderate, or severe MSD. Accordingly, CAS is not by definition, a severe SSD and it has the potential for successful treatment. The upshot of these findings

is that the outlook (prognosis) for CAS is more positive than previously indicated for at least some children, and persistence CAS is not inevitable. A lightly edited version of what Shriberg, Kwiatkowski et al. (2019) said, follows.

*On the **rarity** of Childhood Apraxia of Speech (CAS), although there is no international consensus on the criteria for rare diseases and disorders, the common epidemiological criterion for a rare disorder is a lifetime prevalence of one in 2,000 persons. This [exceeds the] prevalence rate for idiopathic CAS [of] one in 1,000 children, [which is] approximately the same as the population prevalence rate estimated in the present study for Childhood Dysarthria (CD). On the issue of **severity**, CAS studies of children at the ages of the current samples [4.4— 7;8] indicate that rather than always expressed as a severe disorder, CAS can be expressed as only mild to moderate in severity (Murray & Iuzzini-Seigel, 2017; Shriberg & Strand, 2018, p. 28). Last, on the **persistence** of CAS, trends in treatment research include a variety of find-*

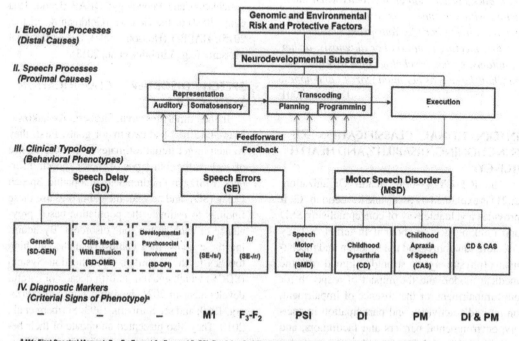

I. Etiological Processes (Distal Causes)

Genomic and Environmental Risk and Protective Factors

II. Speech Processes (Proximal Causes)

Neurodevelopmental Substrates

Representation | Transcoding | Execution
Auditory | Somatosensory | Planning | Programming

Feedforward
Feedback

III. Clinical Typology (Behavioral Phenotypes)

Speech Delay (SD) | Speech Errors (SE) | Motor Speech Disorder (MSD)

Genetic (SD-GEN) | Otitis Media With Effusion (SD-OME) | Developmental Psychosocial Involvement (SD-DPI) | /s/ (SE-/s/) | /r/ (SE-/r/) | Speech Motor Delay (SMD) | Childhood Dysarthria (CD) | Childhood Apraxia of Speech (CAS) | CD & CAS

IV. Diagnostic Markers (Criterial Signs of Phenotype)[a]

— — — M1 F3-F2 PSI DI PM DI & PM

[a] M1: First Spectral Moment; F3 - F2: Format 3 - Formant 2; PSI: Precision-Stability Index; DI/DSI: Dysarthria Index/Dysarthria Subtype Indices; PM: Pause Marker

Figure 2.2 Estimates of the prevalence of motor speech disorders in children with idiopathic speech delay, Shriberg et al., 2019 / with permission from Taylor and Francis.

ings indicating efficacious treatment of children with idiopathic CAS (*e.g.*, Murray & Iuzzini-Seigel, 2017).

Drawing on epidemiological studies of SD conducted in Australia (Eadie et al., 2015), in Southwest England (Wren et al., 2016; see Shriberg & Wren, 2019) and in the United States (e.g., Shriberg et al., 1999), Shriberg, Kwiatkowski et al. (2019) provided an estimate of 82.2% for the population prevalence of idiopathic SD (see Table 2.3, column 3). Then, having analysed audio-recorded speech samples from the 415 recruits, they were able to chronicle population prevalence estimates for the four motor speech disorders (MSD) in children aged 4-to-8 with idiopathic speech delay (SD).

They determined five classifications within **Speech Disorders**, with three under **Speech Delay (SD)**, viz. **SD-GEN**, **SD-OME**, and **SD-DPI**, and two under **Speech Errors (SE)**, namely **SE-/s/** and **SE-/r/**. In the SD category, SD-OME and SD-DPI are currently considered *risk factors* for SD. While their concurrent validity has been supported in small-scale studies reported over several decades, neither have been cross validated as an etiological subtype of SD in larger scale research using SDCS classification methods and measures.

The remaining four classifications were within **Motor Speech Disorder (MSD)**, namely **Speech Motor Delay (SMD)**, **Childhood Dysarthria (CD)**, **Childhood Apraxia of Speech (CAS)**, and **CD & CAS**, plus a fifth category, **No Motor Speech Disorder (No MSD)**. The framework is displayed in Figure 1 of Shriberg, Kwiatkowski et al. (2019). The article is freely available via https://phonology. waisman.wisc.edu or from https://doi.org/10.1080/0 2699206.2019.1595731

Table 2.3 Abbreviations, Behavioural Phenotypes used in the Speech Disorders Classification System (SDCS) Research; Prevalence and Incidence of CAS, CD, CD & CAS, SD, SD & MSD, and SMD.

1. BEHAVIOURAL PHENOTYPE ABBREVIATION	2. BEHAVIOURAL PHENOTYPE	3. POPULATION PREVALENCE*	4. BEHAVIOURAL PHENOTYPE INCIDENCE**
CAS	Childhood Apraxia of Speech	2.4%	2.4 children
CD	Childhood Dysarthria	3.4%	1 child
CD & CAS	Childhood Dysarthria & CAS	—	0/415 children
CND	Complex Neurodevelopmental Disorders		
DI	Dysarthria Index		
DSI	Dysarthria Subtype Indices		
MSD	Motor Speech Disorder		
No MSD	No Motor Speech Disorder		
NSA	Normal(ized) Speech Acquisition		
PM	Pause Marker		
PMI	Pause Marker Index		
PSD	Persistent Speech Delay		
PSE	Persistent Speech Errors		
SD	Speech Delay	82.2%	
SD-GEN	SD-Genetic		
SD-OME risk factor	SD-Otitis Media with Effusion		
SD-DPI risk factor	SD-Developmental Psychosocial Involvement		
SD & MSD	SD & Concurrent Motor Speech Disorder	17.8%	
SDCS	Speech Disorders Classification System		
SDCSS	SDCS Summary		
SE	Speech Errors		
SE-/s/	Speech Errors involving /s/		
SE-/r/	Speech Errors involving /r/		
SMD	Speech Motor Delay	12%	4 children

*POPULATION PREVALENCE = Percentage of children within the Speech Disorders population at one time
**INCIDENCE = Number of children with the behavioural phenotype per 1,000 children with idiopathic SD

The abbreviations and terminology used to characterise the behavioural phenotypes in the SDCS/CDCSS research are displayed in Table 2.3. in the first and second columns respectively. The population prevalence figures for Childhood Apraxia of Speech (2.4%), Childhood Dysarthria (3.4%), Speech Delay (82.2%), Speech Delay and Concurrent Motor Speech Disorder (17.8%), expressed as percentages, are in column in 3., and the incidence of CAS (2.4/1,000), CD (1/1,000), CD & CAS (0), and SMD (4/1,000) is in column 4.

The finding for CAS cross-validates a prior prevalence estimate for Childhood Apraxia of Speech of 1–2 children per 1,000. Shriberg, Kwiatkowski et al. (2019) point out that studies by other research groups using the SDCS measures and other measurement modalities (e.g., neurologic, physiologic, kinematic) are required to cross-validate and extend their initial prevalence findings. With the cross-validation caveats in mind, the team offered five conclusions in the following order.

I. The prevalence of motor speech disorder (MSD)s in children with idiopathic Speech Delay (SD) is theoretically and clinically substantial. If cross-validated, this has implications for research, clinical training, and service delivery. The findings support the need for increased development of the knowledge base in childhood MSD that guides assessment and treatment, with implications for research in prevention.

II. Idiopathic Speech Motor Delay (SMD) is a prevalent clinical entity. Shriberg, Kwiatkowski et al. (2019, p. 699) speculated that

…a significant proportion of children inappropriately identified and treated for CAS may meet criteria for SMD. That is, due to speech, prosody, and voice features common to both CAS and SMD (e.g., vowel distortions, slow rate, inappropriate stress, voice quality deficits), some percentage of children with SD who are false positives for CAS may be true positives for SMD (cf., Shriberg, Campbell et al., 2019; Shriberg & Wren, 2019). Preliminary discussions consider treatment implications of SMD as an execution deficit (Shriberg, Campbell et al., 2019) and CAS as a transcoding deficit

(Shriberg et al., 2019).

III. Findings are interpreted to support an idiopathic subtype of Childhood Dysarthria.

IV. Findings cross-validate a prior prevalence estimate for CAS of 1 child per 1,000.

V. The finding of 0% CD & CAS in children with idiopathic SD needs cross-validation.

Using the SDCS terminology of the day, Shriberg (2006) estimated 'clinical prevalence' figures, noting that SD-GEN accounted for 56% of referrals, SD-OME accounted for 30% of referrals, SD-DPI accounted for 12% of referrals, and SD-AOS (latterly CAS) accounted for fewer than 1% of referrals. Clinical prevalence percentages for SD-DYS (latterly CD), SE-/s/, and SE-/r/ were not included in the 2006 presentation.

Readers who have followed the evolution of the CDCS will notice important differences in the behavioural phenotype descriptors, their abbreviations, and the team's interpretation of their data, particularly since 2010.

Changes to the CDCS

- The placeholder term Motor Speech Disorder Not Otherwise Specified (MSD-NOS), which was added to the SDCS in 2009 (Shriberg et al., 2010), is now called Speech Motor Delay (SMD). Typically, children considered to have SMD have idiopathic SD or Complex Neurodevelopmental Disorders (CND) such as Down syndrome, Fragile X syndrome, Galactosemia, or Velo-Cardio-Facial syndrome (VCFS). Psychometric and substantive research findings for SMD are available for children with SMD in the context of idiopathic SD (Mabie & Shriberg, 2017; Shriberg, Strand et al., 2019) and for individuals with SMD in the context of several types of CND (Shriberg & Mabie, 2017), Down syndrome (Wilson et al., 2019), Galactosemia (Finestack et al., 2022; Shriberg et al., 2011), and VCFS (Baylis & Shriberg, 2018).
- Both Undifferentiated Speech Delay (USD), and Undifferentiated Speech Sound Disorder (USSD) have been removed from the Speech Errors (SE) category.
- Speech Delay Apraxia of Speech (SD-AOS) has been rebadged as Childhood Apraxia of Speech (CAS).

- Speech Delay-Dysarthria (SD-DYS) is now called Childhood Dysarthria (CD).
- A new category, Childhood Dysarthria & Childhood Apraxia of Speech (CD & CAS) has been added to the Motor Speech Disorder (MSD) category.
- Speech Errors-Sibilants has been replaced by Speech Errors-/s/ (and still abbreviated SE-/s/); and
- Speech Errors-Rhotics is now Speech Errors /r/ (with the same abbreviation, SE-/r/).

Clinical Utility of the SDCS

Explaining the rationale for the SDCS, Shriberg et al., 2010, p. 799 said:

> ...classification by aetiology, a so-called medical model of classification, is needed for speech sound disorders (SSD) to participate in the continuing advances in genomic and other biomedical sciences. Specifically, the assumption is that next-generation personalized medicine for assessment, treatment, and eventual prevention of diseases and disorders will require international classification systems based on biological phenotypes. (p. 796) ...the current aetiologic classification terms are not intended to be used in clinical practice until validated by empirical findings.

The original intention of Shriberg and his co-developers in constructing the CDCS was that it should be a research tool. It has continued in this vein, with Shriberg stressing this point regularly over the decades. Commentators have amplified the message that the system has limited applicability as a clinical framework also (e.g., Bauman-Waengler, 2020, pp. 10–13; Waring & Knight, 2013). The CDCS does, however, provide clinicians with a well-organised picture of subtypes of SSD while linking their signs and symptoms to proximal and distal causes (defined in Table 2.2). I have observed, in presenting Continuing Professional Development (CPD) events nationally and internationally that clinicians welcome the addition of MSD-NOS in 2009 (Shriberg et al., 2010) and its further refinement and name-change to Speech Motor Delay: SMD

(Shriberg, Kwiatkowski et al., 2019) as practical and widely applicable to children on their caseloads with Complex Neurodevelopmental Disorders (CND) whose presentation does not comfortably fit CD (dysarthria) or CAS (apraxia). While the CDCS may have limited utility clinically, SLPs/SLTs do well to be familiar with it, and its ongoing development, as it enhances our capacities for critical and clinical thinking (Stoeckel, A25.) and hence clinical decision-making.

4. THE DIFFERENTIAL DIAGNOSTIC CLASSIFICATION SYSTEM: DDCS

The genesis of Dodd's DDCS can be found in Leahy and Dodd (1987) and Dodd et al. (1989), and the beginnings of Core Vocabulary Therapy in Dodd and Iacono (1989). In the early research papers, the children with inconsistent phonological disorder, aka inconsistent speech disorder, were said to make 'inconsistent deviant' errors, with 'deviant' signalling that the errors deviated from typical developmental errors.

> Little difficulty was encountered in diagnosing the inconsistent deviant group. since there were many examples of a word, or a phonological feature, being pronounced differently within the one speech sample, and attempted process analyses could not account for error patterns.
> Dodd et al., 1989

Dodd (1995, pp. 54–57) proposed a four-part classification system of subtypes of functional speech disorders comprising 1) Articulation disorder, 2) Delayed phonological acquisition, 3) Consistent deviant disorder, and 4) Inconsistent disorder. By the time the Diagnostic Evaluation of Articulation and Phonology: DEAP (Dodd, Hua et al., 2002) was published in the UK, a fifth category, Developmental Verbal Dyspraxia (DVD), as CAS was called in Britain at the time, was added (see p. 33 of the 2002 DEAP Manual). This had been advised by panel of clinicians assisting the DEAP research team. They said a DVD category was needed as most therapists thought that inconsistent errors were *the* criterion for DVD. Over the ensuing decade, terminology had changed somewhat (Dodd, personal correspondence November 2021), and this is reflected in the descriptions of the DDCS in Dodd, 2005, 2014.

There is a variation in research articles and textbooks in the title given to Dodd's approach to classification. Dodd (2014) called it the *Differential Diagnosis Model: DDM*, McLeod and Baker (2017) employed the term *Differential Diagnosis System: DDS*, and Ttofari Eecen et al. (2019) referred to it as *Dodd's Model for Differential Diagnosis*. Barbara Dodd's preference is *Differential Diagnostic Classification System; DDCS* (personal correspondence, December 2021). It is a differential diagnosis model with psycholinguistic foundations, based chiefly on linguistic profiling and descriptions of the subtypes. In it, the subtypes, numbered 1-to-5 below, are matched to discrete areas of psycholinguistic difficulty or breakdown that are 'testable' or 'differentially diagnosable'.

The development of the DDCS was driven by a desire to provide a surface-level classification of *idiopathic* speech difficulties that SLPs/SLTs could use to make clinical decisions about individual children's intervention needs and provide clear pathways to suitable intervention (e.g., an Inconsistent Phonological Disorder diagnosis points to Core Vocabulary Therapy). Its five clinical subtypes Dodd (2005, 2014; Dodd et al., 2018) are

1. **Articulation disorder:** in which children have a difficulty at the phonetic level and are unable to produce perceptually acceptable phones (usually [s] and/or [ɹ]). They exhibit identical substitutions or distortions of the 'problematic' sound(s) in isolation, words, and sentences, during imitation, elicitation, and spontaneous speech tasks. In children whose first language (L1) is English, this group accounts for 12.5% of referrals (Broomfield & Dodd, 2004). The following %-referrals, from the 2004 study, also relate to L1 English learners.
2. **Phonological delay:** in which children have a phonemic difficulty and all phonological rules or processes evident in output are attested in typical development but are characteristic of children chronologically younger than the child in question. This, the largest group, accounts for 57.5% of referrals.
3. **Consistent phonological disorder**: in which children have a phonemic difficulty with co-occurring non-developmental or unusual errors *and* developmental rules or processes, with the presence of unusual processes signalling that the child has impaired understanding of the target phonological system. Children in this group comprise 20.6% of referrals.
4. **Inconsistent phonological disorder also called inconsistent speech disorder**: in which children have a phonemic difficulty and exhibit delayed *and* non-developmental error types and variability of production of single-word tokens equal to or greater than 40%. Dodd notes that multiple error forms for the same lexical item must be observed since variability between correct-and-incorrect realisations may reflect a maturing system. This group consists of the remaining 9.4% of referrals.
5. **Childhood apraxia of speech:** in which children have difficulty at the motor planning, programming, and execution levels, exhibiting multiple deficits involving phonological planning, phonetic programming, and motor programming implementation.

Comparing children with consistent versus inconsistent phonological disorder, Crosbie et al. (2009) noted that the two groups had differentiating output characteristics. Those with *consistent* output had greater difficulty with executive functions (EF) in the areas of rule abstraction and cognitive flexibility than those whose speech production was *inconsistent*. In A6, Waring & Dodd look at the speech processing abilities of children with SSD aged 3;6 to 5;11 relative to the executive functions of short-term and phonological working memory, rule abstraction, and cognitive flexibility (Torrington-Eaton & Ratner, 2016; Waring et al., 2017, 2018) and their bearing on clinical practice.

While fine-tuning the DDCS, Dodd and co-workers developed assessments and intervention methodologies that tied in with the classification system. Among these are the Diagnostic Evaluation of Articulation and Phonology: DEAP (Dodd, Hua et al., 2002; Dodd et al., 2006) which is widely used by SLPs/SLTs, and Core Vocabulary intervention for inconsistent phonological disorder (Crosbie et al., 2005).

Commenting that 'Dodd's Model for Differential Diagnosis' was the first SSD classification system to be applicable to both clinical and community cohorts, Ttofari Eecen et al. (2019) provide openly accessible validation of the model. Their data analysis using descriptive statistics, revealed the following percentages of children across Dodd's diagnostic subgroups: suspected atypical speech motor control (10%); inconsistent phonological disorder (15%); consistent atypical phonological disorder (20%); phonological delay (55%); and articulation disorder alone (0%). These findings are in keeping with known prevalence of these subgroups in clinical populations, providing robust support for SLPs/SLTs to use this system in clinical practice for differential diagnosis of and targeted intervention for SSD in children.

Dr. Rebecca Waring has more than 30 years' experience as a paediatric speech pathologist working across Australia and Singapore. Since graduating from La Trobe University, Rebecca has enjoyed working in early intervention, pre-schools, and primary schools, at the Royal Children's Hospital (Melbourne, Australia), university clinics and her own private practices in Melbourne, Sydney and Singapore. Rebecca is currently a lecturer in Speech Pathology at the University of Melbourne and a leading researcher in investigating the association between executive function and childhood SSD.

Dr. Barbara Dodd is currently an honorary professor at the Murdoch Children's Research Institute in Melbourne and at the University of Queensland in Brisbane. She is a researcher and teacher who has worked in departments of psychology, linguistics, and speech-language pathology, at Universities in Australia and the United Kingdom. Her research has focused on the relationship between spoken and written phonological development and cognition in typically developing children and its implications for differential diagnosis of subtypes of speech disorders. She has written seven books and developed three standardised assessments.

Q6. Rebecca Waring and Barbara Dodd: Speech Sound Disorders and Executive Functions

Paediatric speech sound disorder (SSD) is often attributed either to children's poor auditory discrimination of some speech sounds (Hearnshaw et al., 2018), or an impaired motor ability to articulate speech sounds (Terband et al., 2017). Consequently, intervention strategies typically target speech sound perception or production skills. In contrast, recent research has identified deficits in domain of general cognitive processes, providing a more comprehensive account of the range of deficits that can underlie SSD (Torrington-Eaton & Ratner, 2016). Investigations of the speech processing abilities of children with SSD aged 3;6 to 5;11 implicate the executive functions (EF) of short-term and phonological working memory, rule abstraction, and cognitive flexibility (Torrington et al., 2016; Waring et al., 2017, 2018). These findings raise important clinical issues:

- How might executive functions impair speech output when speech perception and speech motor abilities are intact?
- Do all children with SSD show the same profile of executive function performance?
- What intervention strategies might effectively target deficits in executive function?
- What would clinical assessment look like?

A6. Rebecca Waring and Barbara Dodd Thinking Outside the Speech Processing Chain: Executive Function and SSD

How might limitations in executive function performance impair speech output?

Young children are active pattern learners (Plante & Gomez, 2018). When learning to talk, children attend to phonemic structures to recognise similarities and to experiment with and formulate sound pattern rules (Ingram, 1976). Thus, the abilities to abstract speech sound rules (e.g., subconsciously identify in English that /ts/ is possible in word final but not word initial position) and be cognitively flexible (i.e., formulate new rules rather than adhere rigidly to mistaken ones) appear integral to phonological development. Additionally, dynamic construction and rapid modification of phonological representations requires the EF processes of working memory and inhibition control (Diamond, 2013). These key domain-general cognitive processes may interact with the speech processing chain to influence speech development, which brings us to the question: how might this play out in real time?

Consider Lucy, a four-year-old with typical speech and resolving cluster reduction. She attends to spoken words containing two-element consonant clusters (e.g., /s/ clusters /sl/, /sm/, /sn/, and /sw/ and the adjuncts, /st/, /sp/, and /sk/), holds these words in her phonological short-term memory, perceptually analyses the words, and lays down each word's phonological representation in her mental lexicon. Next, supported by phonological working memory, Lucy subconsciously abstracts rules by comparing, and contrasting her existing phonological representations, to determine her own phonological rules about what sounds can be combined and what phonological constrains exist (e.g., /s/ deletes in /s/ + C clusters in word initial position). When Lucy is unintelligible to her listener, or receives direct feedback via modelling and correction, she employs cognitive flexibility (see Clark, 2020), inhibition control (to override her prepotent [or automatic] response that occurs even when it is no longer relevant), phonological working memory and rule abstraction skills (e.g., compares 'old' /s/ deletes in /s/ + C clusters with 'new' rule /s/ before /l/, /t/ in clusters) to revisit realisation rules and phonological plans.

In contrast, Ben continues to reduce consonant clusters beyond the age indicted by normative data. Like Lucy, he attends to words with consonant clusters, but has difficulty holding words in his phonological short-term memory (STM). He is then unable to manipulate the word in working memory to derive how consonant clusters are constructed. Thus, he is unable to reorganise his phonological system and continues to say 'pot' for 'spot'.

Another child, Miriam, demonstrates a different deficit pattern. Unlike Ben, she can hold and manipulate words in her phonological memory, but she struggles to derive correct rules. While comparing/contrasting words held in her phonological working memory, she incorrectly focuses only on manner (i.e., the distinctive frication of /s/ cluster production), missing the importance of place and number of sounds in consonant clusters. She then derives a rule that dictates 'all words starting with a consonant cluster are marked by /f/– so that *spoon* becomes /f ʉːn/ (in Miriam's variety of Australian English), *stick* becomes /fɪk/ and *slip* becomes /fɪp/'. Thus, because she is unable to work out and shift to the correct rule (without assistance), her phonological system remains frozen. These cases illustrate how EF profile variations might lead to different surface error patterns.

Do All Children with SSD Show the Same Executive Function Performance Profile?

Growing evidence suggests that when children with SSD are divided into homogeneous subtypes, within Dodd's (1995, 2005) **linguistic subtypes and speech profiling** classification system, different EF profiles emerge. Children with **phonological disorder** demonstrate distinct domain-general rule abstraction and cognitive flexibility deficits (e.g., Crosbie et al., 2009; Dodd, 2011; Waring, 2019). Further, results suggest children with phonological disorder also have specific difficulty manipulating information in phonological working memory in the context of intact short-term memory performance (Waring et al., 2018).

Conversely, children with **phonological delay** demonstrate phonological short term and phonological working memory deficits (Waring et al., 2017) with intact rule abstraction and cognitive flexibility performance (Crosbie et al., 2009; Waring, 2019). Notably, reduced phonological working memory performance seems to be due to a shorter STM span rather than difficulty manipulating verbal information per se. That is, children with delayed phonological development can 'manipulate' the same number of items that they can hold but they can 'hold' fewer items than expected.

Children with **articulation disorder** do not appear to have EF performance deficits (Kropp, 2020), performing similarly to their age-matched peers with typically developing speech on a range of EF tasks including phonological legality knowledge (Dodd et al., 1989). This is unsurprising given that the basis

Table A6.1 Executive function profile by subgroup.

	Phonological Delay	Phonological Disorder	Articulation Disorder	Inconsistent Disorder
Phonological short-term memory ('hold')	✗	✓	✓	✓
Phonological working memory ('hold' and 'manipulate')	✗	✗	✓	✗
Cognitive flexibility: rule abstraction	✓	✗	✓	✓
Cognitive flexibility: shift	✓	✗	✓	✓

for articulation disorder lies in motor output/execution and not in central linguistic processing. Similarly, children with **inconsistent phonological disorder** demonstrate intact rule abstraction and cognitive shift executive functions (Crosbie et al., 2009); knowledge of phonological legality (Dodd et al., 1989) and phonological awareness (Holm et al., 2008), usually performing as well as peers with typically developing speech. Again, this evidence supports deficits lying outside of central linguistic processing and at the level of phonological planning. Table A6.1 provides a visual summary of the four SSD subtype EF profiles.

What SSD Intervention Strategies Might Effectively Target Executive Function Deficits?

Mounting evidence supports matching therapy approaches to SSD subtypes (Crosbie & Holm, 2017). For instance, 'best clinical practice' for children with phonological disorder (who have distinct and significant EF deficits) appears to be one-to-one, SLP/SLT delivered treatment targeting generalised non-verbal and verbal (including phonological) rule learning (Claessen et al., 2017; Crosbie & Holm, 2017). 'Rule learning' activities include games that allow the clinician to demonstrate and explain patterns, and sorting tasks that require children to detect, describe, and manipulate patterns of increasing complexity such as matching cups and saucers by size/colour and sorting patty pans by size/pattern/colour as part of a tea-party/baking game.

The advantage of these intervention strategies is that they can be employed with children from two years and simultaneously address speech and potential literacy concerns while requiring significantly less time specifically targeting speech output compared to phonological contrast therapy (Dodd, 2015). Further, these tasks potentially represent the next paradigm shift in targeting phonological disorder.

Children with phonological delay seem to require less direct teaching of rules than children with phonological disorder. Best clinical practice for children with phonological delay is a broader range of approaches (e.g., *Metaphon*: Howell & Dean, 1994; minimal contrast therapy: Crosbie & Holm, 2017; enriched language therapy: McIntosh et al., 2008; and phonological awareness: Gillon et al., 2019) that immerse children in a structured, language-rich environment where they can independently develop a heightened sensitivity to rule learning.

Children with articulation disorder and inconsistent phonological disorder are unlikely to benefit from EF strategies given the basis of their speech difficulties most likely lies further down the speech processing chain. The most appropriate approaches for these subgroups are based on the principles of motor learning: PML (Morgan & Gunther, 2017) and core vocabulary therapy (Crosbie et al., 2010), respectively.

What Would Clinical Assessment Look Like?

A *tailored* SSD assessment approach, where the child's presenting surface level errors and suspected diagnosis drive assessment protocols, is suggested. Extending current assessment batteries (that typically focus on surface-level analyses) to include EF tasks for children with phonologically based SSD, may ensure the intricacies of each child's cognitive-linguistic profile are more fully understood before initiating treatment. Profiling may impact discharge planning (e.g., surface-level speech errors may resolve but underlying EF deficits may not), treatment selection (e.g., rule-based therapy versus contrast therapy), and counselling of families and carers around potential long-term prognosis (e.g., ongoing literacy difficulties).

Minimally, rule abstraction and cognitive flexibility assessment is suggested for children diagnosed with phonologically based SSD. A more detailed SSD assessment battery could incorporate phonological short term and working memory tasks. To that end, Carlson (2005) provides a comprehensive summary of appropriate age-based EF assessment tasks. Additionally, individual tasks from EF assessment batteries along with subtests from working memory batteries can be considered.

By thinking outside the speech processing chain and considering domain general cognitive processes, these suggested SSD assessment techniques can be exploited to develop tailored treatments that target underlying deficits, leading perhaps to third-generation intervention approaches.

Independent and Relational Analysis

Stoel-Gammon (1988) considered that an analysis of a child's phonology should involve an independent analysis and a relational analysis. As a mnemonic we can conceptualise the independent analysis as a handful of inventories and the relational analysis as a handful of percentages. The analyses are based on data from a single-word (SW) and conversational speech (CS) sample, of around 200 words if possible. In recording results, it is important to differentiate between what was found in the SW sample, and what was in the CS sample.

For Stoel-Gammon, a completed independent and relational analysis includes:

1. What the child attempted to produce (an independent analysis of adult forms).
2. What the child produced (an independent analysis of child's corpus).
3. What was produced correctly by the child (a relational analysis).
4. What was produced incorrectly by the child (a relational analysis).
5. The nature of the child's incorrect productions (a phonological process analysis and other errors).
6. The extent (percentage of occurrence) of phonological processes and other errors.

Independent Analysis

The independent analysis is a view of the child's unique system without reference to the target (adult) phonology. It consists of a consonant inventory;

vowel inventory; syllable-word shapes or phonotactic inventory; and a syllable–stress patterns inventory. By ascertaining what is not present in the sample, the examiner develops an account of vowel and consonant inventory constraints (absent phones and phonemes); positional constraints (e.g., a sound such as /k/ might not occur word initially in CVC words like cap, although it occurs word finally in CVC words like pack); sequential or phonotactic constraints (the C and V combinations that the child does not use); and syllable stress pattern inventory constraints (e.g., the child might use strong–weak word stress as in dolly) but not weak–strong (as in mistake). Note that in tonal languages an independent analysis of the tones that are present and those that are absent would also be conducted.

Relational Analysis

The relational analysis is a normative comparison that looks at the child's system relative to an idealised version of the target (adult) phonology, as it would be with each sound said 'perfectly' and comprises:

- PCC in SW and CS,
- percentage of vowels correct (PVC) in SW and CS; and
- phonological processes in SW and CS expressed as percentages of occurrence.

Combining elements of SODA analysis (an account of the child's sound [S] substitutions, [O] omissions, [D] distortions, and [A] additions) and place-voice-manner (PVM) analysis (Hanson, 1983; and see Figure 2.1), production errors or mismatches between the child's realisations and the adult target (or 'standard sound') are identified by sound class and position within words.

Errors are described in terms of phonological processes (phonological patterns) (e.g., using the HAPP-3, Hodson, 2004), phonological processes (e.g., via the DEAP, Dodd, Hua et al., 2002), or phoneme collapses (via the SPACS, Williams, 2003, 2006). In tonal languages a relational analysis of tones would be included as required.

The test instruments used will depend on the clinicians' theoretical orientation, the child's assessment needs, and the clinical reality of the test instruments' availability.

Time Allocations for Speech Assessment

In this chapter we have considered speech assessment in terms of, (1) a differential diagnosis model with psycholinguistic roots (Waring & Dodd, A6), and (2) recommendations for useful independent and relational analyses (Stoel-Gammon, A7), while in Chapter 5 we find (3) Schäfer and Fricke (A21) who describe psycholinguistic profiling. Just from these three procedures, it becomes clear that there are varied and often overlapping theoretical approaches and methods available to establish the nature of a child's speech impairment, identify their strengths and challenges, and, based on the data gathered, find an intervention that is the best fit for them, in their situation.

The requirement for SLPs/SLTs to complete gathering and analysing meaningful assessment data within a couple of hours, or fewer, is a genuine but ill-advised reality for practitioners in settings where administrators want to see the bulk of clinician's time with an individual client devoted to intervention – noting that intervention sessions are often limited (also by policymakers and administrators), in duration and frequency. While it is quite possible to assess a mild articulation disorder and screen for other communication difficulties, in voice, language and pragmatics, and fluency, in fewer than 1-to-2 hours, it is an unreasonable and misguided proposition for assessing children with more complex involvement, and where differential diagnosis is not clear-cut.

Unreasonable and misguided are strong words to apply here, but their use is justifiable. This is because, when addressing the needs of children with moderate-to-severe SSD, the more time spent in focused, detailed assessment, analysis, and periodic ongoing assessment and analysis to keep goals current and relevant, the less time is likely to be spent in therapy. This is something the profession needs to impress on those who regulate our time management. Meanwhile, in A7, Carol Stoel-Gammon describes what *can* be done, by way of administering an appropriate, effective, and efficient speech assessment when time is limited to one hour for assessment and one hour for analysis.

Dr. Carol Stoel-Gammon has a PhD in Linguistics from Stanford University and joined the faculty of the Department of Speech and Hearing Sciences at the University of Washington in 1984; she became an ASHA Fellow in 2005 and received Honors from ASHA in 2014.

She is currently a Professor Emerita at the University of Washington. Her many research interests include early linguistic development; cross-linguistic studies of phonological acquisition; early identification of speech and language disorders; phonological acquisition in children with speech and language disorders; relationships between phonological and lexical acquisition; the effects of hearing loss on phonological development; phonological development of children with Down syndrome; and early speech and language development of infants and toddlers with Classic Galactosemia.

Q7.   Carol Stoel-Gammon: Speech Data Collection and Analysis in Two Hours

'*Treatment of speech sounds disorders depends on many factors, one being a valid and reliable assessment from which to derive a treatment plan. Conversational speech (CS) data are potentially representative of a client's everyday speech and in that regard are an ecologically valid basis for planning effective and efficient treatment. A clinician-controlled single-word sample, in comparison, may not elicit a client's typical speech production patterns'*

(Masterson et al., 2005, p. 230)

Considering the unavoidable trade-off between the available time and choosing an appropriate sampling and analysis methodology, how would you guide a clinician with just 1 hour in which to administer a speech assessment for an unintelligible preschooler and 1 more hour to complete the analysis? How can the 2 hours be best spent?

A7.   Carol Stoel-Gammon: Assessment of the Speech of an Unintelligible Preschool Child

Meet 'Brett', 4;9, referred by his preschool teacher, who is concerned about the intelligibility of his speech. His parents, 'John' and 'Vicki', have little difficulty understanding his speech, but know that even close relatives often need them, or Brett's sister 'Dorothy', 3;6, to interpret for them. Brett has received no previous SLP/SLT assessment or intervention when he becomes acquainted with 'Eric', the new graduate SLP/SLT who has just 1 hour to gather speech assessment data and related information.

Eric has reviewed Brett's normal audiogram and tympanogram, the teacher's brief report, and the family's responses to a case history interview. He knows that Brett: (a) is reserved at preschool, seldom talking with peers; (b) shows frustration on the rare occasions that family members ask him to repeat himself, usually responding crossly with 'never mind'; and (c) is sometimes teased by older neighbourhood children because he says *bwett* for *Brett*.

The first 30 minutes of the consultation comprised the case history interview, an unremarkable (but essential) oral muscular examination (see Box 2.1), and a conversation with Brett to establish rapport and gain an impression of his communication skills. The history uncovers nothing of note. Language development is age-appropriate and there are no indications of CAS or dysarthria. Rather, everything points to pho-

nological impairment with the possibility of both phonemic and phonetic issues.

Like many SLPs/SLTs, Eric is equipped with a good-quality audio recorder but does not have video. He has assembled a suitable standardised articulation and phonology assessment (see Fabiano-Smith, 2019) and books, games, and toys so that Eric can gather SW and conversational samples (CS), imitated utterances, and intelligibility and stimulability data. A CS sample provides information that is unavailable from a SW articulation test.

In my view, the most important parts of the assessment are twofold: first, the data collected should reveal the general nature of Brett's speech production patterns; second, the analyses should provide a basis for a treatment plan. The data should show Brett's phonetic inventory in terms of sounds and syllable/word structures; voice quality; prosodic features; consistency of productions at the segmental and word levels; and his stimulability for absent sounds and syllable and word structures.

CS Sample

Potentially, the 10–15-minute conversational speech sample will bring to light Brett's:

1. 'everyday' language abilities in terms of mean length of utterance (MLU) and vocabulary.
2. production patterns in terms of speech rate, phrasal intonation, and fluency.
3. ability to perform revisions and repairs.

Eric will obtain a sample of Brett's conversation with his parents and with Eric himself, and the parents will be asked to repeat any words Eric does not understand. Using the clinician as a conversational partner in sampling should demonstrate how Brett responds when his (relatively unfamiliar) conversational partner does not understand him. Does he simply repeat the utterance, modify it, or refuse to respond?

SW Sample

In SLP/SLT contexts, the SW sample is typically drawn from a phonology or articulation test (see Kirk & Vigeland, 2014). Because Eric knows what the intended targets are in his chosen test, he will be able to perform a relational analysis that displays which aspects of word productions do and do not match the target. Relational analysis is impossible with poorly intelligible CS samples with a high proportion of unknown target words.

Stimulability Assessment

The term stimulability assessment refers to a dynamic evaluation (Strand A31) wherein a clinician provides verbal, visual, tactile, or auditory cues to determine whether the child can adequately produce a sound or syllable structure with clinician support and scaffolding. Having first ascertained from his SW and CS data Brett's sound and syllable structure constraints (absent phonemes and phonotactic combinations), Eric will determine whether Brett can produce, with support, his missing consonants and vowels in isolation, and consonant phonemes in at least two syllable positions (e.g., initially, and finally).

Consistency Assessment

Consistency of production refers to the degree to which the pronunciation of a word (or sometimes a phoneme) remains the same across various productions (Macrae et al., 2014). To assess variability, Eric will have Brett repeat five or six words, produced in error in the SW sample, several times. Then, to determine any effects of utterance length on consistency of production, he will elicit words (both those in error and those produced accurately) in increasingly complex environments. (e.g., by having Brett imitate *ball, basketball, basketball player*, and *big basketball player*).Analysing the Data

The time needed for analysis rests on several factors, including Eric's transcription skills, his familiarity with the analysis measures, and the intelligibility of the sample, but it should be 'doable' within an hour if the SLP/SLT is experienced. Following steps 1 to 5 below can streamline the procedure.

1. SW RELATIONAL ANALYSIS

Real-time data is information – in this case phonetic transcription of single words – is data delivered or recorded immediately after collection. Adopting this method, each word was written down immediately after Brett produced it, using broad transcription and a few helpful diacritics. Let's assume that Eric has gathered and transcribed 45 known words. He will check the accuracy of his real-time transcriptions against his audiotape and make necessary corrections and additions, and then perform a *relational analysis* comparing Brett's productions with the adult targets yielding quantitative measures of Percentage Consonants Correct (PCC), Percentage Vowels Correct (PVC), and percentage CV structure correct. The latter measure allows Eric to quantify the degree to which segment and syllable deletions occur in Brett's speech. In addition, Eric examines the *nature* of Brett's errors in terms of error patterns (often referred to as phonological processes). The error analysis allows Eric to see whether Brett's errors resemble those of younger, typically developing children or are disordered or idiosyncratic. Taken together, these relational measures will give Eric an idea of Brett's accuracy levels in elicited SW productions and of his error-types. He will also examine the accuracy of polysyllabic words, including stress placement, using the words and phrases from the consistency assessment.

2. SW INDEPENDENT ANALYSIS

Now, guided by a checklist, Eric will focus exclusively on Brett's productions without reference to the adult target by noting the presence or absence of certain sound classes and syllable structures. The checklist reveals if there are:

1. stops and nasal at three places of articulation
2. voiced and voiceless stops
3. voiced and voiceless fricatives and/or affricates
4. liquids
5. closed syllables
6. consonant clusters; and
7. three-syllable words.

From this analysis, Eric will be able to determine the number and diversity of consonants and word structures Brett produces in SW productions.

3. CS ANALYSIS

Now Eric listens to the CS sample, glossing (i.e., writing down the words) 50–70 fully or partially intelligible utterances, half from the Brett–parent conversation and half from the Brett–Eric one. He will also record the number of unintelligible (to him) utterances. By dividing the intelligible utterances by the total utterances, and multiplying by 100, Eric gains an idea of Brett's percentage of intelligible utterances in CS. If Brett produces full sentences, yielding a relatively high MLU, a sample of 50 partially or fully intelligible utterances will suffice. Responses such as 'yes' and 'no' should not be included in the utterance count, as they provide little information about Brett's phonological system.

After glossing, Eric listens once again to portions of the CS (about 100–120 utterances in all) and uses the 7-point checklist above to determine presence/absence of the sound classes and word structure forms in Brett's spontaneous speech. This independent analysis will be based on both intelligible and unintelligible utterances, and accuracy of production is not considered. In addition, Eric rates the 'normalcy' of Brett's voice quality, speech rate, lexical stress patterns, sentence rhythm, and prosody. (See McLeod et al., 2015 for a parent-administered intelligibility scale).

4. COMPARING THE SW AND CS ANALYSES

The final step in Eric's analysis (and this should be considered a 'first pass' or 'overview') is to determine how Brett's SW and CS production patterns compare. In many cases, particularly for children who have received SLP/SLT intervention for their speech, SW phonetic inventories are relatively large, word structures are complex, and accuracy of pronunciation may be quite good. In contrast, CS may be characterized by simple CV syllable structures and limited consonant and vowel inventories.

Looking Further

The procedures outlined above can provide a broad, rather than deep, understanding of Brett's

speech. If, for example, the assessment indicated that Brett had significant problems with vowels and multisyllabic words, Eric would later use relevant, more in-depth instruments to gain a more fine-grained analysis. It must be acknowledged that many published SW articulation tests do not assess all the vowels of English and even fewer assess words of more than two syllables; therefore, a full understanding of difficulties in these areas is only possible via additional assessments (see Pollock, A20.).

Interpreting the Analyses

Now, Eric must interpret his findings carefully to plan an effective and efficacious program of treatment. Speculatively, possible outcomes of the analysis and potential treatment approaches are summarized in the following three scenarios.

Scenario 1

Brett exhibits small SW and CS consonant and syllable structure inventories, and consequently a low PCC, low percentage of word structures correct, and of course, limited intelligibility. Accordingly, Eric will consider treatment that focuses on phonetic inventory expansion, across place and manner classes and across syllable structures.

Scenario 2

SW and CS comparisons indicate high PCC scores for Brett's SW productions but a low PCC for spontaneous speech. Eric decides that the focus of intervention must be on transferring Brett's abilities in single words to running speech and talks to John and Vicky about how they can help.

Scenario 3

Brett's SW and CS phonetic inventories are large, and he has a good range of word structures, but he has low accuracy in terms of segments and word structures and is highly inconsistent. So, Eric sets about developing an intervention program to stabilise Brett's productions and encourage segmental and structural accuracy.

Summary

The key points of this assessment are as follows:

1. Assessment data gathering should be broad-based, examining productions in a variety of imitated, elicited, and spontaneous contexts: single words; spontaneous speech; word repetitions; and words/phrases produced with and without clinician support.
2. The analysis should involve both relational and independent approaches and focus on a variety of parameters: segmental accuracy; nature and consistency of segmental errors and word structure errors; vowel inventory and vowel accuracy; presence/absence of sound classes and word structures; stress at the word and sentence levels; and rate, rhythm, and intonation patterns of spontaneous sentence productions.
3. The assessment procedures identified will provide a broad overview of Brett's speech.
4. The time needed for analysis is reduced using a checklist approach. Once preliminary analyses are completed and areas of concern are identified, additional assessments should be performed, as needed.

Oral Musculature Examination (OME)

As a component of swallowing and communication assessment, examination of every client's oral-peripheral mechanism is mandatory. In terms of voice and speech, the purpose of the oral musculature examination is to ascertain whether the structure and the function of the articulators are conducive to age-appropriate voice and speech production. While performing the OME the SLP/SLT will also observe any significant respiratory issues such as shortness of breath or asthma, and nasal structure (e.g., nasal obstruction or septal deviation) and function. Oral structure (speech anatomy) incorporates the proportions (size or dimensions), shape, and symmetry of the articulators, while oral

function concerns articulator movements in terms of range, speed, precision, and coordination. It begins with a screening procedure covering the points in Box 2.1.

Box 2.1   Oral musculature screening examination observations and procedures

A 2-page record form is available to download at: https://www.speech-language-therapy.com/images/omesf2pp.pdf.

ORAL STRUCTURE

On examination, with the aid of a torch (flashlight) and tongue depressor, the SLP/SLT may observe structural irregularities, for example:

- ankyloglossia ('tongue-tie')
- bacterial or viral activity: e.g., tonsillitis usually indicated by redness, swelling, and sometimes halitosis and/or pus around the faucial pillars. The child may feel unwell, although tonsillitis and adenoiditis can be surprisingly 'silent'.
- dental caries
- dysmorphic features potentially related to a congenital disorder, genetic syndrome, or birth defect
- facial asymmetry, e.g., unilateral, or bilateral facial droop
- inflammation: usually associated with red discolouration
- malocclusion; missing teeth (hypodontia) or supernumerary teeth (hyperdontia)
- scarring
- suspected craniofacial anomalies: e.g., submucous cleft palate, signalled by a blue tinge near the midline of the palate

ORAL FUNCTION

In terms of function, the SLP/SLT looks for:
- asymmetrical or sluggish velar movements and/or nasal resonance when the child produces 'ah' [aː] and 'ah-ah-ah-ah' [aʔ-aʔ-aʔ-aʔ] in short bursts
- habitual mouth-open lip posture and/or mouth-breathing
- limited range of movement, uncoordinated movements, or abnormal movement of the articulators
- neurological signs: paralysis, paresis, weakness, or incoordination of the speech musculature; tremor; tongue fasciculations (Choi, 2021)

- poor coordination between respiration and phonation during diadochokinetic (DDK) tasks, or slow DDK

TONGUE FASCICULATIONS

The most common aetiology of fasciculations (spontaneous muscle contractions) in children is benign, leading to a medical diagnosis of benign fasciculation syndrome. Occasionally, a child will need extensive diagnostic investigation by a paediatric neurologist (Choi, 2021). Any individual with fasciculations should be referred to a medical practitioner such as the family doctor who will refer them to a specialist.

DIADOCHOKINESIS (DDK)

In DDK tasks, children should be able to produce nine syllables in roughly three seconds. The SLP/SLT can model [pa]x9 [papapapapapapapapa] or [pata] x5 in a monosyllable task for younger children or children who cannot produce /k/. For older children and even some younger children who can produce /k/, use the more familiar (to us) sequence [pataka] x3 [patakapatakapataka] in a trisyllable task.

Some children approach the task with gusto, inhaling deeply, exhaling exaggeratedly, and then speaking, thereby running out of air. A simple demonstration with visual cues – pictures or objects – to show them they need to BREATHE IN–TALK–BREATHE OUT usually helps. One little trick is to introduce an artificial flower and a 'candle' with an aluminium foil 'flame', that detaches if you 'blow the candle out'. Practise smelling the flower BREATHE IN – saying the DDK string TALK – blowing the candle BREATHE OUT until they remember the IN–TALK–OUT sequence easily.

REFERRALS POTENTIALLY ARISING FROM THE ORAL MUSCULATURE EXAMINATION

Informed observations during the oral musculature examination will assist with SLP/SLT diagnosis, but some issues that might emerge (e.g., apparent dysmorphic features; submucous cleft; abnormal tongue movements such as jerky movements, spasms, writhing or fasciculations) will likely take the clinician beyond the SLP/SLT scope of practice, leading to referral-on (e.g., to a dentist, GP, or medical or dental specialist). On the other hand, certain aspects of structure and function may be part and parcel of what prompted referral to SLP/SLT in the first place.

Assessing Severiy

Having completed the oral musculature examination and analysed and organised a child's speech data (Stoel-Gammon A7), the clinician may want to quantify severity for his or her own information; to inform parents, as part of the process of ensuring appropriate services for the child; or for insurance purposes. The issue of determining and reporting severity of involvement has exercised the research skills of **Dr. Peter Flipsen, Jr**.

Q8.   Peter Flipsen: Assessing and Measuring Severity of SSD

The uncertainty about the best way to rate severity of involvement in child speech disorders persists. As well, it is difficult to get a sense of how it is attempted in current clinical practice, and why clinicians want or even need these ratings. The findings of Flipsen et al. (2005) indicate that the use of impressionistic rating scales for determining severity of involvement in children with speech delay is problematic. What alternative procedures and measures have better clinical utility, and what do you see as the best 'next step' in further investigation of severity measures?

A8.   Peter Flipsen, Jr. Severity and Speech Sound Disorders: A Continuing Puzzle

When we begin discussing severity of involvement, one question my students often ask is 'why do we even need to assess severity? Isn't it enough to just say that the child qualifies for services?' In some instances, it isn't necessary, but sometimes it is. In an era of workforce shortages and expanding demands for SLP/SLT services, we often need to prioritize our time. Where the law permits (not in the United States), children with milder problems may be placed on waiting lists, while those with greater degrees of involvement are given higher priority for services. Severity ratings may also be of value for clinicians who try to improve their efficiency by working with children in groups. A survey by Brandel and Loeb (2011) suggests this is a very common practice in the United States. In such cases, group membership may be determined by level of severity. Finally, some insurance companies may determine the amount of service they will pay for based on severity ratings (i.e., children with milder problems would be entitled to fewer treatment sessions).

Impressionistic Rating Scales

When the situation demands it, my sense is that most clinicians typically rely on impressionistic severity rating scales. But as indicated in the question, such scales are problematic. In our study (Flipsen et al., 2005) we looked at ratings from a group of 10 clinicians with at least 10 years of experience working with children. However, even they did not agree very well on their severity ratings for 17 children with speech delay of unknown origin. Admittedly, the scale we gave the clinicians was just a set of numbers on a line from 1 ('normal') to 7 ('severe'). Besides, we didn't tell them what to think about – we just said: *tell us how severe you think the problem is*. It has been suggested that we should tell clinicians what specifically to focus on when they make their ratings. Some existing rating scales do that, but I cannot honestly say I know whether clinicians agree any more than usual with scales that include detailed instructions. In any event, ratings obtained from rating scales may not be reliable because clinicians may simply be considering different things in their ratings. Assuming we need to focus the clinician's attention on specific things, we then must decide what to tell them to focus on. That was a major goal of our study. Using ratings from the clinicians who agreed the most with each other (we found six who did), we looked at how their ratings correlated with a whole long list of possible severity measures. It appeared that they were considering number, type, and consistency of errors at both the single sound and whole word levels. But as our analysis involved only six clinicians, we don't know if we can generalize these findings to all clinicians. Perhaps more importantly,

we didn't have enough data to allow us to figure out whether any of the things they considered were more important than any of the others. Clearly, a much larger study is needed.

Percentage Consonants Correct (PCC) and PCC-R

So, what's a busy clinician to do? There is not yet a definitive answer, but one measure that continues to show up in the research literature is PCC (Percentage Consonants Correct). Developed in 1982 by Shriberg and Kwiatkowski it was shown to be correlated very nicely with severity ratings of conversational speech samples obtained from a much larger group of clinicians (based on the same scale as in Flipsen et al., 2005). Shriberg and Kwiatkowski showed that if PCC is less than 50% clinicians rated the sample as severe, if it was 50–65% they rated the sample as moderate to severe, if it was 65–85% they rated it as mild to moderate, and if it was greater than 85%, they rated it as mild. That study involved children aged 4;1 to 8;6 (mean = 5;9), so it isn't clear if these severity categories are valid for children outside this age range.

Calculating PCC requires recording a conversational speech sample that includes at least 200 intelligible words. It should be a conversation; it is not clear whether similar severity ratings would be obtained with narrative samples. The sample should then be transcribed using narrow phonetic transcription; it is important to use narrow transcription because the severity categories determined by Shriberg and Kwiatkowski (1982) were based on a definition of PCC which assumes that omissions, substitutions, and distortions (indicated by the presence of diacritics) are all errors (see Table i.1). Using broad transcription ignores distortions, and the resulting measure is called PCC-R (Percentage Consonants Correct – Revised). See Shriberg et al. (1997) for a discussion of different variations on PCC including measures that consider vowels. In any event, once the narrow transcription is completed, all the consonants that were attempted should be examined and a tally made of those which are correct and those which are not (any omissions, substitutions, or distortions). Here's the formula for calculating PCC:

PCC = (# of correct consonants /

total # of consonants attempted) X100

PCC is not perfect, however.

Age Matters

One practical problem with using it clinically is that age differences are not accounted for. If two children (age 3 years and 8 years) both have a PCC score of 75%, would it really mean the same thing for both? Probably not. Error types may not be the same at different ages. That 3-year-old may be producing mostly omission and substitution errors, while that 8-year-old may be producing mostly residual distortion errors (Gruber, 1999). One way to get around the age question (though it doesn't directly address error types) would be to know how PCC normally changes with age.

Although true normative studies don't yet exist, Austin and Shriberg (1996) have developed 'reference data' based on several hundred children with normal or normalized speech (who happened to have been part of various research projects). That report provides means and standard deviations for PCC over a wide range of ages. These PCC data can be freely downloaded as Technical Report 3 from https:// phonology.waisman.wisc.edu/publications-and-presentations/technical-reports The values in that report could be used by American clinicians (since the children all spoke dialects of American English) to estimate how many standard deviations the child is from their age peers. For clinicians in other countries, such reference data could be developed.

The Importance of Assessing Conversational Speech

A related 'concern' with PCC is that it would normally only be considered valid to translate the scores into severity categories if your PCC values come from conversational speech. I refer to this as a concern (and not a problem) only, because many clinicians still fail to assess conversational speech. Several studies over the years (e.g., Andrews & Fey, 1986; DuBois & Bernthal, 1978; Healy & Madison, 1987; Wolk & Meisler, 1998) have shown that performance in single words is usually different from performance in conversation, and thus, conversational speech should be evaluated directly. On the other hand, Masterson et al. (2005) showed that PCC values derived from one particular single-word task were not significantly different from PCC values derived from conversational samples. Arguments from clinicians against evaluating conversational speech are twofold. They say they don't have the time, and they aren't sure they will get a good sample of all the speech sounds. In response to these concerns, Johnson et al. (2004) developed a sentence repetition task that includes a representative sample of the consonants of English, and they showed that PCC scores on their task are not significantly different from PCC scores obtained from conversational speech samples. Administering and scoring the sentence-repetition task is much faster than recording and transcribing conversational speech. The task itself is shown in an appendix of their publication and includes a phonetic transcription and a formula for calculating PCC. Each sentence is read aloud to the child and as the child repeats it, the clinician simply crosses out any consonant phoneme that was not produced correctly (again any omission, substitution, or distortion).

Johnson and colleagues did not, however, directly examine whether severity ratings would be the same on the two tasks. This probably does need to be done as the link from PCC scores on their task to PCC scores from conversation to severity rating from conversation is an indirect one at best. But if you really can't do conversational speech analysis, it may be a place to start.

Assessing Aspects of Speech Processing

There may be a need to administer other, in-depth, assessment tools. This need becomes clear following a thorough assessment – or as thorough as the SLP/SLT can manage given restrictions imposed in workplaces, especially where time spent in intervention sessions is prioritised over time spent in assessment sessions.

Waring and Dodd (A6) explained the rationale and process of applying psycholinguistic principles to speech assessment. Next, Rvachew (A9) and Ingram (A10) discuss procedures that tap a child's psycholinguistic processing, thereby helping with differential diagnosis: first up, Susan Rvachew and the Syllable Repetition Task, followed by David Ingram on Whole Word Measures and the PCC-PWP Intersect.

Dr. Susan Rvachew is Associate Dean and Director of the School of Communication Sciences and Disorders at McGill University, Montreal, Canada. Her longstanding research interests are concentrated on phonological development and disorders leading her to generate an extensive body of evidence and resources, alone or with many collaborators. Within these contexts, she has investigated the role of speech perception development in sound production learning (Rvachew, A18), and speech development in infancy; efficacy of interventions for phonological disorders; and alternative approaches to the treatment of CAS and persistent SSD. In A10., she explores the Syllable Repetition Task (SRT) in terms of its history, applicability, and role in psycholinguistic processing.

Q9. Susan Rvachew: Syllable Repetition Task

'The diagnostic challenge of CAS reflects the complexity of the processes involved given that the acquisition of speech motor control and the tasks used to identify deficits in this area tap multiple linked speech processes and a network of broadly distributed neural networks' (Rvachew & Matthews, 2017). How can the Syllable Repetition Task (Shriberg et al., 2009) help the SLP/SLT to differentiate CAS from other forms of severe speech sound disorder, specifically phonological delay, and inconsistent phonological disorder?

A9. Susan Rvachew: Syllable Repetition Task for Differential Diagnosis

Many nonword repetition tasks are available for use in speech-language pathology assessment (Weismer et al., 2000). Each involves present-

ing the child with a connected series of syllables that make a word-like sequence that is not a meaningful word in the child's language. The child is expected to repeat the nonsense word. Historically, the number of syllables or phonemes repeated correctly has been interpreted as a measure of phonological working memory (PWM), that is, the capacity to hold phonological information in temporary storage long enough to process it, transform it, or transfer it to long-term memory. Children's performance on nonword repetition tasks is often predictive of language skills (Estes et al., 2007). Nonword repetition performance is also considered to be a key feature of heritable language impairment (Bishop & Hayiou-Thomas, 2008) and heritable speech impairment (Shriberg et al., 2005). Therefore, a task to establish nonword repetition accuracy is an important part of the assessment battery when identifying and classifying SSD.

Nonword repetition performance is closely related to the child's speech and language skills because the task requires a range of psycholinguistic processes. First, the child must process the speech sounds in the model that is presented for repetition (phonological processing); then, the child must hold that phonological information in memory long enough to set up a plan for future reproduction of the sequence of sounds (phonological memory and phonological planning); finally, the child must produce the sequence of syllables (motor planning, programming, and execution). When testing children who have an SSD, it is desirable to rule out articulation errors as the source of difficulties when nonword repetition accuracy is low. For this reason, Shriberg et al. (2009) designed the Syllable Repetition Task (SRT) which sequences only simple syllables that consist of one of the consonants /m, n, b, d/ combined with the vowel /ɑ/. The complete task has 18 stimuli for repetition: 8 with two syllables, 6 with three syllables, and 4 with four syllables. Any errors that occur when repeating items such as /mɑdɑ/, /mɑdɑbɑ/, or /mɑnɑbɑdɑ/ are not likely to be caused by an inability to articulate the constituent speech sounds. How can the SLP/SLT know if the child is having difficulty with one or more pre-execution stages of speech processing, however?

Shriberg et al. (2012) developed a series of metrics for identifying subgroups of children with SSD based on the types of errors that the children produced on the SRT. Without detailing the specific coding and scoring procedures (for tutorial, see Rvachew & Matthews, 2017), qualitative analysis and interpretation of error types will be described here. The largest probable subgroup within the population of children with SSDs will present with phonological processing deficits, as measured by phonological awareness tests for example. These children make up at least half of the children referred for speech therapy due to misarticulated speech (Rvachew, 2007; Shriberg et al., 2005). When attempting to repeat the SRT items, these children may have difficulty encoding the features of the speech sounds in the stimulus. Shriberg et al. (2012) hypothesized that this difficulty will manifest as cross-class substitutions; that is the child may produce /mɑdɑ/ → [mɑnɑ]. We have observed that children with phonological processing difficulties sometimes produce a 'favourite sound' especially in place of consonants that occur later in the sequence, such as /mɑdɑ/ → [mɑjɑ] and /mɑdɑbɑ/ → [mɑjɑjɑ] because these later sounds are more difficult to encode fully. In a study of French-speaking children with phonological delay, 20% scored within the normal range on the SRT while just over half scored below expectations for encoding, that is phonological processing of the speech sounds in the stimuli (Brosseau-Lapré & Rvachew, 2017).

Once having recovered the phonological segments from the input string, the child must hold that information in phonological memory. Children who struggle with phonological memory will produce many more errors on three-syllable items than two-syllable items. These children are more likely to have concomitant language impairment than those with phonological processing difficulties alone. Indeed, they *often* have concomitant phonological processing difficulties. We have observed that they may have significant word-finding difficulties. The phonological memory deficit is associated with a phonological planning deficit that produces high within-word inconsistency. In addition to within-word inconsistency (e.g., 'chocolate' → [tɔtɛt], [tɹɔtʃɛ]), the child might also produce phonological or semantic paraphasias (e.g., 'helecopter' → [hɑtdɔg]). Therefore, these children are likely to meet the criteria for Inconsistent Phonological Disorder as described by Dodd (2014).

Finally, motor planning and programming processes are implicated as the child prepares to reproduce the item. Shriberg et al. (2012) identified errors, called transcoding errors, that are highly indicative of Childhood Apraxia of Speech: these are additions that often take the form of nasals at syllable junctions. Examples with spectrographic evidence in Rvachew & Matthews (2017) suggest that some of these errors arise from mistiming of overlapping articulatory gestures. Although we observed nasal additions frequently (/mɑdɑ/ → [bænda]) we also observed addition of stop consonants (/mɑdɑbɑ/ → [nɑdbɑbɑ]) and entire syllables (/dɑbɑmɑ/ → [tɑpɑpɑnɑ]). These transcoding errors usually occur alongside other types of errors and in fact children with the CAS profile demonstrated difficulties with encoding and phonological memory in Shriberg et al. (2012). In Rvachew and Matthews (2019) we also observed that children with transcoding errors demonstrated many symptoms of CAS including poor performance on the oral peripheral examination, the maximum performance tasks, groping, lexical stress errors, and syllable segregation in connected speech.

The Syllable Repetition Task (including recorded speech stimuli) is freely available on the website of the Child Phonology Project at the Waisman Center along with reference data for English-speaking children and adults (Lohmeier & Shriberg, 2011). The task is easy to administer and score although the instructions must be followed carefully, as demonstrated in our written tutorial (Rvachew & Matthews, 2017) and webinar (Mathews, 2020). We discovered that the English reference data are not applicable to children speaking other languages. For example, the phonemes in the stimuli are native to French but the prosody of French is very different from English; in particular, French words are longer and have more even stress patterns. Consequently, French-speaking children with typical speech obtained much higher scores than English-speaking children with typical speech in Brosseau-Lapré and Rvachew (2017).

The Syllable Repetition Task provides one more piece of information that helps to differentiate children with severe phonological delay (most likely caused by deficits in the abstraction of phonological representations from speech) from those with inconsistent phonological disorder (associated with phonological memory and phonological planning deficits). Furthermore, the task helps to differentiate those children whose severe speech impairment reflects a deficit in *phonological* planning from those who have a *motor* planning deficit. This is important because these two latter groups are likely to have inconsistent errors and vowel errors so that they are easily confused with each other. Furthermore, these three diagnostic groups respond differentially to distinct approaches to speech therapy (Dodd & Bradford, 2000; Moriarty & Gillon, 2006; Rvachew & Matthews, 2019). For this reason, it is essential to use all the tools available to us to identify the underlying processing deficits that explain children's speech impairments before developing a treatment plan.

Case Study

TASC20 was a girl aged 4;5 who was referred to participate in a trial of interventions for the treatment of severe speech sound disorders associated with inconsistent speech errors. She presented with above-average verbal and nonverbal intelligence and passed a screening assessment of her oral-motor function. She was able to produce [pataka] accurately but slowly and only after multiple attempts. Groping and syllable segregation were not observed in her connected speech although instances of dysprosody were common. A complete Diagnostic Evaluation of Articulation and Phonology (DEAP) was administered revealing borderline normal scores for articulation accuracy given misarticulation of the consonants [j, g, ŋ, θ, ð, ʧ, ʤ, l, ɹ] and an overall Percent Consonants Correct of 82% and Percent Vowels Correct of 94%. These errors which generally occurred on phonemes that are not expected to be mastered at her age, including instances of weak syllable deletion and cluster reduction, would not typically raise much concern except for the inconsistency of the errors and the atypical nature of the errors. For example, liquids might be produced as glides or stops or nasals. She produced 63% of words on the Word Inconsistency Assessment differently upon repetition, for example, 'vacuum cleaner' → [bætum klaɪnɚ], [bækjum kidɚ], and [bæfrum kɪdɚ]. The child's performance on the Syllable Repetition Task confirmed the impression of phonological planning problems, providing evidence of difficulties with encoding and memory but not transcoding. First, she produced many cross-class phoneme substitutions (e.g., [bada] → [bama]). Even though she had difficulty with two-syllable items, she had significantly more difficulty with three- and four-syllable items, with percent consonants correct being approximately 63, 44, and 19 across the three parts of the test. Finally, she produced addition/transcoding errors on only two items, whereas a threshold of 4 indicates probable CAS. In Rvachew and Matthews (2019), this child responded best to an intervention meant for children with phonological planning disorders and modelled on the core vocabulary approach developed for children with inconsistent speech disorder, although in this case we taught the children nonsense words in a meaningful context. Specifically, she was taught to produce the novel words by relying on visual symbols that cued the place of articulation for the sounds in each word during the pre-practice portion of each treatment session. During the subsequent high intensity practice part of the session, she was reminded to refer to the cue cards, when necessary, to achieve a correct production. This treatment helps the child learn to set up the phonological plan for words independently. The traditional 'watch me and listen carefully' approach provides too much information so that the child does not have enough practice with this crucial phonological planning step. This treatment approach works well when the child is stimulable for the misarticulated speech sounds and the goal of the intervention is consistency of word production. The Syllable Repetition Task, administered along with a comprehensive assessment, can help to identify children who will benefit from this approach.

Delay and Disorder in the DDCS, SDCS, and PCC-PWP Intersect

In Dodd's Differential Diagnostic Classification System (DDCS) there are separate categories, and different diagnostic indicators for children with phonological delay and those with phonological disorder. The DDCS has a clinical focus, and it is widely used by SLP/SLT clinicians. By contrast, Shriberg's Speech Disorders Classification System (SDCS) is primarily intended as a research tool, but it may help to inform clinicians' differential diagnosis. In the SDCS, Speech Disorders is the umbrella heading for three categories of Speech Delay (SD). The three are Speech Delay – Genetic (SD-GEN), Speech Delay – Otitis Media with Effusion (SD-OME), and Speech Delay – Developmental Psychosocial Involvement (SD-DPI), as shown in Table 2.3. David Ingram has developed a way, that differs from Dodd's and Shriberg's, to distinguish speech delay from speech disorder with a whole-word assessment procedure that examines the complexity of *target words* and the complexity of the *child's productions*.

Dr. David Ingram was introduced at the top of A4, and readers will recall that from 1972 to 1998 he was a professor at the University of British Columbia, and then at Arizona State University until his retirement in 2018. The 1976 publication of his groundbreaking *Phonological Disability in Children* saw 'Ingram' become a household name, and 'phonology' a household word for SLPs/SLTs and clinical phonologists (see Müller and Ball A3). Numerous linguists and SLPs/SLTs were excited to bridge the gap between linguistics research in children's phonological, morphological, syntactic, and cross-linguistic acquisition, and apply it in clinical practice. The impact of Dr. Ingram's work on developing theoretically sound and evidence-driven methodologies in working with children with SSD is incalculable.

Q10.   David Ingram: Whole Word Measures

As measures of correct production of whole words, percentage of correct consonants (pCC) and Proportion of Whole-word Proximity (PWP) differ. PCC is a measure Consonant Correctness only, while PWP covers Consonant Correctness, Consonant Substitutions and Vowel Usage. How do the data of these measures intersect to allow the clinician to distinguish speech delay from speech disorder?

A10.   David Ingram: Whole-Word Measures: Using the PCC-PWP Intersect to Distinguish Speech Delay from Speech Disorder

Overview

Determining the severity of phonological impairment in children can be pursued across a continuum from a simple assessment of the percentage of correct consonants (pCC) to much more complex (and time consuming) analyses of phonological patterns, an enterprise requiring a background in linguistics in general and phonological analysis particularly. I have been a proponent over the years of the latter (Ingram, 1976, 1981). In more recent years, however, I have also examined ways to do insightful assessment of a much simpler nature referred to as whole word assessment (Ingram, 2002). The present discussion will be a comparison of measures of whole measure assessment with the assessment of consonant correctness.

Whole word assessment involves measures that consider three aspects of the child's speech productions, that is, consonant correctness, consonant substitutions, and vowel usage. Notice that whole word assessment includes the consideration of *consonant correctness*, so it values of importance of this aspect of speech but is at the same time more inclusive. When only consonant correctness is measured, differences between children regarding incorrect consonants are missed. It is possible for children to have similar rates of consonant correctness but differ in their rate of consonant deletion versus *consonant substitution* for non-acquired consonants. In whole word assessment, children who have high rates of consonant deletions receive lower scores than children who predominantly use consonant substitutions. A similar difference can be found when *vowel usage* is considered. Children may have similar rates of consonant correctness but differ in their use of vowels. It has been known for a long time (e.g., Ingram, 1981) that some children prefer monosyllabic words, e.g., *cat, dog*, while either avoiding or deleting syllables in longer words. Other children, however, do well at the production of longer words, and in some cases at the expense of consonant correctness.

These differences can be shown by taking a very simple example of four hypothetical children's productions of the word 'banana' as follows: Child 1 [nan], Child 2 [nana], Child 3 [mana], and Child 4 [bamama]. If only consonant correctness is considered, Children 1 and 2 do best with 2 correct consonants (67%), followed by Children 3 and 4 who have a single correct consonant (33%). When substitutions are considered, Child 4 does better than Child 3 because he or she produces 3 consonants rather than just 2 consonants. When vowels are considered, Child 2 does better than Child 1 because the former child produces two syllables rather than just one.

In summary, I have identified three aspects of a child's productions that are simple to identify, and measure, consonant correctness, consonant substitutions, and vowel usage. Only one of these, consonant correctness, has been commonly used in speech assessment, both in articulation tests and in the assessment of conversational samples (Shriberg, 1982). It may be that in some instances, this aspect is sufficient to gain an initial impression of speech severity. That said, it takes relatively little further effort to include an assessment of consonant substitutions (versus deletions), and vowel usage. Further, these may identify speech patterns missed by consonant correctness alone. As will be discussed shortly, their inclusion also leads to complexity measures for both the child's productions and their target words that are lacking in assessments examining just consonant correctness. They further allow a measure of proximity between the child's words and their targets that allows for a distinction of two kinds of children with phonological disorders, a topic to be discussed after a more explicit description of the whole word measures.PCC versus pCC

As mentioned, whole word assessment includes a measure that considers the rate of consonant correctness, using the acronym 'pCC'. This measure needs to be distinguished from the popular measure of consonant correctness referred to as PCC or (PCC-R), described in A8, by Peter Flipsen Jr. PCC differs from pCC in at least two ways. First, PCC has been developed for use in conversational samples, not single word assessment. The whole word measurement of pCC has not restricted its use in this manner. Secondly, PCC has been recommended for usage with all the tokens in a conversational sample. Whole word assessment, on the other hand, has been used by me and my colleagues for sampling lexical types and not tokens. If a lexical type (word) is used several times, the child's most typical production is used. This is an important point for it means that a comparison of studies using PCC versus pCC may show different rates of consonant correctness. No comparison of the difference, to my knowledge, has been conducted. It should be noted that these decisions to use the measures on consonant correctness in this manner are not inherent in the measures, but in the decisions on how they have been applied. Both PCC and pCC can be calculated by the same formula, described by Flipsen (A8) as follows:

pCC / pCC = number of consonants / total number of consonants attempted , X 100

Phonological Mean Length of Utterance

The central point of whole word measurement is that the assessment considers word complexity, both in terms of the complexity of the *target words* and the *child's productions*. Words are considered simple when they have a small number of consonants and vowels, and more complex when these numbers increase. The measure of word complexity begins with the target words. The complexity of an individual word is determined by the simple calculation of scoring 2 points for each consonant, and 1 point for each vowel. Since this is a measure that has the same intent for speech assessment as the calculation of mean length of utterance (MLU) has for language assessment, I refer to it as the *phonological mean length of utterance* (pMLU). The formula is as follows:

Target pMLU = C(2) + V / W
(Where C = number of consonants,
V = number of vowels,
and W = number of words.)

Simple words like 'cat' (2 consonants and 1 vowel) will receive a score of 5, while a longer word such as 'banana' (3 consonants, 3 vowels) receives a score of 9. Children using very simple words at the early stages of lexical development have Target pMLUs in the range of 3 to 5. These scores increase as the lexicon increases in size though no normative data are yet available.

The next step in whole word assessment is to determine the pMLU of the child's productions. This is done similarly as in the Target pMLU by assigning points to the child's productions, in this instance using the three aspects of children's speech productions discussed earlier. Correct consonants receive 2 points each, while consonant substitutions and vowels receive 1 point each. These are then totalled, and an average score is determined as done for the Target pMLU by dividing the sum of these counts by the total number of words. The formula is as follows:

Child pMLU = CC (2) + CS + V / W
(Where CC = number of correct consonants,
CS = number of consonant substitutions.)

The Child pMLU values will be higher when rates on consonant correctness, consonant substitutions, and vowel usage increase, and they will be lower when these values decrease. An example of this for a simple word would be the following productions of 'cat', [kat], [tat], [ta], which would have Child pMLU scores of 5, 3, and 2 respectively. Another example for a longer word is the four productions for 'banana' given earlier, [nan], [nana], [mana], [bamama], which would receive Child pMLU scores of 5, 6, 5, 7. Notice the discrepancy between these scores and the pCC values, where the fourth form has the highest Child pMLU score, but the

lowest pCC score. It is due to examples such as these that I have recommended that whole word assessment be used in conjunction with pCC. The Target pMLU and Child pMLU scores provide an idea of whether the child is both producing and/or attempting words with either high or low complexity. Along the way, a score of consonant correctness is also determined.

Whole Word Proximity (PWP)

Once the pMLU scores have been calculated, there is one further measure to be applied, this being the *Proportion of Whole Word Proximity* (PWP), or more simply *Proximity*. This proportion is obtained by dividing the Target pMLU into the Child pMLU, measuring the closeness of child's productions to their targets. The formula is as follows:

PWP = Child pMLU / pMLU

The assessment of Proximity for typically developing two-year-old English-speaking children has found values usually around 65% or above. Single word examples would be .67 (or 67%) for 'banana' [nana] (6/9), and .80 (or 80%) for 'cat' [tat] (4/5). We have found these values to be somewhat higher for similarly aged Spanish-speaking children (Hase et al., 2010). Conversely, we have found Proximity score for children assessed with speech sound disorders to be lower, often at 50% or below. In Ingram & Ingram, 2001, we provide a discussion of how these measures can be utilised in the planning for phonological intervention.

PCC, PWP Intersect

More recently, I have been involved in two further developments in the elaboration of these measures for whole word assessment and consonant correctness. One of these improvements is the consolidation of the Proximity measure and the pCC measure into a single measure referred to as the pCC, PWP Intersect. This development was the result of research conducted by Elena Babatsouli and Dimitrios Sotirpoulos in Greece who have demonstrated mathematically that pCC and PWP are in a linear relationship. A child's PCC score will predict the range of possible PWP scores. When children show high rates of consonant deletion and low vowel usage, pCC scores and PWP scores are relatively close together, though PWP will always be higher since it scores more than consonant correctness. Conversely, when children show low rates of consonant correctness, but high rates of consonant substitutions and vowel usage, the scores are much further apart.

The second development occurred when we began using the Intersect measure to assess phonological samples from both typically developing children and children with speech sound disorders. It turned out (not surprisingly!) that the Intersect measure was being influenced by word complexity, particularly by word-length, and syllable complexity, particularly in words with consonant clusters. After much trial and error, the decision was made to divide children's words for assessment into the following four categories along two dimensions of monosyllables versus multi-syllables, and words with clusters versus words without clusters:

> Monosyllabic Words with only Singleton Cs, e.g., 'go', 'eat', 'cat'
> Monosyllabic Words with at least one Consonant Cluster, e.g., 'grape', 'lamp' 'cramp'
> Multisyllabic Words with only Singleton Cs, e.g., 'mama', 'ticket', 'banana', 'telephone'
> Multisyllabic Words with at least one Consonant Cluster, e.g., 'spigot', 'aardvark'

Two Patterns of Acquisition Based on Word Complexity

The following preliminary results have been found.

- First, with typically developing two-year-old children, these categories fall into a linear relation, where words with monosyllables tend to have higher pCC and PWP scores than words with multi-syllables, and words without clusters have higher scores than words with clusters. That is, consonant correctness correlates with word complexity, the simpler the word, the higher the rate of consonant correctness.
- Second, the results obtained from analyses of children with speech sound disorders have identified two distinct patterns.

- For one set of children, the results are like those just described for young typically developing children. That is, these children show a correlation between word complexity and consonant correctness, and in this sense look like younger typically developing children. I have identified this pattern as one of **speech delay**.
- The second group of children, however, does not show this correlation. For this group, consonant correctness does not noticeably increase across the four categories of word complexity. For these children, their difficulty in producing non-acquired speech sounds is stable and not impacted by word complexity. I have used the term **speech disorder** for this group, since it is not the pattern found in typically developing children. Their PWP scores are influenced by the complexity of the words they produce, however, since longer words with more vowels and substitution increase PWP values. Values can also increase if cluster errors involve substitutions rather than deletions.

Concluding Remarks

The results just discussed indicate the pCC assessments are good predictors of phonological acquisition for typically developing children and children with speech sound disorders who show the pattern of speech delay. The pCC assessment alone, however, is not as helpful for the children with the pattern of speech disorder, where pCC values vary little across categories of word complexity. For these children, the more inclusive whole word measure of Proximity more explicitly the impact of consonant substitutions and vowel usage within the categories.

The identification of the two kinds of speech disorders through the pCC, PWP Intersect measure also consequently has important implications for assessment and treatment. For assessment, it has implications for the usage of articulation tests, since they vary in the number of test-words used across the four categories discussed. For treatment, it suggests that different goals may be necessary for the two types of children. One possibility is that children with speech delay may be more responsive to interventions based on maximal contrasts (Morrisette, 2021) or partly based on maximal contrasts (Williams, A20.), while children with speech disorder may be less so. Treatment studies will be needed to examine this and other possible differences in treatment options for these two kinds of children. More recent studies on the distinction between speech delay and speech disorder are Ingram et al. (2018), and an overview in Ingram (2020).

How Do Children Doing Naming Tests Use Prompts and Cues?

In the final Q&A in this chapter, Deb James looks closely at the psycholinguistic processing aspects of naming a sequence of pictures. In essence, she interrogates what children with speech and language 'do' with the prompts, cues, and forced choices the SLP/SLT provides to help them complete picture-naming tasks. The answers lead her to explore implications for clinical practice.

Dr. Deb James is a close-to-retiring speech pathologist specialising in children's functional communication, speech, and language difficulties. She has delivered speech pathology services across a wide variety of private and public services in health, education, and disability domains. She has taught about paediatric communication, speech and language in speech pathology and teacher education university programs. Her research interests involve paediatric oral and written speech and language problems, centring on children's development of speech and language, especially their productions of polysyllabic words. Her governance interests are reflected in her memberships of Ministerial Advisory Panels, her Directorships of not-for-profit services providing services for people with disabilities and as an accreditor of Australian University Speech Pathology programs. Recently, she has been establishing new University Speech Pathology programs. As an Associate Professor and the inaugural Course (Program) Chair of Speech Pathology at Victoria University (VU) in Melbourne, Australia, she designed and implemented a Speech Pathology program using the VU Block Model design, an Australian first. As an Associate Professor of Speech Pathology, she has also contributed to the design of the inaugural Speech Pathology program at the University of Southern Queensland in Ipswich, Australia.

Q11. Deb James: Prompts, Clues, Hints, and Test-Picture Naming

Children in the 5-to-8-year age range who are referred to SLPs/SLTs because their parents and teachers have concerns about their progress in oral language and literacy are frequently reported by SLPs/SLTs to return scores that are within normal limits on language and speech tests such as the CELF (Semel et al., 2017) and DEAP (Dodd, Hua et al., 2002) respectively. Such tests include picture-naming or so-called confrontation naming tasks, and there is provision in their protocols for clinicians to provide prompts, cues, and sometimes forced-choice alternatives. Might explicit consideration of how these prompts and cues are used, by children and SLPs/SLTs, provide greater insight into the children's phonological processing and provide an explanation for their difficulties with oracy (speaking and listening), reading, and spelling?

A11. Deb James: Prompts that Help Children When Picture-Naming; Does Their Consideration Add Value to Clinical Decision-Making?

Have you experienced the conundrum in which a child returns scores that are within normal limits on language and speech tests, such as the CELF and DEAP respectively, but whose conversational speech is not 'quite right' and reports of literacy difficulties exist? I have. I have also noted that sometimes these same children take longer to complete tests, such as the DEAP, than is usual in my clinical experience. Utilising the generic picture-naming test instructions of seeking children's most spontaneous rendition of words (e.g., Dodd, Hua et al., 2002; James, unpublished; James et al., 2008, 2016) such children seem to need more prompting across a greater number of items than their peers, increasing test administration time. They stall more frequently but notably, if prompted with cues such as picture description and/or the first sound or syllable of the word, they not only returned the correct name, but they also returned it with accurately articulated speech sounds (SSs). Sometimes, circumlocution was present which, in effect, 'bought' time to formulate their response by saying; 'Oh I know it, it's a..., it's a jungle animal and you see them in the water at the zoo, it's a giraffe, no, not a giraffe, it's a hip, it's a hippopotamus'; again, the right name with accurate SSs. Sometimes, they merely stayed silent for what seemed a long time but then gave the right name, again with accurate SSs. These children with their longer response times, when judged for SS accuracy performed as well as their peers with (typical) short response times and, yet clinically, they seemed qualitatively different. It simply felt wrong to 'pass' these children with what I will call slow responses.

These clinical scenarios led me to the following question: Are these slow picture-naming responses a clue to untangling this conundrum? When children like these ones present with age-appropriate SSs on a picture-naming test, should we ignore their slow responses in our clinical decision making, especially when they exhibit oracy and literacy concerns? I contend that we should not because they could provide insight into children's psycholinguistic speech processing that, in turn, may provide clues to their literacy difficulties.

Psycholinguistic Speech Processing Defined

Psycholinguistic speech processing is a broad term that captures the psychological, linguistic, and motor aspects of recognition, understanding, and production of spoken and written linguistic information (Stackhouse & Wells, 1997; van Haaften et al., 2019; and see Schäfer & Fricke A21; Waring & Dodd A6). Psycholinguistic speech processing typically has three components: receiving spoken and written linguistic information (input), remembering,

and storing that information (lexical representation) and producing it (output) (Dodd, 2005; Stackhouse & Wells, 1997a, 1997b). Psycholinguistic speech processing is inclusive of phonological processing which is the conscious or explicit use of the knowledge of speech sounds in one's language or languages (i.e., phonemes) to process spoken and written language (Wagner & Torgesen, 1987). Phonological processing comprises three components of:

1. *phonological awareness (the ability to reflect on and manipulate SSs);*
2. *phonological working memory (the ability to hold SSs in short-term memory to manipulate them);* and
3. *phonological retrieval (the ability to retrieve SSs from long-term memory).*

As van Haaften et al. (2019, p. 2142) eloquently noted '...picture naming taps into the whole chain of speech processes [psycholinguistic speech processing]'. So, thinking about the international practice of using picture-naming to assess children's SSs (McLeod & Verdon, 2014) in psycholinguistic speech processing terms, coupled with the patterns of prompting that SLPs/SLTs provide, and children use during picture-naming enables us to take a glimpse into children's psycholinguistic speech processing status.

The Insights into Psycholinguistic Speech Processing Status that Interrogation of Children's Picture-Naming Responses May Offer
The usual picture-naming instruction is asking 'What's this?' for each picture (e.g., Dodd, Hua et al., 2002; James, unpublished; James et al., 2008, 2016). It is important to note that this instruction does not provide the name of the picture: and I will return to this point. So, answering this question in the absence of a name means children draw little on the first component of psycholinguistic speech processing; the input. Rather, answering the question requires activating a complex cross-modal process that draws more on the other two components of psycholinguistic speech processing; stored linguistic knowledge and output. Assuming the word is established in the child's lexicon, picture-naming draws on the pre-lexical processes of perceptually registering the picture and recognising it (Katz, 1986) and then accessing, utilising, and retrieving the linguistic knowledge in

the lexical representation: the semantics, phonology, and the motor program (Stackhouse & Wells, 1997a; van Haaften et al., 2019). Once the picture is recognised, the key retrieval tasks relate to phonological processing; the retrieval of *the* phonological representation and motor program from long-term memory (Wagner & Torgesen, 1987). *I contend that it is this aspect of retrieval that is critical to consider in unravelling the conundrum.* Finally, picture-naming depends on output processing, that is, the post-lexical psycholinguistic speech processing skills of motor functioning, enabling all the phonemes to be translated into motor gestures, culminating in a prosodically and articulatory accurate word that includes all the SSs in the correct sequence. Thus, unsuccessful picture-naming may result from a breakdown in any one of these processes. I contend that considering children's output in terms of SS accuracy coupled with their use of prompts can help unravel where the breakdown may occur, which I now exemplify.

One picture-naming response children may make is to describe pictures, or the operation or function of the pictured object, rather than name them, such as saying 'You put it up when it's raining' when presented with item 2 in the DEAP: a picture of an *umbrella*. This accurate picture description suggests sufficient visual-conceptual processing for recognition of this picture (Stackhouse & Wells, 1997a; van Haaften et al., 2019) and the presence of an underlying lexical representation that contains semantic information. The absence of the name could reflect a lexical representation underspecified for the phonology and/or the motor program (Stackhouse & Wells, 1997). The absence of a name also means there is no execution information regarding the SSs in *umbrella*. Taken together, this response implies a lexical representation specified for semantics but underspecified the phonology and/or the motor program. No judgement, therefore, can be made about the accuracy of the SSs in the intended word.

If the SLP/SLT prompts the same child, saying 'Yes you do (put it up when it's raining), so now, can you tell me the name?' and the child succeeds, albeit via a circumlocutory response or after a seemingly long silence, then this correct response is inconsistent with the previous hypothesis of underspecification. Rather, the presence of accurate SSs in the object's name indicates (1) a lexical representation specified for the phonology and (2) the motor program as well as (3) intact output skills. However, what this response does indicate is a sluggish retrieval of the phonology and/or the motor program and this sluggishness has implications for the conundrum. This sluggish response may give a clue to the *quality* of phonological representation. It may be specified at a gross level, not a fine level, and this, in turn, may provide an inkling into children's phonological awareness, another component of phonological processing. Phonological awareness can be at two levels. The gross and more holistic one is the syllable level whereby children can segment words into (written) syllables – 'um-bre-la' – or even the syllable into its onset 'br' and rime 'e'. Phonological awareness can be at a fine level: the level of the phoneme or phonemic awareness, where children can break the syllable up into its constituent phonemes, such as breaking a consonant cluster onset like /bɹ/ into its phonemes of /b/ and /ɹ/. So, a child with sluggish responses may have an imprecise, or fuzzy, underlying phonological representation that lacks sufficient detail to drive the motor program to say the word in a timely fashion, yielding circumlocutory or delayed responses, when asked to name a picture. When thinking about the conundrum, its detail may be enough to allow children to articulate the word and all its SSs accurately but not enough to spell it accurately. Spelling requires a more fine-grained phonological representation than saying the same word, giving rise to the situation of accurate speech but poor spelling. So, if this same child is asked to spell 'umbrella', the underlying phonological representation may contain too little information for the child to 'look it up' to then 'sound it out' and place into working memory – another phonological processing component – while they spell it, thereby resulting in spelling problems. It is for this reason that I contend that we should not 'pass' children who take a long time to complete tests such as the DEAP.

Alternatively, if the previous request for naming failed but the same child named the word accurately in response to a follow-up prompt, or model, of the first syllable [ʌm] of the word, then this response can further pinpoint the phonological representation weakness. It suggests difficulties with the retrieval of the phonological representation rather than the motor program because once the phonological representation is triggered, then the rest of the 'speech chain' is liberated, resulting in a correctly articulated name.

Finally, if the prompt of providing the first syllable failed but the same child named the word accurately in response to a request for imitation, then the imitated response provides quite different information about psycholinguistic speech processing than spontaneous picture-naming. This is so because a request for imitation changes the nature of psycholinguistic speech processing involved in picture-naming because the item name is provided, unlike in spontaneous picture-naming. As noted above, spontaneous picture-naming draws on the retrieval of *the* phonological representation and motor program from long-term memory, whereas imitation does not draw on these skills to the same extent. Imitation is also less reliant on the visual-conceptual skills because of less need for picture recognition, as the item is named. However, imitation is more reliant on the auditory input processing skills of listening and processing the incoming information than spontaneous picture-naming. Imitation, like spontaneous picture-naming, involves output processing skills of motor programming and motor planning to compile the motor program and motor plan (Stackhouse & Wells, 1997a) to execute the word. If all the SSs are correct in an imitated response, then the processes are inferred to be relatively intact.

Is There a Relationship?

So, it seems that examination of these prompts has the capacity to provide information about the status of psycholinguistic speech processing. Prompts that do not rely on imitation may yield information about the ability to retrieve the phonological representation and the motor program, which are skills on which spelling also draws (Stackhouse & Wells, 1997a). If so, then an association should be present between prompts that secure a non-imitated picture name and spelling in the developmental period. Brooker (2019) and James and Brooker (2021) conducted a pilot study to explore this association in 19 typically developing 6- to 8-year-olds with verified typically developing speech. They found a significant negative correlation such that lower spelling scores occurred with more picture-naming prompts. As far as they could determine, this was the first evidence they could locate to support this hypothesis.

Implications for Clinical Practice

The implications for clinical practice are as follows. When assessing children's SS accuracy via picture-naming, it is recommended that consideration of their need for prompts is factored into clinical decision-making. As part of that, an imitation prompt is considered the prompt of last resort when a child's literacy skills are slow or low in development, as imitation draws on a different set of psycholinguistic speech processing skills from spontaneous picture-naming. As such, imitation obviates the need to retrieve information from long-term memory; a skill upon which spelling draws. So, given the longstanding and strong evidence that eliciting SSs via spontaneous picture-naming or imitation makes no difference to SS accuracy (McLeod & Masso, 2019), then it seems sensible to opt for spontaneous picture-naming whenever possible when there are literacy concerns because of its potential to reveal information about retrieval of the phonological representation and motor program as well as its possible predictive capacity of children's spelling.

Communicating with Clients

In a much-thumbed chapter on terminology, Kenneth Scott Wood (1971, p. 3) wrote:

> All areas of scientific study are afflicted with a certain amount of ambiguity, duplication, inappropriateness, and disagreement in the use of terms. Like other sciences, speech pathology, audiology, and the entire cluster of studies

associated with the production and perception of speech have been developing over the years a terminology and nomenclature that leave much to be desired in logic and stability. Many terms and their meanings are not well crystallized because the subject matter is always changing; concepts themselves are often tentative and fluid, and many writers have liberally coined new terms whenever they felt a need to do so. This growth of speech pathology and audiology, stimulated as it has been by so many workers, has generated hundreds of terms, some of which are interchangeable, some of which have different meanings to different people, some of which are now rare or obsolete, and some of which for various reasons have had only a short literary life.

If Wood were to drop by unexpectedly today, might he puzzle over what happened to *articulation defects, dyslalia, dysenia, diglossia,* and *the defective in speech* (Wood, 1971)? What on earth would he make of *apps, complex targets, constraint-based nonlinear phonology, electropalatography, linguistic universals, psycholinguistic processing, SIWI SIWW SFWW* and *SFWF, teletherapy,* and *visual biofeedback*?

Technical language can be irksome at times, but it is essential. It enables precise delineation of matters under discussion, potentially helping unambiguous communication within our profession, with other professions, and with consumers: clients and their families. Although it creates circumstances in which SLPs/SLTs must clarify, explain, or simplify terms, in general our terminology serves us well.

Conveying technical information, with or without the burden of jargon, can be challenging. The information itself may be distressing. It is not necessarily easy, for instance, to explain the prognostic implications of a severe motor speech disorder to a troubled parent, or to say, 'You are correct: something's not right'. The information's recipient may be upset, unprepared, or have difficulty absorbing or accepting it. The situation in which the information is delivered may be unfavourable and the available time may be too short to allow helpful discussion and reflection. And the way the information is conveyed may be problematic: written reports, for example, with no face-to-face verbal explanation, may be alienating and overly confronting.

Many of us have experienced unsuccessful attempts to explain complex concepts and issues, for clients or caregivers, without oversimplifying the message. At the same time, we know that, for some consumers, the use of correct terminology is a sign (to them) that professionals willingly share information transparently and respectfully, taking *them* seriously, without making condescending judgements about their capacity to understand, accommodate and 'use' such information. Indeed, numerous families (and clients, if they are old enough) prefer to be told the correct name of a disorder, symptom, anatomical feature, assessment procedure or therapy technique – especially if they want to look it up or seek another opinion.

On the other hand, the last thing many families of children with communication difficulties want is to be inundated with incomprehensible jargon. This is particularly true in the early stages of diagnosis and at times when they are apprehensive. They want facts, but until they are confidently engaged in a constructive program for their child, most can do without the complications of grappling with the differences between, for example, the disconcerting number of 'speech pathology words' that start with 'phon' or 'dys'!

People deal with the information we present in different ways and at different rates. In situations where one parent brings a child to consultations, and the other parent receives information by proxy, it is common for the accompanying parent to reach a degree of acceptance and insight into the child's difficulties ahead of their partner. In such a situation, the parent who meets with the clinician may be more prepared to 'trust' the information conveyed. These and other issues around terminology, classification, description, assessment and 'breaking the news' are often prominent in our engagement with families and the 'special populations' of children described in Chapter 3.

References

American Speech-Language-Hearing Association. (1983). Definition of language. *Asha, 25*(6), 44.

American Speech-Language-Hearing Association. (n.d.). Speech sound disorders: Articulation and phonology [Practice Portal]. https://www.asha.org/practice-portal/clinical-topics/articulation-and-phonology

Andrews, N., & Fey, M. E. (1986). Analysis of the speech of phonologically impaired children in two sampling conditions. *Language, Speech, and Hearing Services in Schools*, *17*(3), 187–198. https://doi.org/10.1044/0161-1461.1703.187

Apel, K. (2014). Clinical scientists improving clinical practices: In thoughts and actions. *Language, Speech, and Hearing Services in Schools*, *45* (2),104–109.https://doi.org/10.1044/2014_LSHSS-14-0003

Austin, D., & Shriberg, L. D. (1996). *Lifespan reference data for ten measures of articulation competence using the Speech Disorders Classification System (SDCS)* (Tech. Rep. No. 3). Phonology Project, Waisman Center, University of Wisconsin-Madison.

Bauman-Waengler, J. (2020). *Articulatory and phonological impairments: A clinical focus* (6th ed.). Pearson.

Baylis, A. L., & Shriberg, L. D. (2018). Estimates of the prevalence of speech and motor speech disorders in youth with 22q11.2 Deletion syndrome. *American Journal of Speech-Language Pathology*, *28*(1), 53–82. https://doi.org/10.1044/2018_AJSLP-18-0037

Bernhardt, B. M., Másdóttir, T., Stemberger, J. P., Leonhardt, L., & Hansson, G. Ó. (2015). Fricative acquisition in English- and Icelandic-speaking preschoolers with protracted phonological development. *Clinical Linguistics and Phonetics*, *29*(8–10), 642–665. https://doi.org/10.3109/026992 06.2015.1036463

Bishop, D. V. M., & Hayiou-Thomas, M. E. (2008). Heritability of specific language impairment depends on diagnostic criteria. *Genes, Brain and Behavior*, *7*(3), 365–372. https://doi.org/10.1111/j.1601-183X.2007.00360.x

Bowen, C. (1996). Evaluation of a phonological therapy with treated and untreated groups of young children (Unpublished doctoral dissertation). Macquarie University. http://hdl.handle.net/1959.14/304812

Bowen, C. (1998). *Developmental phonological disorders: A practical guide for families and teachers*. The Australian Council for Educational Research.

Bowen, C. (2015a). Parents and children together in phonological intervention. In C. Bowen, *Children's speech sound disorders* (2nd ed., pp. 414–451). Wiley-Blackwell. https://doi.org/10.1002/9781119 180418

Brandel, J., & Loeb, D. F. (2011). Program intensity and service delivery models in the schools: SLP survey results. *Language, Speech, and Hearing Services in Schools*, *42*(4), 461–490. https://doi.org/10.1044/0161-1461(2011/10-0019

Brooker, A. (2019). *The assessment of children's speech using picture-naming tests: An exploration of the information generated by prompting* (Unpublished Honours thesis). Southern Cross University, Coolangatta, Queensland, Australia.

Broomfield, J., & Dodd, B. (2004). The nature of referred subtypes of primary speech disability. *Child Language Teaching and Therapy*, *20*(2), 135–151. https://doi.org/10.1191%2F0265659004ct267oa

Brosseau-Lapré, F., & Rvachew, S. (2017). Underlying manifestations of developmental phonological disorders in French-speaking pre-schoolers. *Journal of Child Language*, *44*(6), 1337–1361. https://doi.org/10.1017/S0305000916000556

Carlson, S. (2005). Developmentally sensitive measures of executive functions in preschool children. *Developmental Neuropsychology*, *28*(2), 595–616. https://doi.org/10.1207/s15326942dn2802_3. PMID: 16144429.

Choi, H. W. (2021). Fasciculation in children. *Pediatric Neurology*, *125*(2021), 40–47. https://doi.org/10.1016/j.pediatrneurol.2021.08.008

Claessen, M., Leitäo, S., & Fraser, C. (2017). Intervention for a young child with atypical phonology. In B. Dodd & A. Morgan (Eds.), *Intervention case studies of child speech impairment* (pp. 275–291). J&R Press.

Clark, E. (2020). Conversational repair and the acquisition of language. *Discourse Processes*, *57*(5–6), 441–459. https://doi.org/10.1080/01638 53X.2020.1719795

Crosbie, S., & Holm, A. (2017). Phonological contrast therapy for children making consistent phonological errors. In B. Dodd & A. Morgan (Eds.), *Intervention case studies of child speech impairment* (pp. 275–291). J&R Press.

Crosbie, S., Holm, A., & Dodd, B. (2005). Intervention for children with severe speech disorder: A comparison of two approaches. *International Journal of Language & Communication Disorders*, *40*(4), 467–491. https://doi.org/10.1080/136828205 00126049

Crosbie, S., Holm, A., & Dodd, B. (2009). Cognitive flexibility in children with and without speech disorder. *Child Language Teaching & Therapy*, *25*(2), 250–270. https://doi.org/10.1177%2F0265659009102990

Crosbie, S., Holm, A., & Dodd, B. (2010). Intervention for children with severe speech disorder: A comparison of two approaches. *International Journal of Language & Communication Disorders*, *40*(4), 467–491. https://doi.org/10.1080/13682820500126049

Diamond, A. (2013). Executive functions. *Annual Review of Psychology*, *64*(1), 135–168. https://doi.org/10.1146/annurev-psych-113011-143750

Dodd, B. (Ed.). (1995). *Differential diagnosis and treatment of children with speech disorder*. Whurr Publishers.

Dodd, B. (Ed.). (2005). *Differential diagnosis and treatment of children with speech disorder* (2nd ed.). Whurr Publishers.

Dodd, B. (2011). Differentiating speech delay from disorder: Does it matter? *Topics in Language Disorders*, *31*(2), 96–111. https://doi.org/10.1097/TLD.0b013e318217b66a

Dodd, B. (2014). Differential diagnosis of pediatric speech sound disorder. *Current Developmental Disorders Report*, *1*(3), 189–196. https://doi.org/10.1007/s40474-014-0017-3

Dodd, B. (2015). Assessment and intervention for two-year-olds at risk for phonological disorder. In C. Bowen, *Children's speech sound disorders* (2nd ed., pp. 88–94). Wiley-Blackwell.

Dodd, B., & Bradford, A. (2000). A comparison of three therapy methods for children with different types of developmental disorder. *International Journal of Language and Communication Disorders*, *35*(2), 189–209. https://doi.org/10.1080/136828200247142

Dodd, B., Crosbie, S., Zhu, H., Holm, A., & Ozanne, A. (2002). *Diagnostic evaluation of articulation and phonology (DEAP)*. Psychological Corporation.

Dodd, B., Hua, Z., Crosbie, S., Holm, A., & Ozanne, A. (2006). *Diagnostic evaluation of articulation and phonology* (DEAP, US Edition). Harcourt Assessment.

Dodd, B., & Iacono, T. (1989). Phonological disorders in children: Changes in phonological process use during treatment. *British Journal of Disorders of Communication*, *24*(3), 333–352. https://doi.org/10.3109/13682828909019894

Dodd, B., Leahy, J., & Hambly, G. (1989). Phonological disorders in children: Underlying cognitive deficits. *British Journal of Developmental Psychology*, *7*(1), 55–71. https://doi.org/10.1111/j.2044-835X.1989.tb00788.x

Dodd, B., Ttofari-Eecen, K., Brommeyer, K., Ng, K., Reilly, S., & Morgan, A. (2018). Delayed and disordered development of articulation and phonology between four and seven years. *Child Language Teaching and Therapy*, *34*(2), 87–99. https://doi.org/10.1177%2F0265659017735958

DuBois, E., & Bernthal, J. E. (1978). A comparison of three methods of obtaining articulatory responses. *Journal of Speech and Hearing Disorders*, *43*(3), 295–305. https://doi.org/10.1044/jshd.4303.295

Duchan, J. F. (2001 to date). *A History of Speech-Language Pathology*. http://www.acsu.buffalo.edu/~duchan/new_history/overview.html

Eadie, P., Morgan, A., Ukoumunne, O. C., Ttofari Eecen, K., Wake, M., & Reilly, S. (2015). Speech sound disorder at 4 years: Prevalence, comorbidities, and predictors in a community cohort of children. *Developmental Medicine and Child Neurology*, *57*(6), 578–584. https://doi.org/10.1111/dmcn.12635

Engel, G. L. (1977). The need for a new medical model: A challenge for biomedicine. *Science*, *196*(4286), 129–136. https://doi.org/10.1126/science.847460

Estes, K. G., Evans, J. L., & Else-Quest, N. M. (2007). Differences in the nonword repetition performance of children with and without specific language impairment: A meta-analysis. *Journal of Speech, Language, and Hearing Research*, *50*(1), 177–195. https://doi.org/10.1044/1092-4388(2007/015)

Fabiano-Smith, L. (2019). Standardized tests and the diagnosis of speech sound disorders. *Perspectives of the ASHA Special Interest Groups*, *4*(1), 58–66. https://doi.org/10.1044/2018_PERS-SIG1-2018-0018

Finestack, L. H., Potter, N., VanDam, M., Davis, J., Bruce, L., Scherer, N., Eng, L., & Peter, B. (2022). Feasibility of a proactive parent-implemented communication intervention delivered via telepractice for children with Classic Galactosemia. *American Journal of Speech-Language Pathology*, *31*(6), 2527–2538. https://doi.org/10.1044/2022_AJSLP-22-00107

Flipsen, P., Jr., Hammer, J. B., & Yost, K. M. (2005). Measuring severity of involvement in speech delay: Segmental and whole-word measures. *American Journal of Speech-Language Pathology*, *14*(4), 298–312. https://doi.org/10.1044/1058-0360(2005/029)

Gierut, J. A. (1998). Treatment efficacy: Functional phonological disorders in children. *Journal of*

Speech, Language and Hearing Research, 41(1), S85–S100. https://doi.org/10.1044/jslhr.4101.s85

Gillon, G., McNeill, B., Scott, A., Denston, A., Wilson, L., Carson, K., & Macfarlene, A. (2019). A better start to literacy learning: Findings from a teacher-implemented intervention in children's first year at school. *Reading and Writing*. https://link.springer.com/article/10.1007/s11145-018-9933-7

Gillon, G. T. (1998). The speech-literacy link: Perspectives from children with phonological speech disorders. *New Zealand Speech-Language Therapists Association Biennial Conference Proceedings*, Dunedin, 14–17 April 1998. Supplementary (1), pp. 1–6.

Goldman, R., & Fristoe, M. (2015). *Goldman-Fristoe test of articulation* (3rd ed.). Pearson Clinical Assessment.

Gruber, F. A. (1999). Probability estimates and paths to consonant normalization in children with speech delay. *Journal of Speech Language and Hearing Research, 42*(2), 448–459. https://doi.org/10.1044/jslhr.4202.448

Grunwell, P. (1983). Phonological development in phonological disability. *Topics in Language Disorders, 3*(3), 62–76.

Grunwell, P. (1987). *Clinical phonology* (2nd ed.). Williams & Wilkins.

Grunwell, P. (1989). Developmental phonological disorders and normal speech development: A review and illustration. *Child Language Teaching and Therapy, 5*(3), 304–319. https://doi.org/10.1177%2F026565908900500305

Hanson, M. L. (1983). *Articulation*. W. B. Saunders Co.

Hase, M., Ingram, D., & Bunta, F. (2010). A comparison of two phonological assessment tools for monolingual Spanish-speaking children. *Clinical Linguistics & Phonetics, 24*(4–5), 346–356. https://doi.org/10.3109/02699201003587020

Healy, T. J., & Madison, C. L. (1987). Articulation error migration: A comparison of single word and connected speech samples. *Journal of Communication Disorders, 20*(2), 129–136. https://doi.org/10.1016/0021-9924(87)90004-9

Hearnshaw, S., Baker, E., & Munro, N. (2018). The speech perception skills of children with and without speech sound disorder. *Journal of Communication Disorders, 71*, 61–71. https://doi.org/10.1016/j.jcomdis.2017.12.004

Hodson, B. (2004). *HAPP-3: Hodson assessment of phonological patterns* (3rd ed.). Pro-Ed.

Holm, A., Farrier, F., & Dodd, B. (2008). The phonological awareness, reading accuracy, and spelling ability of children with inconsistent phonological disorder. *International Journal of Language and Communication Disorders, 43*(3), 467–486. https://doi.org/10.1080/13682820701445032

Howell, J., & Dean, E. (1994). *Treating phonological disorders in children: Metaphon—theory to practice* (2nd ed.). Whurr.

ICD10-CM Diagnosis Code F80.0. (2022). Phonological disorder. https://www.icd10data.com/ICD10CM/Codes/F01-F99/F80-F89/F80-/F80.0

Ingram, D. (1976). *Phonological Disability in Children*. Edward Arnold.

Ingram, D. (1981). *Procedures for the Phonological Analysis of Children's Language*. University Park Press.

Ingram, D. (2002). The measurement of whole-word productions. *Journal of Child Language, 29*(4), 713–733. https://doi.org/10.1017/S0305000902005275

Ingram, D. (2020). Ingram's contributions to the study of first language acquisition according to Ingram. In E. Babatsouli (Ed.), *On under-reported monolingual child phonology* (pp. 25–51). Multilingual Matters.

Ingram, D. & Ingram, K. (2001). A whole word approach to phonological intervention. *Language, Speech, and Hearing Services in Schools, 32*(4), 271–283. https://doi.org/10.1044/0161-1461(2001/024)

Ingram, D., Williams, A. L., & Scherer, N. (2018). Are speech sound disorders phonological or articulatory? A spectrum approach. In E. Babatsouli & D. Ingram (Eds.), *Phonology in protolanguage and interlanguage* (pp. 27–48). Equinox.

James, D. G. H. (unpublished). *Assessment of children's articulation and phonology*. ICPLA.

James, D. G. H., & Brooker, A. (2021, June 23–25). Exploring the relationship between the prompts children use to name speech-test pictures and spelling. In J. Cleland (Chair), *Conference of the international clinical phonetics and linguistics association*, University of Strathclyde, Glasgow, UK, ICPLA. https://www.strath.ac.uk/humanities/psychologicalscienceshealth/speechlanguagetherapy/icpla2020

James, D. G. H., Ferguson, W. A., & Butcher, A. R. (2016). Assessing children's speech using picture-naming: The influence of differing phonological variables on some speech outcomes. *International*

Journal of Speech-Language Pathology, 18(4), 364–377. https://doi.org/10.3109/17549507.2015.1101159

James, D. G. H., van Doorn, J., McLeod, S., & Esterman, A. (2008). Patterns of consonant deletion in typically developing children aged 3 to 7 years. *International Journal of Speech-Language Pathology, 10*(3), 179–192. https://doi.org/10.1080/17549500701849789

Johnson, C. A., Weston, A. D., & Bain, B. A. (2004). An objective and time-efficient method for determining severity of childhood speech delay. *American Journal of Speech-Language Pathology, 13*(1), 55–65. https://doi.org/10.1044/1058-0360 (2004/007)

Katz, R. B. (1986). Phonological deficits in children with reading disability: Evidence from an object naming task. *Cognition, 22*(3), 225–257. https://doi.org/10.1016/0010-0277(86)90016-8

Kirk, C., & Vigeland, L. (2014). A psychometric review of norm-referenced tests used to assess phonological error patterns. *Language, Speech, and Hearing Services in Schools, 45*(4), 365–377. https://doi.org/10.1044/2014_LSHSS-13-0053

Kropp, B. (2020). *Exploring the Role of Executive Functions in Phonological and Motor-based Speech Sound Disorder: A Case Series* (Unpublished honours thesis). Australian Catholic University, Queensland.

Laing, R. D. (1971). *The politics of the family and other essays.* Tavistock Publications.

Leahy, J., & Dodd, B. (1987). The development of disordered phonology: A case study. *Language and Cognitive Processes, 2*(2), 115–132. http://dx.doi.org/10.1080/01690968708406353

Limbrick, N., McCormack, J., & McLeod, S. (2013). Designs and decisions: The creation of informal measures for assessing speech production in children. *International Journal of Speech-Language Pathology, 15*(3), 296–311. https://doi.org/10.3109/17549507.2013.770552

Lohmeier, H. L., & Shriberg, L. D. (2011). *Reference data for the Syllable Repetition Task (SRT).* Phonology Project, Waisman Center, University of Wisconsin-Madison, https://www2.waisman.wisc.edu/phonology/pubs-tech.html

Mabie, H. L., & Shriberg, L. D. (2017). Speech and motor speech measures and reference data for the Speech Disorders Classification System (SDCS). (Technical Report No. 23). *Phonology Project, Madison: Waisman Center, University of Wisconsin–Madison.* https://phonology.waisman.wisc.edu

Macrae, T., Tyler, A. A., & Lewis, K. E. (2014). Lexical and phonological variability in preschool children with speech sound disorder. *American Journal of Speech-Language Pathology, 23*(1), 27–35. https://doi.org/10.1044/1058-0360(2013/12-0037)

Masterson, J. A., Bernhardt, B. H., & Hofheinz, M. K. (2005). A comparison of single words and conversational speech in phonological evaluation. *American Journal of Speech-Language Pathology, 14*(3), 229–241. https://doi.org/10.1044/1058-0360 (2005/023)

Mathews, T. (2020). Administering and scoring the syllable repetition task. A Webinar produced by the Child Phonology Laboratory. Online Courses | IALP: International Association of Communication Sciences and Disorders (IALP). https://ialpasoc.info/online-courses

McIntosh, B., & Dodd, B. J. (2008). Two-year-olds' phonological acquisition: Normative data. *International Journal of Speech-Language Pathology, 10*(6), 460–469. https://doi.org/10.1080/17549500802149683

McLeod, S., & Baker, E. (2017). *Children's speech: An evidence-based approach to assessment and intervention.* Pearson.

McLeod, S., Crowe, K., & Shahaeian, A. (2015). Intelligibility in context scale: Normative and validation data for English- speaking preschoolers. *Language, Speech, and Hearing Services in Schools, 46*(3), 266–276. https://doi.org/10.1044/2015_LSHSS-14-0120

McLeod, S., & Masso, S. (2019). Screening children's speech: The impact of imitated elicitation and word position. *Language, Speech, and Hearing Services in Schools, 50*(1), 71–82. https://doi.org/10.1044/2018_LSHSS-17-0141

McLeod, S., & Verdon, S. (2014). A review of 30 speech assessments in 19 languages other than English. *American Journal of Speech-Language Pathology, 23*(4), 708–723. https://doi.org/10.1044/2014_AJSLP-13-0066

McLeod, S., & Verdon, S., & International Expert Panel on Multilingual Children's Speech. (2017). Tutorial: Speech assessment for multilingual children who do not speak the same language(s) as the speech-language pathologist. *American Journal of Speech-Language Pathology, 26*(3), 691–708. https://doi.org/10.1044/2017_ajslp-15-0161

Morgan, A., & Gunther, T. (2017). Clinical management of articulation impairment in children. In B. Dodd

& A. Morgan (Eds.), *Intervention case studies of child speech impairment* (pp. 9–30). J&R Press.

Moriarty, B. C., & Gillon, G. T. (2006). Phonological awareness intervention for children with childhood apraxia of speech. *International Journal of Language & Communication Disorders*, *41*(6), 713–734. https://doi.org/10.1080/13682820600623960

Morrisette, M. L. (2021). Complexity approach. In A. L. Williams, S. McLeod, & R. J. McCauley (Eds.), *Interventions for speech sound disorders in children* (2nd ed., pp. 91–110). Paul H. Brookes Publishing Co.

Murray, E., & Iuzzini-Seigel, J. (2017). Efficacious treatment of children with childhood apraxia of speech according to the international classification of functioning, disability, and health. *Perspectives of the ASHA Special Interest Groups*, *2*(2), 61–76. https://doi.org/10.1044/persp2.SIG2.61

Patchell, F., & Hand, L. (1993). An invisible disability – Language disorders in high school students and the implications for classroom teachers. Independent Education. https://eric.ed.gov/?id=ED425601

Plante, E., & Gomez, R. (2018). Learning without trying: The clinical relevance of statistical learning. *Language, Speech, and Hearing Services in Schools*, *49*(3S), 710–722. https://doi.org/10.1044/2018_lshss-stlt1-17-0131

Robbins, S. D. (1947). Principles of nomenclature and of classification of speech and voice disorders. *Journal of Speech Disorders*, *12*(1), 17–22. https://doi.org/10.1044/jshd.1201.17

Ruscello, D. M. (1993). A motor skill learning treatment program for sound system disorders. *Seminars in Speech and Language*, *14*(2), 106–118. https://doi.org/10.1055/s-2008-1064163

Ruscello, D. R. (2008). *Treating articulation and phonological disorders in children*. Elsevier.

Rvachew, S. (2007). Phonological processing and reading in children with speech sound disorders. *American Journal of Speech-Language Pathology*, *16*(3), 260–270. https://doi.org/10.1044/1058-0360 (2007/030)

Rvachew, S., & Brosseau-Lapré, F. (2018). *Developmental phonological disorders: Foundations of clinical practice* (2nd ed.). Plural Publishing, Inc.

Rvachew, S., & Matthews, T. (2017). Using the Syllable Repetition Task to reveal underlying speech processes in Childhood Apraxia of Speech: A tutorial. *Canadian Journal of Speech-Language Pathology and Audiology*, *41*(1), 106–126. http://www.cjslpa.ca/detail.php?ID=1207&lang=en

Rvachew, S., & Matthews, T. (2019). An N-of-1 randomized controlled trial of interventions for children with inconsistent speech sound errors. *Journal of Speech, Language, and Hearing Research*, *62*(9), 3183–3203. https://doi.org/10.1044/2019_JSLHR-S-18-0288

Scarborough, H. S., & Brady, S. A. (2002). Toward a common terminology for talking about speech and reading: A glossary of the 'phon' words and some related terms. *Journal of Literacy Research*, *34*(3), 299–336. https://doi.org/10.1207/s15548430jlr3403_3

Semel, E., Wiig, E. H., & Secord, W. A. (2017). *Clinical evaluation of language fundamentals, Australian and New Zealand* (5th ed.). Pearson.

Shelton, R. L. (1993). Grand rounds for sound system disorder. Conclusion: What was learned? *Seminars in Speech and Language*, *14*(12), 166–177. https://doi.org/10.1055/s-2008-1064168

Shriberg, L. D. (1980). Developmental phonological disorders. In T. J. Hixon, L. D. Shriberg, & J. S. Saxman (Eds.), *Introduction to communicative disorders* (pp. 262–309). Prentice Hall.

Shriberg, L. D. (1982). Diagnostic assessment of developmental phonological disorders. In M. Crary (Ed.), *Phonological intervention, concepts and procedures* (pp. 35–60). College-Hill Inc.

Shriberg, L. D. (1993). Four new speech and prosody-voice measures for genetics research and other studies in developmental phonological disorders. *Journal of Speech and Hearing Research*, *36*(1), 105–140. https://doi.org/10.1044/jshr.3601.105

Shriberg, L. D. (2006, June). *Research in idiopathic and symptomatic childhood apraxia of speech*. Paper presented at the 5th International Conference on Speech Motor Control Nijmegen, the Netherlands.

Shriberg, L. D. (2010). Childhood speech sound disorders: From post behaviourism to the postgenomic era. In R. Paul & P. Flipsen, Jr. (Eds.), *Speech sound disorders in children: In honour of Lawrence D. Shriberg* (pp. 1–33). Plural Publishing.

Shriberg, L. D., Austin, D., Lewis, B. A., McSweeny, J. L., & Wilson, D. L. (1997). The percentage of consonants correct (PCC) metric: Extensions and reliability data. *Journal of Speech, Language, and Hearing Research*, *40*(4), 708–722. https://doi.org/10.1044/jslhr.4004.708

Shriberg, L. D., Campbell, T. F., Mabie, H. L., & McGlothlin, J. H. (2019). Initial studies of the phenotype and persistence of Speech Motor Delay (SMD). *Clinical Linguistics & Phonetics, 33*(8), 737–756. https://doi.org/10.1080/02699206.2019.1595733

Shriberg, L. D., Fourakis, M., Hall, S., Karlsson, H. K., Lohmeier, H. L., McSweeny, J., Potter, N. L., Scheer-Cohen, A. R., Strand, E. A., Tilkens, C. M., & Wilson, D. L. (2010). Extensions to the speech disorders classification system (SDCS). *Clinical Linguistics & Phonetics, 24*(10), 795–824. https://doi.org/10.3109/02699206.2010.503006

Shriberg, L. D., & Kwiatkowski, J. (1982). Phonological disorders III: A procedure for assessing severity of involvement. *Journal of Speech and Hearing Disorders, 47*(3), 256–270. https://doi.org/10.1044/jshd.4703.256

Shriberg, L. D., Kwiatkowski, J., & Mabie, H. L. (2019). Estimates of the prevalence of motor speech disorders in children with idiopathic speech delay. *Clinical Linguistics & Phonetics, 33*(8), 679–706. https://doi.org/10.1080/02699206.2019.1595731

Shriberg, L. D., Lewis, B. A., Tomblin, J. B., McSweeny, J. L., Karlsson, H. B., & Scheer, A. R. (2005). Toward diagnostic and phenotypic markers for genetically transmitted speech delay. *Journal of Speech, Language, and Hearing Research, 48*(4), 834–852. https://doi.org/10.1044/1092-4388(2005/058)

Shriberg, L. D., Lohmeier, H. L., Campbell, T. F., Dollaghan, C. A., Green, J. R., & Moore, C. A. (2009). A nonword repetition task for speakers with misarticulations: The Syllable Repetition Task. *Journal of Speech, Language and Hearing Research, 52*(5), 1189–1212. https://doi.org/10.1044/1092-4388(2009/08-0047)

Shriberg, L. D., Lohmeier, H. L., Strand, E. A., & Jakielski, K. J. (2012). Encoding, memorial and transcoding deficits in Childhood Apraxia of Speech. *Clinical Linguistics & Phonetics, 26*(5), 445–482. https://doi.org/10.3109/02699206.2012.655841

Shriberg, L. D., & Mabie, H. L. (2017). Speech and motor speech assessment findings in eight complex neurodevelopmental disorders. (Technical Report No. 24). *Phonology Project, Madison: Waisman Center, University of Wisconsin–Madison.* https://phonology.waisman.wisc.edu

Shriberg, L. D., Potter, N. L., & Strand, E. A. (2011). Prevalence and phenotype of childhood apraxia of speech in youth with galactosemia. *Journal of Speech, Language, and Hearing Research, 54*(2), 487–519. https://doi.org/10.1044/1092-4388(2010/10-0068)

Shriberg, L. D., & Strand, E. A. (2018). *Speech and Motor Speech Characteristics of a Consensus Group of 28 Children with Childhood Apraxia of Speech.* (Technical Report No. 25). Phonology Project, Madison, WI: Waisman Center, University of Wisconsin–Madison. http://www.waisman.wisc.edu/phonology

Shriberg, L. D., Strand, E. A., Jakielski, K. J., & Mabie, H. L. (2019). Estimates of the prevalence of speech and motor speech disorders in persons with complex neurodevelopmental disorders. *Clinical Linguistics & Phonetics, 33*(8), 707–736. https://doi.org/10.1080/02699206.2019.1595732

Shriberg, L. D., Tomblin, J. B., & McSweeny, J. L. (1999). Prevalence of speech delay in 6-year-old children and co-morbidity with language impairment. *Journal of Speech, Language, and Hearing Research, 42*(6), 1461–1481. https://doi.org/10.1044/jslhr.4206.1461

Shriberg, L. D., & Wren, Y. E. (2019). A frequent acoustic sign of speech motor delay (SMD). *Clinical Linguistics & Phonetics, 33*(8), 757–771. https://doi.org/10.1080/02699206.2019.1595734

Stackhouse, J., & Wells, B. (1997a). *Children's speech and literacy difficulties: A psycholinguistic framework (Book 1).* Wiley.

Stackhouse, J., & Wells, B. (1997b). *Children's speech and literacy difficulties: A psycholinguistic framework.* Whurr Publishers.

Stoel-Gammon, C. (1988). *Evaluation of phonological skills in pre-school children.* Thieme Medical Publishers.

Terband, H., Maassen, B., & Maas, B. (2017). Towards a model of pediatric speech sound disorders (SSD) for differential diagnosis and therapy planning. In P. van Lieshout, B. Maassen, & H. Terband (Eds.), *Speech motor control in normal and disordered speech: Future developments in theory and methodology* (pp. 81–110). American Speech-Language-Hearing Association.

Torrington-Eaton, C., & Ratner, N. (2016). An exploration of the role of executive functions in preschoolers' phonological development. *Clinical Linguistics & Phonetics, 30*(9), 679–695. https://doi.org/10.1080/02699206.2016.1179344

Ttofari Eecen, K., Eadie, P., Morgan, A. T., & Reilly, S. (2019). Validation of Dodd's model for differential diagnosis of childhood speech sound disorders: A longitudinal community cohort study. *Developmental Medicine and Child Neurology*, *61*(6), 689–696. https://doi.org/10.1111/dmcn.13993

van Haaften, L., Diepeveen, S., van den Engel-Hoek, L., Jonker, M., de Swart, B., & Maassen, B. (2019). The psychometric evaluation of a speech production test battery for children: The reliability and validity of the computer articulation instrument. *Journal of Speech, Language & Hearing Research*, *62*(7), 2141–2170. https://doi.org/10.1044/2018_JSLHR-S-18-0274

Wagner, R. K., & Torgesen, J. K. (1987). The nature of phonological processing and its causal role in the acquisition of reading skills. *Psychological Bulletin*, *101*(2), 192–212. https://doi.org/10.1037/0033-2909.101.2.192

Waring, R. (2019). *An Investigation of the Cognitive-linguistic Profile of Children with Phonological Delay and Phonological Disorder* (Unpublished doctoral dissertation). The University of Melbourne, Victoria. http://hdl.handle.net/11343/233288

Waring, R., Eadie, P., Rickard Liow, S., & Dodd, B. (2017). Do children with phonological delay have phonological short-term and phonological working memory deficits? *Child Language Teaching & Therapy*, *33*(1), 33–46. https://doi.org/10.1177/0265659016654955

Waring, R., Eadie, P., Rickard Liow, S., & Dodd, B. (2018). The phonological memory profile of preschool children who make atypical speech sound errors. *Clinical Linguistics & Phonetics*, *32*(1), 28–45. https://doi.org/10.1080/02699206.2017.1326167

Waring, R., & Knight, R. (2013). How should children with speech sound disorders be classified? A review and critical evaluation of current classification systems. *International Journal of Language and Communication Disorders*, *48*(1), 25–40. https://doi.org/10.1111/j.1460-6984.2012.00195.x

Weiner, F. (1981a). Treatment of phonological disability using the method of meaningful contrast: Two case studies. *Journal of Speech and Hearing Disorders*, *46*(1), 97–103. https://doi.org/10.1044/jshd.4601.97

Weiner, F. (1981b). Systematic sound preference as a characteristic of phonological disability. *Journal of Speech and Hearing Disorders*, *46*(3), 281–286. https://doi.org/10.1044/jshd.4603.281

Weismer, S. E., Tomblin, J. B., Zhang, X., Buckwalter, P., Chynoweth Jan, G., & Jones, M. (2000). Nonword repetition performance in school-age children with and without language impairment. *Journal of Speech, Language, and Hearing Research*, *43*(4), 865–878. https://doi.org/10.1044/jslhr.4304.865

Wells, B., Stackhouse, J., & Vance, M. (1999). La conscience phonologique dans le cadre d'une evaluation psycholinguistique de l'enfant [Assessment of phonological awareness within a psycholinguistic framework]. *Re-education Orthophonique*, *197*, 3–12.

Williams, A. L. (2003). *Speech disorders: Resource guide for preschool children*. Thomson Delmar Learning.

Williams, A. L. (2006). A systemic perspective for assessment and intervention: A case study. *Advances in Speech-Language Pathology*, *8*(3), 245–256. https://doi.org/10.1080/14417040600823292

Wilson, E. M., Abbeduto, L., Camarata, S. M., & Shriberg, L. D. (2019). Estimates of the prevalence of speech and motor speech disorders in adolescents with Down syndrome. *Clinical Linguistics & Phonetics*, *33*(8), 772–789. https://doi.org/10.1080/02699206.2019.1595735

Wolk, L., & Meisler, A. W. (1998). Phonological assessment: A systematic comparison of conversation and picture naming. *Journal of Communication Disorders*, *31*(4), 291–313. https://doi.org/10.1016/S0021-9924(97)00092-0

Wood, K. S. (1971). Terminology and nomenclature. In L. E. Travis (Ed.), *Handbook of speech pathology and audiology* (pp. 3–29). Prentice-Hall.

World Health Organization. (2021). International Classification of Functioning, Disability and Health (ICF). https://www.who.int/standards/classifications/international-classification-of-functioning-disability-and-health

World Health Organization (WHO Workgroup for development of version of ICF for Children & Youth). (2007). *International classification of functioning, disability, and health – Version for children and youth: ICF-CY*. Geneva: World Health Organization.

Wren, Y., Miller, L. L., Peters, T. J., Emond, A., & Roulstone, S. (2016). Prevalence and predictors of persistent speech sound disorder at eight years old: Findings from a population cohort study. *Journal of Speech, Language, and Hearing Research*, *59*(4), 647–673. https://doi.org/10.1044/2015_JSLHR-S-14-0282

Chapter 3

Working with Families and Special Populations of Children

Chapter 3 begins with questions families often ask when they are considering assessment, or intervention, and when their child is receiving services for their SSD. Possible answers to those questions are expressed with as little jargon as possible. Readers might like to share the questions and answers (Q&A) with families, 'as is', or modified to suit them.

One Q&A set is in Boxes 3.1 to 3.6 all headed **Plain-English Explanations for Families**. Their topics are Box 3.1 *What is language?* Box 3.2 *What do phoneme, phone, phonetics, and morpheme mean, and what are syntax, semantics, and pragmatics?* Box 3.3 *What is speech?* Box 3.4 *What is a speech sound disorder?* Box 3.5 *How do articulation, phonological, and motor speech disorders differ?* Box 3.6 *What are the red flags and risk factors for SSD?* Although primarily geared towards non-speech-language-professionals, SLP/SLT students and assistants have commented that they have found the explanations in Boxes 3.1 to 3.6 and Boxes 3.7 to 3.10 personally informative.

Interspersed throughout the chapter is information about the prevalence of SSD; three types of screening (population, triage, and formal screening); speech assessment; audiology assessment; diagnostic evaluations; and factors in assessment and intervention related to a child with SSD's temperament, personality, and behaviour. The five expert essays here are about 'special populations' of children. The topics are listed below with the authorities' names in paratheses. The children they write about have SSD and:

1. hearing impairment (Asad, Fairgray, Teagle, and Purdy, A13)
2. 'difficult' behaviour (Bitter, A14)
3. co-occurring conditions (Stoeckel, A15)
4. language impairment (McCauley, A16)
5. craniofacial anomalies including cleft palate (Golding-Kushner, A17)

A second Q&A set of boxes (Boxes 3.7 to 3.10) is headed **The Questions Families Ask**. They contain commonly posed questions about SSD, and answers in relatively technical language for SLPs/ SLTs to modify if necessary for individual families. Their topics are: Box 3.7 *Severity: How serious is my child's problem?* Box 3.8 *Prevalence and comorbidities: Do many children have this problem? Do they have difficulties with schoolwork?* Box 3.9a Aetiology: *What caused this problem?* Box 3.9b *Aetiology: Case example.* Box 3.10 *Prognosis: What does the future hold?*

Web Questions

From 1998 to 2015, my website (Bowen, 1998) attracted around 14 000 emails containing questions and requests for advice from over 1 000 000 unique site visitors scattered worldwide, at the rate of 10 to 20 weekly. About half were from SLP/SLT practitioners, assistants, and students and the rest were from families, adults with communication disorders, professionals in other disciplines, and interested others. For this chapter, the questioners have been anonymised while the questions are unchanged.

Many asked about classification and terminology. For example, seven-year-old Michael's father, in Ireland, wrote that his son had seen his first SLT in an early intervention program and had been seeing his second for two years. He explained that Michael had a repaired cleft palate and hearing, language and literacy, speech, and voice quality (resonance) issues and said:

> *I know when our SLTs talk about "language" and "speech" they mean different things, but I'm unsure of the distinction. I tried looking it up, but oh my goodness.*
>
> KEVIN (see Boxes 3.1 and 3.3)

He emailed again weeks later, hoping to better understand more terms, including 'phoneme', 'morpheme', and 'syntax', and querying the use of the word 'pragmatics':

> *Hi, back again! Our SLT says Michael's pragmatics are good, and that that is a real plus, but I'm unclear what that means. I don't want to confess that I don't know these things after all this time. The SLT might think I've been bluffing my way through our many conversations about Michael.*
>
> KEVIN (see Box 3.2)

Writing from Canada, the mother of an unintelligible 4-year-old asked:

> *Can you tell me, please, the difference between a speech sound disorder, a disorder of articulation and a phonological disorder; how can you tell them apart? I think my daughter Natasia suffers from one of these.*
>
> JODI (see Box 3.4)

A couple from South Africa wrote:

> *Six weeks ago, Sajna our 5-year-old was assessed for a 2nd opinion by a PhD speech and language pathologist in Joburg who diagnosed a phonological disorder or phonological impairment. But our speechie in Boksburg says she has "a phonological PROCESSING disorder" and needs a lot of "ARTIC WORK". We are so, so confused: help!*
>
> VIKAS AND MEKA (see the two notes in Box 3.5)

Justin in New Zealand said:

> *Our Cameron is a great little guy. He is a bright boy, but his speech is usually impossible for anyone outside the family to understand, including his teacher and the lady who runs his swimming lessons. We're also a bit worried that he shows no interest in being read stories or in reading. In truth, his teacher is quite concerned about that, but we haven't forced the issue. We've taken him to two Ministry of Ed speech-language therapists, but they both couldn't persuade him to cooperate. He went from Dr. Jekyll to Mr. Hyde the instant they wanted him to do something, followed by an epic meltdown each time (two months apart). At home school, and swimming you wouldn't know he was capable of that. I am writing to ask your advice. Is there a type of therapy he should have, as well as, or instead of speech therapy? Cameron has just turned 6.*
>
> JUSTIN (see Bitter, A.14)

Ethics and Time

The questions raised ethical and time-related issues. It would be unethical to provide any advice or input about a child I had not assessed and/or who was someone else's client; besides the prospect of answering all 14 000 emails individually was formidable. The questions, however, stimulated the idea that SLPs/SLTs might value web-based, plain English explanations of some of our concepts, terms, and processes. Perhaps they could point their clients to them, saving time and facilitating parent-to-practitioner discussions with the child's *own* SLP/SLT.

Meanwhile, I could provide questioners with links to relevant pages, with the strong suggestion that they discuss the content and its relevance (or not) to their child, with the treating clinician acquainted with the child, the family, and 'the history'. I would also remind questioners of the disclaimer, present on the site since its inception, '*The information provided on speech-language-therapy dot com is designed to support, not to replace, the relationship that exists between a client/site visitor and their speech-language pathologist (SLP) / speech and language therapist (SLT)*'.

So, the 'web questions' drove the development of certain not-too-technical information on my website. Variations of the information are shown in Boxes 3.1 to 3.10. They are intended as guides to what practitioners might say in response to typical questions from families, or to prompt reflection around how they might answer in their own words, to match the needs of families on their caseloads. Multilingual SLP/SLT clinicians have translated the content for clients to read and discuss in their preferred language(s). For some clients, the 'plain English' will not be plain enough. As well, some clients do not want explanations – plain-English or otherwise – or to be 'educated', they simply want their child's speech-language issues addressed.

Box 3.1   Plain-English explanations for families

What is language?

Human language is partly innate (inborn) and partly learned from interactions with the people in our world. The 'learned' part is like a code or a set of systematic rules that enable us to communicate ideas and express wants and needs. Reading, writing, spelling, gesturing including signing, and speaking are all forms of language. For convenience, we can think of language as having two main divisions: receptive language, or understanding what

is said, read, or signed; and expressive language, or speaking, writing, and spelling, or signing. Key aspects of language are phonology, morphology, syntax, semantics, and pragmatics. Note particularly that phonology, and hence phonological disorder come under the heading of language.

Phonology concerns speech sounds in languages and the rules for how those sounds combine to form words 'legally', without breaking the rules, and how they are said. It is one component of language, along with semantics (vocabulary), morphology (grammar), syntax (sentence structure), and pragmatics (the non-verbal social rules). Two types of SSD are considered phonological in nature: phonological disorder (phonological impairment) and inconsistent speech disorder (inconsistent phonological disorder) see Figures i1 and 3.1.

The explanation of 'language' in Box 3.1 may lead some family members to ask for clarification of some or all the terms used, such as phoneme, phone, phonetics, morpheme, syntax, semantics, and pragmatics.

Box 3.2   Plain-English explanations for families

What is meant by the terms: phonology, phoneme, phone, phonetics, morphology, morpheme, syntax, semantics, and pragmatics?

Phonology is the study of the sound system of languages, involving close inspection of the phonemes and phones that are present in the language being studied (e.g., the phonology of Danish, the phonology of French, etc.) The **phoneme** is the smallest unit within a language that can distinguish meanings between words, while a **phone** or individual 'speech sound', is the smallest unit of speech.

Phonetics is the study of the physical characteristics of phones. Linguists describe the phonemes that are used in the languages they have chosen to study, pinpointing the rules that govern how they are combined into words and longer utterances. In the process, they apply their knowledge of phonetics and phonology, often using **phonetic symbols** to transcribe (write down) speech.

Morphology is the study of the structure of words. **Morphemes** are the smallest meaningful units within a language. For example, 'white' and 'green' in the sentence 'I like white, and green

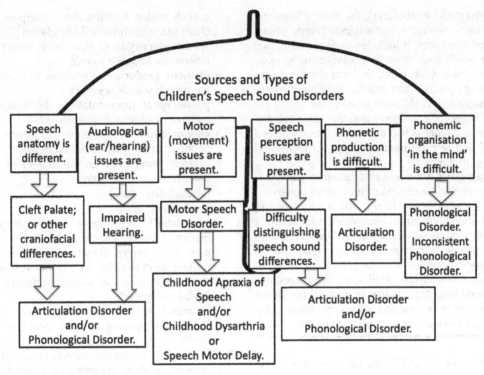

Figure 3.1   The SSD Umbrella showing the sources and types of children's speech sound disorders, with plain(er)-English labels. © Caroline Bowen 2023.

together' have one morpheme (one unit of meaning) each and are 'monomorphemic'. The words 'whites' and 'greens' as in 'The wallpaper's whites and greens changed the room from uncolourful to colourful'. 'Whites' and 'greens' are bimorphemic with two morphemes, the **root morphemes** (or base form that has just one meaning) white and green and the **bound morpheme** 's' which is an inflection that indicates number. The three types of bound morphemes are added to root morphemes to make more complex words. They are **prefixes**, **suffixes**, and **inflections**.

○ **Prefixes** change the meaning of the word but not the grammatical class; for example, 'un—' changes the verb 'cover' to the verb 'uncover'; 'il—' changes the adjective 'logical' to the adjective 'illogical'; and 'nano—' changes the noun 'technology' to 'nanotechnology'.
○ **Suffixes** change meaning and grammatical class. For example, '—er' changes 'lead' (verb) to 'leader' (noun); '—ant' changes 'vigil' (noun) to 'vigilant' (adjective); and '—ly' changes 'slow' (adjective) to 'slowly' (adverb).

Uncolourful, in 'The wallpaper's whites and greens changed the room from uncolourful to colourful', above is trimorphemic, with three morphemes: colour (root), un (prefix), ful (suffix).
○ **Inflections** provide information about grammatical categories such as number (e.g., lion – lions), case (e.g., Ruth – Ruth's), verb tense (e.g., jump – jumps, jumping, jumped), comparatives (e.g., quick – quicker), and superlatives (quicker – quickest).

<u>Syntax</u> concerns the arrangement of words and phrases into grammatical sentences that follow the syntactic rules of a given language. For example, 'Leo **is parking** their car at the station every weekday' is grammatically correct in German, but not strictly correct in English where you would say, 'Leo **parks** their car at the station every weekday'. In French the word choices in 'I **live** in Ankara since last year', and 'I can't stay for dinner. **I do my** study' are correct, but in English they would change to something like 'I**'ve lived** in Ankara since last year' and 'I can't stay for dinner. **I must** study' or 'I can't stay for dinner **because I must** study'.

Semantics (vocabulary) is the study of linguistic meaning, covering the meanings of words, phrases, and sentences. It includes understanding that some words have more than one meaning (e.g., cricket, lock, stall, ham), or have similar meanings (e.g., precise, and exact), or different meanings signalled by different word-stress – e.g., the verb 'ob**ject**' ('to protest') and the noun '**ob**ject' ('a thing'), re**bel** (verb) and **re**bel (noun), re**cord** (verb) and **re**cord (noun), and **pro**ject (verb) and pro**ject** (noun).

Pragmatics is the area of language function that embraces the use of language in social contexts – knowing what to say, how to say it, and when to say it; modifying our communication for different listeners and social situations; and how to 'be' with other people. It includes all the nonverbal aspects of communication like facial expression, turn-taking (you talk – I listen – I talk – you listen), gestures and body language, choices of words, how formal or informal to be, and relating appropriately to the situation and the person or people present.

The ways SLPs/SLTs use the terms **speech** and **language**, **speech disorder** and **language disorder**, can be mystifying for some of our clients and colleagues, and the 'what is speech?' and the 'what is the difference between speech and language?' questions occur a lot. Some people hesitate to ask these questions, out of embarrassment or because they think they should know the answer, but *not* understanding the distinctions adds to the confusion experienced by families and others who have difficulty comprehending the jargon in our verbal explanations and in our written reports.

Box 3.3   Plain-English explanations for families

What is speech?

Speech is the spoken (oral) medium of language. The ability to speak clearly enough for others to comprehend us relies on interrelated factors, including satisfactory:

- ○ **speech anatomy**: the articulators and vocal tract
- ○ **speech physiology**: respiration, phonation, and articulation/resonance systems
- ○ **hearing**: with or without a hearing aid(s) or cochlea implant(s)

- ○ **speech motor function** that underpins precisely planned and timed articulation
- ○ **speech perception** to allow us to detect fine differences between sounds
- ○ **phonetic production**: the ability to articulate the speech sounds we need
- ○ **phonological representation**: the system of contrasting phones stored mentally
- ○ **phonotactics**: to assemble sequences of phones that form syllables and words
- ○ **prosody**: word-tones, grammatical-tones, rhythm, stress, and intonation
- ○ **intelligibility**: the degree to which a speaker can be understood
- ○ **acceptability**: the 'appropriateness' or **pragmatics** of an individual's speech, in terms of their age, gender, status, and culture, that enables them to participate in society (e.g., at home, school, and a variety of informal and formal gatherings).

- The **motor** (motoric) aspect of speech deals with the movements of the articulators (larynx or 'voice box', tongue, lips, and palate).
- The **phonetic produc**tion aspect of speech takes care of articulation: the motor act of producing phones (vowels and consonants) so that we have a repertoire of all the sounds we need.
- The **phonological representation** aspect is the component of language function that oversees the phonemes. It involves the 'brainwork' that sees to organising the phones into patterns of sound contrasts.
- **Phonotactics** is to do with arranging speech segments – phones in syllables and words – into the correct order.
- **Prosody** makes our speech 'expressive'; in tonal languages it includes word and grammar tones, and in all languages, it involves rhythm, strong and weak word stress (e.g., **pro**ject versus pro**ject**), and intonation or variations in the pitch of the voice (e.g., 'You need one of these.' versus 'You need one of these?').

While simple with impossibly discrete levels, the SSD Umbrella in Figure i.1 is useful in explaining to SLP/SLT students new to the topic, and to clinicians in need of a refresher, on how the components dovetail and interact. The version of the SSD Umbrella displayed in Figure 3.1 in Box 3.4, is intended for parents and other important people in the life of a child with SSD and contains slightly less jargon.

Box 3.4   Plain-English explanations for families

What is a speech sound disorder (SSD)?

> *Children with speech sound disorders experience any mixture of problems with speech perception, speech motor function/articulation, and/or phonological representation of phones (consonants and vowels), phonotactics, and prosody that may impact speech intelligibility and acceptability.*

Sources and Types of Children's Speech Sound Disorders (SSD)

Figure 3.1 begins with an umbrella heading 'Sources and Types of Children's Speech Sound Disorders'. The top row of 'boxes' (rectangles) holds six potential sources of SSD: anatomic, audiologic, motoric, perceptual, phonetic, and phonemic issues. These lead to six underlying causes of SSD: craniofacial differences, hearing impairment, motor speech disorder, speech perception difficulties in distinguishing differences between speech sounds (e.g., not distinguishing the difference between *rabbit* and *wabbit*, *sum* and *thumb*, or *catch* and *cash*), articulation disorder, and phonological disorder. Finally, there are three boxes that indicate that craniofacial differences, hearing impairment, and perception issues can all be implicated in articulation disorder and/or phonological disorder, while motor speech disorder can be in the form of childhood apraxia of speech (CAS) and/or childhood dysarthria.

The most frequent 'frequently asked questions' from www.speech-language-therapy.com visitors have been about distinguishing between the different types of SSD. Around one third of these questions have come from parents, foster parents, home schooling parents, and grandparents of children diagnosed with or suspected to have SSD, another third from SLP/SLT students, and the remainder from SLP/SLT clinicians, other health, and education professionals (e.g., doctors, psychologists, school counsellors, social workers, teachers), journalists, young people through to adults with SSD or SSD histories, and secondary school students aspiring to pursue SLP/SLT as a career.

Box 3.5   Plain-English explanations for families

How do articulation, phonological, and motor speech disorders differ?

It is important to remember that SLPs/SLTs make a distinction between **speech** and **language** (see Boxes 3.1 and 3.3). One way of understanding the difference between articulation disorders and phonological disorders is to think of articulation difficulties (phonetic production difficulties) as happening 'in the mouth' or 'on the lips', and phonological difficulties (phonemic organisation difficulties) as happening 'mentally' or 'in the mind' (Grunwell, 1989).

Articulation Disorder

This is a **speech disorder** that adversely affects phonetic production so the child has difficulty saying certain consonants and vowels. Children with typical anatomy and normal hearing may have articulation disorders, and so can children with 'craniofacial' (head and face) differences such as cleft palate, as well as children with hearing impairment. Articulation (phonetic production) issues and phonological disorder often co-occur in the same child. Also, a sizable proportion of children with articulation disorders have difficulty discriminating between certain speech sounds (e.g., recognising that *'ride'* and *'wide'* start with different sounds and sound different from each other).

> ○ **NOTE 1 in response to the question from Vikas and Meka**
>   SLTs/SLPs to refer, accurately, to intervention for **articulation disorder** as 'articulation therapy/intervention', or 'artic therapy/intervention' and to children as having problems with 'articulation' or 'artic'. Confusion arises for clients and others when SLPs/SLTs use the term 'articulation disorder' as a cover term for *all* speech sound disorders (SSD), or as a cover term for articulation *and* phonological disorders. It is common to hear SLPs/SLTs say things like, 'she needs work on her artic' when it would be more accurate to say, 'her phonology needs work'.

Phonological Disorder

Odd as it may seem, phonological disorder is a language disorder that affects phonemic organisation, therefore affecting speech. A way of expressing this is to say that *phonological disorder is a speech sound disorder with linguistic (language) foundations*. The child can either already say the phones (vowels and consonants), or can be taught to relatively easily, but they have difficulty organising them into consistent patterns of contrasts. There are two types of phonological disorder:

1. **phonological impairment** (also called **phonological disorder**), and
2. **inconsistent speech disorder** (also called **inconsistent phonological disorder**).

As with articulation disorder, children with phonological disorders may have typical anatomy and normal hearing; or they may have 'craniofacial' (head and face) differences such as cleft palate; and/or they may have impaired hearing. Many children with phonological disorder and normal hearing have difficulty recognising the difference ('discriminating'), by listening, between certain speech sounds, as in the *'ride'* and *'wide'* example above.

> ○ **NOTE 2 Also in response to the question from Vikas and Meka**
> Unfortunately, some SLPs/SLTs modify the term phonological disorder, calling it: *phonological processing disorder, phonological process disorder,* or *phonological processes disorder*. While these made-up 'diagnoses' are commonly used – on the internet, in informational handouts, and in SLP/SLT reports – they are inaccurate and are not suitable alternatives to the well-defined terms 'phonological disorder' or 'phonological impairment'.

Motor Speech Disorders (MSD)

Motoric or 'motor speech' disorders are speech disorders. There are two main types of MSD that can co-occur in the same child.

Childhood Apraxia of Speech (CAS)

The first main type of MSD, which is comparatively uncommon, but not as rare as once thought (Shriberg, Kwiatkowski et al., 2019), is **childhood apraxia of speech** (CAS), also called **developmental verbal dyspraxia** (DVD), although use of the term DVD is dwindling. Children with CAS have difficulty planning and programming the movements required for speech reliably and smoothly with normal prosody (see Box 3.3).

Childhood Dysarthria

The second main type of MSD, which is particularly common in children with cerebral palsy, is **childhood dysarthria** (also called **developmental dysarthria**). Children with childhood dysarthria have difficulty making the movements required for speech, and often have difficulties performing the movements necessary for eating and drinking (sucking, chewing, and swallowing). There are several types of childhood dysarthria, so some authorities refer to them a 'the dysarthrias'. They are spastic dysarthria, flaccid dysarthria, ataxic dysarthria, hyperkinetic dysarthria, and mixed dysarthria. An additional type, hypokinetic dysarthria, mainly occurs in Parkinson's disease in adults. The dysarthrias in children and young people have many different causes, including cerebral palsy, neonatal stroke, and traumatic brain injury (TBI). In childhood dysarthria the speech mechanism, including the muscles of respiration (breathing), may be paralysed, weak, or poorly co ordinated. The dysarthrias can affect all motor speech processes – breathing, phonation (making speech sounds), articulation, resonance, and prosody.

Speech Assessment: Expectations

In numeric terms, there are two major SSD subgroups on typical SLP/SLT caseloads. First, poorly unintelligible preschoolers and children below age 9;0 with low percentages of consonants correct (PCCs) and multiple errors; and second, acceptably intelligible 'older' school-aged students with high PCCs and residual errors. Residual errors are those that have persisted beyond 9 years of age and into adulthood (Shriberg et al., 1997; Van Borsel et al., 2007). In practice, clinicians often reserve the terms 'articulation disorder' and 'functional articulation disorder' for the reasonably intelligible children of all ages, with one or just a few speech production difficulties, characteristically involving /s/, /z/, /l/ and /ɹ/ and, in some settings, /θ/ and /ð/ also.

Prevalence of SSD

According to surveys conducted in the United Kingdom, some 6.5% of all children have SSD (Broomfield & Dodd, 2004) and Pring et al. (2012) found that 82% of surveyed paediatric SLTs served children with speech difficulties. Broomfield and Dodd (2004) reported that of 1 100 children referred to a mainstream paediatric speech and language therapy service over a period of 15 months, 12.5% of children had articulation disorder and no children in their cohort had CAS. The remaining 87.5% had a phonological disorder. Using Dodd's classification, the *Differential Diagnostic Classification System; DDCS*, described in Chapter 2, of the 87.5%, 57.5% had phonological delay, 20.6% had consistent phonological disorder, and 9.4% had inconsistent phonological disorder.

Shriberg, Kwiatkowski et al. (2019) confirmed earlier studies that determined the prevalence rate for idiopathic CAS to be one in 1 000 children which is less than 1% of the SSD caseload (see Table 2.3). Also in Table 2.3 are the Shriberg, et al. population prevalence figures for CAS (2.4%), Childhood Dysarthria (3.4%), Speech Delay (82.2%), Speech Delay and Concurrent Motor Speech Disorder (17.8%), and Speech Motor Delay (12%).

Speech Assessment

Recapping the information in Chapter 2, speech assessment involves careful, informed observations and hypothesis testing. It normally begins with the referral, collecting an account of what prompted the referral, gathering basic identifying information, and a brief case history interview, followed by a preliminary, informal screening procedure in which the SLP/SLT listens to and watches the child speak.

Referral to Audiology

If, in the clinician's expert view, speech or language concerns are present, consultation with an audiologist is recommended. In some clinical and education settings, children are not seen for initial consultation *unless* they have had an audiogram, or at least have an appointment for one booked within a week or so. In such settings, audiology referral is therefore mandatory. The audiologist decides which tests to administer, but usually they

will proceed with pure tone audiometry (a hearing test with headphones) and tympanometry (to check middle ear and eustachian tube function). In more developed countries (in the minority world) and in various other countries it is routine for a child with a speech and/or language disorder to have these important tests. The audiometry results are displayed as a graph called an audiogram (see Figure 3.2) and the tympanometry results are displayed in a graph called a tympanogram (Figure 3.3).

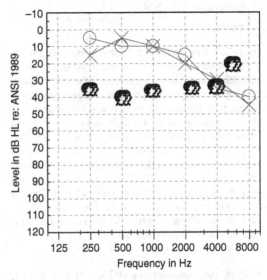

Figure 3.2 Pure tone audiogram showing mild bilateral, high-frequency hearing loss. Circles=right ear; crosses=left ear hearing thresholds. Normal hearing thresholds are in the range −10 to +15 dB HL. The dB HL scale represents hearing levels relative to hearing of young 'otologically normal' 18–30-year-olds. Face symbols on some graphs represent average speech level in each frequency region for conversational speech (59 dB SPL at 1 m spoken by an adult female). Even with mild hearing loss, high-frequency speech sounds (e.g., /s/) are close to hearing threshold, and may not be audible. The term 'speech banana' is used to refer to the speech spectrum since speech is softest for very low and high frequencies and loudest at low-mid frequencies, producing a banana shape plotted on the audiogram. Hearing thresholds of 16–25 dB HL=slight hearing loss, 26–40 dB= mild, 41–55 dB=moderate, 56–70 dB=moderate-severe, 71–90 dB= severe, and >90 dB=profound (Adapted from (American Speech-Language-Hearing Association, 2015)).

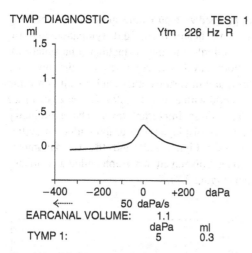

TYMP DIAGNOSTIC   TEST 1
  ml   Ytm 226 Hz R

EARCANAL VOLUME: 1.1
                       daPa   ml
TYMP 1:   5   0.3

Figure 3.3 This is a normal 'Type A' tympanogram. The ear canal volume of 1.1 mL is estimated based on the admittance at +200 daPa pressure, when the eardrum is clamped with positive pressure and there is reduced energy flow through the middle ear. The peak occurs close to zero pressure, at 5 daPa, with a normal peak admittance value of 0.3 mL. 'Admittance' refers to flow of energy through a mechanical system (eardrum, middle ear space, and middle ear ossicles). Peaks that occur below −100 daPa ('Type C' tympanograms) indicate negative middle ear pressure. Flat 'Type B' tympanograms indicate either a perforation in the eardrum (if volume is high) or a blocked middle ear (if volume is low), usually due to OME.

- **Pure tone audiometry (PTA).** PTA is used to measure hearing sensitivity. Tones are presented via earphones. If a loudspeaker is used with young children only the 'better' ear is tested. The softest levels at which tones are detected are hearing thresholds (measured in dB HL). In preschoolers, PTA is accomplished using conditioned play that turns the test into a game of putting a block or peg into a hole when a sound is heard. In children 6–24 months **visual reinforcement audiometry (VRA)** is used. Infants turn their heads in response to sounds, and this is reinforced by the sounds being accompanied by an illuminated, moving mechanical puppet (Northern & Downs, 2002).
- **Tympanometry.** Tympanometry is used to measure middle ear function. The tympanometer probe inserted into the ear contains a pressure pump, tone generator, and microphone to measure sound levels. As ear canal pressure changes

from positive to negative, the eardrum is 'clamped' by the pressure, then released, then clamped again. This causes a peak in the tympanogram near normal air pressure, as shown in Figure 3.3. The peak indicates maximum middle ear admittance (energy flow through the system); this should be close to 0 decaPascals (daPa) pressure, indicating normal eustachian tube aeration of the middle ear

Essential Collaboration between Audiologists and SLPS/SLTS

An SLP's/SLT's grasp of typical speech and language development, and what can go wrong with them, is critical to understanding an individual child's language and/or speech disorder. It is underpinned by research and practice information from the sciences of audiology, dentistry, linguistics, medicine, neurology, psychology, speech-language pathology itself, and related disciplines. The reliance on knowledge from kindred professional disciplines is nowhere more evident than in SLPs'/SLTs' frequent collaboration with audiologists. In affluent countries and parts of the developing world, most children, with or without typical hearing, who see an SLP/SLT will see, or have already seen an audiologist. In A13, SLTs Areej Asad and Liz Fairgray, and audiologists Holly Teagle and Suzanne Purdy discuss the assessment and management of the 'special population' of children who wear hearing aids and children fitted with cochlea implants.

Dr. Areej N. Asad is a Speech Language Therapist and a Postdoctoral Research Fellow in Audiology at the University of Auckland, New Zealand. In 2008, Areej completed her postgraduate degree with honours and worked as a Speech Language Pathologist, in the Center for Phonetics Research, Speech and Hearing Clinic at the University of Jordan. She completed a PhD at the University of Auckland in 2016. Her research interests include speech sound disorder, hearing loss, the narrative abilities of children with hearing loss, dynamic assessment, the use of communication assistive technology with children with autism, paraprofessional collaborative work (e.g., psychologists, audiologists, and speech-language therapists), emotional and behavioural challenges for children with communication disorder, bilingualism, and optimal speech-language therapy approaches for monolingual and bilingual children.

Liz Fairgray is a Speech Language Therapist and Clinical Educator at The University of Auckland where she had worked since 2007. For the past 35 years, her area of clinical interest and expertise has been combined speech pathology and audiology. In 1998, she became the founding therapist for *The Hearing House*, a centre for oral communication in children with profound hearing loss and cochlear implants. Liz was the first New Zealander to become a Certified Auditory Verbal Therapist and combines AVT techniques with SLT when working with children. Liz uses a family-centred approach, ensuring that collaboration with parents equips them to conduct follow-up activities at home and practice the targets in a natural setting. Liz also provides clinical education to students, supervises projects and lectures in the programme for Master of Speech Language Therapy Practice.

Dr. Holly F. B. Teagle is a clinical audiologist who has provided patient care and collaborated in clinical research related to cochlear implantation for many years. Holly has published over 60 peer-reviewed articles, authored 13 chapters for academic textbooks or conference proceedings and has presented at local, national, and international conferences. Currently, Holly is an Associate Professor in Audiology at the University of Auckland, New Zealand, and is the Clinical Director of Audiology and Habilitation at The Hearing House in Auckland. She provides classroom instruction for graduate audiology students, supervises research projects, and oversees The Hearing House clinical team. Research interests include cochlear implant outcomes, focusing on device efficacy and clinical management issues.

Dr. Suzanne C. Purdy, CNZM, is Professor and Head of School at the University of Auckland's School of Psychology and principal investigator in the Centre for Brain Research and the Brain Research New Zealand Centre of Research Excellence. Suzanne trained as a clinical audiologist at the University of Melbourne in 1981 after completing a master's in psychology. After a period of clinical work, she began researching hearing aid fitting and electrophysiological assessment of hearing for infants, prior to completing a PhD at the University of Iowa in 1990. With colleagues, she has established audiology and speech language therapy master's programmes at the University of Auckland. Her research interests encompass the disciplines of speech-language, hearing, and psychology and include communication disorders, electrophysiological assessment of hearing, auditory processing disorder, and neurological conditions. In the 2021 Queen's Birthday Honours, Purdy was appointed a Companion of the New Zealand Order of Merit (CNZM), for services to audiology and communication science.

Q13. Areej Asad, Liz Fairgray, Holly Teagle, and Suzanne Purdy: Children with Hearing Loss

What are the essential ingredients in assessing and treating the speech perception and production of children who were fitted with cochlear implant/s (CIs) and or hearing aid/s (HAs)? What are the key points SLPs/SLTs should cover in discussion with the child's audiologist(s) when preparing to intervene with this population? How would SLP/SLT intervention for CI(s) users and HA(s) differ from what happens with children who have speech sound disorder and normal hearing (CWSSD)?

A13. Areej N. Asad, Holly F.B. Teagle, Liz Fairgray, and Suzanne C. Purdy : Speech Perception and Production in Children with Hearing Loss: Assessment and Management

Advancements in hearing technologies, including high-end digital hearing aids (HAs), cochlear implant (CI) systems, and other hearing assistive technologies, enable audiologists to optimise children's use of sound. Access to sounds across the speech spectrum affords progress in receptive and expressive spoken language, and makes possible cascading impacts of good hearing, among them peer-to-peer social engagement and academic progress. Beyond early identification of hearing loss and appropriate fitting of hearing devices, several other factors affect communication outcomes that are unique to each deaf or hard of hearing child, including hearing history, aetiology, anatomy of the cochlea and status of the auditory nerve, and (re)habilitation and family support.

Children with mild-to-moderate hearing losses with sufficient residual hearing can access the speech spectrum through HAs. Carefully programmed HAs provide access to speech by selectively amplifying sound to targeted intensity levels, using evidence-based algorithms that optimise access to speech and listening comfort. Through HA programming software, the audiologist applies signal processing features that compress sound, both in intensity and frequency, into the child's comfortable listening dynamic range (softest audible to maximum comfortable sound). Compression ensures speech is accessible but introduces sound distortion that can influence discrimination of speech sounds.

HAs acoustically amplify sound which travels through the outer and middle ear to stimulate the cochlea and auditory nerve. CIs, which are recommended for severe to profound sensorineural hearing losses, bypass the outer and middle ear and stimulate the auditory nerve directly. CIs are designed to detect, convert, code, and transmit salient features of acoustic signals into electrical signals that are delivered to the cochlea. Critical features of pitch, loudness, and timing that make speech intelligible are coded by CI software that converts acoustic signals into electrical signals, with speech features coded by number and location of electrodes and type, rate, and amplitude of electrical stimulation.

Other assistive hearing technologies such as remote microphones or streaming functions from audio and video sources (i.e., phones, television, computers) that improve access in complex listening environments become increasingly essential as a child progresses through school. These technologies improve speech perception by overcoming problems of distance and poor signal-to-noise ratio. The child's use of additional technology such as remote microphone hearing aid systems (RM-HAs) in the classroom or at home necessitates liaison between the SLP/SLT and audiologist to optimise use of the technology and troubleshoot listening difficulties (Muñoz & Blaiser, 2011). Regular audiological care is essential to monitor hearing levels, maintain and update hearing technologies as a child grows, and assess progress, ensuring each child's access to sound allows them to achieve their potential for communication. Hearing device use must be consistent; studies of device use, whether HAs or CIs, strongly support full-time use (Park et al., 2019; Walker et al., 2015).

Communication and Collaboration between SLPS/SLTS and Audiologists

In child- and family-centred intervention approaches, the audiologist, SLP/SLT, Early Interventionist and other team members work alongside one another and with the family (Moeller et al., 2013). The audiogram, hearing technology, amplification, and RMHAs (previously referred to as frequency modulation/FM systems) are key topics that SLPs/SLTs discuss with audiologists (Schafer & Sweeney, 2012). SLPs/SLTs should request the child's audiogram and information about hearing technology to develop therapy goals and support the child's Individualized Education Program (IEP). The audiogram provides information about the degree and configuration of hearing loss and will show which speech sounds (if any) the child can access without amplification. When aided, if a child is not able to repeat sounds from the Ling six-sound test (Ling, 2002), auditory only, during a behavioural listening check, SLPs/SLTs should refer the child to the audiologist to check CI mapping and/or HA settings.

Audiologists can support the SLP/SLT and Early Interventionist by providing instructions on how to clean/troubleshoot/maintain hearing devices, in an accessible format that can be shared with teachers, family, and other professionals. Even with amplification and additional assistive technology such as RMHAs, Children with Hearing Loss (CWHL) can struggle to localise sound and understand speech in noisy learning environments, hence it is important that SLPs/SLTs work collaboratively with Early Interventionists and/or Itinerant Teachers of the Deaf (ITOD) to evaluate and monitor the child's use and progress with hearing technology.

Speech Assessment for CWHL

SLPs/SLTs evaluate the speech of CWHL by conducting an orofacial examination, using standardised speech assessments, and collecting conversational or spontaneous speech samples (Bauman-Waengler, 2020) to identify facial anomalies and speech errors. The speech of CWHL should be assessed using standardized assessments such as the Diagnostic Evaluation of Articulation and Phonology (DEAP) (Dodd et al., 2002), Goldman-Fristoe Test of Articulation (GFTA-3) (Goldman & Fristoe, 2015), and the Hodson Assessment of Phonological Patterns-Third Edition (HAPP-3) (Asad et al., 2018; Ching & Dillon, 2013; Hodson, 2004; St John et al., 2020). It is not known which assessment provides SLPs/SLTs with the most relevant, detailed information about the type of speech errors of CWHL. For example, the HAPP-3 and DEAP Articulation subtests both examine vowel inventory, but vowels are not included in the GFTA-2. The DEAP provides clinicians with information about the type of speech errors (developmental or unusual patterns) and the extent of the identified phonological delay. The HAPP-3 is also used to rate speech severity and describe types of phonological patterns.

Contemporary studies indicate that standardized speech assessments do not provide SLPs/SLTs with a sufficiently comprehensive evaluation and many recommend adding supplementary data such as using additional words (Kirk & Vigeland, 2015). No single test covers the consonant inventory in onset and coda position, consonant accuracy in onset and coda position, and developmental and non-developmental phonological processes; hence several assessments are needed to encompass the range of effects of hearing loss on speech for CWHL.

Speech Perception in CWHL

Speech perception (and hence production) for children using HAs and CIs relies on the integrity of surviving neural elements, but HA success also depends on surviving hair cells within the cochlea. Outer hair cells amplify cochlear responses to soft sounds and intact inner hair cells across a range of frequencies are needed to transmit the amplified signal delivered by the HA to the auditory nerve. Although audibility of speech sounds is critical for the development of speech, the ability to resolve speech sounds based on loudness, pitch and timing is also important. Beyond the cochlea and the nerve, central auditory processes affect speech perception and functional use of sound. Central auditory abilities such as pitch and temporal discrimination are needed for discrimination of speech sounds that differ in frequency content (e.g., /ʃ/ vs /s/) or temporal features such as duration or voice onset time (e.g., /pa/ vs /ba/).

Audiologists typically measure speech perception using open- or closed-set lists of words or sentences, with the child responding by selecting objects or pictures or repeating what they heard. Such measures are useful for monitoring overall progress but not informative for setting SLP/SLT intervention goals. A meta-analysis of consonant and vowel identification in CI users measured using nonsense words (Rødvik et al., 2018) found the most common consonant confusions were those with same manner of articulation, for example, confusion between /k/ and /t/, /m/ and /n/, and /p/ and /t/. Vowel perception primarily relies on low-frequency first and second formant frequency cues between 200 Hz and 2500 Hz and hence may depend on length of the electrode insertion in CI users. Activation of low-frequency nerve fibres in the apex of the cochlea requires full electrode insertion, which may be compromised due to congenital cochlear anomalies or, ossification post-meningitis, as examples. Speech perception varies more amongst HA users due to variations in amplified hearing and signal processing strategies. High-frequency hearing loss impacts the audibility and discriminability of consonants with energy above 3000–4000 Hz (/s/, /ʃ/, /t/, /z/ and /ʒ /), and speech contrasts such as /p/-/t/-/k/ may be discriminable in quiet but not in noise (Phatak et al., 2009). A perceptual basis for speech sound disorders is likely in CWHL, especially those with greater degrees of hearing loss for whom HAs fail to enable full audibility of speech sounds or provide distorted access. Their speech perception abilities are then further compromised when background noise is present.

SLP/SLT Intervention for CWHL vs. CWSSD

Despite advances in hearing technologies, early intervention is required for the child to learn to actively listen and interpret the auditory signal. Actively embedding information into the auditory cortex is essential for CWHL to commence their journey to clear speech. A comparison between therapy for CWHL and CWSSD shows that there are many similarities. Importantly, some differences relate to the sequencing of interventions rather than to different techniques. CWSSD may present with idiosyncratic processes, whereas CWHL tend to have a combination of delayed and disordered productions. An auditory verbal therapy (AVT) approach now falls under the global certification domain of Listening and Spoken Language Specialists (LSLS) under the auspices of the AG Bell Academy. It is widely used with CWHL and relies on the child receiving good access to speech sounds through hearing technology that is optimised for the child's hearing loss. This approach emphasizes listening as the primary mode of communication, early identification of hearing loss, and optimal amplification to enhance access to speech and discrimination of speech sounds. Acoustic highlighting is a key element, involving significant use of suprasegmental pitch, duration, and rhythm features of speech, and is an important element of the therapy process for CWHL. Consistent with LSLS principles, signal-to-noise ratio is optimized by sitting close to the child's better hearing ear (aided) and minimising noise in the therapy environment.

For CI users, the tonotopic arrangement of the electrode array, which ensures better stimulation of high-frequency than low-frequency nerve fibres, means that children are particularly sensitive to the high-frequency fricatives /s, z, ʃ, f, ʒ / and the affricate /tʃ/. These phonemes can be acquired early in children with CIs but may be inaudible or not discriminated in children with moderate-severe hearing loss fitted with HAs. In CWSSD, fricatives are often produced inaccurately due to the persistent retention of phonological processes such as stopping, and cluster reduction. More commonly a CWHL may have persistent final consonant deletion, nasalisation, a favoured sound, and use of glottal replacements for velars.

We see these error-types in the case of Bobby, summarised below. His intervention included many techniques used for CWSSD, but in a different order. The therapy briefly outlined here for Bobby can be provided by paediatric SLPs/SLTs and is ideally augmented by Auditory Verbal Techniques which emphasize listening (Estabrooks et al., 2016). Bobby had bilateral CIs activated at 15 months. He produced ten words but only the open vowels /a/ and /æ/, /ʌ/ and /ɪ/ were recognisable, so other vowels were targeted. Early intervention initially included protowords (e.g., 'Oh-ooh. It broke', Step-wise pitch rise 'Up, up, up, whee down', Long duration 'Nigh-nigh') to highlight suprasegmentals (of stress, intonation and duration) that CWHL may struggle to hear (Most & Peled, 2007).

The low-frequency bilabials were established and presented with words featuring maximum contrasts in their acoustic features. As the Ling sound check showed that Bobby had full access to the long-duration, high-frequency speech sound /ʃ/, his therapist targeted fricatives (contrasting voiceless fricatives with voiced stops). The /ʃ/ was contrasted with a short-duration low-frequency repeated /b-b/ with some verbal instructions ('Lips together'), and less emphasis on techniques such as visual mirror information and tactile cues typically used in CWSSD. Principles embedded in AVT were augmented with evidence-based speech therapy approaches such as maximal oppositions (Gierut, 1989). High auditory contrast was used so that he heard the speech sound differences more readily, for example, shoe/Ben, sheet/bib, sharp/bin.

Speech sounds were targeted in the following sequence: fricatives, stops, alveolars, velars, and finally affricates. Even though affricates are motorically complex sounds to produce, Bobby achieved these easily as the auditory signal was readily accessible and a tactile air puff reinforced this. Bobby presented with developmental (e.g., cluster reduction) and non-developmental (e.g., glottal replacement) errors.

Different evidence-based speech therapy approaches including multiple oppositions (Williams et al., 2010), minimal pairs (Baker, 2021), the 'aspiration trick' for prevocalic voicing of /k/ (https://www.speech-language-therapy.com/pdf/k-aspiration-trick.pdf), /t/ and /p/ (https://www.speech-language-therapy.com/pdf/t-aspiration-trick.pdf and https://www.speech-language-therapy.com/pdf/p-aspiration-trick.pdf respectively), were combined with AVT principles. These encompass acoustic highlighting, focus on listening, optimised hearing technology ideal signal-to-noise ratio and parent involvement in therapy. Bobby (now seven) received weekly or fortnightly 60-minute speech language therapy sessions for four years. Fifteen minutes daily homework occurred. All phonological targets were presented in the context of daily language, with an emphasis on verbs rather than nouns whenever possible. Language intervention occurred concurrently from the start of the intervention (Kaipa & Danser, 2016). Reading was taught at school using a phonics-based approach. The sound-letter relationship was reinforced during work addressing the speech sound errors. Bobby's persisting errors involve the low-frequency nasals, /m/ and /n/ with errors in both directions (e.g., hammer → ['hænə]; tiny → ['taɪmi]). Despite these, he is readily intelligible to familiar and unfamiliar listeners.

Three Types of Screening

This section is an adaptation, used by permission, of Roulstone (2015, pp. 76–80), with thanks to Susan Roulstone. The term 'screening' is used in different ways in SLP/SLT and more widely in health and education services. Commonly, it indicates a level of assessment offering a pass/fail outcome, denoting whether a child has a communication difficulty requiring more comprehensive, confirmatory assessment. There are points in the diagnostic pathway at which 'screening' might be used, including the following three.

5. ***Early identification screening of at-risk populations***

Early identification screening, or 'population screening', is a public health process in which children within a defined population are tested, to identify those at risk for speech and language problems and refer them for further diagnostic testing. The aim of population screening is to provide early identification, preferably before symptoms appear, to provide appropriate treatment as early as possible.

6. ***Informal SLP/SLT triage screening***

Informal triage screening is conducted by an SLP/SLT at the first assessment of child following referral. Pickstone (2007) described this as a 'triage' process whereby the proficient SLP/ SLT makes informed judgements about the priority status of a newly referred child to make best use of resources and monitor the urgency and needs of those being referred. This screening does not involve a standardised test and may be as simple as making observations of the child in conversation during a play or hand activity (e.g., building with Lego®; completing a puzzle; or drawing a picture), with the therapist or with a parent, sibling, or peer. With chatty children, asking them to describe what they're doing, or having them name a few objects or pictures, or imitate a few words and sounds may elicit enough speech for a usable sample.

7. ***Formal screening assessment***

Formal screening sees SLPs/SLTs take 5–10 minutes, or sometimes slightly longer, to administer a screening assessment to gather a quick indication of speech output that reveals whether further investigation is justified. The screening procedures of the DEAP (Dodd et al., 2002), HAPP-3 (Hodson, 2004), the Phoneme Factory Phonology Screener (Wren et al., 2006) The Quick Screener (Bowen, 1996), The Quick Vowel Screener (Bowen, 2010), or The Quick Screener for Teachers (Bowen, 2006a) might be used. So too might the GFTA-2 (Goldman & Fristoe, 2000) because its speedy administration in fewer than 15 minutes means it meets screener criteria. Typically, children doing the DEAP, HAPP-3, Phoneme Factory, and Quick Screener screening assessments enjoy the procedures, finding them fun.

The three distinctive types of screening represent the gradual focusing-in of the identification and diagnostic stages, at the same time eliminating or confirming the presence of other voice, fluency, language, and literacy concerns. To decide *who* could or should administer screening, it can be beneficial to establish the stage in the process the investigations have reached, and the purpose of screening at that point.

In the minority, more affluent world, the first type, *early population screening* falls within the public health remit and is executed by health and education professionals. They might be health visitors, teachers, SENCOs, and nursery staff (in the UK) and in other settings around the world teachers, day care and pre-school staff who work in primary care, and paraprofessionals in some community settings, trained for a particular procedure (Pickstone et al., 2002). A health visitor is a registered nurse or midwife who has undertaken post-registration training to qualify as a member of a primary healthcare team. The promotion of health and the prevention of illness across the lifespan are central to the role of the health visitor.

Population screening is rarely conducted directly by British SLTs, but they may advise on the procedures to use and train the other professionals involved. Occasionally, when ascertaining the needs of a population, (e.g., establishing a new service in a school or preschool), SLTs might do population screening themselves. Later, the screening and referral process is handed back to people in regular contact with the child and the SLT's role is to provide materials and training. In the UK, triage screening and formal screening assessment for speech and language impairment are the job of registered SLTs, perhaps supported by an SLT assistant within some constrained contexts. Pickstone (2007) reported the use of more experienced therapists in the triage process, to utilise their expertise in decision making.

Usually without discussion or collaboration, experienced SLPs/SLTs everywhere draw on the screening data they have gathered, to formulate tentative explanations, or hypotheses, about the nature of any apparent difficulties with a view to conducting further investigations if needed.

Software: Phoneme Factory Phonology Screener (after Roulstone, 2015)

As described above, a person who is not an SLP/SLT may be called upon to conduct initial speech screening and it may involve the use of computer software (McLeod et al., 2017). For example, the engaging 66-picture computerised Phoneme Factory Phonology Screener, developed in the United Kingdom (Wren et al., 2006) and Australia (Wren & Roulstone, 2013), is designed for teachers to administer to children whom they suspect have speech sound difficulties, before referring them to SLT services for assessment. The teacher listens as the student names the pictures, writing down alphabetically or phonetically the child's production of one sound per word.

The software generates a report, based on the teacher's record, specifying the errors and patterns revealed, with normative comparisons and an indication of whether the child's speech difficulties are 'developmental' or 'disordered'. Any recommendation to refer to speech therapy is based on this report. The report also guides the teacher to appropriate activities to use in an associated Phoneme Factory software title, the Phoneme Factory Sound Sorter (Wren, et al., 2006).

In testing the software, 408 children were assessed on the screener by a teacher–researcher and by an SLT using the DEAP's phonology subtest (Dodd et al., 2002). These two measures of the children's speech were used to determine the screener's sensitivity (71%), specificity (99%), and positive predictive values (81%). The order of testing was randomised (i.e., sometimes the children were assessed first by the teacher and sometimes first by the SLT) to control for order effects.

Culturally Sensitive Practice

Appropriate screening, assessment, and intervention reflect the SLP's/SLT's sensitivity to cultural and linguistic diversity, and the extent to which they pursue cultural humility. Cultural humility involves regular self-reflective practice on how our background and the background of others (clients, colleagues, students, etc.) impact our clinical practice, teaching, learning, research, creative activity, leadership, etc. In family-centred practice

(Davies et al., 2019; Jensen de López et al., 2021; Klatte et al., 2020; Melvin et al., 2020; Sugden et al., 2018, 2019; Watts Pappas et al., 2016), which is by no means universal, there is collaboration around the nature and conduct of further assessment. The SLP/SLT provides pertinent information, but the family decides whether to proceed, who should give more detailed case history information, who should be present in assessment sessions, and so on.

Diagnostic Evaluation

Child speech assessments for the purpose of diagnosis are prompted by:

1. referral, including referral by a child's family, or a health or education professional.
2. a child's medical, sensory, or developmental status, for example, the speech of children with cleft palate (Golding-Kushner, A16) and the speech and language progress of children fitted with hearing aids or cochlea implants, is routinely assessed in most of the industrialised world; or
3. 'failing' a speech–language screening.

Diagnostic evaluations are conducted by credentialed SLPs/SLTs, working individually or as members of collaborative teams that may include the child, family, and others. Speech assessments are administered to children as needed, requested, or mandated or where there are signs that individuals have articulation and/or phonology impairments associated with their body structure and/or function and/or communication activities and participation (McLeod, A2).

Joining

> *Therapeutic relationships start with the first contact that practitioners have with clients. Even though it may be impractical in some cases, I recommend that counselors either make their own appointments or personally call clients after appointments have been made to answer initial questions and give clients a sense of what to expect when they come. Even on the phone, clients will communicate a lot through their tone of voice, the language they use to describe their situations, and the types of concerns they express.*
>
> Bitter, 2021, p. 469

Evaluations generally build on the information gathered in the initial contact and in the case history interview (see below). The clinician actively and respectfully 'joins' with the family, building a connection (and ideally, rapport) with each member, to initiate and maintain a therapeutic alliance. 'Joining' is a structural family therapy process (Minuchin, 1974), also prominent in strategic family counselling (Haley, 1976). In its original definitions it involved the therapist accepting and accommodating the family or family members to win their confidence, make them feel comfortable, and circumvent resistance. Strategic models have evolved into more collaborative approaches since the 1970s, so the process of joining as a *partnership* has become increasingly central (Bitter, 2021; Lappin, 2018).

Having laid the groundwork for a working relationship with the family, and gained the child's trust and cooperation, the SLP/SLT can usually embark without delay on formal assessment, which a parent, or parents, may choose to observe. Some parents prefer to leave the child with the clinician because they feel that the child will perform better, with more compliant behaviour, if they are not there. Contingent on the setting, they have, or do not have this option.

Depending on the presenting picture, the clinician normally does an oral musculature examination (see Chapter 2) and examines the phonetic, phonological, perceptual, phonotactic, prosodic, speech motor, and intelligibility aspects of the child's speech, and screens for difficulties in other areas (at a minimum: language, pragmatics, voice, and fluency). In evidence-based practice (E^3BP), the test battery's composition depends on the child's presentation, the educated preferences and theoretical orientation of the clinician, and well-informed clients'/patients' values, wishes, and preferences.

The Case History Interview and 'Red Flags'

The case history interview and/or a history questionnaire provide helpful information about the child and the family that may assist the therapist to manage the assessment and intervention process sensitively and appropriately. Ideally, information gathering is conducted with an eye to the potential 'red flags' for speech impairment (summarised in Box 3.6), including family history (Stein et al., 2011); the risk and protective factors (Harrison & McLeod, 2010) that alert the clinician to a range of important inherent **parent** and **family** risk factors, risk factors intrinsic to the **child**; and 'leads' to pursue. Importantly, red flags do not signal the inevitable; risk factors and protective factors are not prophecies; and 'leads' sometimes come to nought.

- **Risk factors**

  Harrison and McLeod (2010) reported that among 4-and 5-year-olds, the consistent and significant **child factors** for risk of speech and language impairment were:
  - maleness,
  - ongoing hearing problems, and
  - having a less persistent, less sociable, and more reactive temperament.

  The more influential **parent factors** were:
  - family history of speech and language problems and
  - maternal low educational level.

  The **family factors** included:
  - having low socioeconomic status (SES), and
  - the presence of older siblings, noting that having older siblings is a potential risk or protective factor.

  Drawing on their own and others' research, the factors Harrison and McLeod recognised as *not* posing significant risks (while acknowledging contrary research) were postnatal factors, multiple births, medical conditions, intelligence, minority status or race, having younger siblings, and support for children's learning at home.

- **Protective factors**

  Harrison and McLeod found that significant protective factors were:
  - the child having a more persistent temperament, and
  - parental proficiency in the home language.

Red Flags (Warning Signs), Risk Factors, and Leads

A procedure I have found helpful is to use the information in Box 3.6 to guide discussion with the caregivers who are providing history data. I have often given them tailored (to the reader) variations of the 'Red Flags' information *before* the session to prepare them for the topics we may cover, and to get them thinking.

Box 3.6   Plain-English explanations for families

What are the potential 'red flags' and risk factors for SSD?

These are some of the red flags (warning signs) and risk factors speech-language pathologists/ speech and language therapists will look out for when a child has a speech and language assessment and 'leads' they will pursue. Not all of them will apply to every child or family. Remember, red flags and warning signs do not signal the inescapable or predict the future; risk factors are not prophecies; and although 'leads' must be investigated, as every detective will tell you, they may be irrelevant.

POTENTIAL RED FLAGS FOR SPEECH SOUND DISORDERS

POTENTIAL RED FLAGS	BACKGROUND INFORMATION
Failure to babble or late onset of canonical babbling	Infants begin producing canonical (speech-like) consonant-vowel (CV) and vowel-consonant (VC) strings of babble at around 7 months. All infants should be producing canonical babble, at least some of the time, before their first birthday. Canonical babbling may go together with many other perfectly normal baby noises including strange vocalisations, shrill shrieks, squeals, and gurgles. Babble and real speech overlap for months, with the baby producing both. **Failure to babble**, and **late onset of canonical babble**, are both associated with (1) hearing impairment and (2) motor speech disorder (MSD). Late babbling may predict late language development.

POTENTIAL RED FLAGS FOR SPEECH SOUND DISORDERS

POTENTIAL RED FLAGS	BACKGROUND INFORMATION
Otitis media with effusion (OME) or 'Glue ear' or 'Middle ear disease'	OME / 'glue ear' /middle ear disease between 12 and 18 months is associated with speech delay. Audiologists and SLPs/SLTs are alert to this in children with grommets (PE tubes), especially if they were inserted at age 1–3 years.
Glottal replacement	**Glottal replacement** is the use of a 'glottal stop' [ʔ] in place of certain consonants when it is inconsistent with the home dialect. It alerts SLPs/SLTs to the risk of SSD.
Initial consonant deletion (ICD)	**ICD** is not attested in first language learners of English, alerting us to the possibility of moderate and severe SSD. **NOTE:** It occurs in typical development in some languages, e.g., French, Finnish, Maltese, Spanish, and Thai.
Small phonetic inventory	Small repertoire of sounds (just **a few consonants** and/or just **a few vowels**) may signal moderate and severe SSD.
Inventory constraints	**Six missing consonants** or **six consonants in error** across three manner categories signal severe SSD, e.g., two stops missing/erred, e.g., /k, g/, two fricatives missing/erred, e.g., /f, ʃ/, and two liquids missing/erred, e.g., /l, ɹ/.
Backing of obstruents: *Stops* /b, p, t, d, k, g/ *Fricatives* /f, v, θ, ð, s, z, h, ʃ, ʒ/ *Affricates* tʃ, dʒ Shriberg et al., 2003	Backing of obstruents is a diagnostic marker for speech delay associated with otitis media with effusion. 'Backing' involves consonants made at the front of the mouth, or just behind the alveolar ridge being replaced by sounds made further back in the mouth. The sounds that will be 'backed' will include some, but rarely all of these: /b, p, t, d, k, g, f, v, θ, ð, s, z, ʃ, ʒ, tʃ, dʒ/. **ARTICLE** www.waisman.wisc.edu/phonology/pubs/PUB15.pdf
Vowel errors 'Wandering' vowels Eisenson & Ogilvie, 1963; Gibbon, 2013; Pollock, 2013; Pollock & Berni, 2003	Prevalent or inconsistent vowel errors are a diagnostic marker for CAS. Children with CAS and those with moderate/severe phonological disorder frequently experience difficulties producing vowels. Vowel errors may occur in as many as 50% of children with these diagnoses. 24–65% typically developing children below 35 months have a high incidence of vowel errors, but by 35 months errors are far less prevalent (0–4%).
Persisting Final Consonant Deletion (FCD)	Prevalent FCD (e.g., 'bike' pronounced as 'by') coming up to the third birthday alerts the clinician to the possibility of SSD. Typically, FCD is eliminated by about age 2;10–3;3.
Beginning readers' conversational Percentage of Consonants Correct (PCC) <50% Shriberg & Kwiatkowski, 1982	PCC below 50% when reading instruction starts (at about age 5;6) is associated with literacy acquisition difficulties. **Conversational PCC – Based on a sample of at least 200 Utterances** (Shriberg & Kwiatkowski, 1982). PCC Severity scale for children 4;1–8;6 >85% Mild SSD 65–85% Mild–moderate SSD 50–64% Moderate–severe SSD <50% Severe SSD
Critical age hypothesis Bishop & Adams, 1990	The critical age hypothesis is that literacy acquisition is likely to be compromised if children are not intelligible by the age of 5;6, especially if they also have SPEECH SOUND DISORDER and SEMANTIC and SYNTACTIC difficulties.
Mild speech production difficulties >6;9 Nathan et al., 2004	Persistent, mild speech production errors, beyond the age of 6;9, are associated with literacy acquisition difficulties affecting reading and/or writing, and/or spelling.

POTENTIAL RED FLAGS FOR SPEECH SOUND DISORDERS

POTENTIAL RED FLAGS	BACKGROUND INFORMATION
'Losing words' 'Dropping words'	If parents are concerned that their child 'loses words', it may be significant, but it is not a 'CAS indicator'/'SSD indicator'. The 'losing words' phenomenon occurs in early *typical* development (Nelson, 1973). However, it may indicate language regression (Shinnar et al., 2001) due to epilepsy (e.g., Landau–Kleffner syndrome) or autism, so it is essential to take heed.
Intellectual disability Shriberg & Widder, 1990	Children and adults with cognitive impairment are likely to have speech sound errors. The most frequent error type is likely to be deletion of consonants. Errors are likely to be inconsistent. The pattern of errors will probably be like that of very young children or children with idiopathic SSD.
Hearing impairment Chin et al., 2003; Ertmer, 2008; Flipsen & Parker, 2008	Children with hearing loss (H/L) develop intelligible speech more slowly than typically developing peers. Speech of children using CIs or hearing aids contains developmental and non-developmental (unusual) phonological patterns.
Potential risk factors Harrison & McLeod, 2010	**Child factors** Being male Having ongoing hearing problems Having a less persistent temperament Having a less sociable temperament Having a more reactive temperament [A more persistent temperament may be protective] **Parent factors** Family history of speech and language problems Low level of maternal education [Parental home language proficiency may be protective] **Family factor: SES** Low socioeconomic status **Family factor: Siblings** Having an older sibling is a risk or protective factor.

Temperament and Personality

A pertinent finding for clinicians is that children of four and five years of age who exhibit a less persistent, less sociable, and more reactive temperament are at risk for speech and language impairment (Harrison & McLeod, 2010). Any SLP/SLT who gave a silent groan or empathetic sigh of recognition on reading the tale of Cameron at the top of this chapter will have thought about the link between temperament and behaviour. They will also relate professionally to the list, 1–8 below, from Vassallo and Sanson (2013) with its mentions of behavioural and emotional adjustment problems, learning and behavioural difficulties, shyness, irritability, troubles with peers, high anxiety *or* depression, and genetic factors. With our academic and clinical backgrounds in SLP/SLT it is almost impossible *not* to make connections between children's temperament, personality, and behaviour on one hand, and communication impairment – including speech and language impairment – on the other. Almost impossible too, *not* to think of memorable children on our caseloads troubled by age-inappropriate emotional expression and modulation, and/or a volatile temperament style characterised by acting-out behaviour.

<u>Temperament</u> is the foundation of personality, usually assumed to be biologically determined and present early in life, including such characteristics as energy level, emotional responsiveness, demeanour, mood, response tempo, behavioural inhibition, and willingness to explore.

<u>Personality</u> is the enduring configuration of characteristics and behaviour that comprises an individual's unique adjustment to life, including major traits, interests, drives, values, self-concept, abilities, and emotional patterns. Personality is generally viewed as a complex, dynamic integration or totality shaped by many forces, including hereditary and constitutional tendencies; physical maturation; early training; identification with significant individuals and groups; culturally conditioned values and roles; and critical experiences and relationships. Various theories explain the structure and development of personality in different ways, but all agree that personality helps determine behaviour.

American Psychological Association (n. d.)

Researchers responsible for The Australian Temperament Project (ATP) followed a large group of individuals from the first months of life to their late 20s when they began following *their* children, with an eventual plan to follow *their* children (the third ATP generation) from 2012. Vassallo and Sanson (2013) reported key findings. The eight most relevant to understanding children with SSD are listed below, with the author's italics.

1. Temperament is relatively stable over time, with many children showing small changes but very few children changing radically.
2. More 'difficult' infant temperament characteristics can lead to ***behavioural and emotional adjustment problems*** in early childhood and beyond, particularly if there are other risks in a child's life.
3. Temperament can be modified through experiences such as the style of parenting a child receives.
4. ATP research confirms the importance of identifying children with ***learning and behavioural difficulties*** as early as possible, to prevent them from persisting across development.
5. ATP research also shows that children can recover from early learning problems.
6. ***Shyness, irritability, and troubles with peers or parents*** may increase the risk of young people experiencing ongoing problems with anxiety or depression.
7. Children with ***high anxiety or depression*** may be more likely to overcome their symptoms if they develop good social skills, have better parent and peer relationships and more positive school experiences.
8. ***Genetic factors*** appear to increase the risk of anxiety and depression for some people, along with a range of other influences.

Speech Sound Disorders and Behaviour

There are promising indications in the literature that it is possible to reduce behaviour difficulties by targeting communication skills (e.g., Law et al., 2012). Anecdotally, clinicians and parents, have recounted improvements in children's behaviour, confidence, mood, and overall happiness, as their intelligibility builds, and this is often attributed to a corresponding reduction in communicative frustration. Conversely, some parents say their child's behaviour became more difficult, disruptive, and forceful when their taciturn offspring came out of their shell, becoming more assertive and 'verbal'.

For example, my client Harriet who presented at 4;0 with a percentage of consonants correct (PCC) of 35% was a passive, 'good' little girl whose mother said compensated for her intelligibility difficulties by being 'everybody's helper' to the point where she earned the family nickname 'Helpful Harry'. By 5;6 her speech approached normal expectations and she began 'answering back' – usually piercingly – with, '*No! Why should I?*' '*You can't make me!*' and the like when asked to do something. Prior to her intelligibility improving, she had been accustomed to holding the floor at home and when visiting friends and relatives because people close to her dreaded 'inhibiting' her further speech progress. If anyone hinted that it might be someone else's turn to talk, she would react heatedly ('*You don't CARE what I think!*', '*You NEVER let me talk*', and so on). Around this time her mother called me, sounding shocked, '*I never thought I would tell Harry to "shut up" – but I just did!*' We talked about the factors involved, and over two or three months, Harry's speech normalised, and her behaviour improved. It is not always so easy to deal with children's difficult behaviour – and it was a relief to call on what I learned in a 2-year diploma in family therapy, after 15 years in SLP practice.

There is a small, expanding literature for SLPs/SLTs to draw on when faced with oppositional, acting-out or disruptive child behaviour. Chow (2018), Chow and Wallace (2021), Chow et al. (2021), Halle et al. (2006), Holland and Nelson (2020), Keller-Bell and Short (2019). But there are three groups of children with SSD whose behaviour is beyond most SLPs'/SLTs' remit, requiring the expert help of and/or appropriate referral to a professional counsellor. The three are:

1. Children like Cameron who can demonstrate cooperation and good rapport with adults in other situations who exhibit 'difficult' behaviour, including refusal to cooperate in assessment and intervention; or those who cooperate in the treatment room coupled with flat refusal to do homework.
2. Children who are unable to demonstrate cooperation and good rapport with adults in speech assessment and intervention settings, and in other situations. These children may present for SLP/SLT assessment and intervention with parents 'expecting' the SLP/SLT to manage both the difficult behaviour and the speech disorder. Some conscientious SLPs/SLTs make themselves miserable by trying unsuccessfully to handle behavioural issues with no relevant background in social work, psychology, family therapy, counselling and so on.
3. Children who do not have the potential for speech who are referred by their families. Young, inexperienced, or newly qualified SLPs/SLTs, especially those in private practice, often have difficulty talking to parents openly about children who are more suited to AAC – or indeed, may not have the capacity even to benefit from simple, low-tech augmentative devices – and the parents themselves may assert that if they elect to bring the child to therapy, then the SLP/SLT is obliged to work with the child.

Dr. James Robert Bitter is Professor of Counseling and Human Services at East Tennessee State University in Johnson City, TN. A Diplomate in Adlerian Psychology and the former Editor of the Journal of Individual Psychology, Dr. Bitter has served as the President of the North American Society of Adlerian Psychology. He has authored or co-authored four books: most recently Theory and Practice of Couples and Family Counseling (Bitter, 2021) – and over 100 journal articles, chapters, and videos. The companion website, https://www.jamesrobertbitter.com, for the 2021 book houses a collection of counselling resources. During his career, Dr. Bitter has worked with the late pioneer of family therapy, Virginia Satir, as well as the master Adlerian family therapists, Manford Sonstegard and Oscar Christensen.

Q14.   James Bitter: Working with Professional Counsellors

Thinking about the above three groups of children and their families, can you explore for the reader the reasons why these behaviours might manifest, the first steps in setting counselling goals that an SLP/SLT might take, basic management strategies, indicators as to when to refer to a specialist in counselling, and ways that SLPs/SLTs who are not normally engaged in multi- or trans-disciplinary teams can liaise productively with such specialists?

A14.   James Bitter: Counselling and SSD: Systemic Interventions for Speech-Language Professionals

Despite Western culture's emphasis on individuality, all humans are relational beings (Gergen, 2009). Human life is social, purposeful, subjective, and interpretive in nature (Sweeney, 2019). Without this orientation to life, and the social, physical, and emotional nurturing provided by adults, no infant would survive. Moreover, the quality of attachment experienced by a child plays a significant role in the child's development across the lifespan (Bowlby, 1988/2015; Johnson, 2019).

When individuals choose to couple, they hope to build a better life together than either of them might have had separately. Individuals or couples who choose parenthood usually want a happy, *healthy* child with whom they can bond and travel through life. What happens when the dream of a happy, healthy child does not occur at birth or is derailed by the revelation of protracted or atypical speech development? Initially, the family experiences shock (Holland & Nelson, 2020).

The Reality of Diagnosis

Diagnosis of a significant speech sound disorder (SSD) shocks the family system, forcing its members to deal with a new reality, with the SSD becoming the focus of everyone's attention. Many families are in chaos at this point and unable to mobilise the internal and external resources needed to deal constructively with the problems they face. This is not a good time for the SLP/SLT to give family members information about the SSD and its implications, because their shock and chaos will prevent them from absorbing it or even hearing it. Indeed, when information is provided prematurely, many family members will later say that they never received any information about the disorder.

Acknowledgment and acceptance take time. A significant SSD constitutes the *loss* of the dream of a healthy child, and that process of loss is well documented (Goldberg, 2006; Kabat-Zinn, 2009; Kleinman, 1988; Kubler-Ross, 1969). Commonly, the initial shock of diagnosis slowly evolves into a realisation that the problem will not be *wished* away, easily remediated, or evaporate with time. This realisation often results in a *retreat*, into some combination of denial, prayer, bargaining, depression, or anger. Family members will react differently from each other, too often leaving individuals feeling alone or disconnected. All of this can be happening while the SLP/SLT endeavours to help the child and the family address the reality of a significant SSD.

Listening

The first step, therefore, in counselling an individual client or a client family is to stay present and *listen*. Staying present means staying in the moment, asking what it is like to hear difficult news, and remaining alert to how people are feeling; it means employing *reflection* or *active listening*. Active listening is paraphrasing to clients what you hear them say and what you empathically believe they might be feeling. 'Hearing that Beatrice is developing speech that is quite different from others her age, and from what she will need as an adult, is hard. You must be worried about all that lies ahead of you'. Notice that these two sentences avoid the use of technical language and focus on what the family feels. Active listening will likely promote further sharing, and the SLP/SLT continues paraphrasing – perhaps for quite some time. This kind of presence and connection creates a safe, holding space and parallels the kind of presence that you want the parents to provide for the child. Attachment is all about emotional attunement. It is listening with the heart.

Acknowledgment changes the family system at multiple levels. It focuses on the *family atmosphere*, and it influences the way *mistaken goals and mistaken interactions* develop. These are considered separately below, even though they develop concurrently and have recursive effects on each other.

Family Atmosphere

In each family, an atmosphere or climate develops that can be said to characterise how the family members relate to each other. Let's say that a child is born with an unexpected cleft palate, requiring surgery with the anticipation of years of speech therapy. The initial experience of cleft palate throws the family into shock. Initially, the parents are incapable of hearing any important information. The key professional attributes that an SLP/SLT can bring to a first meeting with the family are patience, presence, empathy, and active listening skills. It is by staying present and listening empathically that shock and retreat eventually give way to realization and acknowledgment (Holland & Nelson, 2020). When these latter stages occur, professional information is more easily received. This informational delivery will affect the development of the family atmosphere over many years. Over time, the family will evolve into some version of a 'cleft palate' family as the craniofacial anomaly significantly influences who they are. It may pull the parents together or push them apart. The family may feel supported or abandoned in the frustration of dealing with doctors, insurers, parents, and children of other families, social support systems, and other agencies including school and advocacy groups. The family atmosphere emerges within the domain of the disorder, impacting who takes charge and who retreats; the emotions expressed with whom and towards whom; the expectations developed for the child with the cleft compared to typically developing children. These aspects contribute to the model the child receives for handling life.

A debilitating family atmosphere results when parents lapse into feeling sorry for both themselves and their child. Such an atmosphere robs family members of courage, removes confidence, blocks resilience, and may lead to pampering or over-protection. In intervention sessions, these parents will want to hover, intervene, and/or block sadness, challenge, or discomfort in the child. This counterproductive stance, relative to their child and the disorder, emanates from the belief that the child has already suffered enough and should experience no additional difficulties. The family has not yet come to terms with what Holland and Nelson (2020, p. 6), quoting Kabat-Zinn (2009, p. 5), call the full catastrophe: '...*it is not a disaster to be alive just because we feel fear and we suffer...* [to understand] *that there is joy as well as suffering, hope as well as despair, calm as well as agitation, love as well as hatred, health as well as illness...*'.

Part of the work of the SLP/SLT is to help the family develop psychological muscle, to build on their strengths, and to reinforce optimism and resilience. This sounds like a lot, but it really starts with listening for the strengths already in the family, naming those strengths, acknowledging their presences, and validating their use. Rasmussen and Schuyler (2020) describe four essential pillars to psychological muscle. They are:

1. Taking responsibility for self and family.
2. Connection and cooperation with external resources of which the SLP/SLT is one.
3. Respect for self and others.
4. Courage to face the challenges and burdens – as well as the courage to be imperfect, merely human (p. 312).

Naming and appreciating these attributes, acknowledging, and validating their use, builds a family cohesiveness that supports on-going resilience.

Mistaken Goals of Children's Misbehaviour

Some children with SSD also exhibit challenging and disrupting behaviours. When such conduct interrupts or overwhelms therapeutic practices, addressing the behaviours per se must become an explicit therapy goal. Dreikurs (1940a, 1940b) first delineated four goals of children's misbehaviour as a motivational typology for the everyday behaviours of children. These goals are attention getting, power struggle, revenge, and a demonstration of inadequacy (also called an assumed disability and signifying the goal of withdrawal). Dreikurs (1948, 1950) and Dreikurs and Soltz (1964) described the behaviours associated with these four goals and these are displayed in Table A14.1.

Table A14.1 Identifying the mistaken goals of children's misbehaviour.

Mistaken goals	Observed behaviour	Adult response	What the child does when corrected
Attention getting	Model child, cute and charming, pest and nuisance, lazy	Irritated, annoyed, frustrated	Stops for a short while when corrected–even just a few moments or minutes
Power struggle	Rebellious, argues and fights, stubborn, passive-aggressive	Angry, challenged, defeated	Keeps going even when told to stop and may even intensify the misbehaviour
Revenge	Vicious or violent vandalism, meanness, violent passivity	Hurt	Intensifies the misbehaviour, and the misbehaviour becomes mean
Assumed disability	Acts hopeless, gives up, is discouraged, acts incompetent	Despair, helplessness	Limited or no interaction, adults start to give up too, won't try

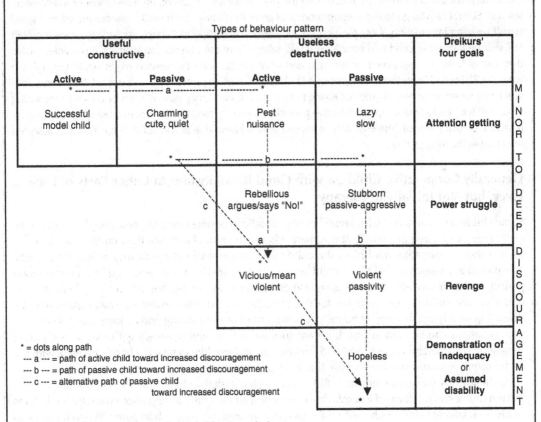

Figure A14.1 Dreikurs' four goals of children's misbehaviour.

There are two ways in which an SLP/SLT can determine the goal of a child's misbehaviour. First, by observing what happens when a child is corrected; and second by asking what the adult feels during the misbehaviour. These indicators are noted by goal in Figure A14.1.

Applications to Specific Situations

As a profession, SLP/SLT has its own set of best practices, ethical codes, and goals and objectives. Training in counselling does not seek to turn SLPs/SLTs into professional counsellors. Rather, the goal is to learn enough about the counselling process and systemic development to aid clients and families with the transition into effective therapy for the presenting communication disorder. To this end, let's look at three separate situations involving children with SSD:

1. Children who are generally cooperative and have good relations in other parts of their lives, but not initially in therapy.
2. Children who generally demonstrate a lack of cooperation in most settings.
3. Children or families without the potential for SLP/SLT intervention and who need to be referred.

Some Basics

The first goal is always to form a positive relationship with the child and the family. If the service delivery model requires the child to be separated from the parents for all, or part of, an assessment or intervention session, SLPs/SLTs who go to the waiting room and greet the family in a friendly manner are off to a good start. Providing information about the process facilitates a transition to therapy, including where the SLP/SLT will be taking the child and how long it will take; where the parents can wait, or if possible, where they can observe the assessment or therapy; and what the goals for the session might be. In general, we want the SLP/SLT to leave the waiting room with the child, parting from the parents even if the parents, too, will leave for separate viewing room. During this process, parents may raise worries or concerns regarding what will happen to their child. An effective transition is usually facilitated via active listening followed by reassurance that parental concerns will be more easily addressed after the SLP/SLT has met and assessed the child in the therapy room.

Generally Cooperative Children with Good Relationships in Other Parts of Their Lives, but Not Initially in Therapy

Some children can initially be frightened in new situations or when meeting new people. This is especially true for children in a family atmosphere where parents feel sorry for their child or are trying to protect them from further hardships. The child's non-cooperative behaviour may reflect the parents' apprehension as much as that of the child. Some children are fine for several sessions, a honeymoon period, and then suddenly become upset. When children start to cry, the SLP/SLT may hear the parents coax the child or make excuses for the behaviour or express surprise or embarrassment ('She doesn't generally act this way at home'). A statement of understanding goes a long way: 'You know, new situations can be hard at first, but I am sure we will be fine when we get to know each other [engaging with the child at eye level and smiling]. Would you like to take my hand and walk with me to the room, or would you like to walk like a big girl on your own?'

In the therapy room, take time to build a relationship with the child. Even in a 30-minute session, 5–10 minutes can be devoted to exploring the room with the child, asking about what the child likes or dislikes, talking calmly with each other, and perhaps even playing a short game. When it is time to engage in a task, say clearly what the task is, have only that task in front of the child, and then notice what the child does in response and what feelings emerge in you (the SLP/SLT). Is the child seeking attention, power, or revenge (the three most common)? If the child is seeking attention, the SLP/SLT will only want to provide it for on-task behaviour: ignore the rest. If the child is seeking power or revenge, the SLP/SLT, having explained what is required in the task, can say, 'Let me know when you are ready to begin' and then stay quiet. If the child moves towards the door, the SLP/SLT might move to sit quietly in front of the door. If the child lets the SLP/SLT know that s/he is ready to cooperate, the SLP/SLT begins the process again provided the child stays on task. End the session with a game or joint play. It may take a whole session to build rapport, and this is time well invested.

Whether parents participate in assessment and intervention sessions or stay in a waiting room, it is important to update them on the process of therapy and to answer their questions readily. This builds cooperation between the family and the therapist. As the parents relax about the process, the child will also tend to do so.

Children Who Generally Demonstrate a Lack of Cooperation in Most Settings

An SLP/SLT working with a child who is uncooperative in most settings is forced into pitting control against power. But let's be clear about what the therapist can control. Therapists can control themselves and the situation, but not the child. Indeed, the child is probably out of control because the family has used ineffective responses in attempting to control him or her. The SLP/SLP must first control the room. Remove or secure any items or objects that will not be a direct part of either the therapy task or a single play event. A general rule is: if you don't want it damaged, don't have it in the room. In the therapy room, prepare for a child to throw a temper tantrum that might include yelling, crying, falling on the floor, pounding on doors or windows, and attempts at hitting or kicking. Bring a book or something else to occupy you during periods of temper. If a temper tantrum starts (whining counts), say, 'Let me know when you are ready to work'. Say this once and sit in a chair in front of the therapy room door. Read, do your crossword, or pursue some other peaceful activity, stay calm, and stay quiet.

Sometimes, SLPs/SLTs must invest two to three therapy sessions in winning a child over. It is useful to assure the parents that this has happened before, and that the SLP/SLT expects to catch up rather quickly once the child loses steam and becomes cooperative. Taking an indirect approach, the SLP/SLT models for the parents the setting of limits with the child. Children do what works, and they will eventually stop what does not work. When SLPs/SLTs work with a very uncooperative child they can expect the child to try everything that has worked at home. Behaviour will get worse before it gets better. Riding it out can seem difficult, but it seldom takes more than three half-hour sessions, after which the child and the parents tend to be much more cooperative. Children will test SLPs/SLTs subsequently. The child may cooperate for several sessions and then come into a session with anger and rage flying. It is important that the therapist set their practice goals aside and return to waiting the child out, calmly requesting that the child let the SLP/SLT know when he or she is ready to work.

Children or Families without the Potential for SLP/SLT Intervention, Requiring Appropriate Referral Elsewhere

There are two general types of families who may need referral. First, there are the families whose psycho-social-behavioural problems overwhelm any treatment possibilities. Second, those families with a child who has a speech-sound disorder that requires outside services, or who has no speech and no apparent capacity for speech, again requiring appropriate referral. Parents sometimes bring their children who have severe cognitive challenges to the SLP/SLT thinking the child can be 'taught to speak'. It is surprising how often these families can slip through the screening process and arrive at the office of the SLP/SLT as inappropriate referrals.

In the first category are children whose misbehaviour is consistently aimed at a goal of revenge or a demonstration of inadequacy (extreme withdrawal). The former includes consistent attempts to hit, bite, kick, or hurt as well as acts of vandalism or vicious attacks on pets or other humans. The latter will most likely be expressed in extreme feelings of anxiety, depression, encopresis or enuresis, or phobic reactions. Under such circumstances, referral to a child psychologist or family therapist should become a pre- or co-requisite for speech services.

In the second category are children with SSD that may need additional referrals for assessment and treatment planning, perhaps to an ENT specialist. Further, there may also be a need for referral when speech therapy will be coupled with either medical (as in cleft palate) or audiology (say, for hearing aids) services – or when the child and family are more appropriately seen by a clinician from a totally different profession. Referral is nothing more than the involvement of other professionals in service to the child and the family. Having a fully developed, local referral list is essential to good practice.

A Family with a Speech Sound Disorder

In general, the more severe and chronic the disorder, the greater the impact will be on family dynamics. As in any serious medical illness (for example, cancer or heart problems), families tend to coalesce around family members who have special needs. When these special needs are severe and ongoing, it is not a child with a speech sound disorder; it is a family with a speech sound disorder. In larger communities, there are usually support groups for all sorts of difficulties. Even in smaller communities, there are professional counsellors and social workers who can help families set new goals and priorities and still live a life characterised by acceptance, happiness, success, and fulfilment.

Referral

When meeting with a family in need of a referral, it is important to take the process in steps. Ideally, preparation would see the SLP/SLT with a choice of options for any referral or set of referrals that might be made. This includes a written list of the specialists and agencies including addresses and phone numbers. Meeting the family starts with a simple inquiry about how people are doing and how they are feeling. The SLP/SLT should respond with active listening. When the family is ready, the SLP/SLT calmly reviews what has been learned and where the child and family 'are' in the process of facing the tasks ahead. The SLP/SLT thereby lays the foundation for why a referral is necessary and potentially useful – and ultimately, the likely next steps following the referral. It is important to check that the information is understandable to the family and to ask how they feel about it. Provision of additional information or further planning may be needed at this point, usually requiring more active listening.

Towards the end of the referral session, the SLP/SLT ascertains whether the child and the family need support in enacting the referral. Do they need letters or paperwork from the SLP/SLT? Do they know where they need to go and how they will get there? Do they need phone or video calls or other support services? What can the family do if other service agencies are not meeting their needs? An effective referral is one in which all parties see the need, have a plan, and have the possibility of enacting the plan. Finally, SLPs/SLTs who sets a time to follow up with the family after the referral date are more likely to ensure treatment adherence and prevent treatment interruption and derailment.

Not all children and their families will be difficult clients. Many will fall right into speech therapy and benefit greatly from it. My aim here has been to identify ways of understanding and working with children and families who may not accept therapy interventions quite so smoothly. Because individuals, children, and adults, are always in relationship, always part of systems, learning to interact with and treat the whole family is the surest way to support positive outcomes in therapeutic practice with less than cooperative client.

Children with SSD and Additional Developmental Concerns

For SLPs/SLTs, fundamental aspects of child-centred dynamic assessment and therapy delivery within family-centred practice frameworks are the provision of accurate and timely information. There is also an obligation for us to communicate empathically, and clearly in a manner that 'fits' the needs, capacities, cultures, value systems and beliefs, levels of acceptance, and emotional landscapes of the family and their significant others. In each unique and changing situation that arises around multiply involved, minimally verbal or highly unintelligible children with major SSD, such as severe CAS, we have both an educative and a counselling role.

Dr. Ruth Stoeckel is a speech-language pathologist. She recently retired from clinical practice and has ongoing involvement in research work. For her PhD at the University of Minnesota, she investigated development of phonological knowledge in young children. She was employed at the Mayo Clinic in Rochester, Minnesota, where she evaluated and treated young children with a range of speech-language difficulties, including motor speech disorders. She continues to present her work at professional conference and CEU events locally and nationally in the United States and internationally.

Q15. Ruth Stoeckel: Counselling Families of Children with SSD Plus

Many of our families, endlessly striving to do the best they can for their children, are influenced by information about the nature and management of their children's issues that is variously unscientific, misleading, time-wasting, worrying, or downright dangerous.

This is of particular concern in cases of children who may indeed have CAS, and for whom its treatment becomes a raison d'etre for their parents, but who have a range of other challenges impacting progress. It is also of concern to parents of children with complex communication needs (CCN) who do not have, and may never have, a definite speech-language disorder or other diagnosis. Misinformation can come from the immediate and wider circle of family and friends, where inevitably there will be a self-styled, often critical or denying, child development expert at hand! It can also come from our SLP/SLT and other professional colleagues and friends, and from faceless but ostensibly authoritative Internet 'experts' and 'e-friends'.

There are no easy answers, but how would you educate the educators and counsel the counsellors charged with these important and demanding SLP/SLT educative and counselling tasks?

A15. Ruth Stoeckel: Discussing Appropriate Treatment Options for Children with SSD and Comorbid Conditions

Mrs. Smith's 4-year-old son, Timmy, runs around the room, opens every door and drawer, impulsively picks up and drops toys, and produces a constant stream of unintelligible jargon. He does not look at you or his mother, even when you try to get his attention so that you can work with him. Attempts to have him sit quietly for a moment result in resistance and screaming. Mrs. Smith has told you that Timmy has diagnoses of delayed language, speech sound disorder, and sensory issues. His progress in prior speech therapy was slow. Mrs. Smith is asking for a second opinion about diagnosis and treatment strategies. She expresses an expectation that if Timmy can communicate more effectively, his behaviour will be much improved as well. How would you approach discussion of communication and behaviour as it relates to Timmy?

Precious, a 5-year-old girl with Down syndrome comes for therapy with her father, Mr. Sanchez. Precious expresses herself mainly with single words and a few 2-word combinations, mostly 'I want' plus a noun. She follows one-step directions easily but still needs help to follow two-step directions. Mrs. Sanchez has heard from a fellow parent in the preschool program that Precious attends about a vitamin regimen 'proven' to help improve a child's speech. He wants an opinion about the best dosage for Precious. How would you provide 'in the moment' counselling about cognitive, linguistic, and speech motor contributions to his daughter's communication disorder, and address his desire to try this 'proven' vitamin regimen?

Sigrid is the 22-month-old daughter of Mr. & Mrs. Happel. She was born nearly 6 weeks premature and has been slow to achieve developmental milestones. Sigrid began walking at 19 months. She had difficulty sucking as an infant, and currently chokes on foods other than thickened cereals. Babbling is limited to 'ah' either as a single syllable or in repeated syllable strings. She is just beginning to point to objects out of her reach and to manipulate toys rather than put them in her mouth. Her parents realise that she is delayed in several areas and have been searching for answers to why she does not yet talk. They tell you that Sigrid 'fits all the signs' of childhood apraxia of speech that they found on one internet site. They have decided that Sigrid requires a specific approach after reading testimonials about how well it has worked for other children. They are requesting that you begin intensive therapy immediately, employing this approach. Based on your work with this child, you disagree both with the request for intensive individual therapy at this point and with the requested therapy approach. How do you maintain a collaboration with the parents that focuses on the needs of this child considering the disagreement about intervention?

Ten-year-old Abdi was given a diagnosis of childhood apraxia of speech by a paediatrician when he was 3 years old because he was unintelligible. You have been working with him during the last school year to resolve a residual distortion of /ɹ/. Abdi has struggled with learning to read; he is far behind others in his class although he does well in other academic areas. He struggles to grasp information that he has read and to sound out words that he doesn't already know. His parents are frustrated. They have read that, children who have apraxia may have difficulty learning to read and ask you to intensify your efforts to 'fix his apraxia' in hopes that he will catch up to his peers. How would you include support for literacy in your work with Abdi? How would you explain to that while his history of speech impairment is a risk factor for later literacy issues, his current difficulty may need to be treated as a related, but separate area of need?

Looking at the 'Whole Child' in Context

What the above scenarios have in common is a child with a speech disorder and additional developmental concerns, with parents asking for help. Some parents recognise their child's speech disorders as just one of multiple challenges. Others may focus on speech as the core problem, which, when treated, they hope will result in improvements in all areas. There will be parents hoping for an easy answer to their child's needs. At the moment that they are asking these types of questions, it is critical for the SLP/SLT to be an empathetic listener to hear the concern behind the question and to be conscious of responding within the scope of practice specified by our respective professional associations, e.g., ASHA (American Speech-Language-Hearing Association, 2016), IASLT, NZSTA, RCSLT, SACOAC, and SPA. Our job as clinicians includes not only evaluation and treatment of speech and language disorders but also helping parents to understand the relative contribution of these issues within the context of the 'whole child'. With respect to the examples above, that may mean discussing the influence of other developmental concerns on prognosis for change in the child's speech sound disorder. It may require discussion of the parents' priorities, with pros and cons of specific interventions they are requesting. At times, it may lead to incorporating parent suggestions. At other times, the request may go beyond our scope of practice (e.g., nutritional changes, significant behavioural issues) and require referral to, or additional consultation with, other professionals.

Responding

When responding to questions and concerns at the moment, empathetic listening means being sensitive both to what the parents are asking and what they are ready to hear (Luterman, 2016). Parents can be invited to engage *with* us to identify both strengths and needs. Miron (2012) found that for parents of children with speech sound disorders, emotional stress was influenced by a perception of receiving inadequate services. Positive interactions and confidence in service providers facilitated positive outcomes. Responding to parent questions from a basis of empirical evidence (when available) without negating parent concerns may help to build trust and forge the way forward to a plan that will maximise benefit to the child.

Even when parents and clinicians share a common understanding of diagnosis and intervention, perspectives about outcomes may potentially differ. Several groups of researchers (McCormack et al., 2010; Rusiewicz et al., 2018; Thomas-Stonell et al., 2009) have interviewed parents and clinicians about expected outcomes of treatment. Their questions were based on the areas identified in the World Health Organization's (WHO) International Classification of Functioning, Disability, and Health – Child and Youth Version: ICF-CY (2007). A common finding was that while clinicians and parents agreed that verbal communication was an area of concern for children with SSD, there was a difference in perceived priority of factors such as social relationships and community participation. Parents valued activities and participation goals, such as peer relationships, to a greater degree than clinicians, who tended to prioritise intelligibility. The broader view suggested by the WHO model potentially influences the way we respond to parent requests and inquiries.

Parents can find a wealth of information about speech-language disorders through a variety of sources, including seminars, stories in the popular press, and Internet sites that run the gamut from general information to product advertisements. Well-meaning friends and relatives may offer their own advice or experience. The availability of many sources of information can facilitate the parents' ability to learn about their child's disorder and more actively participate in both assessment and treatment. However, critical evaluation of this information to recognise content that may be incomplete, incorrect, or even irresponsible is essential. There can be bias even in information presented as research. As clinicians, when responding to parents' questions, we have a responsibility to be aware of credible sources of information and to guide parents to those resources. Parents bring deep knowledge of their children to the discussion. Honouring their contribution

while providing education to tease out reputable information can foster greater trust and a more collaborative approach to establishing goals for intervention. On occasion, that may mean helping parents to obtain a second opinion about the child's communication disorder for reassurance and possibly to identify other options for intervention.

Ethical practice demands that we operate within our scope of practice. SLPs/SLTs are the professionals with knowledge and expertise to diagnose and treat speech and language disorders. When these disorders occur in the context of comorbid disorders, other professionals will be involved or should become involved via referral. There will be times with 'in the moment' questions about unproven or unfamiliar treatments when the most helpful response will be 'I don't know, but let's look into it together.' Seeking information from trustworthy sources and knowledgeable professionals can be of benefit to all involved: parents, clinicians, and most of all, the child.

Children with SSD and Language Impairment

Continuing the subject of multiply involved children with SSD, Rebecca McCauley discusses a client population that is prominent on most paediatric SLP/SLT caseloads: children with speech, language, and communication needs. Like Stoeckel in A15 above, she emphasises evidence-based, family-centred practice where partnerships with parents, and collaborative teamwork with other professionals prevail.

Dr. Rebecca McCauley is Professor in the Department of Speech and Hearing Science at the Ohio State University. She is a Fellow and Honors Recipient of the American Speech-Language-Hearing Association. Her primary interests are speech sound disorders in children, especially severe speech disorders such as childhood apraxia of speech, and the description of interventions for evidence-based practice. Publications related to these topics include 12 books, of which three especially relevant volumes are *Interventions for speech sound disorders in children (2nd ed.)*, co-edited with A. Lynn Williams and Sharynne McLeod (Williams et al., 2021), *Treatment of language disorders in children (2nd ed.)*, co-edited with Marc Fey and Ron Gillam, and *Treatment of autism spectrum disorders (2nd ed.)*, coedited with Patricia Prelock, published in 2021, 2019, and 2022 respectively.

Q16.　Rebecca Mccauley: Children with Co-Occurring Speech and Language Concerns

In day-to-day practice, SLPs/SLTs must often decide how treatment should be prioritised for children who have severe language impairments including, Developmental Language Disorder (Ebbels et al., 2018; McGregor, 2020), as well as an SSD. How would you set about prioritising and implementing speech and language treatment; and in what ways would you involve parents and the wider family in the intervention team? When parents' or team members' perception of the SLP/SLT needs of the child and their expectations of the focus therapy is at odds with the speech-language clinician's findings and recommendations, how would you approach the task of information sharing and reaching a consensus on treatment priorities and goals?

A16.　Rebecca J. McCauley: Involving a Child's Family When Speech *and* Language are Areas of Need

Children with severe language delays and disorders who also show evidence of speech sound disorders represent a large heterogeneous group with diagnoses such as developmental language disorder: DLD (also known as specific language impairment: SLI), autism, or developmental delay (called 'learning disability' in the UK). Almost invariably, these children find it difficult to make themselves understood in everyday communication – in fact, usually, that is the reason they have been found eligible for intervention. In addition, such children may exhibit co-occurring or core challenges in attention or behaviour (e.g., tantrums or withdrawal) that negatively affect their lives at home and at school. Prioritising intervention goals for children whose needs span speech, language, communication – and sometimes management of problem behaviours – represents a delicate balancing act.

That balancing act is both facilitated, in the long run, and complicated, in the short run, by the involvement of teams of educators, SLPs/SLTs and other allied health professionals, and families. Intensified interest in promoting more effective collaborations among SLPs/SLTs, educators, and health professionals has occurred relatively recently through the promotion of interprofessional education and practice (e.g., Geiss & Serianni, 2018; Johnson, 2016; Prelock et al., 2017) and is likely to contribute significantly to team interactions for children with speech and language needs. Nonetheless, parents or other primary caregivers will continue to play a central role in the teams constituted to address the child's communication needs (McLeod & Baker, 2014), especially in the context of early intervention (Woods et al., 2011).

Teamwork

Within a philosophy of family-centred practice (Committee on Hospital Care and Institute for Patient- and Family-Centered Care, 2012; Watts Pappas et al., 2007), parents' expertise about, investment in and access to the child are recognized as invaluable resources. To help establish a strong alliance among all team members – professional or familial, I find it helpful to introduce at least three concepts:

- *speech production*
  the sounds, and sequences of sounds that were used and whether they were used for communicative purposes.
- *language*
  words and larger units of meaning that were understood or attempted in production.

- **communication**
  verbal and nonverbal means of sharing and receiving information.

Ideally, I incorporate examples from our shared observations of the child to illustrate these concepts and their interrelationships. In addition, using plain English and avoiding jargon will facilitate exchanges for all participants on the team. For children exhibiting challenging behaviours, I would also point out that such behaviours probably represent efforts to communicate that can be replaced when more conventional communications are identified, learned, and rewarded (Halle et al., 2006; and see Bitter, A14).

To the extent that all members of the child's team share a common understanding of *speech, language*, and *communication*, they are in a better position to react to any plan that I might propose based on evaluation results and my knowledge of what research evidence exists to support a given set of intervention goals and strategies. Team collaboration on such a plan facilitates changes ranging from subtle refinements to everyday interactions with the child, to major modifications that more effectively incorporate knowledge of the child, his surroundings (including his or her family's needs and values), and team members' abilities to contribute.

Strategies and Intervention Methods

Plans for children with significant speech and language needs often incorporate two kinds of strategies: (a) augmentative alternative communication (AAC) strategies for optimising the child's current communicative effectiveness and (b) specific intervention strategies for improving the child's more specific speech and language skills.

Initially, parents are sometimes reticent about using AAC strategies (e.g., a communication board or signing) because of fears that it represents a lowering of expectations and may hamper speech and language development. However, reassurance on two fronts usually allays those fears. First, available evidence

suggests that the use of AAC is more likely to facilitate than retard advances in other forms of communication (Branson & Demchak, 2009; King et al., 2013; Schlosser & Wendt, 2008; Speech Pathology Australia, 2020). Second, the child's becoming a more effective communicator can be expected to produce immediate improvements in the quality of his life and the lives of those around him – a valuable outcome independent of future effects, although one that requires additional research for validation.

Intervention methods used for speech and language facilitation vary depending on the child's level of development in each area, but often include those described by Prezas et al., A5. and Strand, A31., as well as a variety of methods described in McCauley et al. (2017) and in Prelock and McCauley (2022).

Involving Parents and the Wider Family in Intervention

How I involve parents and significant others in implementing an intervention plan depends on their interest and resources. Often, at the outset of therapy for a child who is seen outside of the context of Early Intervention, I will suggest that we start small and consider their greater involvement as we go. At the most basic level, I ask that parents keep me abreast of times when they see advancement or suspect special unanticipated challenges that might affect the course of our work. Most parents are also happy to reward the spontaneous use in the home setting of target behaviours that I can let them know are emerging in treatment sessions.

For children whose communication and language are in relatively early stages of development, parent-implemented programs are especially appropriate and well supported by evidence if parents are interested and able to take the time. In such programs, parents are taught several facilitating strategies to use in play and/or book reading with their child (e.g., Weitzman et al., 2017). For other parents with similar children but less time, capacity, or interest, I might teach them a specific strategy (e.g., focused stimulation; Ellis Weismer et al., 2017). Yet another area in which parents and I have had success is in approximating stimulability activities such as those described by Miccio and Williams (2021) or phonemic awareness activities, such as those discussed by Bowen, 2019; McNeill, A22., and Neilson, A49., A50.

Maintaining Focus

Working with parents and other professionals in a team context can be an immensely satisfying process, even as it is challenging. The team's diverse perspectives not only produce a better plan for the child but also help me do my job better. When children have many missing speech and language skills, it is very easy to get lost in the 'trees' of their many potential goals. Other team members, especially parents and significant others, can help us all keep track of the 'forest', that is, the child's overall communicative effectiveness.

Children with SSD and Craniofacial Differences

The final 'special population' in this chapter is children with SSD and cleft palate and/or other craniofacial anomalies. **Dr. Karen Golding-Kushner** is well known for her roles as the past Executive Director of the Velo-Cardio-Facial Syndrome Educational Foundation, Inc. and former Clinical Director of the Center for Craniofacial Disorders at the Montefiore Medical Center, Bronx, NY. She is currently owner of the Golding-Kushner Speech Center, LLC and Golding-Kushner Consulting, a private practice New Jersey, USA. As well, she is a consultant for the Virtual Center for VCFS/22q and Other Craniofacial Disorders. Dr. Golding-Kushner was a founder and the inaugural Associate Coordinator of ASHA SIG18 (Telepractice). An ASHA Fellow, she has specialised in craniofacial disorders, cleft palate, and velopharyngeal function for over 40 years.

Q17. Karen Golding-Kushner: Children with Craniofacial Anomalies

For the generalist SLP/SLT and others who are inexperienced with craniofacial disorders (Alighieri et al., 2021), cleft palate, and velopharyngeal function, what are the important issues in speech development, assessment, and intervention? Can these issues be addressed when in-person services are not possible, such as occurred during the COVID-19 pandemic? Are there circumstances in which the generalist is best advised to step back and recommend to families that they seek experienced, expert guidance?

A17. Karen Golding-Kushner: Issues in Speech Development, Assessment, and Intervention for Children with Craniofacial Disorders, Cleft Palate, and Velopharyngeal Dysfunction

Soon after a new baby with a cleft is born, and prior to any surgery, the SLP/SLT should meet baby and parents, providing information on normal communication, stimulating oral sound development, and feeding. Every child with a cleft palate or craniofacial disorder requires thorough speech and language evaluation by age 12 months. In the industrialised world, cleft palate is usually repaired at around 12 months, and because of this population's propensity for otitis media, pressure-equalising tubes (ventilation tubes or 'grommets') are frequently surgically inserted then too. Importantly, middle-ear health and hearing must be closely monitored. Provided these things happen in a timely manner, most children with cleft lip only, or non-syndromic cleft palate, demonstrate typical speech and language progress. For some 20% of children with cleft palate and for children with craniofacial disorders associated with certain syndromes, language, speech, voice, and resonance may be compromised by risks. These risks relate to associated anomalies potentially affecting hearing, cognition, morphological (anatomic) structure, physiology (function or movement of structures), and dentition (Golding-Kushner, 2001). Further, some syndromes are associated with specific patterns of articulation, voice, resonance, and language disorders.

Hearing

The association between palatal clefts, even submucous clefts, and middle ear disease is strong, because the levator veli palatine, tensor palatine, and other palatal and pharyngeal muscles are abnormally positioned and oriented. The eustachian tube, designed to ventilate the middle ear, leads from each middle ear to the back of the throat. The tensor palatini is responsible for opening the eustachian tube orifice, and its abnormal placement and function limits or prevents ventilation. Sometimes, the eustachian tube itself may be angled or positioned abnormally. To exacerbate matters, the belly of the levator veli palatini often elevates to fill the eustachian tube's opening, occluding it during speech and swallowing, preventing it from ventilating and equalising pressure on either side of the middle ear cavity. This tends to improve with age. Some syndromes, e.g., Treacher Collins syndrome, are associated with severe conductive hearing loss. Others are associated with sensorineural hearing loss. For affected infants and toddlers, early detection, medical or surgical treatment, and, if appropriate, amplification, are essential (see Asad et al., A13.).

Associated Syndromes

Over 400 syndromes are associated with cleft palate, and some, including velo-cardio-facial syndrome (VCFS, 22q11.2 deletion) and foetal alcohol spectrum disorder (FASD), are associated with cognitive impairment, language delays or disorders, and/or significant hearing loss. These risks, caused by the same genetic defect responsible for the cleft, are inherent to the syndrome under consideration. Further,

some syndromes, such as VCFS, caused by a microdeletion on chromosome 22 in the 22q11.2 region, are associated with syndrome-specific patterns of speech and language disorders (Golding-Kushner, 2020).

Voice

Vocal quality, pitch, and volume each reflect activity at the level of the larynx. Although cleft palate is not a direct risk factor for any of these features, individuals with borderline velopharyngeal competence may exhibit degrees of hyperfunctional voice use, vocal fold changes, and dysphonia (hoarseness), due to attempts to compensate for loss of intraoral air pressure. Some syndromes are associated with laryngeal anomalies, resulting in voice disorders. For example, among the characteristics of VCFS are unilateral vocal fold paralysis and laryngeal asymmetry which may cause hoarseness; and, laryngeal web, which may cause elevated vocal pitch and loss of volume (loudness) (Golding-Kushner, 2020). Vocal loudness also may be reduced in speakers with conductive hearing loss and increased in speakers with sensorineural hearing loss, both of which might be associated with specific syndromes.

Oral Resonance

Very severe oral crowding or hypertrophy (enlargement) of the gingival tissue, or, more commonly tonsillar hypertrophy, can cause oral damping of the acoustic signal and muffled resonance. Enlarged tonsils may or may not appear to be infected but, usually, removal and pathology analysis reveals they are bacteria laden. Infection aside, their presence can cause a muffling referred to as 'potato-in-the-mouth' or cul-de-sac resonance. Extremely hypertrophied tonsils in toddlers acquiring speech are also associated with habitual forward tongue carriage as the child works to open the airway by maintaining an anterior tongue posture. Tonsil size appears different, 60% of the time, when viewed looking in the mouth, versus looking into the airway (Golding-Kushner, 2005). Therefore, in many cases, diagnosis is based on imaging the vocal tract via nasoendoscopy or, if that is unavailable, lateral fluoroscopy with a good barium coat. It cannot be based on *only* an oral view of the tonsils. Oral resonance abnormalities typically require physical management (e.g., tonsillectomy) and are not amenable to speech therapy.

Hyponasality

Too little nasal resonance may result from adenoid hypertrophy, deviated septum, other nasal anomalies, or obstruction of the nasopharynx following pharyngoplasty (secondary surgery to eliminate VPI). Because hyponasality can co-occur with hypernasality, both should be rated separately during evaluation. While the treatment of hyponasality is usually medical or surgical, increasing the duration of nasal consonants during connected speech and especially in the context of nasal-oral consonant clusters (/sn/, /sm/, /ŋk/) may effectively reduce the perception of hyponasality. For example, with /ŋ/ omitted, /ˈmʌŋki/ → [ˈmʌki].

Hypernasality

Excessive nasal resonance during vowel production, due to communication between the oral and nasal cavities, is among the greatest risks associated with cleft palate. Hypernasality, the consequence of VPI, is best diagnosed by a trained listener and not instrumentally, because it is *only* of significance if it is perceptible. Conversely, velopharyngeal dysfunction (VPD) can *only* be diagnosed using instrumentation to visualise the region. Hypernasality permeates connected speech and occurs when the speaker is unable to fully separate the oral and nasal cavities at the right time during connected speech due to a physical inability to effect velopharyngeal closure, timing errors, or both. Hypernasality is a vowel phenomenon but commonly co-occurs nasal emission, which is nasal air escape through the nose during speech that is most apparent during production of pressure consonants. Nasal air escape is an obligatory error that occurs in the presence of VPI.

Velopharyngeal Insufficiency / Velopharyngeal Dysfunction

VPI: velopharyngeal insufficiency (or VPD: velopharyngeal dysfunction) has several causes including deficient velar tissue, abnormal or asymmetric movement of the velum, lateral pharyngeal walls, or posterior pharyngeal wall, tonsillar hypertrophy (Shprintzen et al., 1987), and errors in learning. If present, an oronasal fistula may exacerbate the effects of VPI (Isberg & Henningsson, 1987). Compensatory articulation errors may also exacerbate VPI (Golding-Kushner et al., 1990; Henningsson & Isberg, 1986). Neuromotor problems may also cause VPI, but cleft palate is not a risk factor for neuromotor problems and motor speech disorders (MSD) occur rarely in children with cleft palate. Other than when caused by errors in learning, treatment of VPI requires physical management.

Treatment efficacy always rests on accurate diagnosis, and diagnosis of VPI requires direct visualisation of velopharyngeal function during unimpeded connected speech. Best practice for assessing velopharyngeal closure is direct visualisation using both flexible fibreoptic nasopharyngoscopy to analyse anatomy and airway patency (openness), and multiview videofluoroscopy to view pharyngeal wall and velar motion and tongue activity during speech. Unfortunately, many clinicians rely on indirect measures like pressure-flow techniques or nasometry to diagnose disorders of resonance and VPI. They confuse data that appear 'objective' with an assessment that is valid (relevant). Indirect assessment techniques provide no information about the location, configuration, consistency, or cause of VPI, so their value in treatment planning is debatable (Peterson-Falzone et al., 2017).

People often ask, 'Why not do trial therapy to see if hypernasality reduces without surgery?' There is no therapy technique to eliminate velopharyngeal closure when VPI is consistently present. Other than for errors of learning, speech therapy is ineffective in eliminating VPI. Nevertheless, clinicians persist with non-evidence-based NS-OME (Ruscello & Vallino, 2020; Lof, A24.).

Errors in Learning

Some children, with or without clefts, exhibit adequate velopharyngeal closure on all but one phoneme or sound class, typically involving a nasal snort or nasal fricative substitution for one or more fricative or affricate sounds /s, z, f, v, ʃ, ʒ, tʃ, dʒ/. Occluding the nares during stimulability testing results in production of /k/ or silence, and the speaker may exhibit discomfort duets the inability to emit air. Such errors in learning are easily treatable with speech therapy, and physical management is inappropriate and unwarranted. (In contrast, a speaker with nasal emission, that is, passive loss of air through the nose, sounds better with the nares occluded because he or she was directing air orally and closing the nose eliminated the passive 'leak.') When this nasal fricative, or nasal snort, occurs in people without history of structural anomalies, it is known as 'phone-specific' or 'sound-specific' VPI. Unfamiliar clinicians are sometimes baffled by this phenomenon and refer the client for ENT assessment. However, when nasal production is isolated to a single sound or single group of sounds, clearly therapy is the appropriate treatment.

Articulation

Articulation errors in children with cleft palate, VPI, and craniofacial syndromes may be obligatory, maladaptive, developmental, or compensatory. Of these, all but developmental errors may be related to malocclusion, palatal fistulae, VPI, severe oral crowding, or hearing loss. Children with cleft palate do not typically have CAS, oral-motor weakness, dysarthria, or other MSD. Regrettably, they are regularly misdiagnosed with these disorders, leading to inappropriate interventions (Golding-Kushner, 2020), including NS-OME, which are bereft of evidence and never indicated (Ruscello & Vallino, 2020), and see Lof, A24; Ruscello, A38.

Concerning children who are not known to have a cleft or VPI: the mouth may appear normal on oral examination but occult submucous cleft or VPI cannot necessarily be ruled out. A decision tree can be helpful. If you hear hypernasality and all speech errors are obligatory, refer to velopharyngeal imaging. If you hear nasal airflow on only one sound, one cognate pair, or one sound class, but nasal airflow is appropriate on other sounds, the problem is likely nasal snorting (also called nasal fricative or phone-specific VPI), treatable with speech therapy only, and referral to a craniofacial team is unnecessary. Physical management would not remediate that error. Nasal airflow can be detected easily by holding a sensitive mirror beneath the nares while the child produces words without /m, n, ŋ/, or by holding one end of a drinking straw at the edge of a nostril and the other end of the straw to your ear. If you are not sure, pinch the nose and see if speech (excluding nasal sounds /m, n, ŋ/) seems better. If it is better, the airflow was likely obligatory. If it sounds the same or even worse, the error was likely phone-specific, requiring speech therapy. If unsure, referral to an SLP/SLT with appropriate expertise, to a craniofacial team, or both, is recommended. While the basic therapy procedures are those used in 'traditional' articulation therapy, an SLP/SLT with applicable expertise may offer special techniques and 'tricks' to the treating clinician (Vallino et al., 2019; Golding-Kushner & Shprintzen, 2011; Ruscello, A38.).

Expert Guidance

Before treatment starts, it is incumbent on SLPs/SLTs to distinguish aspects of the SSD that are and are not amenable to therapy. Unfortunately, most SLPs/SLTs lack specific training in cleft palate and VPI. If the client is followed by a cleft palate team the clinician can ask the team's SLP/SLT for guidance. I can report good outcomes working with children (and their parents) who live far away using videoconferencing (Golding-Kushner, 2020; Golding-Kushner & Scherer, 2020). While tele-evaluation and teletherapy have been available for years, they abruptly and globally became the only service delivery option during the COVID-19 pandemic (see Williams, Thomas & Caballero, A46.). In addition to providing direct therapy services to remote locations, telepractice enables SLPs/SLTs with less experience in treating specific disorders, and families, to consult with specialists (Shprintzen & Golding-Kushner, 2012).

The Specific Questions Families Ask about SSD and *Their* Child

No matter the child's age, once the speech assessment is complete, parents, caregivers, or the client in the case of an adolescent or young adult are provided with a report. This may be a verbal report in some cases, but often it is a written report; and in various settings, reports in writing are mandatory. The questions parents ask their SLP/SLT, and often *keep* asking, arising from such reports, are ordinarily related specifically to *their* child, not children in general, and the answers the SLP/SLT gives will be focused on that child.

For example, Box 3.4 contains an answer to the question *'What is a speech sound disorder?'* and the explanation is illustrated with a metaphorical 'SSD umbrella' in Figure 3.1. Figure 3.1 is less busy version of the SSD umbrella, with plain(er)-English labels than in Figure i.1, which SLPs/SLTs may prefer to use with some clients. Either provides a broad overview of the possible bases for the different types of SSD (anatomic, audiologic, motoric, perceptual, phonetic, and phonemic issues, or a combination of these), probable underlying causes (craniofacial differences, hearing impairment, motor speech disorder, speech perception difficulties, articulation disorder and phonological disorder, singly or in combination), and how the disorders can overlap and co-occur.

When answering questions about an individual client, the emphasis shifts to talking primarily about the aspects of SSD *specific to them*. If the child has a reasonably straightforward articulation disorder, for example, parents are unlikely to want a detailed account of all the other speech issues that might have arisen.

The questions parents are likely to ask about *their* child's SSD are displayed in Box 3.7. They will probably revolve around **severity** ('How serious is my child's problem?'), **prevalence** ('Do many children have this problem?' 'Is it a common problem, or rare?') and **comorbidities** (e.g., 'Do children with SSD have difficulties with schoolwork?'), **aetiology** ('What caused this problem?' 'Is it something we did wrong?'), **classification** ('What kind of speech sound disorder is it?'), **prognosis** ('Can the problem be corrected?' 'How long will it take?' 'How often will we need to come?'), **intervention** ('What are you, or we, going to do about the problem?'), **target selection and goal setting** ('Where do we start working on the problem?' 'And then what?'), and the **family's role in intervention** ('Is there something we can do at home?').

Box 3.7   The questions families ask

Severity: How serious is my child's problem?

Subjective Estimates

SLPs/SLTs will often provide an informal estimate of the severity of a child's SSD that is based on their experience with a similar child or children. They may do so without necessarily explaining that the severity rating is based on personal professional experience, or whether their view is influenced by

- any **red flags** for SSD in the child's history, see Box 3.6
- the **frequency** of the SSD, for example, whether it is common or rare in the overall population; and/or whether it is common or rare on the clinician's own caseload.
- the **impact** of the SSD, for example, whether it is likely to be easy or difficult for the child and family to tolerate, or for the child to overcome; how it might affect the child's participation in society, their quality of life, society's perception of them; and whether it might affect their chances in life.
- the **persistence** of the SSD, for example, whether it can likely be eliminated, or perhaps persist in a modified form as the child grows older.
- the SSD's likely **sequelae** and/or **comorbidities:** whether there are any, and if so, what they are like in terms of frequency, impact, and persistence.
- the **characteristics of the child** with the SSD including temperament, personality, behaviour, attention span, task persistence, cooperation, stimulability; and the **family characteristics and resources** including the support they can provide, and their insight into the child's situation.

Objective Measures

There are three simple-to-use aids available to help in answering questions about severity, each based on objective measures. The three: **PCC, percentage of occurrence of processes or patterns**, and **normative data** can be used in combination, alongside

informal intelligibility ratings and the SLP's/SLT's **impressionistic severity rating** (discussed above).

Percentage of consonants correct (PCC)

Despite its limitations (Flipsen, A9), PCC provides a useful impression of 'severity of involvement' to parents. It is important to explain to them that not everything to do with speech impairment can be neatly classified in terms of severity, and that the severity increments (Mild–Normal, Mild–Moderate, Moderate–Severe and Severe) suggested by Shriberg and Kwiatkowski (1982) for PCCs of >85%, 65–85%, 50–65% and <50% respectively, as displayed in Table i.1 and Box 3.6. Important too, to be aware that they cannot be reliably applied with children below age 4;1 or above age 8;6, and that they are derived from connected speech samples (not single-word naming tasks, for example). Also, the descriptors (Mild–Normal, Mild–Moderate, Moderate–Severe, and Severe) relate to children with *SSD in general*, not to specific diagnoses under the SSD umbrella heading. This means that a child with a PCC below 50 can be said to have a 'severe SSD'. If that same child had a diagnosis of phonological disorder, it would be incorrect to say that the child had a 'severe phonological disorder'. Similarly, if the child had a PCC below 50 and a diagnosis of CAS it would be incorrect to say that he or she had 'severe CAS'.

An advantage of using a scale of 0 to 100 percent is that it can illustrate progress (or lack of progress) over time, to families. As well, some children, from the age of about 4;0, particularly those who are entranced by numbers or who like to see progress represented graphically, enjoy and are encouraged by seeing their PCCs rise. Simple imagery using a drawing of a ladder, mountain, flight path, or train journey (with a PCC of 50 shown at the half-way mark and 100 or thereabouts at the summit or destination and gradations between) can provide pleasure and motivation.

Percentage of occurrence of processes or patterns

Similarly, when the occurrence of phonological patterns or phonological processes is expressed in percentage terms (e.g., Cluster Reduction 100%) in initial reporting to parents, it provides a straightforward way for them to appreciate their child's therapy gains as the percentages drop. Again, this can be conveyed to those children who are spurred on by performance feedback (e.g., verbal praise: 'well done', 'great progress', etc.; non-verbal praise: a thumbs-up sign, and the like) and extrinsic reinforcers (e.g., stamps, stickers, award certificates, progress graphs, etc.).

Normative data

Phonetic acquisition norms (Tables 1.2 and 3.1) and ages of elimination of processes (Tables 2.1 and 3.2) may be helpful for parents, allaying anxiety in those who tend to expect too much too soon, like the parents who worry unnecessarily about gliding off liquids and interdental /s/ and /z/ in 3-year-olds!

Informal intelligibility ratings

The speech and language therapist who is an 'expert' listener may not be the best judge of a child's intelligibility overall. The views of others, including parents/carers, teachers/ assistants, and peers, need to be sought to establish a child's functional intelligibility

Speake et al., 2012, p. 294

Table 3.1 Developmental schedules in the United States (1993; 2020), and internationally (2018).

Order of acquisition * Shriberg, 1993 USA children	Order of acquisition** Crowe & McLeod, 2020 USA children ***	Order of acquisition* McLeod & Crowe, 2018 English-speaking children***
Early 8	Early 2;0–3;11	Early 2;0–3;11
m n j b w d p h	b, n, m, p, h, w, d, g, k, f, t, ŋ, j	p, b, m, d, n, h, t, k, g, w, ŋ, f, j
Middle 8	Middle 4;0–4;11	Middle 4;0–4;11
t ŋ k g v tʃ dʒ	v, dʒ, s, tʃ, l, ʃ, z	l, dʒ, tʃ, s, v, ʃ, z
Late 8	Late 5;0–6;11	Late 5;0–6;11
ʃ ʒ l ɹ s z ð θ	ɹ, ð, ʒ, θ	ɹ, ʒ, ð, θ

Table 3.2 Typical ages-of-elimination of phonological processes (Grunwell, 1987).

Phonological process / Phonological pattern	Approximate age of elimination in years; months
Context-sensitive voicing	3;0
Word-final devoicing	3;0
Final consonant deletion	3;3
Velar fronting	3;9
Palatal fronting	3;9
Consonant harmony/consonant assimilation	4;0
Weak syllable deletion	4;0
Cluster reduction	4;0
Gliding of liquids	5;0
Stopping	
/f/ /s/	3;0
/v/ /z/	3;6
/ʃ/ /tʃ/ /dʒ/	4;6
/θ/ /ð/	5;0

* Data source: monosyllabic words in conversational speech samples
** Data source: single words; 90%–100% acquisition criteria averaged across eight studies
***McLeod & Crowe list consonants in age of acquisition order, from youngest to oldest

Intelligibility ratings are notoriously unreliable, but they have considerable clinical utility, as they are informative for parents. It can be a useful exercise for clinicians to ask parent(s) or a significant other, such as a grandparent or preschool teacher, for impressionistic intelligibility ratings on a 5-point scale:

1. *Completely intelligible*
2. *Mostly intelligible*
3. *Somewhat intelligible*
4. *Mostly unintelligible*
5. *Completely unintelligible*

Those doing the rating are asked, 'How intelligible is [the child's name] in day-to-day conversation. How much of what [the child's name] says do you understand?' They then select a point on the scale. Sometimes they will qualify their ratings, for example, by observing that the child is less intelligible when tired, unwell, or rushed, or that intelligibility often seems better when the child speaks on the telephone, and this is useful information for the clinician to have. Reviewing the original intelligibility ratings for the child and comparing them with current ratings, once intervention is underway and progress is evident, can provide a boost for parents, which they may convey to their child receiving

therapy. Occasionally, it is enlightening to ask children how intelligible they believe they are by getting them to rate a familiar adult as a listener ('How well does dad understand your words?' and 'How well does he understand—'s [naming another child or adult] words?').

Recall from Table 2.2 how prevalence and incidence differ. **Prevalence** refers to the total number (or percentage) of cases of a disease or condition in a population at one time. By contrast, **incidence** refers to the number of new cases of a disorder or disease during a given time interval, usually per annum. Incidence is expressed as *Incidence Proportion (Risk)* or as *Incidence Rate*, both of which are defined in Table 2.2.

Box 3.8 The questions families ask

Prevalence and comorbidities: Do many children have this problem? Do they have difficulties with schoolwork?

We know from **quantitative research** that the short answer to these questions is yes, SSD is a high prevalence disorder in children, either by itself, or

comorbidly with language impairment. Quantitative research deals with data that are numerical or that can be converted into numbers. It involves systematic scientific enquiry into quantifiable (measurable) properties and phenomena and their relationships, using statistical techniques. Such techniques, applied appropriately, allow the organisation, analysis, interpretation, and presentation, of the numerical data generated. A potential pitfall of statistical analysis is that it may be executed on data with poor appreciation of the most suitable statistical tests to use and how to apply them correctly. A benefit of quantitative research in SLP/SLT is that it can provide numerical data to help address the questions that regularly arise in everyday practice.

There is much variation in the research rigour of the slew of studies that tell us that SSD is a high prevalence disorder in children. Confusingly, disparities are found in

- the **definition of SSD**: e.g., whether normative comparisons were made that might explain certain errors or error patterns in younger children, or not.
- the **age-ranges** of children: e.g., just preschoolers aged 3;0 to 5;0 vs. vs. 5;0 to 8-year-olds vs. 8;0-year-olds vs. children 0–14;0 years.
- the **data collection method**: e.g., standardise testing vs. parent and teacher questionnaires vs. prevalence on clinical caseloads reported by SLPs/SLTs.
- the **population sampling** methods including the geographical distribution of the sample: e.g., all babies born in a certain health district or hospital followed over time vs. a school district population sample vs. a population sample across a state, county, or province vs. country-wide sampling.
- the sample size.
- the standardised test cut-off points: e.g., Eadie et al., 2015 used the 10th percentile, whereas Beitchman et al., 1986 who used the 16th percentile.

Sifting through the one hundred of more prevalence studies, it becomes clear that the best estimates to use when informing families, administrators, and ourselves are epidemiological studies based on the most acceptable quantitative methods overall, taking account of the SSD definition, children's ages and age-range, data collection and population sampling methods, numbers of children studies, and test cut-offs.

Four well-designed studies fulfilled these criteria. Two epidemiological studies looked at kindergarten-aged children: Beitchman et al. (1986) considered 5-year-olds in Canada, and McLeod and Harrison (2009) studied 4-and-5-year-olds in Australia. They found a prevalence of approximately 11–12% for SSD incorporating children with speech impairment only (≈6%) and speech impairment comorbidly with language impairment (≈5%). A comorbid condition is a health or developmental problem (in this case, language impairment) that co-occurs with the primary health or developmental problem (in this case, SSD).

The children in the third study, Roulstone et al. (2009) were 8-year-olds in the UK, followed longitudinally with case-control comparisons at 2, 5, and 8 years. At each time-point, Roulstone et al. counted any type of SODA error (errors of substitution, omission, distortion, and omission) finding that at 8 years 18% had persistent speech errors. In the fourth study, Wren et al. (2016) examined and reanalysed the data from the same UK cohort at 8;6 concluding that the prevalence of persistent SSD was 3.6%.

From the range of well-designed prevalence studies, it is known that:

- About 11–12% of 5-year-olds have SSD. Of them, ≈6% have SSD only, and ≈5% have SSD plus language impairment.
- About 18% of 8-year-olds have persistent speech errors.
- Compared with individuals without speech sound disorder, adolescents with SSD at age 8 have twice the risk of reporting self-harm with suicidal intent, even when other important predictors are considered (McAllister et al., 2023).
- A large proportion of children who are treated for SSD as preschoolers continue to produce speech errors into adulthood.
- It is not certain that stuttering (stammering) and SSD are comorbid among preschoolers, but they often co-occur in students on school SLP/SLT caseloads.
- Language, including literacy, disorders are frequently comorbid with SSD.
- Children who have a preschool history of SSD are predisposed to reading difficulties in third grade, if (note *if*):
  - ○ the SSD persists into the school-age period and/or
  - ○ there is comorbid language disorder and/or
  - ○ there is a family history of speech, language, or reading disability.
- Adults diagnosed with moderate phonological disorder when they started school, and whose difficulties with literacy skills persisted, restricting their educational and vocational options,

report life satisfaction comparable with adults without speech impairment histories (Felsenfeld et al., 1994).

- Children with CAS may overcome the disorder, but it appears that many become young people with CAS and eventually, adults with CAS. They may benefit from brief bursts of intensive intervention for speech, language, and literacy, coupled with multi-disciplinary management for psychological issues such as anxiety, particularly performance anxiety around speaking (McCabe, A34).

Aetiology: The Study of Causes or Origins

Not only do the speech, language and reading impairment phenotypes change over time but the proximal and distal factors associated with these phenotypes vary in magnitude at different epochs in development. The notion that phenotypes and the factors that influences them change is a positive one because it allows for the possibility of improvement and recovery. Clearly, the phenomenology of these developmental disorders makes the practical enterprise of identifying children at risk for these disorders and predicting their outcomes a significant challenge.

Taylor & Zubrick, 2009, p. 341

In classification systems for SSD that are based on a medical model, such as the SDCS (Shriberg, Kwiatkowski et al., 2019), causal factors for SSD are frequently described as **proximal (downstream) causes or risk factors** and **distal (upstream) causes or risk factors** (see Table 2.2). 'Proximal' comes from the Latin, *proximus*, or nearest, and 'distal' is derived from the English word, *distant*. The use of the adjectives 'downstream' and 'upstream' constitutes a streamflow metaphor that does not always 'work', is sometimes overly simplistic, and can confuse the way we think about aetiology.

The distal cause or distal risk factor is typically considered to be the 'actual' (real) reason something occurred or might occur or the 'actual' aetiology. It works well in anatomy, where it is from, but in human functioning, disability, and health the

proximal-distal divide is contentious. Krieger (2008) argued that viewing aetiology as a distal-to-proximal, far-to-near, sequence is not necessarily the right way to conceptualise drivers of health, because influences flow in both directions. She found the proximal-distal paradigm, and the downstream-upstream metaphor problematic because it insinuates that the only relationships are causal ones that flow from distal factors to proximal factors. That may be true to an extent, but it does not automatically hold for all the factors.

In the paradigm, proximal and distal causes interact with each other over time; with the child's characteristics (e.g., temperament, personality, sociability, cognitive capacity, wellbeing, etc.); and with the child's environment (e.g., support for the child's learning at home, outside intervention, etc.). These interactions are unique to each child – family – milieu combination, neatly explaining the individual variation and differing developmental trajectories of different children who are diagnosed with the same communication impairment, combination of impairments, or SSD subtype.

Proximal causes are located **downstream**, near, or within a child, and they **directly** affect their body function, health, and/or development. In SSD, such causes might be observed as problems with input processing and/or phonological processing and/or output processing. Proximal causes **explain** the types of speech errors the child produces in terms of the underlying speech process that is impaired.

Distal causes are located **upstream**, far from the child, and **indirectly** affect their body function, health, and/or development. The distal cause is the aetiology, or origin of the underlying speech process that is impaired. For example, family history of speech impairment, developmental language disorder, or reading difficulties (Lewis et al., 2006) imply a genetic or inherited origin.

Box 3.9a   The questions families ask about aetiology

Explaining to families the likely aetiology of a child's SSD when it has a known cause or organic cause is more straightforward – but still potentially complicated – than explaining the likely aetiology of the so-called 'speech disorders of unknown origin' or functional speech disorders. Indeed, many parents come to an initial assessment more conversant with their child's identified condition or syndrome than the practitioner, giving SLPs/SLTs an opportunity to learn from them. These well-informed parents may have acquired their knowledge via medical and developmental specialist consultations (e.g., with audiologists, paediatricians, genetic counsellors, or clinical psychologists), from reading, and from contact with other parents or support groups. As a group, they tend to be the ones who want clear-cut information about aetiology that is as precise and detailed as possible. But it may be challenging or impossible for the SLP/SLT to provide the desired precision and detail because of the many interacting factors that may exist in an individual situation, and because of gaps in the aetiological literature on children's speech.

1. What caused this problem?

The Aetiology of a Speech Sound Disorders with a <u>Known</u> Cause
Known causes of SSD include:

- **Cognitive/Intellectual impairment:** e.g., Down syndrome, Fragile-X syndrome
- **Craniofacial differences**: e.g., cleft palate, velo-cardio-facial syndrome: VCFS (Golding-Kushner, A16)
- Genetic chromosomal conditions/genetic syndromes: e.g., Down syndrome
- **Genetic metabolic conditions:** e.g., Galactosaemia, Phenylketonuria: PKU
- **Hearing impairment**: e.g., sensorineural hearing loss
- **Neurodevelopmental disorders:** e.g., Foetal Alcohol Spectrum Disorder: FASD, Autism spectrum disorder: Autism
- **Neuromotor impairment**: e.g., cerebral palsy

Although we can list known aetiologies, things can become complicated. This is because, often the distal cause of the original problem may have brought about another problem (a proximal cause). The proximal cause may be responsible for maintaining the problem while the distal cause may or may not still be operating, as illustrated in the anonymised case example of Shane in Box 3.9b.

2. What caused this problem?

The Aetiology of a Speech Sound Disorders with an <u>Unknown</u> Cause
Explaining to families – or to anybody – the likely aetiology of a child's SSD that has an unknown cause or a less obvious cause is more complicated. Some families appear content with *'We don't know for sure'* or some other *'It's just one of those things we can't explain'* kind of response, but others find them unacceptable. Fortunately, nowadays we can answer the aetiological and risk factor questions in a more satisfactory manner and answer related questions about prognosis objectively.

Recall from Table 2.3 that Shriberg, Kwiatkowski et al. (2019) provide **population prevalence** figures for CAS (2.4%), Childhood Dysarthria (3.4%), Speech Delay (82.2%), Speech Delay and Concurrent Motor Speech Disorder (17.8%), and Speech Motor Delay (12%). Thirteen years earlier, Shriberg (2006) used the 2006 SDCS nomenclature to report the **clinical prevalence** (percentage of referrals to SLP/SLT) of SD-GEN 56%, SD-OME 30%, SD-DPI 12%, and SD-AOS now called CAS <1%. In the 2019 update of the SDCS, the three subtypes of the large idiopathic Speech Delay (SD) group with its population prevalence of 82.2% were as follows:

- **SD-GEN**, a heritable SSD comprising **56%** of SSD referrals. The proximal cause of SD-GEN, SD-OME, and SD-DPI relates to impaired phonological representations. Two processes, operating singly or in combination, potentially explain the impaired phonological representations (or underlying representations: UR).
  - First, some children may have an auditory-perceptual impairment that makes it difficult for them to transform the speech they hear into clear URs. This is sometimes referred to as having 'fuzzy' representations, something Kyrie suspected when Shane was 4;5.
  - Second, some children may have difficulty with phonological memory processes that disrupt the proper storage and retrieval of

phonological representations when perceiving speech, and during speech production.

- ◦ Third – and this generally applies to children in the severe SD range who *will* have language impairment too – some children may have pervasive difficulties with auditory-perceptual encoding *and* phonological memory.

There is good evidence to support the heritability of SD-GEN. Affected children mostly have a family history of difficulties with speech, language, and/or literacy acquisition (Lewis et al., 2006). Moreover, there is evidence of overlap between the genetic underpinning of SSD and reading disability (Eicher et al., 2015). Many investigators have demonstrated, via robust behavioural, neuroimaging, and genetics studies, that the proximal cause common in SSD *and* reading impairment is difficulty with phonological processing (e.g., Claessen & Leitão, 2012; Larrivee & Catts, 1999; Rice et al., 2020; Unger et al., 2021).

- **SD-OME**, comprises 30% of SSD referrals. Otitis Media with Effusion (OME) is a risk factor but not necessarily a cause of SSD as a direct causal link is not clear.
- **SD-DPI** comprises 12% of SD referrals. Like OME above, Developmental Psychosocial Involvement (DPI) is a risk factor, but not necessarily a proximal cause of SSD, because a direct causal link is not established.

The case example of Shane in Box 3.9b shows how the distal and proximal causes of current difficulties can change. His story also serves to introduce another topic: the potential hazards of taking too-narrow a focus on the case history and assessment process.

Box 3.9b   Case example: Shane

Shane was diagnosed at birth with a non-syndromic unilateral cleft palate necessitating several surgeries. Eustachian tube dysfunction was suspected early and at 16 months It was found that both his eustachian tubes were narrow with medial to lateral compression and poor elasticity. When Kyrie, his SLP enquired, Shane's parents Conor and Siobhan reported no family history of craniofacial anomalies, hearing impairment, or speech and language difficulties.

As a capable and key member of a cleft palate team, Kyrie had a special interest in infants, toddlers, and preschoolers born with cleft lip and palate, and in working on any of their feeding issues, cleft speech characteristics: CSCs (Alighieri et al., 2020, 2022; Golding-Kushner, A16; Ruscello, A38) and cooccurring difficulties. These were areas where she had extensive experience as a clinician and published researcher. Colleagues valued her expertise, often consulting her for second opinions.

Shane and his mother first met with Kyrie soon after his birth and before they were discharged from hospital, for feeding advice. After four difficult weeks, Shane routinely finished a (bottle) feed in 30 minutes, thrived, and proceeded to solid foods at 6 months. He had no subsequent feeding difficulties.

Continuing to support the family, Kyrie monitored his voice, speech, and language progress closely and at 2;9 administered the 37-word *Toddler Phonology Test* (McIntosh & Dodd, 2011) noting typical nasal resonance, atypical phonological patterns, and an inconsistency score of 54%, potentially heralding an SSD. A year later at 3;9, Kyrie reviewed the case history information that Conor and Siobhan had provided when Shane was an infant, confirming that there was no known family history of craniofacial anomalies, or difficulties with hearing, speech, or language. She then reassessed his speech and language progress, recording a primary diagnosis of phonological disorder with articulatory and auditory-perceptual difficulties, good stimulability for singleton consonants, poor stimulability for CVs and VCs, and low receptive and expressive vocabularies. His consonantal phonetic inventory was sparse (lacking /t, d, ŋ, s, z, ʃ, ʒ, θ, ð, f, v, tʃ, dʒ, ɹ/ and /l/) while his vowel inventory was complete. Typical phonological patterns were present: final consonant deletion (with no word final/syllable final glottal replacement), stopping of fricatives, cluster reduction, and weak syllable deletion. He also had the unusual patterns (for English) of extensive initial consonant deletion, deletion of alveolar stops and nasals, and gliding of the fricatives /f and /v/ word initially (e.g., *win* for *fin*) and syllable initially within words (e.g., [ˈwʌniˌweɪ] for funnyface). His intelligibility was low, but in Kyrie's opinion his speech output, voice and resonance did not reflect his cleft history.

In her report, and in discussion with Conor and Siobhan, Kyrie emphasised that while his speech and language difficulties were quite marked, Shane 'ticked all the boxes' for a hopeful prognosis. She highlighted to them Shane's sociable, friendly personality and his persistence during difficult tasks and when asked to repeat utterances – often several times – due to his poor intelligibility. She counselled that these were important attributes because they were identified as 'protective factors' by Harrison and McLeod (2010). She also stressed the value of their unfailing support for Shane's development and learning.

Distal and proximal factors in Shane's SSD

Shane's **craniofacial anomalies** – cleft palate and narrow, obstructed eustachian tubes – were the **distal cause** of his SSD. The distal cause likely led to eustachian tube dysfunction involving poor middle ear aeration. He had continual bouts of otitis media with effusion (OME) from the ages of 6–18 months (see Box 3.6) and beyond. During these episodes, Conor and Siobhan saw that Shane was noticeably hard of hearing, and by 3;9 – when the SSD diagnosis was made – his audiologist, ENT specialist, and Kyrie hypothesised that the **proximal factor** in his speech delay was intermittent conductive hearing loss – bearing in mind that OME is a risk factor for SSD rather than a direct cause (Shriberg, Kwiatkowski et al., 2019).

Fortunately for Shane, successful cleft palate surgeries, which began when he was a year old, yielded a satisfactory cosmetic outcome and his orofacial anatomy, including his dental anatomy, and palate function were adequate for normal voice and speech development. However, bilateral myringotomies and insertion of tympanostomy tubes at 24 and 30 months did not solve his conductive hearing difficulties because the tubes fell out, both times, shortly after they were introduced. At 4;0 he had ear surgery for a third time, successfully, and regular reviews by his audiologist showed that his hearing acuity was within normal limits, and stable.

Kyrie saw him for intervention, with one or other parent participating in the sessions, once weekly. Progress was gradual and at 4;5 his speech remained largely unintelligible with a PCC of 38%, putting his SSD in the severe range on the Shriberg and Kwiatkowski (1982) scale displayed in Box 3.7. Kyrie noted again that he performed poorly on

tests of stimulability and auditory discrimination, and that he had semantic and syntactic difficulties. Thinking about his speech, she postulated that Shane might have fuzzy, poorly developed underlying representations (URs) of phonemes, arising from his longstanding suboptimal hearing (now resolved). By now, his hearing impairment was becoming thought of as the *new* distal cause of his SSD, and his unreliable underlying representations as the *maintaining* proximal cause now that his orofacial structures were functionally adequate.

After a slow start, Shane progressed gradually in intervention with a well-reasoned combination (Alighieri et al., 2022) of a **motor-phonetic–based approach** (Sand et al., 2022) including **stimulability intervention** (Miccio, A17), **phonological intervention** in the form of multiple oppositions intervention (Williams, A19), and speech **perception training** (Hearnshaw et al., 2018; Rvachew, A18). These approaches were integrated with work on his receptive and expressive **vocabulary** and **grammar**, supported by diligent home-practice in quiet, conducive surroundings (i.e., good listening conditions) with Conor and/or Siobhan. Although his language difficulties persisted, at 5;9 he had a PCC of 75%, equating to a mild-to-moderate SSD.

An enthusiastic, sociable student, Shane was popular with his peers, loved school, and was usually intelligible to strangers by the time he was 6;1 and engaged in formal reading instruction. He discontinued his SLP intervention around then because Conor and Siobhan were content with his speech progress and wanted him to 'concentrate on schoolwork'. However, he returned for a review assessment with Kyrie at 7;5 because his teacher was concerned about his slow reading, spelling, and written expression progress, and poor performance on phonological awareness (PA) tasks (McNeill, A22; Neilson, A49).

Kyrie found that he had mild speech difficulties with rhotics and three voiced fricatives. He replaced /ɹ/ with [w] and stopped /v/ with [b] and /ʒ/ and /ð/ with [d] (see the late-4 acquired consonants at 5;0 to 6;11 determined by McLeod & Crowe, 2018 in Table 1.2). His PCC was 90%, and his receptive and expressive vocabularies, and syntax were below age expectations (16th percentile). He resisted a reading task, saying '*Reading makes me feel stupid*', and abandoning the task when the first 'tricky word' occurred. Kyrie was disheartened: this was so out of character for Shane.

So, almost seven and a half years after meeting in a neonatal unit, Kyrie recommended assessment, with a view to further therapy with Dhin, a speech-language clinician and former primary school teacher (i.e., a junior school, elementary school, or grade-school teacher of 5- to 11-year-olds) who visited the school to work with children with speech, language, and literacy difficulties.

When Dhin had supplemented Kyrie's assessment with further procedures including a brief trial of evidence-based reading and spelling intervention (Snow, 2016, 2021) he met with Conor and Siobhan who warmed to him immediately, willingly engaging in a *third* SLP/SLT case history interview. Afterwards, Dhin and Kyrie talked. Inevitably, the topic of aetiology arose in the handover process. With great assurance, Kyrie stressed Shane's hearing history as a distal cause, and the probable cooccurrence of SSD and low or slow reading acquisition, particularly given Shane's persistent mild speech, semantic and syntactic difficulties. When she finished, Dhin asked a question that had been bothering him since meeting with Shane's parents.

Dhin: *Did they tell you about the family history of dyslexia?*
Kyrie (stunned):   *What?*
Dhin: On Siobhan's side. Her father, an uncle and one of her two brothers. Her other brother read just fine, but his 8-year-old daughter struggles with literacy.
Kyrie: How did I miss that red flag! Did you say the family history, in combination with his speech, semantic and syntactic problems was significant?
Dhin: I did. They said it answered a lot of questions for them. Conor is a funny guy, isn't he? He told me they'd always blamed Shane's plumbing for his speech and language disorders, but now they saw it was down to a combination of plumbing and wiring! I didn't say that what with downstream and upstream we can do without more metaphors – but I thought it!
Dhin (finally noticing Kyrie's discomfort): Don't worry. They're still your number one fans. I have big shoes to fill.

Kyrie was dismayed. She had 'missed' a likely contributor to Shane's language and literacy problems. She realised she had focussed too narrowly on her clinical and research area – craniofacial anomalies – as the aetiology of Shane's speech, language, and literacy difficulties, to the exclusion of other aspects of his history. She prided herself an taking careful, detailed histories, and staying abreast of research literature, so it was hard for her to put her oversight down to experience and move on.

Horses, Not Zebras

When you hear hoofbeats behind you, don't expect to see a zebra.
    Theodore E. Woodward, MD (1914–2005),
                          cited by Sotos, 1991

Whether conducting informal (triage) screening, formal screening assessment, or formal diagnostic assessment, SLPs/SLTs are mindful of the prevalence figures for the various types of SSD. Good judgment dictates that the process of zeroing in on a diagnosis will *probably* point, progressively, to one, or a combination of, the more common speech sound disorders: articulation disorder or phonological disorder. It could *possibly* point to CAS, alone, or in the mix but that would be relatively infrequent finding. There is a wisdom in taking this common-sense, 'expect horses, not zebras' approach to speech assessment that starts with the expectation of identifying 'the usual'. That is not to say that we should doubt our own judgement, or feel we are complicating the situation unnecessarily, when we notice pointers to an infrequent, alternative diagnosis, or to unusual co-occurring concerns. Rather, we must follow them up to rule them 'in' or 'out'.

The inspiration for the title *Zebra Cards: An aid to obscure diagnosis* (Sotos, 1991) was the quote from Woodward, above. Sotos writes (https://www.zebracards.org)

Zebra Cards is about patients who surprise us. It's about listening to the patient, looking at the patient, and knowing that the human body is subtle in its wiles. It's an inoculation against clinical hubris and impatience.

At the time of Kyrie's first contact with Shane, Siobhan and Conor, the prospect of future reading difficulties was far from everyone's thoughts. An authority on cleft palate in infants, toddlers and preschoolers, Kyrie was consulted *because* of her special expertise, and her case history questions were centred around orofacial anomalies, hearing impairment, and speech and language development. She had taken the sensible step of a case history review at 3;9 but crucially, did not ask: *Do you have a history of reading problems or learning problems in either of your families*? Even when Shane was 7;5 with his teacher reporting problems with PA, reading, spelling, and written expression, neither Kyrie nor the teacher asked. It was not until Dhin, coming freshly to the situation, with generalist knowledge of clefts, OME, and conductive hearing loss, and extensive knowledge of the science of language and reading (Snow, 2021) identified the questions that needed asking, receiving relevant and helpful replies.

Two Simple Rules

In making the diagnosis of the cause of illness in an individual case, calculations of probability have no meaning. The pertinent question is whether the disease is present or not. Whether it is rare or common does not change the odds in a single patient. … If the diagnosis can be made based on specific criteria, then these criteria are either fulfilled or not fulfilled.

Harvey et al. (1979)

I am a veteran of hundreds of 'second' opinions (for which read second, third, fourth…opinion, in many instances), and many transfers of clients to me from previous therapists. Arising from this experience, I suggest, when presenting SSD continuing professional development events, two simple rules to employ when assessing 'new' clients. The rules are unoriginal, unexciting, and important. They apply whether the client and family are new to SLP/SLT, new on your caseload having received SLP/SLT services previously, or a newly referred sibling of a child or children you have seen.

1. **Take a detailed history**

   Even if time is short, avoid relying on telephone intake information, a history provided by a previous therapist, or by the person who referred the client to you, or details in a pen-and-paper or online case history questionnaire. Gather necessary information yourself, in a face-to-face interview. In some workplaces, where one clinician assesses and another delivers intervention, this may mean going through the assessor's history entries in the file to double-check and augment where necessary. Ask *before* the interview if parents are comfortable with the child's presence in the interview, and if not, ensure that arrangements are made to have the child minded while they are out of the room (e.g., they might bring a willing friend or relative).

   Rationale

   A case history interview is an opportunity for you to join with the family, start getting to know them, and learn what is important to them, so initiating a collaborative working relationship. Conversely, it is their opportunity to get to know you as an ally in helping their child. Some parents (and clinicians) prefer children *not* to be present at these interviews because they don't want the child to hear themselves being 'discussed', but if they are there, it is an opportunity for the child to see their parents interacting positively and cooperating with this 'new' grown-up, and possibly for you to explain simply to the child what the interview is about.

2. **Do an oral musculature examination**

   Every time you add a new client to your caseload, perform an oral musculature examination (also called intraoral examination, oral peripheral examination, oral inspection, and oral examination). Don't be lulled by the thought that someone else (e.g., their GP, ENT, Paediatrician, or a previous SLP/SLT) has already done so. Perhaps they have, but you need to look for yourself. If the child is uncooperative – as frequently, and understandably occurs with children who are very young, or cautious with new people, or who need time to 'warm-up' in new situations – make a note in their file to try again when the time is right.

   Resource

   The components of and procedure for performing an oral musculature examination are described in Box 2.1 where there is an example of a form for collecting oral inspection data. The two-page form is available, copyright free, for clinicians to use and adapt; see https://www.speech-language-therapy.com/images/omesf2pp.pdf

Rationale

Systematic examination of each client's oral-peripheral mechanism is an obligatory component of SLP/SLT assessment. Its purpose is to establish whether the structure (anatomy) and the function of the speech articulators will allow the production of age-typical speech output. Oral structure embraces the anatomic proportions, shape, and symmetry of the articulators, while oral function concerns movements of the organs of speech in terms of range, speed, precision, and coordination. In the diagnostic process, observations drawn from the oral musculature examination allow SLPs/SLTs to rule-in, rule-out or query any structure related or function related issues that might be causing or contributing to clients' difficulties.

My second opinion and client-handover experiences have taught me those intraoral examinations are sometimes *not* performed, only partially completed, and not repeated as longer-term clients grow and develop. This can happen easily. For example, very young or apprehensive children often refuse to 'open wide' or 'show me what you had for breakfast' so the clinician (wisely) backs off, intending to return to the task when the child has adjusted to the situation and is more forthcoming. When this happens, it is important to record in the child's file that the examination was omitted, or incomplete.

Various scenarios may follow for example, the clinician forgets to do the oral exam; or the clinician moves to a different post and his or her successor, in the absence of a verbal report or case note, may *assume* the procedure was carried out; or, with clients who attend for a long time it can be overlooked that their oral musculature examination may be out-of-date. My experience had included discovering ankyloglossia, submucous clefts, a tiny hard palate fistula (once), and significant dental caries in children who had returned normal results at younger ages.

Box 3.10   The questions families ask

Prognosis: What does the future hold?

Questions about the anticipated duration of intervention, dosage and intensity of service delivery, and the eventual prognosis – with and without intervention – are couched in a variety of ways. They include *'How much treatment does my child need?'* (this may sound like an enquiry about the probable cost in money and time) to a more direct, *'Will my child's speech be normal by school-entry age?'* and *'Will my child's speech improve to the point that no one would know there was ever a speech difficulty?'* to *'What happens if you don't treat, and hope they'll grow out of it?'* Such questions are commonly asked early in the therapeutic engagement, often prior to assessment or intervention, so too soon in most cases for SLPs/SLTs to give reasoned answers. Reasoned answers will usually become more available once the clinician has completed an assessment, initiated intervention, observed early progress (or not), and started to know the child in terms of cooperation and interest in therapy, temperament (especially the protective factors of persistence and sociability identified by Harrison & McLeod, 2010), ability and willingness to stay on-task, and has developed a realistic expectation of the level of support they will receive at home. If some questions come too soon, the most logical answers will be along the lines of: *'Let me get to know you and* [child's name] *a little before I give you an answer'* or *'It's a bit too early to tell. I need to work with you and* [child's name] *before I can give you a sensible reply'* and *'What I can tell you at this early stage is that, for most children with SSD, the outlook is optimistic'* (Gierut, 1998; Kamhi, 2006; Shriberg, 1997).

'WHAT HAPPENS IF YOU DON'T TREAT? WON'T THEY GROW OUT OF IT?'

Normalisation without treatment

Normalisation of SSD without intervention depends on the child's stimulability and intelligibility. If children are stimulable for all their erred consonants in CV nonsense syllables, and their intelligibility to caregivers is high, according to the *Intelligibility in Context Scale* (https://www.csu.edu.au/research/multilingual-speech/ics) their median age of no-treatment normalisation is 6.59 years of age (To et al., 2022). To and colleagues reported that those with atypical error patterns, and those with expressive language difficulties did not necessarily take longer to normalize. They also noted that current research yields differing findings on the no-treatment prognosis for children with cooccurring SSD and Developmental Language Disorder (DLD) so it is uncertain whether low expressive language ability is a risk factor for persistent SSD.

Normalisation with treatment

If diagnosis is early, and intervention is early (with older 3s and possibly younger 4s) the short-term prognosis for speech normalisation appears comparatively positive (e.g., Webster et al., 1997 who followed 45 children whose average age was three). Bear in mind, however, that overdiagnosis of SSD in 3-year-olds is probably higher than it is with 4s and 5s, and that a proportion of diagnosed 3-year-olds might have achieved typical phonology without intervention (Glogowska et al., 2000).

When children are diagnosed towards the end of their time at preschool (as often happens) or once they begin school, age-typical speech in the short-term – where short-term means within two years of diagnosis or by the 6th birthday according to Shriberg et al. (1994) – is less probable. Shriberg et al. (1994) followed 54 four-year-olds whose SSDs were, on average, severe and only 18% displayed short-term normalisation. Subsequently, Shriberg (1997) reported that about 75% of children with speech delay had normal range speech performance by age of six (with or without SLP/SLT intervention), and that the remainder (25%) normalised by nine, with just a few children showing residual errors, typically involving /s/, /ɹ/ and /l/.

A decade later, Dodd et al. (2018) monitored 93 children with SSD from age 4 to age 7. These children exhibited less severe SSDs than the Shriberg et al., 1994 cohort. Of them, 58% of the children attained normal speech production abilities. Applying Dodd's classification, the DDCS (Dodd, 2005; Leahy & Dodd, 1987; Waring & Dodd, A7) described in Chapter 2, short-term normalisation was most likely for the children with Phonological Delay (67%), less so for those with consistent phonological disorder (45%) and least likely for those with inconsistent speech disorder (0%).

Prioritising children with SSD for treatment

Epidemiological studies aid us in the sometimes-sensitive process of prioritising children for speech and language services, based on their presentation at the time of initial assessment and/or initial diagnosis. Rvachew and Rafaat (2014) appraised a selection of carefully designed, published reports, concluding that immediate SLP/SLT intervention should be offered when SSD under the following conditions:

1. The child is aged from 4 to 6 years, inclusive
2. There is a family history of speech, language, or fluency disorder
3. There is a comorbid language disorder
4. The SSD significantly impacts activities of daily living

Rvachew and Rafaat further concluded that if none of the four risk factors were present, a longer period could be left between diagnosis and services. To et al. (2022) advised that children with low intelligibility and poor stimulability should take priority for SLP/SLT services due to the unlikelihood of their speech errors resolving naturally.

Questions Posed to E3BPforSSD Members

When writing Chapter 3, I asked the members of the E3BPforSSD private Facebook Group to share questions their clients had put to them. It was interesting to see the variety of questions, some of them familiar, and some unusual, and to consider possible answers.

- Are there apps we can buy to use instead of coming to speech?
- Can we see you more often?
- Could he have the SSD because he's a middle child?
- Do we need to come for very long? How long?
- Does thumb-sucking cause SSD?
- Does not being breast fed cause SSD?
- Does drinking from a sippy cup cause SSD?
- Everyone says I talk too fast, and I'm scared that causes SSD. Does it?
- Has anyone found a causal link between SSD and eating a limited variety of food textures, especially

having a diet of mainly soft food that requires little chewing?

- How long will it take for the SSD to be fixed and for speech to be normal?
- I don't really want to have a break from coming; can we keep seeing you?
- If adults around the child wear face masks, will it affect speech development?
- Is SSD due to (a child's) laziness?
- Might the SSD have developed because we don't read to him? He hates stories!
- My in-laws think the SSD is because I couldn't breast feed. Could that be right?
- Please can you suggest a workbook we can get to help with speech?
- We want to know if the SSD is because we speak two languages at home.
- What can we do to help at home?
- Where can we find some special mouth exercises that will help?
- Will SSD cause spelling problems?
- Which method do you use?

Which Method Do You Use?

Choosing the right approach to treatment is paramount to success in speech sound therapy.
Farquharson and Tambyraja (2022)

It is quite usual for parents to ask their new therapist the final question on the list, '*Which method do you use?*' especially if they have been advised – perhaps by a non-SLP/SLT – that a particular method is desirable or even 'the method' of choice. There is, of course, a range of evidence-based treatment approaches for SSD available and these are described in Chapters 1 (CPPA), 3 (intervention for children with craniofacial anomalies), 4 and 5 (phonetic, stimulability, perceptual, and phonological approaches, and more), 7 (Phonotactic Therapy), and 8 (intervention approaches for motor speech disorders in children: Childhood Apraxia of Speech: CAS and Childhood Dysarthria).

Since CAS, and speech motor delay (SMD) associated with Down syndrome appear to be the SSDs that stimulate the most activity among the

people who produce interventions with little regard for evidence or peer-reviewed publication (Bowen & Snow, 2017), the parents' 'which method' question is discussed at the end of Chapter 8. But first, let's move on to Chapters 4 and 5, which bristle with treatment choices.

References

Alighieri, C., Bettens, K., Bruneel, L., D'haeseleer, E., Van Gaever, E., & Van Lierde, K. (2020). Effectiveness of speech intervention in patients with a cleft palate: Comparison of motor-phonetic versus linguistic-phonological speech approaches. *Journal of Speech, Language, and Hearing Research, 63*(12), 3909–3933. https://doi.org/10.1044/2020_jslhr-20-00129

Alighieri, C., Bettens, K., Bruneel, L., Perry, J., Hens, G., & Van Lierde, K. (2022). One size doesn't fit all: A pilot study towards performance-specific speech intervention in children with a cleft (lip and) palate. *Journal of Speech, Language, and Hearing Research, 65*(2), 649–686. https://doi.org/10.1044/2021_JSLHR-21-00405

Alighieri, C., Bettens, K., Verhaeghe, S., & Van Lierde, K. (2021). From excitement to self-doubt and insecurity: Speech-language pathologists' perceptions and experiences when treating children with a cleft palate. *International Journal of Language & Communication Disorders, 56*(4), 739–753. https://doi.org/10.1111/1460-6984.12624

American Psychological Association. (n.d.). *APA dictionary of psychology.* https://dictionary.apa.org

American Speech-Language-Hearing Association. (2015). Type, degree, and configuration of hearing loss. *Audiology Information Series.* https://www.asha.org/siteassets/ais/ais-hearing-loss-types-degree-configuration.pdf

American Speech-Language-Hearing Association. (2016). *Scope of practice in speech-language pathology [Scope of Practice].* www.asha.org/policy

Asad, A. N., Purdy, S. C., Ballard, E., Fairgray, L., & Bowen, C. (2018). Phonological processes in the speech of school-age children with hearing loss: Comparisons with children with normal hearing. *Journal of Communication Disorders, 74,* 10–22. https://doi.org/10.1016/j.jcomdis.2018.04.004

Baker, E. (2021). Minimal pairs intervention. In A. L. Williams, S. McLeod, & R. J. McCauley (Eds.), *Interventions for speech sound disorders in children* (2nd ed., pp. 33–60). Brookes.

Bauman-Waengler, J. (2020). *Articulatory and phonological impairments: A clinical focus* (6th ed.). Pearson Education, Inc.

Beitchman, J. H., Nair, R., Clegg, M., Patel, P. G., Ferguson, B., Pressman, E., & Smith, A. (1986). Prevalence of speech and language disorders in 5-year-old kindergarten children in the Ottawa-Carleton region. *Journal of Speech and Hearing Disorders*, *51*(2), 98–110. https://doi.org/10.1044/jshd.5102.98

Bishop, D. V. M., & Adams, C. (1990). A prospective study of the relationship between specific language impairment, phonological disorders and reading retardation. *The Journal of Child Psychology and Psychiatry*, *31*(7), 1027–1050. https://doi.org/10.1111/j.1469-7610.1990.tb00844.x

Bitter, J. R. (2021). *Theory and practice of couples and family counseling* (3rd ed.). American Counseling Association.

Bowen, C. (1996). *The quick screener*, speech-language-therapy dot com. www.speech-language-therapy.com

Bowen, C. (1998). speech-language-therapy dot com. https://www.speech-language-therapy.com

Bowen, C. (2006a). *The quick screener for teachers*, speech-language-therapy dot com. www.speech-language-therapy.com

Bowen, C. (2010). *The quick vowel screener*. Speech-language-therapy dot com. www.speech-language-therapy.com

Bowen, C. (2019). Phonological and phonemic awareness. In J. S. Damico & M. J. Ball (Eds.), *The SAGE encyclopedia of human communication sciences and disorders* (pp. 1366–1370). Sage Publications.

Bowen, C. (2023). The Speech Sound Disorders Umbrella with Plain English Labels. https://www.speech-language-therapy.com/images/cssd3efig3_1umbrella.png

Bowen, C., & Snow, P. (2017). *Making sense of interventions for children with developmental disorders*. J & R Press.

Bowlby, J. (2015). *A secure base*. Routledge. (Original work published 1988).

Branson, D., & Demchak, M. (2009). The use of augmentative and alternative communication methods with infants and toddlers with disabilities: A research review. *Augmentative and Alternative Communication*, *25*(4), 274–286. https://doi.org/10.3109/07434610903384529

Broomfield, J., & Dodd, B. (2004). The nature of referred subtypes of primary speech disability. *Child Language Teaching and Therapy*, *20*(2), 135–151. https://doi.org/10.1191%2F0265659004ct267oa

Chin, S. B., Tsai, P. L., & Gao, S. (2003). Connected speech intelligibility of children with cochlear implants and children with normal hearing. *American Journal of Speech-Language Pathology*, *12*(4), 440–451. https://doi.org/10.1044/1058-0360(2003/090)

Ching, T. Y. C., & Dillon, H. A. (2013). Major findings of the LOCHI study on children at 3 years of age and implications for audiological management. *International Journal of Audiology*, *52*, S65–S68. https://doi.org/10.3109/14992027.2013.866339

Chow, J. C. (2018). Comorbid language and behavior problems: Development, frameworks, and intervention. *School Psychology Quarterly*, *33*(3), 356–360. https://doi.org/10.1037/spq0000270

Chow, J. C., & Wallace, E. S. (2021). Speech-language pathologists' behavior management training and reported experiences with challenging behavior. *Communication Disorders Quarterly*, *42*(2), 67–72. https://doi.org/10.1177%2F1525740119887914

Chow, J. C., Zimmerman, K. N., & Senter, N. (2021). Tailoring effective behavior management strategies for speech-language pathologists. *Language, Speech, and Hearing Services in Schools*, *52*(1), 260–272. https://doi.org/10.1044/2020_lshss-20-00073

Claessen, M., & Leitão, S. (2012). Phonological representations in children with SLI. *Child Language Teaching and Therapy*, *28*(2), 211–223. https://doi.org/10.1177%2F0265659012436851

Committee on Hospital Care and Institute for Patient- and Family-Centered Care. (2012). Patient-and Family-centered care and the pediatrician's role. *Pediatrics*, *129*(2), 394–404. https://doi.org/10.1542/peds.2011-3084

Crowe, K., & McLeod, S. (2020). Children's English consonant acquisition in the United States: A review. *American Journal of Speech-Language Pathology*, *29*(4), 2155–2169. https://doi.org/10.1044/2020_AJSLP-19-00168

Davies, K. E., Marshall, J., Brown, L. J. E., & Goldbart, J. (2019). SLTs' conceptions about their own and parents' roles during intervention with preschool children. *International Journal of Language & Communication Disorders*, *54*(4), 596–605. https://doi.org/10.1111/1460-6984.12462

Dodd, B. (Ed.). (2005). *Differential diagnosis and treatment of children with speech disorder* (2nd ed.). Whurr Publishers.

Dodd, B., Hua, Z., Crosbie, S., Holm, A., & Ozanne, A. (2002). *Diagnostic evaluation of articulation and phonology: DEAP*. Pearson Education.

Dodd, B., Ttofari-Eecen, K., Brommeyer, K., Ng, K., Reilly, S., & Morgan, A. (2018). Delayed and disordered development of articulation and phonology between four and seven years. *Child Language Teaching and Therapy, 34*(2), 87–99. https://doi.org/10.1177%2F0265659017735958

Dreikurs, R. (1940a, November). The importance of group life. *Camping Magazine*, 3–4, 27.

Dreikurs, R. (1940b, December). The child in the group. *Camping Magazine*, 7–9.

Dreikurs, R. (1948). *The challenge of parenthood*. Duell, Sloan, & Pearce.

Dreikurs, R. (1950). The immediate purpose of children's misbehavior, its recognition and correction. *Internationale Zeitschrift für Individual-psychologie, 19*, 70–87. https://www.adlerpedia.org/bibliographies/9804

Dreikurs, R., & Soltz, V. (1964). *Children: The challenge*. Hawthorn.

Eadie, P., Morgan, A., Ukoumunne, O. C., Ttofari Eecen, K., Wake, M., & Reilly, S. (2015). Speech sound disorder at 4 years: Prevalence, comorbidities, and predictors in a community cohort of children. *Developmental Medicine and Child Neurology, 57*(6), 578–584. https://doi.org/10.1111/dmcn.12635

Ebbels, S. H., McCartney, E., Slonims, V., Dockrell, J. E., & Norbury, C. (2018). Evidence based pathways to intervention for children with language disorders. *International Journal of Language and Communication Disorders, 54*(1), 3–19. https://doi.org/10.1111/1460-6984.12387

Eicher, J. D., Stein, C. M., Deng, F., Ciesla, A. A., Powers, N. R., Boada, R., Smith, S. D., Pennington, B. F., Iyengar, S. K., Lewis, B. A., & Gruen, J. R. (2015). The DYX2 locus and neurochemical signaling genes contribute to speech sound disorder and related neurocognitive domains. *Genes, brain, and behavior, 14*(4), 377–385. https://doi.org/10.1111/gbb.12214

Eisenson, J., & Ogilvie, M. (1963). *Speech correction in the schools*. Macmillan.

Ellis Weismer, S., Venker, C. E., & Robertson, S. (2017). Focused stimulation approach to language intervention. In R. J. McCauley, M. E. Fey, & R. B. Gillam (Eds.), *Treatment of language disorders in children* (2nd ed., pp. 121–154). Paul H. Brookes Publishing Co.

Ertmer, D. J. (2008). Speech intelligibility in young cochlear implant recipients: Gains during year three. *Volta Review, 107*(2), 85–99. http://dx.doi.org/10.17955/tvr.107.2.585

Estabrooks, W., MacIver-Lux, K., & Rhoades, E. A. (2016). *Auditory-verbal therapy for young children with hearing loss and their families and the practitioners who guide them*. Plural Publishing, Inc.

Farquharson, K., & Tambyraja, S. (2022). Introduction: Innovations in treatment for children with speech sound disorders. *Language, Speech, and Hearing Services in Schools, 53*(3), 627–631. https://doi.org/10.1044/2022_LSHSS-22-00065

Felsenfeld, S., Broen, P. A., & McGue, M. (1994). A 28-year follow-up of adults with a history of moderate phonological disorder: Educational and occupational results. *Journal of Speech and Hearing Research, 37*(6), 1341–1353. https://doi.org/10.1044/jshr.3706.1341

Flipsen, P. J., & Parker, R. G. (2008). Phonological patterns in the conversational speech of children with cochlear implants. *Journal of Communication Disorders, 41*(4), 337–357. https://doi.org/10.1016/j.jcomdis.2008.01.003

Geiss, S., & Serianni, R. (2018). Interprofessional practice in schools: Part 3. *Perspectives of the ASHA Special Interests Groups: SIG, 16*(3), 88–94. https://doi.org/10.1044/persp3.SIG16.88

Gergen, K. (2009). *Relational being: Beyond self and community*. Oxford University Press.

Gibbon, F. (2013). Therapy for abnormal vowels in children with speech disorders. In M. J. Ball & F. E. Gibbon (Eds.), *Handbook of vowels and vowel disorders* (pp. 429–446). Psychology Press.

Gierut, J. (1989). Maximal opposition approach to phonological treatment. *Journal of Speech and Hearing Disorders, 54*(1), 9–19. https://doi.org/10.1044/jshd.5401.09

Gierut, J. A. (1998). Treatment efficacy: Functional phonological disorders in children. *Journal of Speech, Language, and Hearing Research, 41*(1), S85–S100. https://doi.org/10.1044/jslhr.4101.s85

Glogowska, M., Roulstone, S., Enderby, P., & Peters, T. (2000). Randomised controlled trial of community-based speech and language therapy in preschool children. *British Medical Journal, 321*, 923–928. https://doi.org/10.1136/bmj.321.7266.923

Goldberg, S. (2006). Shedding your fears: Bedside etiquette for dying patients. *Topics in Stroke Rehabilitation, 13*(1), 63–67. https://doi.org/10.1310/F9XR-U2AT-CACK-0PV3

Golding-Kushner, K. J. (2001). *Therapy techniques for cleft palate speech and related disorders.* Singular.

Golding-Kushner, K. J. (2005). Speech and language disorders in velo-cardiofacial syndrome. In K. Murphy & P. Scambler (Eds.), *Velo-cardio-facial syndrome: A Model for understanding microdeletion disorders* (pp. 181–199). Cambridge University Press.

Golding-Kushner, K. J. (2020). Communication in velo-cardio-facial syndrome. In D. Landsman (Ed.), *Educating children with velo-cardio-facial syndrome, 22q11.2 deletion syndrome, and Digeorge syndrome* (3rd ed., pp. 101–132). Plural Publishing.

Golding-Kushner, K. J., Argamaso, R. V., Cotton, R. T., Grames, L. M., Henningsson, G., Jones, D. L., Karnell, M. P., Klaiman, P. G., Lewin, M. L., Marsh, J. L., & Skolnik, M. (1990). Standardization for the reporting of nasopharyngoscopy and multiview videofluoroscopy: A report from an International Working Group. *Cleft Palate Journal, 27*(4), 337–347. https://doi.org/10.1597%2F1545-1569_1990_027_0337_sftron_2.3.co_2

Golding-Kushner, K. J., & Scherer, N. (2020). *Family-centered speech-language services via telepractice for individuals with craniofacial anomalies.* American Speech-Language-Hearing Association. http://tiny.cc/wgmwtz

Golding-Kushner, K. J., & Shprintzen, R. (2011). *Velo-cardio-facial syndrome volume 2: Treatment of communication disorders.* Plural Publishing, Inc.

Goldman, R., & Fristoe, M. (2000). *Goldman-Fristoe test of articulation-2 (GFTA-2).* American Guidance Service.

Goldman, R., & Fristoe, M. (2015). *Goldman-Fristoe test of articulation-3 (GFTA-3).* PsychCorp.

Grunwell, P. (1987). *Clinical phonology* (2nd ed.). Williams & Wilkins.

Grunwell, P. (1989). Developmental phonological disorders and normal speech development: A review and illustration. *Child Language Teaching and Therapy, 5*(3), 304–319. https://doi.org/10.1177%2F026565908900500305

Haley, J. (1976). *Problem solving therapy.* Harper.

Halle, J. W., Ostrosky, M. M., & Hemmetter, M. L. (2006). Functional communication training: A strategy for ameliorating challenging behavior. In R. J. McCauley & M. E. Fey (Eds.), *Treatment of language disorders in children* (pp. 509–546). Paul H. Brookes Publishing Company.

Harrison, L. J., & McLeod, S. (2010). Risk and protective factors associated with speech and language impairment in a nationally representative sample of 4 to 5-year-old children. *Journal of Speech, Language, and Hearing Research, 53*(2), 508–529. https://doi.org/10.1044/1092-4388(2009/08-0086)

Harvey, A. M., Bordley, J., II, & Barondess, J. (1979). *Differential diagnosis* (3rd ed.). W.B. Saunders.

Hearnshaw, S., Baker, E., & Munro, N. (2018). The speech perception skills of children with and without speech sound disorder. *Journal of Communication Disorders, 71*, 61–71. https://doi.org/10.1016/j.jcomdis.2017.12.004

Henningsson, G., & Isberg, A. (1986). Velopharyngeal movements in patients alternating between oral and glottal articulation: A clinical and cineradiographical study. *Cleft Palate Journal, 23*(1), 1–9. PMID: 3455897.

Hodson, B. W. (2004). *Hodson assessment of phonological patterns (HAPP- 3)* (3rd ed.). Pro-ed.

Holland, A. L., & Nelson, R. L. (2020). *Counseling in communication disorders: A wellness perspective* (3rd ed.). Plural.

Isberg, A., & Henningsson, G. (1987). Influence of palatal fistulas on velopharyngeal movements: A cineradiographic study. *Plastic and Reconstructive Surgery, 79*(4), 525–530. https://doi.org/10.1097/00006534-198704000-00001

Jensen de López, K. M., Lyons, R., Novogrodsky, R., Baena, S., Feilberg, J., Harding, S., Kelić, M., Klatte, I. S., Mantel, T. C., Tomazin, M. O., Ulfsdottir, T. S., Zajdó, K., & Rodriguez-Ortiz, I. R. (2021). Exploring parental perspectives of childhood speech and language disorders across 10 countries: A pilot qualitative study. *Journal of Speech, Language, and Hearing Research, 64*(5), 1739–1747. https://doi.org/10.1044/2020_JSLHR-20-00415

Johnson, A. (Ed.). (2016). Interprofessional education and interprofessional practice in communication sciences and disorders: An introduction and case-based examples of implementation in education and healthcare settings. American Speech-Language-Hearing Association. https://www.asha.org/Practice/IPE-IPP-Activities-and-Collaborations

Johnson, S. (2019). *Attachment theory in practice: Emotionally focused therapy (EFT) with individuals, couples, and families.* Guilford.

Kabat-Zinn, J. (2009). *Full catastrophe living: Using the wisdom of your body and mind to face stress, pain, and illness* (15th anniversary ed.). Delta.

Kaipa, R., & Danser, M. L. (2016). Efficacy of auditory-verbal therapy in children with hearing impairment: A systematic review from 1993 to 2015. *International Journal of Pediatric Otorhinolaryngology*, *86*, 124–134. https://doi.org/10.1016/j.ijporl.2016.04.033

Kamhi, A. G. (2006). Treatment decisions for children with speech-sound disorders. *Language, Speech, and Hearing Services in Schools*, *37*(4), 271–279. https://doi.org/10.1044/0161-1461(2006/031)

Keller-Bell, Y., & Short, M. (2019). Positive behavioral interventions and supports in schools: A tutorial. *Language, Speech, and Hearing Services in Schools*, *50*(1), 1–15. https://doi.org/10.1044/2018_LSHSS-17-0037

King, A. M., Hengst, J. A., & DeThorne, L. S. (2013). Severe speech sound disorders: An integrated multimodal intervention. *Language, Speech, and Hearing Services in Schools*, *44*, 195–210. https://doi.org/10.1044/016101461(2012/12-0023)

Kirk, C., & Vigeland, L. (2015). Content coverage of single-word tests used to assess common phonological error patterns. *Language, Speech and Hearing Services in Schools*, *46*(1), 14–29. https://doi.org/10.1044/2014_LSHSS-13-0054

Klatte, I. S., Lyons, R., Davies, K., Harding, S., Marshall, J., McKean, C., & Roulstone, S. (2020). Collaboration between parents and SLTs produces optimal outcomes for children attending speech and language therapy: Gathering the evidence. *International Journal of Language & Communication Disorders*, *55*(4), 618–628. https://doi.org/10.1111/1460-6984.12538

Kleinman, A. (1988). *The illness narratives: Suffering, healing, and the human condition*. Basic Books.

Krieger, N. (2008). Proximal, distal, and the politics of causation: What's level got to do with it?. *American Journal of Public Health*, *98*(2), 221–230. https://doi.org/10.2105/ajph.2007.111278

Kubler-Ross, E. (1969). *On death and dying*. Macmillan.

Lappin, J. (2018). Joining in structural family therapy. In J. Lebow, A. Chambers, & D. Breunlin (Eds.), *Encyclopedia of couple and family therapy*. Springer. https://doi.org/10.1007/978-3-319-15877-8_971-1

Larrivee, L. S., & Catts, H. W. (1999). Early reading achievement in children with expressive phonological disorders. *American Journal of Speech-Language Pathology*, *8*(2), 118–128. https://doi.org/10.1044/1058-0360.0802.118

Law, J., Plunkett, C. C., & Stringer, H. (2012). Communication interventions and their impact on behaviour in the young child: A systematic review. *Child Language Teaching and Therapy*, *28*(1), 7–23. https://doi.org/10.1177%2F0265659011414214

Leahy, J., & Dodd, B. (1987). The development of disordered phonology: A case study. *Language and Cognitive Processes*, *2*(2), 115–132. http://dx.doi.org/10.1080/01690968708406353

Lewis, B. A., Freebairn, L. A., Hansen, A. J., Stein, C. M., Shriberg, L. D., Iyengar, S. K., & Taylor, H. G. (2006). Dimensions of early speech sound disorders: A factor analytic study. *Journal of Communication Disorders*, *39*(2), 139–157. https://doi.org/10.1016/j.jcomdis.2005.11.003

Ling, D. (2002). *Speech and the hearing-impaired child: Theory and practice*. Alexander Graham Bell Association for the Deaf and Hard of Hearing.

Luterman, D. M. (2016). *Counseling persons with communication disorders and their families* (6th ed.). Pro Ed.

McAllister, J., Skinner, J., Hayhow, R., Heron, J., & Wren, Y. (2023). The Association Between Atypical Speech Development and Adolescent Self-Harm. *Journal of Speech, Language, and Hearing Research*, *66*(5), 1600–1617. https://doi.org/10.1044/2023_JSLHR-21-00652

McCauley, R. J., Fey, M. E., & Gillam, R. B. (Eds.). (2017). *Treatment of Language Disorders in Children* (2nd ed.). Paul H. Brookes Publishing Co.

McCormack, J., McLeod, S., Harrison, L. J., & McAllister, L. (2010). The impact of speech impairment in early childhood: Investigating parents' and speech-language pathologists' perspectives using the ICF-CY. *Journal of Communication Disorders*, *43*(5), 378–396. https://doi.org/10.1016/j.jcomdis.2010.04.009

McGregor, K. K. (2020). How we fail children with Developmental Language Disorder. *Language, Speech, and Hearing Services in Schools*, *51*(4), 981–992. https://pubs.asha.org/doi/10.1044/2020_LSHSS-20-00003

McIntosh, B., & Dodd, B. (2011). *Toddler phonology test*. Pearson.

McLeod, S., & Baker, E. (2014). Speech-language pathologists' practices regarding assessment, analysis, target selection, intervention, and service delivery for children with speech sound disorders. *Clinical Linguistics & Phonetics*,

28(7–8), 508–531. https://doi.org/10.3109/02699 206.2014.926994

McLeod, S., Baker, E., McCormack, J., Wren, Y., Roulstone, S., Crowe, K., Masso, S., White, P., & Howland, C. (2017). Cluster randomized controlled trial evaluating the effectiveness of computer-assisted intervention delivered by educators for children with speech sound disorders. *Journal of Speech, Language, and Hearing Research, 60*(7), 1891–1910. https://doi. org/10.1044/2017_JSLHR-S-16-0385

McLeod, S., & Crowe, K. (2018). Children's consonant acquisition in 27 languages: A cross-linguistic review. *American Journal of Speech-Language Pathology, 27*(4), 1546–1571. https:// doi.org/10.1044/2018_AJSLP-17-0100

McLeod, S., & Harrison, L. J. (2009). Epidemiology of speech and language impairment in a nationally representative sample of 4- to 5-year-old children. *Journal of Speech, Language, and Hearing Research, 52*(5), 1213–1229. https://doi. org/10.1044/1092-4388(2009/08-0085)

Melvin, K., Meyer, C., & Scarinci, N. (2020). What does "engagement" mean in early speech pathology intervention? A qualitative systematised review. *Disability and Rehabilitation, 42*(18), 2665–2678. https://doi.org/10.1080/09638288.2018.1563640

Miccio, A. W., & Williams, A. L. (2021). Stimulability approach. In A. L. Williams, S. McLeod, & R. J. McCauley (Eds.), *Interventions for speech sound disorders in children* (2nd ed., pp. 279–304). Paul H. Brookes Publishing Co.

Minuchin, S. (1974). *Families and Family Therapy.* Harvard University Press.

Miron, C. (2012). The parent experience: When a child is diagnosed with childhood apraxia of speech. *Communication Disorders Quarterly, 33*(2), 96–110. https://doi.org/10.1177/1525740110384131

Moeller, M. P., Carr, G., Seaver, L., Stredler-Brown, A., & Holzinger, D. (2013). Best practices in family-centered early intervention for children who are deaf or hard of hearing: An international consensus statement. *Journal of Deaf Studies and Deaf Education, 18*(4), 429–445. https://doi. org/10.1093/deafed/ent034

Most, T., & Peled, M. (2007). Perception of suprasegmental features of speech by children with cochlear implants and children with hearing aids. *Journal of Deaf Studies and Deaf Education, 12,* 350–361. https://doi.org/10.1093/deafed/enm012

Muñoz, K., & Blaiser, K. (2011). Audiologists and speech-language pathologists: Making critical cross-disciplinary connections for quality care in early hearing detection and intervention. *Perspectives on Audiology, 7*(1), 34–43. https://doi. org/10.1044/poa7.1.34

Nathan, L., Stackhouse, J., Goulandris, N., & Snowling, M. J. (2004). The development of early literacy skills among children with speech difficulties: A test of the "Critical Age Hypothesis". *Journal of Speech, Language and Hearing Research, 47*(2), 377–391. https://doi.org/10.1044/1092-4388(2004/031)

Nelson, K. (1973). Structure and strategy in learning to talk. *Monographs of the Society for Research in Child Development, 38*(1/2), 1–135. Stable URL: https://www.jstor.org/stable/1165788

Northern, J. L., & Downs, M. P. (2002). *Hearing in children* (5th ed.). Lippincott, Williams, and Wilkins.

Park, L. R., Gagnon, E. B., Thompson, E., & Brown, K. D. (2019). Age at full-time use predicts language outcomes better than age of surgery in children who use cochlear implants. *American Journal of Audiology, 28*(4), 986–992. https://doi.org/10.1044/ 2019_AJA-19-0073

Peterson-Falzone, S. J., Trost-Cardamone, J. E., Karnell, M., & Hardin-Jones, M. A. (2017). *The clinician's guide to treating cleft palate speech.* Mosby.

Phatak, S. A., Yoon, Y.-S., Gooler, D. M., & Allen, J. B. (2009). Consonant recognition loss in hearing impaired listeners. *The Journal of the Acoustical Society of America, 126*(5), 2683–2694. https://doi. org/10.1121/1.3238257

Pickstone, C. (2007). Triage in speech and language therapy. In S. Roulstone (Ed.), *Prioritising child health* (pp. 35–40). Routledge.

Pickstone, C., Hannon, P., & Fox, L. (2002). Surveying and screening preschool language development in community-focused intervention programmes: A review of instruments. *Child: Care Health & Development, 28*(3), 25–264. https://doi.org/10. 1046/j.1365-2214.2002.00270.x

Pollock, K. E. (2013). The Memphis vowel project: Vowel errors in children with and without phonological disorders. In M. J. Ball & F. E. Gibbon (Eds.), *Handbook of vowels and vowel disorders* (pp. 260–287). Psychology Press.

Pollock, K. E., & Berni, M. C. (2003). Incidence of non-rhotic vowel errors in children: Data from the Memphis Vowel Project. *Clinical Linguistics & Phonetics, 17*(4–5), 393–401. https://doi. org/10.1080/0269920031000079949

Prelock, P. A., & McCauley, R. J. (Eds.). (2022). *Treatment of autism spectrum disorder: Evidence-based intervention strategies for communication and social interactions* (2nd ed.). Paul H. Brookes Publishing Co.

Prelock, P. A., Melvin, C., Lemieux, N., Melekis, K., Velleman, S., & Favro, M. A. (2017). One team: Patient, family, & healthcare providers – An IPE activity providing collaborative and palliative care. *Seminars in Speech and Language, 38*(5), 350–359. https://doi.org/10.1055/s-0037-1607071

Pring, T., Flood, E., Dodd, B., & Joffe, V. (2012). The working practices and clinical experiences of paediatric speech and language therapists: A national UK survey. *International Journal of Language and Communication Disorders, 47*(6), 696–708. https://doi.org/10.1111/j.1460-6984.2012.00177.x

Rasmussen, P. R., & Schuyler, E. J. (2020). Life tasks and psychological muscle. *Journal of Individual Psychology, 76*(4), 308–327. https://doi.org/10.1353/jip.2020.0032

Rice, M. L., Taylor, C. L., Zubrick, S. R., Hoffman, L., & Earnest, K. K. (2020). Heritability of specific language impairment and nonspecific language impairment at ages 4 and 6 years across phenotypes of speech, language, and nonverbal cognition. *Journal of Speech, Language, and Hearing Research., 63*(3), 793–813. https://doi.org/10.1044/2019_JSLHR-19-00012

Rødvik, A. K., von Koss Torkildsen, J., Wie, O. B., Storaker, M. A., & Silvola, J. T. (2018). Consonant and vowel identification in cochlear implant users measured by nonsense words: A systematic review and meta-analysis. *Journal of Speech, Language, and Hearing Research, 61*(4), 1023–1050. http://doi.org/10.1044/2018_JSLHR-H-16-0463

Roulstone, S. (2015). Screening for speech impairments. In C. Bowen, *Children's speech sound disorders* (2nd ed., pp. 76–80). Wiley-Blackwell.

Roulstone, S., Miller, L. L., Wren, Y., & Peters, T. J. (2009). The natural history of speech impairment of 8-year-old children in the Avon Longitudinal Study of parents and children: Error rates at 2 and 5 years. *International Journal of Speech-Language Pathology, 11*(5), 381–391. https://doi.org/10.1080/17549500903125111

Ruscello, D. M., & Vallino, L. D. (2020). The use of nonspeech oral motor exercises in the treatment of children with cleft palate: A re-examination of available evidence. *American Journal of Speech-Language Pathology, 29*(4), 1811–1820. https://doi.org/10.1044/2020_AJSLP-20-00087

Rusiewicz, H. L., Maize, K., & Ptakowski, T. (2018). Parental experiences and perceptions related to childhood apraxia of speech: Focus on functional implications. *International Journal of Speech-Language Pathology, 20*(5), 569–580. https://doi.org/10.1080/17549507.2017.1359333

Rvachew, S., & Rafaat, S. (2014). Report on benchmark wait times for pediatric speech sound disorders. *Canadian Journal of Speech-Language Pathology and Audiology, 38*(1), 82–96. https://cjslpa.ca

Sand, A., Hagberg, E., & Lohmander, A. (2022). On the benefits of speech-language therapy for individuals born with cleft palate: A systematic review and meta-analysis of individual participant data. *Language, Speech, and Hearing Services in Schools, 65*(2), 555–573. https://doi.org/10.1044/2021_JSLHR-21-00367

Schafer, E. C., & Sweeney, M. (2012). A sound classroom environment. *ASHA Leader, 17*(4), 14–17. https://doi.org/10.1044/leader.FTR2.17042012.14

Schlosser, R. W., & Wendt, O. (2008). Effects of augmentative and alternative communication intervention on speech production in children with autism: A systematic review. *American Journal of Speech Language Pathology, 17*(3), 212–230. https://doi.org/10.1044/1058-0360(2008/021)

Shinnar, S., Rapin, I., Arnold, S., Tuchman, R. F., Shulman, L., Ballaban-Gil, K., Maw, M., Deuel, R. K., & Volkmar, F. R. (2001). Language regression in childhood. *Pediatric Neurology, 24*(3), 183–189. https://doi.org/10.1016/s0887–8994(00)00266-6

Shprintzen, R., & Golding-Kushner, K. J. (2012). International use of telepractice. *Perspectives on Telepractice, 2*(1), 16–25. https://doi.org/10.1044/tele2.1.16

Shprintzen, R. J., Sher, A. E., & Croft, C. B. (1987). Hypernasal speech caused by hypertrophic tonsils. *International Journal of Pediatric Otorhinolaryngology, 14*(1), 45–56. https://doi.org/10.1016/0165-5876(87)90049-8

Shriberg, L. D. (1997). Developmental phonological disorders: One or many? In B. W. Hodson & M. L. Edwards (Eds.), *Perspectives in applied phonology* (pp. 105–132). Aspen.

Shriberg, L. D. (2006, June). Research in idiopathic and symptomatic childhood apraxia of speech. *Paper presented at the 5th International Conference on Speech Motor Control Nijmegen*, The Netherlands.

Shriberg, L. D., Austin, D., Lewis, B. A., McSweeny, J. L., & Wilson, D. L. (1997). The speech disorders classification system (SDCS): Extensions and lifespan reference data. *Journal of Speech, Language, and Hearing Research, 40*(4), 723–740. https://doi.org/10.1044/jslhr.4004.723

Shriberg, L. D., Campbell, T. F., Mabie, H. L., & McGlothlin, J. H. (2019). Initial studies of the phenotype and persistence of Speech Motor Delay (SMD). *Clinical Linguistics & Phonetics., 33*(8), 737–756. https://doi.org/10.1080/02699206.2019.1 595733

Shriberg, L. D., Kent, R. D., Karlsson, H. B., McSweeny, J. L., Nadler, C. J., & Brown, R. L. (2003). A diagnostic marker for speech delay associated with otitis media with effusion: Backing of obstruents. *Clinical Linguistics and Phonetics, 17*(7), 529–547. https://doi.org/10.1080/0269920031000138132

Shriberg, L. D., & Kwiatkowski, J. (1982). Phonological disorders III: A procedure for assessing severity of involvement. *Journal of Speech and Hearing Disorders, 47*(3), 256–270. https://doi.org/10.1044/jshd.4703.256

Shriberg, L. D., Kwiatkowski, J., & Gruber, F. A. (1994). Developmental phonological disorders II: Short-term speech-sound normalization. *Journal of Speech and Hearing Research, 37*(5), 1127–1150. https://doi.org/10.1044/jshr.3705.1127

Shriberg, L. D., Kwiatkowski, J., & Mabie, H. L. (2019). Estimates of the prevalence of motor speech disorders in children with idiopathic speech delay. *Clinical Linguistics & Phonetics, 33*(8), 679–706. https://doi.org/10.1080/02699206.2019.1595731

Shriberg, L. D., & Widder, C. J. (1990). Speech and prosody characteristics of adults with mental retardation. *Journal of Speech and Hearing Research, 33*(4), 627–653. https://doi.org/10.1044/jshr.3304.627

Snow, P. C. (2016). Elizabeth Usher Memorial Lecture: Language is literacy is language: Positioning speech language pathology in education policy, practice, paradigms, and polemics. *International Journal of Speech Language Pathology, 18*(3), 216–228. https://doi.org/10.3109/17549507.2015.1112837

Snow, P. C. (2021). SOLAR: The science of language and reading. *Child Language Teaching and Therapy, 37*(3), 222–233. https://doi.org/10.1177/0265659020947817

Sotos, J. G. (1991). *Zebra Cards: An aid to obscure diagnosis*. Mt. Vernon Book Systems.

Speake, J., Stackhouse, J., & Pascoe, M. (2012). Vowel targeted intervention for children with persisting speech difficulties: Impact on intelligibility. *Child Language Teaching and Therapy, 28*(3), 277–295. http://doi.org/10.1177/0265659012453463

Speech Pathology Australia. (2020). *Augmentative and alternative Communication Clinical Guideline*. Speech Pathology Australia. https://speechpatho logyaustralia.org.au

St John, M., Columbus, G., Brignell, A., Carew, P., Skeat, J., Reilly, S., & Morgan, A. T. (2020). Predicting speech-sound disorder outcomes in school-age children with hearing loss: The VicCHILD experience. *International Journal of Language & Communication Disorders, 55*(4), 537–546. https://doi.org/10.1111/1460-6984.12536

Stein, C. M., Lu, Q., Elston, R. C., Freebairn, L. A., Hansen, A. J., Shriberg, L. D., Taylor, H. G., Lewis, B. A., & Iyengar, S. K. (2011). Heritability estimation for speech-sound traits with developmental trajectories. *Behavioral Genetics, 41*(2), 184–191. https://doi.org/10.1007/s10519-010-9378-5

Sugden, E., Baker, E., Munro, N., Williams, A. L., & Trivette, C. M. (2018). An Australian survey of parent involvement in intervention for childhood speech sound disorders. *International Journal of Speech-Language Pathology, 20*(7), 766–778. https://doi.org/10.1080/17549507.2017.1356936

Sugden, E., Munro, N., Trivette, C. M., Baker, E., & Williams, A. L. (2019). Parents' experiences of completing home practice for speech sound disorders. *Journal of Early Intervention, 41*(2), 159–181. https://doi.org/10.1177/1053815119828409

Sweeney, T. (2019). *Adlerian Counseling and Psychotherapy: A Practitioner's Wellness Approach* (6th ed.). Routledge.

Taylor, C., & Zubrick, S. (2009). Predicting children's speech, language and reading impairment over time. *International Journal of Speech-Language Pathology, 11*(5), 341–343. https://doi.org/10.1080/17549500903161561

Thomas-Stonell, N., Oddson, B., Robertson, B., & Rosenbaum, P. (2009). Predicted and observed outcomes in preschool children following speech and language treatment: Parent and clinician perspectives. *Journal of Communication Disorders, 42*(1), 29–42. https://doi.org/10.1016/j.jcomdis.2008.08.002

To, C., McLeod, S., Sam, K. L., & Law, T. (2022). Predicting which children will normalize without intervention for speech sound disorders.

Journal of Speech, Language, and Hearing Research, *65*(5), 1724–1741. https://doi.org/10.1044/2022_JSLHR-21-00444

Unger, N., Heim, S., Hilger, D. I., Bludau, S., Pieperhoff, P., Cichon, S., Amunts, K., & Mühleisen, T. W. (2021). Identification of phonology-related genes and functional characterization of Broca's and Wernicke's regions in language and learning disorders. *Frontiers in Neuroscience*, *15*(680762). https://doi.org/10.3389/fnins.2021.680762

Vallino, L., Ruscello, D., & Zajac, D. (2019). *Cleft palate speech and resonance: An audio and video resource*. Plural Publishing, Inc.

Van Borsel, J., Van Rentergem, S., & Verhaeghe, L. (2007). The prevalence of lisping in young adults. *Journal of Communication Disorders*, *40*(6), 493–502. https://doi.org/10.1016/j.jcomdis.2006.12.001

Vassallo, S., & Sanson, A. (Eds.) (2013). *The Australian Temperament Project (ATP): The first 30 years*. Australian Institute of Family Studies. https://aifs.gov.au/publications/australian-temperament-project

Walker, E. A., McCreery, R. W., Spratford, M., Oleson, J. J., Van Buren, J., Bentler, R., Roush, P., & Moeller, M. P. (2015). Trends and predictors of longitudinal hearing aid use for children who are hard of hearing. *Ear and Hearing*, *36*, 38S–47S. https://doi.org/10.1097/AUD.0000000000000208

Watts Pappas, N., McAllister, L., & McLeod, S. (2016). Parental beliefs and experiences regarding involvement in intervention for their child with speech sound disorder. *Child Language Teaching and Therapy*, *32*(2), 223–239. https://doi.org/10.1177%2F0265659015615925

Watts Pappas, N., McLeod, S., McAllister, L., & McKinnon, D. H. (2007). Parental involvement in speech intervention: A national survey. *Clinical Linguistics and Phonetics*, *22*(4–5), 335–344. https://doi.org/10.1080/17549507.2017.1356936

Webster, P. E., Plante, A. S., & Couvillion, L. M. (1997). Phonologic impairment and prereading: Update on a longitudinal study. *Journal of Learning Disabilities*, *30*(4), 365–376. https://doi.org/10.1177%2F002221949703000402

Weitzman, E., Girolametto, L., & Drake, L. (2017). Hanen Programs® for Parents: Parent-implemented early language intervention. In R. J. McCauley, M. E. Fey, & R. B. Gillam (Eds.), *Treatment of Language Disorders in Children* (2nd ed., pp. 27–56). Paul H. Brookes Publishing Co.

Williams, A. L., McLeod, S., & McCauley, R. A. (2021). *Interventions for speech sound disorders in children* (2nd ed.). Paul H. Brookes Publishing Co.

Williams, A. L., McLeod, S., & McCauley, R. J. (2010). *Interventions for Speech Sound disorders in Children*. Paul H. Brookes Publishing Co.

Woods, J. J., Wilcox, M. J., Friedman, M., & Murch, T. (2011). Collaborative consultation in natural environments: Strategies to enhance family-centered supports and services. *Language, Speech, and Hearing Services in Schools*, *42*(3), 379–392. https://doi.org/10.1044/0161-1461(2011/10-0016)

World Health Organization. (2007). *International Classification of Functioning, Disability and Health: Children and Youth Version: ICF-CY*. World Health Organization. https://apps.who.int/iris/handle/10665/43737

Wren, Y., Hughes, T., & Roulstone, S. (2006). *Phoneme factory Phonology Screener*. NFER Nelson Publishing Company.

Wren, Y., Miller, L. L., Peters, T. J., Emond, A., & Roulstone, S. (2016). Prevalence and predictors of persistent speech sound disorder at eight years old: Findings from a population cohort study. *Journal of Speech, Language, and Hearing Research*, *59*(4), 647–673. https://doi.org/10.1044/2015_JSLHR-S-14-0282

Wren, Y., & Roulstone, S. (2013). *Phoneme factory sound sorter: Australian Version*. (2nd ed.). Bristol Speech and Language Therapy Research Unit.

Chapter 4
Phonetic, Stimulability, Perceptual, and Phonological Interventions

Even theoretically sound, well-intentioned, and carefully implemented interventions can result in equivocal outcomes. When they do, careful attention to the evidence and willingness to rethink strategy often serves to right the course.

Gillam & Gillam, 2014

Chapter 4 begins with a selected **glossary** of intervention related terms, with further definitions dotted through the chapter. After the glossary are descriptions of **general principles and techniques** for implementing **articulation interventions**, emphasizing the phonetic aspects of speech acquisition; and an account of the **phonological principles** underpinning **phonological interventions** that concern the (linguistic) organization of children's systems of contrastive phones.

Next, are accounts of commonly used intervention approaches. They are: Phonetic Intervention or Articulation Therapy (Bowen, 2019); Stimulability Intervention (Miccio, A17); Perceptual Intervention or Speech Perception Training, (Rvachew, A18); and Minimal Pair Approaches to Phonological Intervention:

- Conventional Minimal Pairs Intervention approaches: **Meaningful Minimal Pairs** and **Perception-Production Minimal Pairs**.
- Complexity Approaches:
  - **Maximal Oppositions** and **Empty Set**.
  - **Multiple Oppositions Intervention** (Williams, A19).
- **Vowel Intervention** (Pollock, A20).

A Selected Glossary of Terms Related to Interventon

The definitions in the glossary are for:

- Service delivery plan
- Intervention
- Intervention agent
- Intervention setting
- Intervention continuity
- Cumulative intensity
- Trials
- Dose
- Dose form
- Dose frequency
- Intervention approach
- Intervention procedure
- Intervention session
- Intervention session duration
- Intervention session frequency
- Intervention duration
- Intervention goal

- Session goal
- Session format
  - Pull-out model
  - Push-in model
- simultaneous scheduling
- SMART goals and aspirational goals
- Goal attack strategies
  - Cyclical
  - Horizontal
  - Vertical
- Generalization,
- Response generalization,
- Phonological response generalization
- Stimulus generalization
- Resources/materials
- Reinforcers/rewards

- **Service delivery plan:** A description of the intervention, and intervention setting, agent, format, continuity and goal, and the session duration and frequency.
- **Intervention** is a goal-directed activity, founded on plans and procedures, conducted by an intervention agent, in an intervention session or sessions. Interventions are designed to ameliorate a presenting problem, to improve a client's wellbeing.
- **Intervention agent** may be an SLP/SLT, SLP/SLT assistant, or a teacher, teacher's assistant, parent/caregiver/significant other, computer software, etc.
- **Intervention setting** is the place that intervention occurs, for example, in a publicly funded SLP/SLT clinic (e.g., community health centre, NHS), private or independent SLP/SLT practice rooms, school, early childhood setting (e.g., daycare, nursery or preschool), the client's home in-person or via telepractice.
- **Intervention continuity and cumulative intensity, trial, and dose**
  - **Intervention continuity** refers to the scheduling of intervention sessions. Typically, sessions may be continuous and open-ended as required, or in a block such as a school term, or a blocks-and-breaks sequence for set times, for example, 10-weeks-on-10-weeks-off-10-weeks-on etc., with the end

point determined collaboratively by the child's parents and the SLP/SLT. In some settings intervention continuity is imposed administratively, often by personnel who are not SLPs/SLTs, without reference to the evidence base or best practice guides. Dose is intertwined with **intervention continuity** and **trials**.
- **Cumulative intervention intensity** is a quantitative account of the extent of target practice. It is calculated as: session dose expressed as trials × dose frequency per time unit × intervention duration. If a child performed 80 production practice trials, twice weekly, for 15 sessions, cumulative intervention intensity would be 80×2×15=2,400 production practice trials.
- **Trials / trial:** A trial is the number of times an intervention target is repeated, in response to stimuli, in a session. For example, in some instances, where a child's SSD has mild-to-low-moderate severity (see Table i.1), a minimum dose of at least 50 production trials in 30-minutes may suffice for intervention to be effective. For a more severely involved child, greater dose intensity might make all the difference, say 70 trials in a session of 30-to-40 minutes, or 100 trials in 40-to-60-minute session. Researchers and research teams that develop and test interventions may provide

guidance around the trial intensity associated with their approach. Using clinical judgement, clinicians can adjust dose intensity. For example, if Child-1 were uncomfortable with 100 trials in 40 minutes, the dose might be dropped to at least 70 trials in 30 minutes; or, if progress monitoring revealed slower than expected gains for Child-2 the dose might go from 60 trials in 30 minutes to 90 in 40 minutes.

- **Dose**: The dose is the number of teaching episodes in one session, or the sum of trials of target practice stimuli in a session (e.g., 100 trials).
- **Dose form:** The kind of activity in which teaching and learning moments occur, for example, as SLP/SLT-directed drill play in a tower-building game.
- **Dose frequency**: The occasions of treatment sessions per time unit, for example, for one client, two sessions weekly: one individually and one in a group.
- **Intervention approach:** An approach is a specific methodology, developed by a researcher or research team, designed to improve children's speech in the context of a specific SSD. The developer usually specifies the assessment procedures, which they may have developed themselves (e.g., *DEAP*, Dodd et al., 2002), that indicate whether their approach is suitable for a child and to monitor progress. They also describe, in journal publications, a book or book chapter, and/or a manual, typical goals, service delivery modalities, and/or the intervention procedures used to address the SSD with guidelines. Trustworthy intervention approaches are well-grounded theoretically and/or are supported by peer-reviewed evidence published in quality scholarly journals.
- **Intervention procedure**: A teaching instruction or action such as a model, performed by an intervention agent designed to promote learning in a child.
- **Intervention session**: A formal clinical encounter between a client and an intervention agent. In SLP/SLT, each consultation ('consult') with a client constitutes a session. A session may have a single objective or several, and the client may be seen in an individual session and/or a group session.

- **Intervention session duration** is the specified time an assessment, treatment, or probe assessment session will last, for example, 30, 40, 60, or 90 minutes.
- **Intervention session frequency** is the number of sessions in each timeframe: for example, one session per week, or two sessions per week, or one pull-out session on school days, or one individual session and one group session each week, etc.
- **Intervention duration** is the entire time-period an intervention will/has run.
- **Intervention goal** (see Table 1.4; Bowen, 1996; Fey, 1985, 1986, 1992). The intervention goal comprises the overall objective of any intervention, including intervention for SSD. The purpose of the goal, and the way it is designed, is to improve a child's wellbeing. The basis for the goal is threefold, founded on a perspective that acknowledges the interaction between the **impairment** itself, the child and family's **social milieu**, and **biopsychosocial** factors. Speech intervention goals are customarily called **intervention targets**. Once the child's and/or parents' aspirational goal is achieved, the child may need no further SLP/SLT intervention.
  - **Session goals**: The behaviours, skills, awareness, or knowledge taught, via intervention procedures, in an intervention activity, in a session.
  - **Session format**: The format is the design of intervention sessions which may occur in-person or online, individually (child, parent(s)/caregiver, and therapist) and/or in a group. The intervention format can also be in the form of parent training, or consultative intervention. Session formats include pull-out and push-in models
  - **Pull-out model:** An intervention agent sees a child for assessment and/or intervention in the clinician's office or dedicated professional 'rooms', etc.
  - **Push-in model:** An intervention agent sees a child in a specially assigned area of a school classroom while their classmates do other activities.
- **Simultaneous scheduling:** The SLP/SLT combines interventions, in each session, to address goals across two or more domains, for example,

phonology *and* fluency; articulation *and* voice; childhood apraxia of speech *and* language with semantic and syntactic targets; speech perception, *and* phonemic awareness *and* reading.

- **SMART goals and aspirational goals**: A goal is the ambition, aspiration, end, intent, objective, or purpose towards which an endeavour is directed. In business, a process of SMART goal setting is sometimes used. The SMART acronym stands for a series of questions interrogating whether potential goals are Specific, Measurable, Attainable, Relevant, and Timely, as follows:
  - **Specific**: What do you want to achieve? Is the goal clear and well defined?
  - **Measurable**: Can progress towards and reaching of the goal be measured?
  - **Attainable**: Is the goal achievable? Is it realistic? Is it *too* 'aspirational'?
  - **Relevant**: Does it fit with client-parent-clinician values and preferences?
  - **Timely**: Is the schedule defined without creating a false sense of urgency?

Also, in business, **aspirational goals** are frequently contrasted with SMART goals because the aspirations they represent may be illogical, reflecting magical thinking (THINKS: *'If I wish for something enough, or if it is important enough, it will happen.'*). Aspirational goals may also lack a timeline, have undefined steps to goal achievement, with the means, mechanism or active ingredient whereby change, and the goal will be achieved, unexplained. The SMART goal conditions can be usefully applied to goal setting for SSD, mindful that *some* aspirational goals will conform to the SMART criteria.

- **Goal attack strategy: cyclical**: Using a cyclical goal attack strategy, the SLP/SLT follows a schedule whereby several targets are addressed, sequentially, in a set timeframe. The client then ceases working on those targets and turns to several other targets, regardless of whether the previous targets are identified, perceived, organized, or produced accurately. Throughout the cycles, the focus is on only one goal per treatment session.
- **Goal attack strategy: horizontal ('training wide')**: Using a horizontal goal attack strategy, the SLP/SLT targets several targets within a session.

- **Goal attack strategy: vertical ('training deep')**: In a vertical goal attack strategy, SLPs/SLTs focus on one or two targets (e.g., phonetic repertoire, speech perception, stimulability, phonemic contrasts, phonological processes, syllable/word shapes (phonotactics), syllable/word stress, prosody) at a time. The targets are addressed until a criterion is reached, before advancing to a new goal.
- **Generalization** is a phenomenon in which intervention for one behaviour (e.g., intelligibility) in one intervention context expedites change in the same behaviour in other nontreatment contexts, and in related behaviours.
- **Response generalization** involves improvement or carryover change in a yet-to-be targeted goal that is related to the targeted intervention goal. In essence, response generalization in SSD is, transfer of learning from the treatment target to another aspect, or to other aspects of a child's phonology.
- **Phonological response generalization**: Enhancement of a client's phonological system beyond the skill level targeted in intervention. The changes may manifest, *apparently* spontaneously:
  - In **untreated words**, for example, for a child with velar fronting, *call, key, cap*, and *cave* are targeted, and production of *corn, keep, can*, and *cape* normalizes.
  - **Across word positions**, for example, final (SFWF) fricatives are targeted and there is phonological response generalization to fricatives SFWW, and SIWI.
  - **Within sound classes**, for example, the voiced stop /g/ is targeted and the voiceless stop /k/ shows improvement (Gierut & Hulse, 2010).
  - **Across sound classes**, for example, affricates are targeted, and fricatives show improvement, or fricatives are targeted, and stops show improvement (Gierut & Hulse, 2010).
  - At **more complex linguistic levels**, for example, a sound is targeted in single words, and when phrases are targeted, the sound quickly establishes; or *while* a sound is targeted in sentences it generalizes to conversation.
- **Stimulus generalization** is transfer of learning from the intervention context to other contexts such as home, school, and sports field. Grunwell (1992, p. 109) called this socioenvironmental generalization. She identified four generalization

types in children in treatment for developmental speech disorders:

3. **Phonological**: (a) from one syllabic position to another; (b) from one target phoneme to another in the same natural class.
4. **Lexical**: from one word to all the others in which the target phoneme occurs.
5. **Syntactic**: from one type of linguistic unit (e.g., single word) to larger linguistic units (phrases, clauses, conversation).
6. **Socioenvironmental**: from the clinic to all environments and types of discourse.

- **Resources/ Materials:** The materials used in intervention, such as books, pictures, objects, equipment, toys, computer software, and games.
- **Reinforcers/Rewards**: Positive behavioural rewards for performance in, and sometimes between sessions (e.g., for 'good' home practice) that appeal to the child.

Resources / Materials

Apps, books, board games, cards, slideshows, stories, 'therapy materials', and web-based resources (free, purchased or by subscription), are employed to support all kinds of SSD intervention. These are used are in combination with materials suited to individual children, particularly things they like (e.g., Barbie and dinosaur activities for Barbie and dinosaur enthusiasts respectively), toys, games, and dressing-up costumes that children bring from home (e.g., Elsa and Anna the royal sisters of Arendelle; Willy Wonka), enjoyable games SLPs/SLTs amass and cherish for their utility in intervention sessions and popularity with children. Among the commercially available games are Ravensburger's *Coco-Crazy*, Game Zone's *Monkey Business* (also available as Early Learning Centre's *Monkeying Around*), Tomy's *Pop-up Pirate*, and *Smart Chute* from Smart Kids. Apart from purchasing materials, SLPs/SLTs have a long history of creating board and card games, magnet games (e.g., magnetic fishing), flash cards, and other resources.

In my own practice, certain toys and books were a hit with many children, value-adding to assessment and intervention sessions. In assessment, a Viewmaster proved handy for story re-telling to gather connected speech samples, as did the book *Pigs in Hiding* by Arlene Dubanevich. Several versions of *Pigs in Hiding*, read aloud, are available in YouTube and Vimeo (e.g., https://vimeo.com/465619358). You can play the video once or twice with the sound on, mute the video and have the client re-tell the story while watching it. Successful intervention toys and games have included a *Smart Chute*, or more accurately, a *succession* of *Smart Chutes*, which a passing parade of enthusiastic preschoolers loved to bits. Pictures of production practice words maintain their 'slip' when glued onto normal playing cards. To play, the child says each word X-times before placing the card in the top of the chute, and again before picking it up at the bottom. Some children would be motivated to perform numerous drill or drill-play trials in exchange for opportunities to twist, pull, knot, and contort *Stretch Armstrong*, and release him to see him return to his original shape.

Reinforcers/Rewards

Children perform production practice (drill) within games (drill play). Cooperation, effort, and successful performance in treatment sessions and homework are rewarded with nonverbal social reinforcers that children like (e.g., smiles, pats-on-the-back, thumbs-up, air punches, etc.); verbal reinforcers such as praise and positive comments; tangible rewards like certificates, tokens (e.g., stars, stickers, and toys), treats and fun activities. Although nonverbal, verbal, and tangible reinforcers are used, it is worth knowing that pitched appropriately, intervention is generally enjoyable (intrinsically rewarding) for all: child, parent, and clinician.

Opinions differ on whether it is preferable to have the child first produce the sound in isolation, e.g., [s], or in a syllable, e.g., *sea* [si] or *ice* [aɪs]; whether it is desirable to use a mirror; and whether feedback toys like *Echo Microphone*, *Tok-Back*, *Toobaloo*, and comparable home-made devices aid listening and perception. The use of mirrors and feedback toys has not been empirically tested, but it can be justified if a clinician observes that they increase individual children's cooperation, enjoyment, interest, and on-task behaviour in sessions, and it must be conceded that some children love 'equipment'.

Articulation / Phonetic Intervention: General Principles

The hallmark of traditional therapy lies in its sequence of activities for: (1) identifying the standard sound, (2) discriminating it from its error through scanning and comparing, (3) varying and correcting the various productions until it is produced correctly, and finally, (4) strengthening and stabilizing it in all contexts and speaking situations.

Van Riper (1978, p. 179)

In principle, separating phonetic approaches from phonemic approaches helps us think clearly about the level at which we are working with a child with SSD. In practice, however, 'phonemic therapy' (phonological intervention), 'phonetic therapy' (articulation intervention) and even 'auditory discrimination training' (perceptual intervention) are not always totally distinct. Phonetic targets are the phones that

- the client is not producing – e.g., /tʃ, dʒ/ are absent from their phonetic inventory.
- the client produces incorrectly – e.g., /s, z/ are produced as [ls, lz] ('lateral-lisp').
- lack true stimulability – e.g., /k/ can be produced in isolation, but not in two syllable positions, e.g., [kiː] and [iːk]; or [kiː] and [ɪki]; or [ɪki] and [iːk].
- the client cannot perceive accurately – e.g., they cannot reliably identify whether the productions ['ɹoʊˌbot], ['woʊˌbot]; [fɹɪdʒ], [fwɪdʒ]; [dʒəˈɹaf/ dʒəˈɹæf]; and [dʒəˈwaf/dʒəˈwæf], for robot, fridge, and giraffe, are correct or incorrect.

The goal of articulation intervention is usually not so much to improve intelligibility, but for clients to achieve speech that matches standard pronunciation for their language. Mostly, the intelligibility of children and adults with articulation disorders is mildly impacted, or not at all.

Sometimes however, comprehensibility is an issue when an error creates listener confusion. For example, if a child who replaces /k/ with [t] said, '*The tar is on the road*' should the listener assume they mean 'The car is on the road', or take what they heard literally, agreeing that the road in question is tarred? How should a listener respond to '*Bel put her tote in her tote*'? Did she put one of her totes inside the other, or did she put her coat in her tote, or wrap her coat in her other coat? Sometimes too, a [t] for /k/ substitution can lead to the child innocently saying a 'rude word' in an ambiguous context ('titty' for 'kitty' may raise eyebrows) or unintentionally saying something that is considered cute ('spartle' for 'sparkle'; 'tuptate' for 'cupcake'), comical ([tʌm ˈtwɪtli] for 'come quickly') or, unpleasant ('rotting horse' for 'rocking horse').

Implementing Articulation / Phonetic Intervention

In articulation or phonetic intervention (Bowen, 2019), sometimes nicknamed 'Van Riper therapy', the therapist guides the client through carefully graded steps, usually one phoneme at a time.

Therapy starts with *perceptual intervention* (also called *ear training* and/or *auditory discrimination training*) to help the client recognize target and error by listening (Hearnshaw et al., 2019). Then, using placement techniques to adjust the client's best *approximations* to the target phone, alongside metalinguistic cues and imagery, client and SLP/SLT (and in many cases, parents too) work together until correct production is achieved.

Stabilizing correct production is accomplished through drill and drill play, until the client produces the target in all linguistic contexts (words, phrases…) and in all speaking situations (home, school, community). Finally, the phone is used in spontaneous conversation, and the emphasis moves to self-monitoring and self-correction by the child. In the stabilizing and final phases, the client may do 'homework' with family help (Davies et al., 2017; Sugden et al., 2018, 2019).

Phonetic Placement Techniques

Placement techniques include *imitation*, *shaping*, *phonetic-placement cues* with *visual and/or auditory imagery*, *motor-kinaesthetic cues*, and *touch cues*, augmented with *metalinguistic cues* (see Table 4.1) tailored to the child's and family's interests and preferences. Phonetic placement techniques are routinely included in SSD treatment, irrespective of the type or combination of types of SSD.

Imitation

To introduce a new phone, or a phone the child is learning in a new syllable position, the clinician provides visual cues *with* verbal cues. For example, to introduce a new phone in the syllable initial word initial (SIWI) position, the therapist might begin with, '*Listen to me and watch what I say.*' and model the target one or more times. This might be

the sound in isolation or in a syllable, e.g., [g] or [guː].

In the next step, the SLP/SLT might say, '*Listen to me, watch what I do, and then say **with** me.*' and model the sound or syllable for the child to say in unison with them. This might be followed by the clinician silently mouthing the sound or syllable while the child says it aloud. Finally, the child is tasked with listening, watching, and repeating the sound or syllable *after* the clinician in a listen-watch-and-say routine. The steps are often in flux, with the clinician back-tracking to a previous, easier level if the child's performance deteriorates (e.g., if they are having a 'bad day' or unwell).

Table 4.1 Examples of metalinguistic cues for a selection of target phones.

Refer to 'your' pop, 'your' windy, etc. so that the child 'owns' the target. Personalize the cues for the child and family.
If the child modifies the imagery name or verbal cue, use *their* preferred words.

TARGET	IMAGERY NAME...	VERBAL CUE...	GESTURE CUE...
The target is modelled in isolation or CV or VC by parent or clinician.	...provided by parent or clinician and possibly modified by the child.	...provided by parent or clinician and possibly modified by the child.	...provided by an ADULT parent / teacher /'helper'.
STOPS AND NASALS			
p, b	Popping sounds Poppers Pop sounds	'Where's your pop?' 'You forgot your pop.' 'Let's hear your pop'	The adult puffs cheeks up with air, and 'plodes' /p/ or /b/ onto the child's hand for them to feel a 'pop'.
t, d	Tippies Tongue ready!	'Use your tippy.' 'Was your tongue ready?'	The adult says the sound, touching his or her philtrum with a straight finger.
k, g	Throaty sounds Throaties Glug-glug sounds	'Where's your throaty?'	The adult makes a 'U' with thumb and index finger, touching the mandible angles.
m	Humming sound Yum-yum sound	'Close your mouth and humm...' or 'mmm mmm.'	The adult hums 'mmm', touching larynx to feel vibration.
n	'N...' sound	'Tongue ready and buzz.'	The adult hums 'nnn' touching the larynx to feel vibration.
ADJUNCTS AND CLUSTERS			
ADJUNCTS st, sp, sk **2-ELEMENT CLUSTERS** sm, sn, sl, fl, sw, tw, kw, shr, pr, br, tr, dr, kr, gr fr, thr	Friendly sounds Friends Twins Two-step sounds Two-steps	'You forgot your friend.' 'Remember its friend.' 'You forgot his/her twin.' 'Remember its twin.' 'Let's hear your two steps' 'Where's your other step?' 'And your next step?'	The adult slides a finger on a surface while saying /s/, ending by tapping the finger silently when the 'friendly sound' is added. Or the adult 'walks' with fingers on a surface or up an imaginary ladder saying the first phone on the first step and the second on the second step.

(Continued)

Table 4.1 (*Continued*)

FRICATIVES AND AFFRICATES			
h	Puppy panting sound Hot puppy sound Open mouth blowy	'Where's your puppy?' 'Remember to blow' 'I didn't feel you blow.'	The adult places a flattened hand just in front of his/her or the child's mouth to feel the air.
f v	Bunny rabbit sound Biting lip blowy Lip-up sound	'You forgot to bite.' 'You forgot your wind' 'Where's your bunny?'	The adult brings their lower lip up to touch the teeth and blows or makes a face like a rabbit.
s z SIWI	Smiley, blowy snake Big snake teeth Buzzy bee	'Show me your teeth' 'Where's your buzzy bee?'	The adult makes a toothy smile and blows, indicating frontal airflow with the fingers.
ʃ	Pouty blowy sound 'Be quiet' noise 'Shh, my baby's asleep'	'Teeth shut and push those lips out' 'Teeth SSHut and puSHH.'	The adult pouts lips and blows, indicating 'be quiet' and then frontal air-flow with the fingers.
tʃ dʒ	Chomping sound Choo-choo train sound Elephant trunk sound	'Make those lips move!' 'Where's the choo-choo?' 'Where's your trunk'	The adult protrudes their lips imaginary trunk while making a chomping or choo-choo sound.
LIQUIDS AND GLIDES			
l	Tower sound Up-down sound Tongue ready la-la	'Open up – tongue up.' 'Tongue ready, and down' 'Touch the top aand down!'	The adult assumes a mouth open posture with the tongue behind their upper teeth, then lowers it to behind the bottom teeth. Use a mirror to rehearse silently first.
ɹ	'Rrr' sound Pirate sound	'Push up on the sides and move your tongue back.'	The adult demonstrates the butterfly position, pushing the sides of the tongue on the teeth.
w	Pouty face. Pouty lips	'OOO-EEE sliding' 'OOO-WEE sliding'	The adult mimes /uː/ with lips protruded, then says /iː/ or /wiː/.
j	Sliding sound Smiley-pouty sound	'EEE-OR sliding.' 'EEE-YOR sliding'	The adult models /iː/ while smiling then a pouty /ɔː/ or /jɔː/.
ALL FINAL CONSONANTS			
Final consonants	Sticky sounds	'Where's your sticky?'	The adult moves their arm left to right starting with an open hand and finishing with a closed hand.

The sequence would be repeated if the SLP/SLT wanted to introduce the same sound, /g/, in a different syllable position (e.g., syllable final word final: SFWF as in 'egg' and 'hug'; syllable initial within word: SIWW as in 'yoga' and 'tiger'; or syllable final within word: SFWW as in 'doghouse' and 'big-end'). The SIWI position is also described as being prevocalic, and the SFWF position as postvocalic. In appropriate contexts, SIWW and SFWW are described as intervocalic. 'Intervocalic' works for words like 'buggy', 'Lego', 'Megan', and 'wagon' where /g/ is preceded *and* followed by a vowel, but not for words like 'hungry', 'jingle', 'penguin', and 'ragtime'; and in rhotic varieties of English where /ɹ/ is pronounced, as in words like 'burger', 'cargo', 'gurgle', and 'organ'.

Ambisyllabic and 'Medial' Consonants

In some words, the so-called 'medial consonant' or within word 'medial cluster' is neither SIWW nor SFWW, but rather, ambisyllabic. An ambisyllabic consonant, or consonant cluster, is simultaneously the final consonant in the coda of one syllable and the initial consonant of the onset of the following syllable. This implies that the consonant in question 'belongs' to both syllables. For this to occur, the vowel in the first syllable must be both *short* and *stressed*, e.g., /k/ in *bicker*, but not /k/ in *baker, barker, beaker, biker,* or *burqa*; /kl/ in *suckling* but not /kl/ in *cycling*; /p/ in *shipping* but not /p/ in *shaping*.

Shaping / Sound Modification

The clinician identifies a sound the client *can* produce and helps him or her to convert it into a new sound. For example, Sally (6;1) could produce [t] and [d]. Her SLT used a well-tried procedure by 'shaping' them into a prolonged [t] and [d] with friction ([tsss], [dzzz]) to target /s/ and /z/.

Phonetic Placement Cues

The clinician describes or demonstrates how a sound is produced, using metaphors and other metalinguistic cues and imagery, models, diagrams, animations and in some specially equipped settings, electropalatography (EPG) and ultrasound tongue imaging (Cleland & Scobbie, A47).

Motor-kinaesthetic Cues

Gloved fingers, objects (e.g., tongue depressors) or foods are used – mindful of allergy precautions – to help the client 'find' and 'feel' the desired place of articulation. Foods may include, with parental permission, confectionary (e.g., lifesavers, lollipops), spreads (e.g., cheese spread) and breakfast cereals (e.g., Froot Loops). For example, the child 'holds' a lifesaver on the alveolar ridge with their tongue to locate and 'sense' alveolar place of articulation.

Touch Cues

The SLP/SLT uses formal tactile cues (e.g., Prompts for Restructuring Oral Muscular Phonetic Targets [Namasivayam et al., 2021]) or informal 'made-up' touch cues (e.g., as in Dynamic Temporal and Tactile Cueing, Strand, A31).

Metalinguistic Tasks and Cues

All intervention for SSD incorporates metalinguistic tasks and cues, including, to a greater or lesser extent, auditory and visual cues, phonetic placement techniques, and imagery cues. Simply asking a child to, '*Watch me and say what I say*' or '*Say these words after me*' constitute metalinguistic tasks.

Metalinguistic cues for /s/ might integrate the adult saying [s], providing an imagery name such as 'the snake sound', a verbal cue such as 'remember your hissy sound' and a gestural cue (e.g., running an index finger along a forearm, or sliding it along a surface, to suggest the snake idea, and the 'long' feature of the sound).

Metalinguistic cueing also encompasses the use of alphabet letters (e.g., 's' for /s/), cue cards (e.g., a bouncing ball with a 'b' caption for /b/), toys representing the target (e.g., a rabbit with prominent upper teeth for /f/), alliterative game, media or storybook characters ('*Vera Violet Vinn is very, very, very awful on her violin*'), and well-chosen Apps to target specific phones; and creatures great and small, real and imagined, for work on vowels (e.g., owl-themed activities for /uː/; mouse-themed activities for /iː/) and consonants (e.g., Miccio's Zippy Zebra for /z/, Coughing Cow for /k/, Rowdy Rooster for /ɹ/, and Shy Sheepy for /ʃ/; see Table A17.1).

In terms of imagery, in the Butterfly procedure for shaping /s/, located at https://www.speech-language-therapy.com/index.php?option=com_content&view=article&id=48 the child is cued to assume the position for /iː/ and to imagine the tongue as a butterfly's wings 'grooving' in the midline (the butterfly's body), and 'bracing' against the teeth. This imagery is combined, playfully, with shaping (converting a prolonged /t/ into /s/, while simultaneously maintaining the tongue-position for /iː/), phonetic placement instructions, and metalinguistic cues.

Drill, Structured-, and Semi-Structured Play

In an award-winning article, Shriberg and Kwiatkowski (1982) explained the configuration of treatment activities within intervention sessions in terms of

- **Drill**

    Highly structured stimulus-response drill comprising an antecedent instructional event followed by the client's (child's) response. Drill sessions involve a high intervention dose with minimal play in sessions that comprises a series of teaching and learning moments. While play is not included within trials, sessions may contain nonverbal (nods, smiles, thumbs-up), verbal (*great, try again, keep going, you're getting there*), and material (tangible) reinforcement (stars, stickers, ticks (check marks), scores to support cooperation, motivation, participation, and persistence. Drill may be more palatable for child and parent (some parents, and indeed some clinicians, dislike 'drilling', sometimes referring to it as 'drill-and-kill') if the child receives a cumulative reward for achieving a goal, e.g., a badge or certificate for every 100 trials. One Canadian school-based S-LP commenting on Byers et al. (2021) said, '*If I'm purely doing drill and kill, I can usually get over 50 [trials]. But I only do it with students I know can handle that kind of therapy. In my experience, it works better with older students.*'

Drill-play

Structured stimulus-response-reward **drill-play** includes an antecedent motivational component (e.g., an activity, directed by the clinician, incorporating board games – such as dominoes, snakes and ladders or lotto; card games; Origami paper finger puzzles; and posting and stacking games). The set-up for drill-play's learning-and-teaching moments may be, for example, that the child takes a turn in a game, or puts a monkey in a palm tree (as in *Coco Crazy*), or adds a predetermined number of Lego pieces, after a specified number of trials. It is desirable for a drill-pay component to extend for 30 minutes containing three or four drill-play activities. Drill play is often used with, enjoyed, or at least well tolerated by three, four, and five-year-old children with SSD.

Structured Play

Structured stimulus-response-reward activities (learning and teaching moments, again) within **structured play** activities are conducted similarly to drill-play except that the clinician presents the activity as a game, without a formal instructional component, and the practice rate is moderate, or less intense than in drill-play. Craft, building, or other quiet hand activities are suitable in structured play. The child may select the game (e.g., dressing paper dolls, loading cargo on a raft, or building a tower) while the clinician structures play by setting the rate of practice, the words to be practiced and the rules. For example, in a doll-dressing activity the clinician and child would take turns to stick the stimulus pictures, from a set predetermined by the SLP/SLT, on the lid of a box containing the paper clothes. When the child has said the stimulus word X number of times, they can remove the lid, take an item of clothing (e.g., a hat), replace the lid, and put the hat on the doll. The game ends when the doll is wearing all the clothes that were in the box. An internet search for 'Printable Paper Doll with Dress Ups Free' leads to various options.

Play (or Child-led Semi-structured Play)

Here, the child experiences the activities as 'free play', whereas the therapist will have 'loaded' the environment, so that targeted-words, singly or in longer utterances occur 'naturally' (from the child's perspective) in play. In Trevor's therapy in Box 4.1, Dave the SLP stacked the room with play items to elicit final consonant inclusion from the preschooler (*Babe, surf, bike, cage*, and *hive*).

To encourage use of the targets the SLP/SLT employs models, personal contributions, phatics, conversational recasts, self-talk, and other devices. (see https://www.speech-language-therapy.com/pdf/adultcommunicativestyles.ppsx). In semi structured play the dose rate is regulated by the child because the activity is not clinician-directed, but child-directed. The teaching and learning moments are scattered through play as openings arise.

For example, Dave and Trevor might have played a car-parking game with a multi-story toy carpark with a hand-car-wash service (search: toy parking garage) using a carpark, vehicles, and figurines (people and/or animals) as final consonant stimuli rather than pictures, to elicit for instance, *park, up, down, back, out*; or *drive, in, brake, wash, wet*; or *Ford, Dodge, Fiat, Jag, Rav*.

Choosing between Drill and Drill Play

Shriberg and Kwiatkowski (1982) reported that drill and drill play, with their higher dose rates, were more effective and efficient than structured play and play. They also found drill and drill play had equal effectiveness and efficiency. SLPs' evaluation of the four alternatives revealed that they intuited that drill play was most effective and efficient for their clients, and that the SLPs preferred it. In the article, Shriberg and Kwiatkowski advocated that the following three factors be contemplated when choosing the configuration of treatment activities in sessions: (1) a general knowledge of the child's personality, (2) the intended target response, and (3) the stage of therapy.

In sociocultural terms, Shriberg and Kwiatkowski's SLPs' preference for drill-play, over drill, may reflect a 1980s US, and possibly middle-class perspective. From personal encounters with CPD participants in professional development events focusing on SSD, this may not reflect current attitudes cross culturally. Participants in (or from) Hong Kong, India, Indonesia, Malaysia, Pakistan, and Singapore, and correspondents from China, Japan, South Korea, and Taiwan, often express surprise when they consider this finding, noting their preference for drill, perceiving it as more effective and efficient. Some participants believed that parents preferred it. For example, after a small group discussion in Singapore, six SLPs/SLTs presented a summary report that included, *the parents don't want to see us playing in the sessions. They want to see their kids working. They themselves did rote-learning at school and believe that's the best way for children to learn. They'd rather see drill, and see you count the trials.* Another group in the same study day reported, *it's not so much that we have a drill-and-kill mentality; it's that the parents expect it, and we know they'll do it [drill] at home whatever we advise or have a nanny do it.*

Comparison Table

Table 4.2 contains a summary for quick reference. It contains a brief comparison between the characteristics, assessment procedures, and intervention approaches for articulation disorder, phonological disorder, and childhood apraxia of speech.

It can be useful to tailor a plain-English, or other language as appropriate, version of Table 4.2 to discuss with interested parents.

Table 4.2 may be particularly helpful when a child is switching from one type of intervention to another, as in the case of misdiagnosed children mistakenly, treated for CAS for a period before commencing a phonological intervention. It helps parents and significant others to see the similarities and differences between these SSDs, why their treatment differs, and where there is overlap.

Children with Limited Stimulability

The aim of stimulability assessment is to discover whether the production of an erred or missing sound is enhanced or made possible when elicitation conditions are simplified. Traditionally, in child speech *assessment*, a child was said to be stimulable for a phone if they produced it in isolation when given auditory and visual models, encouragement, and support, with minimal distractions and linguistic demands.

Table 4.2 Comparing characteristics, assessment, and intervention for articulation disorder, phonological disorder, and childhood apraxia of speech.

Articulation Disorder: phonetic level difficulties

Characteristics

The child (or adult) has difficulty producing one, or a few sounds and may or may not have stimulability to 2 syllable positionsfor the sound(s). Traditionally, error-types in articulation disorder have been called 'SODA' errors: **S**ubstitutions where a sound replaces another ('blue' for 'glue'), **O**missions ('pea' for 'Pete'), **D**istortions (e.g., a 'lateral-s' /ls/), and **A**dditions ('mica' for 'Mike', 'below' for 'blow'). Substitution errors involving /s/ and /z/ ('thing' for 'sing'; 'then' for 'Zen') are popularly called lisps.

Assessment

Articulation (phonetic) assessment: of single words (SW) and connected speech (CS), stimulability assessment, perceptual (auditory discrimination) assessment.

Phonetic Intervention / Articulation Therapy

Targeting the *phonetic level*, the therapist guides the client through carefully graded steps, usually phone by phone starting with *perceptual training* (auditory discrimination) to help them distinguish target from error by listening. Then, using *placement techniques* to vary and correct the client's production attempts, with *metalinguistic cues*, *imagery*, and *feedback*, client, clinician, and often parents too, work jointly until the target is produced correctly, in increasingly challenging contexts. *Stabilizing* the correct phone is achieved through drill. Ultimately, the phone *generalizes* to conversation, and the emphasis moves to self-*monitoring* and self-*correction*.

Phonological Disorder: phonemic level difficulties

Characteristics

Static speech sound system
Variable production without gradual improvement
Persistence of phonological processes
Chronological Mismatch
Idiosyncratic rules/processes
Restricted use of contrast

Diagnostic Signs

The puzzle phenomenon
Unusual errors
Odd marking of contrasts
Error sounds are readily stimulable

Assessment:

Core speech assessment battery
Independent and relational analyses
Additional testing as indicated, e.g., perceptual, stimulability and inconsistency assessment.
Phonological analysis, or analysis of phoneme collapses

Phonological Intervention: 'Minimal Pairs Tx'

Targeting the *phonemic level*, the therapist devises activities based on the systematic nature of phonology, applying **phonological principles**. Activities are *conceptual* rather than motoric, although some work at phonetic and perceptual levels may be appropriate for some children with phonological disorder. The goal of intervention is *generalization*, thereby promoting intelligibility.

Phonological approaches, often called 'minimal pairs therapy' focus on teaching children the function of sounds; that *changing sounds changes meaning*; and that making meaning is needed for communication (to *make sense when we talk*). The guiding principle is that once introduced to a child's system, a distinctive feature contrast will generalize readily to other relevant minimal pairs.

Childhood Apraxia of Speech (CAS/DVD): motoric level difficulties

Characteristics
Segmental Characteristics

Articulatory struggle
Transpositional substitution errors
Marked inconsistency, especially token-to-token
Sound and syllable deletions
Vowel / diphthong errors

Suprasegmental (Prosodic) Characteristics

Inconsistent word and sentence stress
Inconsistent timing of speech and pauses
Inconsistent application of nasal resonance

Diagnostic Signs

Speech motor sequencing difficulties
Prosodic / suprasegmental differences
Receptive-expressive gap

Assessment

Core speech assessment battery:
independent and relational analyses
Motor speech assessment
Speech characteristics rating (prosody in particular)
Additional testing as indicated: e.g., language, perceptual, stimulability, and inconsistency assessment.

PML-based Intervention

Targeting the *motoric level*, the therapist devises activities based on the **principles of motor learning (PML)**, favouring motoric activities rather than conceptual ones, and maximizing *motor drill*.

Children with CAS need 'speech work' at the phonetic level too, and many need work at the perceptual and phonological levels, *and* intervention to address prosody and the receptive-expressive language gap.

Intervention based on the PML has *habituation*, then *automaticity* as its goal, promoting intelligibility. Non-speech oral motor exercises have no place in intervention for CAS (or for any other SSD). Robustly evidence-based intervention approaches include Dynamic Temporal and Tactile Cueing (DTTC), Integral Stimulation, the Nuffield Centre Dyspraxia Programme, and Rapid Syllable Transition Treatment (ReST).

Also traditionally, developers of *treatment* approaches for SSD have had no trouble in persuading clinicians to focus on early developing and stimulable (in isolation) sounds first on the basis that these sounds are easier for children to learn, and easier for the clinician to teach. 'Easier to learn, and easier to teach' were plausible rationales around which to make treatment target selection decisions, remaining unchallenged for decades.

Eventually however, dissenting voices were heard from the mid-to-late 1990s (Miccio et al., 1999; Powell & Miccio, 1996; Rvachew et al., 1999) and into 2020s (e.g., DeVeney et al., 2020). This research cultivated a new appreciation of stimulability data as being of most significance when SLPs/SLTs gathered them from young children with severely restricted phonetic inventories, and of most use to clinicians when analysed for sounds *absent* from a child's inventory. Reading these insights, or hearing about them in professional development events, changed some SLPs'/SLTs' understanding of the term 'stimulable'. 'Stimulable', in the *assessment* literature, became associated with the concept of 'true stimulability' with both terms used to mean that a child is stimulable for a consonant in at least two syllable positions, rather than simply being able to produce it imitatively in isolation. So, for example, a child would be considered stimulable for /k/ if able to produce it in isolation, and in the pre-vocalic and post-vocalic syllable positions (/k/, /ki:/, /a:k/); or in isolation, and in the pre-vocalic and inter-vocalic syllable positions (/k/, /ki:/, /eɪki:/). The child would not need to produce /k/ in a variety of vowel contexts (e.g., /ki:/, /ku:/, /kɔ:/, /ka:/; /ɪk/, /ɒk/, /ʌk/ and /æk/) to demonstrate 'true stimulability'; two syllable positions suffice.

Epenthesis

One practical reason to aim for CVs and VCs when working on stimulability and introducing new phones is that it may obviate a *learned* **epenthesis** (see Table 4.3) or 'schwa insertion' which then must be eliminated, adding a potentially avoidable, step to intervention. Epenthesis, which is unusual in typical English language learners, but common in children with SSD, sees the child introducing a

vowel-like intrusion, a hiatus, a schwa, or a shwa and glottal stop when moving from the isolated phone to using the phone in a syllable or word.

Epenthesis at word level, which may be dialectal, is sometimes called **anaptyxis**, **intrusion**, or **vowel intrusion** (e.g., [ˈæθəˌliːt] for *athlete*, [ˈfɪlˌəm] for *film*, [ˈpæˌvəˈlouˌvə] for *pavlova*), or **consonant intrusion** (e.g., [ˈbɜɡˌjuˌlə] for *burgler*, [ˈfæmˈbliː]/[ˈfæmbəˈliː] for *family*, [haɪtθ] for *height*).

The following examples of epenthetic productions of *choo, coo, foo, goo, sue,* and *shoo*, are commonly found in children with SSD who are first taught to produce a new consonant in isolation – and in at least some cases it is possible that the clinician has inadvertently *taught* the epenthetic intrusions. Examples are [tʃ-uː], [k-uː], [f-uː], [g-uː], [s-uː], and [ʃ-uː] with a hiatus, or [tʃə-uː], [kə-uː], [fə-uː], [gə-uː], [sə-uː], and [ʃə-uː] with a schwa, or [tʃəʔ-uː], [kəʔ-uː], [fəʔ-uː], [gəʔ-uː], [səʔ-uː], and [ʃəʔ-uː] with a schwa and glottal stop. It reduces frustration for the child, saving time, effort, and resources, if productions of this type are avoided.

Stimulability Training, and Pre-practice

Schmidt et al. (2019) defined motor learning, discussed in more detail in Chapter 7, as '*a set of processes associated with practice or experience leading to relatively permanent changes in the capability for movement.*' The precursors to motor learning are: (1) **motivation**, (2) **focused attention** and (3) **pre-practice**. In speech motor learning, pre-practice involves phonetic placement training prior to entering the practice phase; so, for many clients, it is inextricably bound to stimulability training. Irrespective of speech diagnosis, for those clinicians who see their clients infrequently (e.g., on a sporadic consultative basis, or for brief, low intensity therapy blocks of say, six half hour consultations over six weeks), and for those who have virtually unlimited access to their clients, the modern notion of true stimulability for consonants has major implications.

Unfortunately–due to lack of administrative support, personnel, funding, and resources–in many clinical settings worldwide SLPs/SLTs see their clients with speech disorders infrequently. In this regard, there are at least three common service delivery scenarios. First, some SLPs/SLTs working in consultative models may only see a given client briefly, once or twice in a school term. Second, other SLPs/SLTs see children for between 6 and 10 assessment/treatment sessions and then hand over the entire business of intervention to a parent in the form of a home program, or to a teacher, aide, assistant or other non-SLP/SLT as a school program, perhaps reviewing the child's progress at intervals, but possibly not. And third, and literally quite close to home for the me, children attending publicly funded (taxpayer funded) agencies are allocated, by legislation, a total of 10 SLP/SLT appointments. Not 10 per school term or 10 per year: 10 and that's it! Against these inequitable scenarios, SLPs/SLTs are uniquely qualified to make non-stimulable sounds stimulable, whereas most non-SLPs/SLTs probably must rely on luck to achieve success with obstinate obstruents and stubborn sonorants (including vexatious vowels).

When the late **Dr. Adele W. Miccio** (1952–2009) explored the role of stimulability in the treatment of children with SSD in the first edition of this book, she was Associate Professor of Communication Sciences and Disorders and Applied Linguistics and Co-Director of the Center for Language Science at Pennsylvania State University. There, she taught courses in phonetics and phonology and conducted research on typical and atypical phonological acquisition, the relationship between bilingual phonological development and later literacy abilities, bilingual phonological assessment, and treatment efficacy.

Formerly a clinical SLP in Colorado, Dr. Miccio received her PhD in Speech and Hearing Sciences from Indiana University–Bloomington. She was an Associate Editor of the *American Journal of Speech-Language Pathology* and on the editorial board of *Clinical Linguistics & Phonetics*. Her contribution to scholarship in our field was immeasurable and she is sorely missed. Her contribution was included in the second edition of this book, and appears here, in the third, with the kind cooperation and permission of her children, Anthony and Claire Miccio.

Q17.   Adele W. Miccio: Stimulability and Phonetic Inventory Expansion

Should clinicians focus on stimulability training with infrequently seen 'home/school program' clients, and what should the parents' or other helpers' role be in this situation? In other situations, where the clinician has reasonably unfettered access to a client, how would you prioritize and implement work on stimulability?

A17.   Adele Miccio: First Things First: Stimulability Therapy for Children with Small Phonetic Repertoires

Stimulability has been defined several ways since the term first appeared in the speech pathology literature in the 1950s (Carter & Buck, 1958; Milisen, 1954), although Travis (1931) described the concept even earlier. Simply put, stimulability is a client's ability to immediately modify a speech production error when presented with an auditory and visual model (Lof, 1996; Powell & Miccio, 1996).

Stimulability Assessment

Bain (1994) noted that stimulability testing determines the difference between a child's abilities during a highly supportive imitative condition and a typical spontaneous condition where the phonetic environment as well as lexical and syntactic issues may restrict articulatory abilities. To determine stimulability, target sounds are elicited in isolation, syllables and/or words (Carter & Buck, 1958). Earlier studies (Sommers et al., 1967) referred to a child's general stimulability or overall likelihood to self-correct. In other words, if a child's performance improves from that in spontaneous speech, a child is judged to have good stimulability skills – a positive prognosticator for future success in treatment. Thus, treatment is most important for children with poor stimulability skills.

Although more sophisticated phonological assessments that identify patterns of errors and illuminate a child's knowledge of the phonological system have been developed (Bernhardt & Stemberger, 2000; Elbert & Gierut, 1986; Ingram, 1981; Shriberg & Kwiatkowski, 1980) and have increased our understanding of generalization patterns, researchers have also documented a relationship between sound-specific stimulability and generalization (Miccio et al., 1999; Powell et al., 1991). Consequently, stimulability continues to be used to prioritize caseloads. Children who are stimulable for consonants absent from their phonetic inventories will most likely acquire these sounds without treatment. Sounds absent from the child's inventory that are not stimulable are unlikely to be acquired without direct treatment.

Stimulability is also a consideration in treatment target selection. Treating non-stimulable sounds is most likely to result in the acquisition of both treated and non-treated sounds. Non-stimulable sounds tend to be more complex. Targeting more complex sounds promotes system-wide generalization and increases the learnability of less complex sounds (Gierut, 2007; Tyler & Figurski, 1994). Targeting both stimulable and non-stimulable sounds promotes early success (Edwards, 1983; Rvachew & Nowak, 2001).

Furthermore, stimulability testing may also be used to probe for learning during treatment. Adaptations of Carter and Buck's (1958) protocols are still widely used for this purpose (Miccio, 2002; Powell & Miccio, 1996). Glaspey and Stoel-Gammon (2005, 2007) developed the Scaffolding Scale of Stimulability, a hierarchical scale of cues and linguistic environments, to monitor discrete changes in production in response to treatment. This scale also quantifies improved responses to cues as well as the change in the number of cues needed over time.

Targeting Stimulability

Despite the positive aspects of using stimulability for assessment purposes, it has met with resistance, by clinicians, regarding treatment target selection (Fey & Stalker, 1986; Hodson & Paden, 1991; Rvachew, 2005b). This generally relates to the difficulty of teaching non-stimulable sounds, the time involved in instruction or the increased frustration of children who have difficulty imitating sounds absent from their phonetic inventories. These concerns have motivated the development of treatment programs for young children with small phonetic inventories who are not stimulable for production of sounds missing from their inventories (Miccio, 2005; Miccio & Elbert, 1996; Powell & Miccio, 1996).

To target non-stimulable sounds and still achieve early success, Miccio and Elbert (1996) proposed teaching all consonants at once during every session (both stimulable and non-stimulable). The important components of this treatment strategy include directly targeting non-stimulable speech sounds, making targets the focus of joint attention, associating speech sounds with hand/body motions, associating the sounds with alliterative characters of interest to the child, encouraging vocal practice and ensuring successful communicative attempts.

Because the primary goal is to enhance stimulability, speech sounds are taught in isolation (e.g., [s::::::::::]) or in a CV context (e.g., [kʌ]). Each consonant is associated with a character and a hand or body motion. Details regarding the characters and their associated movements are shown in Table A17.1, and they are illustrated in Figure A17.1. Information on how stimulability probes are conducted and generalization data are gathered across sessions may be found in Miccio (2005).

Table A17.1 Stimulus characters and associated motions.

Manner	Consonant	Character	Associated motion
Stop	/p/	Putt-Putt Pig	Glide hands in a skating motion
	/b/	Baby Bear	Pantomime rocking a baby
	/t/	Talkie Turkey	Raise a pretend phone receiver to ear
	/d/	Dirty Dog	Make digging motion with hands
	/k/	Coughing Cow	Place hand near top of throat
	/g/	Goofy Goat	Roll eyes toward ceiling
Fricative	/f/	Fussy Fish	Fussily push hands away from body
	/v/	Viney Violet	Move arms up as a winding vine
	/θ/	Thinking Thumb	Move thumb in a circle
	/s/	Silly Snake	Move finger up arm
	/z/	Zippy Zebra	Zip coat
	/ʃ/	Shy Sheepy	Clutch hands together and push down
Affricate	/tʃ/	Cheeky Chick	Move hand sassily toward cheek
	/dʒ/	Giant Giraffe	Move hand upward in stair steps
Nasal	/m/	Munchie Mouse	Push lips together and rub tummy
	/n/	Naughty Newt	Shake finger in a scolding motion
Liquid	/l/	Lazy Lion	Stretch arms in 'L' shape
	/ɹ/	Rowdy Rooster	Rev motorcycle gears
Glide	/w/	Wiggly Worm	Shiver
	/j/	Yawning Yo-Yo	Yawn and move hand to suppress it
	/h/[a].	Happy Hippo	Laugh and shake shoulders

Adapted from Miccio and Elbert (1996, Table 4.3). Reproduced with permission from Elsevier.

[a] From a phonological perspective, /h/ is considered a glide in English. It has no cognate and patterns as a glide (e.g., is not phonemic in coda position). Thus, all the sounds are listed from the front to the back and by sound class with stops, fricatives, and affricates first, then the nasals, and finally, the liquids and glides. Because /h/ cannot be strictly continuous like the other fricatives, it has a CV motion, [ha].

Case Example

A typical treatment is described below for 'Fiona', age 4;3. Pre-treatment, Fiona's phonetic inventory consisted of [m n p b t d w j h]. None of the English consonants absent from her phonetic inventory were stimulable.

At the beginning of the session, following the administration of a brief stimulability probe, large 5 × 7-inch (13 cm × 18 cm) character cards were reviewed with the associated speech sound and motion. To focus Fiona's attention on each character, the cards were shown one at a time. Doing so ensured that Fiona understood the target sounds and their associated motions. Research on semantic development shows that children are more likely to spontaneously repeat the names of objects that are the focus of joint attention and that were previously labelled for them (Baldwin & Markham, 1989). For this reason, speech sounds are associated with characters of interest to children.

The character cards, shown in greyscale in Figure A17.1, are available (free) in colour at www. speech-language-therapy.com/pdf/miccio4s.pdf. The character for /z/, for example, is Zippy Zebra. Alliterative characters also provide an immediate opportunity to generalize new information to larger linguistic units and to facilitate phonological awareness (PA) and the alphabetic principle that are important for emerging literacy skills (Adams et al., 1998). Each consonant is also associated with a motion. The motion for [z] is zipping up a coat. All fricatives are associated with continuous motions. All stop consonants, on the other hand, are associated with ballistic motions to draw a child's attention to these features of speech sounds. All consonants, including those that are present in the phonetic inventory, are reviewed (worked on), and associated body movements are always used concurrently with speech production.

Fazio (1997) found that children with specific language impairment (SLI) remembered poems after a 2-day delay when the poem was learned with accompanying hand motions. The hand motions

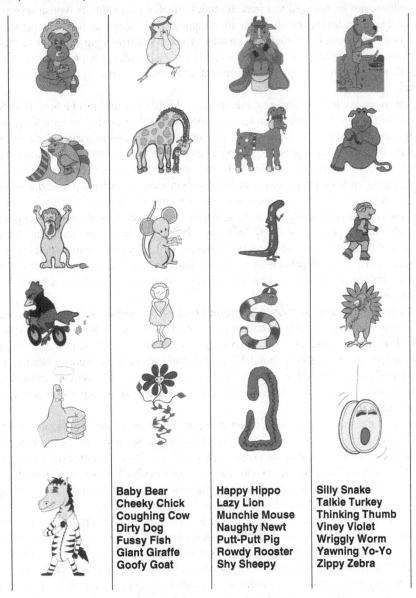

	Baby Bear	Happy Hippo	Silly Snake
	Cheeky Chick	Lazy Lion	Talkie Turkey
	Coughing Cow	Munchie Mouse	Thinking Thumb
	Dirty Dog	Naughty Newt	Viney Violet
	Fussy Fish	Putt-Putt Pig	Wriggly Worm
	Giant Giraffe	Rowdy Rooster	Yawning Yo-Yo
	Goofy Goat	Shy Sheepy	Zippy Zebra

Figure A17.1 Miccio character cards. PICTURES: Caroline Bowen / https://www.speech-language-therapy.com/pdf/miccio4s.pdf; https://www.speech-language-therapy.com/pdf/stimax.pdf

appeared to serve as retrieval cues. To learn new speech sounds, children must be able to retrieve the new articulatory information later and to use the new sounds in words. Multimodal input increases the ability to remember new sounds (Rauscher et al., 1996).

To facilitate speech sound production, treatment was embedded in play-like activities that provided Fiona with multiple opportunities to imitate consonants. Although direct imitation of the correct production of sounds in error is not required in this program, vocal practice is encouraged, and children make verbal requests. For example, Fiona's favourite character was Happy Hippo. She would say, '*I'm happy like Happy Hippo. Ha Ha Ha! Are you happy, too?*' Doing so is an important element for acquisition and generalization to larger linguistic units (Powell et al., 1998; Saben & Ingham, 1991). In this program, children are encouraged to speak through turn-taking activities. A typical session utilizes a maximum of three turn-taking activities that are designed specifically around the target speech sound characters. Both Fiona and the clinician were fully involved in turn-taking activities so that the clinician was constantly modelling the target sounds and Fiona had multiple opportunities to imitate them. Sometimes Fiona's parents participated in treatment activities. They also took turns and modelled the target sounds.

Characters were printed on playing cards to easily facilitate sound production. Fiona's favourite activity was *Go Fish*. In this familiar game, everyone had a set of cards and took turns asking for a desired card. Because both stimulable and non-stimulable sounds were included, Fiona often failed to produce the intended sound when requesting a card. The associated movement, however, provided the clinician with the information needed to identify the intended sound. When Fiona produced [d] but mimed zipping up her coat, for example, the clinician knew the intended sound was [z]. Because the clinician handed Fiona a Zippy Zebra card, Fiona's communication attempt was successful. At the same time, the clinician provided feedback about how to produce [z] while miming zipping her coat: 'Let me see, do I have Zippy Zebra? Zippy Zebra says [z:::::::::]'. When Fiona requested Putt-Putt Pig, a sound she knew, she said [pʌ pʌ] while making a skating motion with her hands (Putt-Putt Pig is wearing roller skates). The clinician provided positive feedback, '*Great! You made the Putt-Putt Pig sound, [pʌ pʌ]*' while making the skating motion. Every time Fiona took a turn, she was free to request any character she wished.

Giving Fiona the freedom to choose any sound enabled immediate success. Successful communication, in turn, encouraged more verbalization (Rescorla & Bernstein Ratner, 1996). Whenever the clinician took a turn, she requested a non-stimulable sound. In this way, Fiona was always assured of successful production attempts with stimulable sounds and had multiple opportunities to attempt non-stimulable sounds. In addition, the clinician had many opportunities to provide instruction without resorting to drill-like activities. Fiona was given an assertive role involving requesting and directing attention to sounds of interest.

Because all characters are alliterative, multiple opportunities arose to indirectly target generalization of newly learned sounds to lexical items and to use them spontaneously. Baby Bear, for example, has a bib and a bottle. Putt-Putt Pig is pink and wears a purple dress. Fiona commented on these characteristics when she requested these characters and again received feedback about the sounds she made with accompanying motions. Fiona, as well as other young children, preferred simple games. Simple games also provide the most opportunities to attempt speech sounds. After playing *Go Fish*, Fiona played a game where she took turns requesting character cards to place in a spaceship. At the end of the session, the spaceship took off and a door opened with a sticker inside for Fiona to wear home. It is important to remember that Fiona was never required to imitate correct production after the clinician. The clinician identified the intended target by the associated motion even when it was produced incorrectly. The clinician drew attention to the correct production through modelling and phonetic placement cues. As Fiona became more comfortable with the clinician and had more successful communicative attempts, she also began to imitate the clinician more frequently and to attempt to correct herself.

The treatment activities provided a supportive framework that encouraged speech production and enhanced Fiona's awareness of the properties of speech sounds. At the end of the session, a short probe of palindromes (dad, mom, pop, bob, etc.) was administered to assess generalization to the coda position. Fiona's parents had a set of character cards at home. At the end of the session, we suggested a few sounds to work on at home. These were always stimulable sounds, for example, [n] and [d], and the parents were advised to always use the corresponding motions. Thus, the parents assisted with generalization but did not force production of sounds that were difficult. At the end of the session, Fiona said, 'Mommy starts with the Munchy Mouse sound'.

Fiona participated in this program twice weekly for 12 weeks. Sessions were 50 minutes in length. Post-treatment, she had added all fricatives, affricates and [ɹ] to her phonetic inventory and was stimulable for [k g l]. Pre-treatment, Fiona produced complete sentences, but with only stops, nasals and glides in her consonant inventory, and she was unintelligible to all but her immediate family. When she began treatment, she substituted [d] for velars, affricates, and voiced fricatives, [h] for voiceless fricatives and [w] for liquids.

Following 12 weeks of treatment to enhance stimulability, she was stimulable for all targeted sounds and produced many of them in simple words or used typical developmental substitutions in more difficult contexts. When Fiona returned to the clinic after a winter break of 4 weeks, she began a minimal pair treatment approach using *Maximal Oppositions* (Williams, A19) to directly target the contrastive nature of speech sounds and to continue to encourage generalization across the phonological system.

Treatment Research

This program to enhance stimulability for speech sound production is based on findings from treatment research. As noted above, non-stimulable sounds are least likely to change without treatment and targeting non-stimulable sounds results in acquisition of the treated non-stimulable sounds as well as untreated stimulable sounds (Miccio et al., 1999; Powell et al., 1991). For children with small inventories, it is important to rapidly increase the size of the phonetic inventory for intelligibility reasons. This program is designed especially for young children with small phonetic inventories who are not stimulable for production of the speech sounds absent from their phonetic repertoires. Once children are stimulable for most consonants, they move on to treatment using a contrastive approach or a combination of stimulability intervention and phonological contrasts. In addition, children are ready for direct phonetic placement training if needed.

Discriminating Error from Target

Just as basic as Miccio's idea that things become easier for children with SSD if they are taught to produce their missing or misarticulated sounds, is an appreciation that they will progress more readily if they can recognize their target sounds and distinguish them from their own erred productions. And that is where Susan Rvachew's perceptual intervention, or speech perception training, comes in.

Readers were introduced to Dr. Susan Rvachew in A9 in Chapter 2 and will remember that she is Associate Dean and Director of the School of

Communication Sciences and Disorders at McGill University, Montreal, Canada. Her research interests are focused on phonological development and disorders. Specific research topics include: the role of speech perception development in sound production learning; speech development in infancy; efficacy of interventions for phonological disorders; and digital media applications in the treatment of phonological disorders and emergent literacy. Current projects include investigations of alternative approaches to the treatment of childhood apraxia of speech and persistent speech sound disorders. Other research is concerned with emergent literacy and especially gender gaps in the acquisition of early literacy skills. In all these studies the use of digital applications to enhance assessment and intervention is explored.

In A18, she explains the process and importance of speech perception training for numerous children with SSD.

Q18.   Susan Rvachew: Speech Perception Training

'Children with expressive phonological delays often possess poor underlying perceptual knowledge of the sound system...' (Rvachew et al., 2004). What are the implications of this research finding for evidence-based clinical practice with children who have SSD?

A18.   Susan Rvachew: Perceptually Based Interventions

Many studies have shown that a large proportion of children with speech sound disorders have difficulty with speech perception in comparison to children of the same age who do not have speech sound disorders. The speech perception difficulties may not be obvious to parents or other people who are talking with the child. However, these difficulties with speech perception have been found in studies using a large variety of assessment techniques and speech stimuli (Cohen & Diehl, 1963; Edwards et al., 2002; Hearnshaw et al., 2018; Hoffman et al., 1985, 1983; Munson et al., 2005, 2006; Rvachew, 2007b; Sherman & Geith, 1967; Shuster, 1998; Sutherland & Gillon, 2007).

A systematic review confirmed that some but not all children with SSD have difficulty with speech perception, especially when assessed with appropriate tasks that target phonemic perception rather than phonetic discrimination (Hearnshaw et al., 2018). These findings imply that attention to children's speech perception abilities may be an important component of a speech therapy program, and indeed this hypothesis has been supported by intervention studies (Jamieson & Rvachew, 1992; Rvachew, 1994; Rvachew et al., 2004, 1999).

Speech Assessment and Interactive Learning System (SAILS)

SAILS is a computer-based tool that can be used to improve children's speech perception skills. SAILS targets commonly misarticulated consonant phonemes in the onset (initial) and coda (final) position of words. The program is based on recordings of naturally produced words. These words were recorded from English-speaking adult talkers with accurate speech, child talkers with accurate speech, and child talkers with a speech sound disorder. The child's task is to listen to each word and indicate whether it is an exemplar of the target word or not an exemplar of the target word. The child responds by pointing to a picture of the target word or to an 'X'. Visual feedback is provided after the child's response.

Typically, the child engages with the SAILS task for 5- to 10-minutes at the beginning or end of each therapy session. In Rvachew (1994), the SAILS program was used as part of a traditional speech therapy program in which phonetic placement, modelling, and drill-play activities were used to help children master a single phoneme in syllables, words, and sentences. In Rvachew et al. (1999) SAILS was provided for three sessions concurrently with phonetic placement targeting 3 phonemes, as a prelude to a 9-week course of group phonological therapy using the 'cycles approach' (Hodson & Paden, 1983). In Rvachew et al. (2004), the child's speech therapist decided whether to use a traditional or phonological approach depending on her perception of the child's needs. The SAILS intervention was provided after each therapy session. In all these studies, children who received the SAILS intervention showed twice as much progress toward the achievement of age-appropriate articulation accuracy than children whose intervention programs did not include a speech perception component.

The SAILS App

The program has recently been implemented as an iPad application ('app') that includes all the original modules in North American English, a French language module, and modules in Australian English developed by Stephanie Hearnshaw (https://apps.apple.com/ca/app/sails/id1207583276).

What are the Conditions under Which the Program Has Been Shown to Be Effective?

In the studies mentioned above, the intervention was provided for only 5 to 10 minutes at the beginning or end of the child's therapy sessions. In these studies, the intervention was provided by a communication disorders assistant or undergraduate student research assistant. These individuals, who had access to a procedural manual if required, received about one hour of training in administering SAILS, all demonstrating that it can be provided very efficiently by non-SLPs/SLTs with minimal training. The children in all these studies were 4- to 5- years of age with moderate or severe speech sound disorders, as determined by a standardized test of articulation accuracy. Other groups of children are known to have difficulty with speech perception and thus may benefit from the intervention (e.g., older children who have residual distortion errors, second language learners, and children with specific language impairment or dyslexia). However, no studies have investigated the effectiveness of SAILS with these groups.

Are There Alternatives to the SAILS Program?

Basic research on optimum procedures for perceptual training indicates that stimulus variability is very important. Therefore, SAILS includes multiple voices and a variety of good and poor exemplars of the target words. Thus, SAILS may be an effective adjunct to these live-voice procedures that usually involve the presentation of exaggerated speech models produced by one or two talkers (e.g., speech therapist and/or parent). However, SAILS cannot be used with children who are not speaking a dialect that matches the modules that are included (i.e., North American or Australian English).

In other language or dialect contexts, live voice procedures may be effective, especially if you can still find ways to introduce multi-talker variability into your treatment. Rvachew and Brosseau-Lapré (2015) used live-voice procedures with French-speaking children when implementing an input-oriented approach to phonological intervention with good results. Variability was included in the program by including two clinicians in the child's treatment and by varying rate and prosody when providing speech input. Additionally, many technologies exist that can be used to develop speech perception tasks for specific clients. For example, if you were working with a group of children who misarticulate /ɹ/ you could use a computer with digital recording software to record the children's efforts to say words that contain this phoneme. If there is variability within the group and within children with respect to their production accuracy, you will have a perfect set of stimuli for teaching identification of correct and incorrect exemplars of the /ɹ/ phoneme. You can insert the recordings and pictures of the target words into power point slides for presentation to your students. Arrange the slides so that there is a random ordering of correct and incorrect exemplars and ask the children to identify the words that are pronounced correctly.

Case Study

Kenny commenced speech therapy for treatment of a moderate speech sound disorder at age 3;8 when he presented with unintelligible speech despite above average receptive language abilities, age-appropriate expressive language skills, and normal hearing and oral structure and function. His error patterns included backing of alveolar stops and nasals, backing of affricates, fronting of palatal fricatives, and gliding of liquids. Initially, his SLP employed a traditional approach to target /l/ in word initial singleton and cluster contexts during weekly one-hour individual speech therapy sessions.

When Kenny was 4;3 he was enrolled in a randomized control trial (Rvachew et al., 2004) and was assigned to receive the SAILS intervention in addition to his regular speech therapy program for 16 weeks. His SLP continued with weekly sessions, targeting /t/, /d/, /ʃ/, and /tʃ/ using a traditional approach and a horizontal goal attack strategy. In addition to these sessions, he also received 15 minutes of the SAILS intervention, administered by his mother under the guidance of a student research assistant. Each week he learned to identify correct and incorrect versions of words that began or ended with a given phoneme, specifically /t, p, m, k, l, ɹ, f, s/ in the word initial position for the first 8 weeks and in word final position for the second 8 weeks of the study (see the published research report for details of the phonemic perception and phonological awareness activities that were implemented by computer for these phonemes). All treatment was discontinued when he was 4;7 and he received no further treatment as a preschooler. It is not known whether he ever received speech therapy in elementary school.

His speech accuracy was assessed at enrolment to the study just as the SAILS intervention was about to begin (pre-treatment assessment), 6 months later (post-treatment assessment) and 12 months later (follow-up assessment). These assessments were conducted by an SLP who was blind to his assigned experimental treatment condition and who was not involved in the regular or experimental portion of his intervention. Kenny's percentile rankings of 5, 10, and 32 on the Goldman-Fristoe Test of Articulation (Goldman & Fristoe, 2000) during the pre-treatment, post-treatment, and follow-up assessments respectively revealed excellent progress.

An examination of the total number of errors on this test showed that his improvement between the pre- and post-treatment assessments was almost twice as great as the improvement that was observed on average for children in the control group who did not receive the SAILS intervention. Kenny's improvement mirrored the results obtained for the entire experimental group. The clinical importance of this outcome is highlighted by the fact that he began first grade with age-appropriate speech (w/ɹ substitutions being the only remaining speech error), an outcome enjoyed by comparatively few children in the control group. These improvements in speech accuracy were also reflected in significantly improved speech intelligibility as illustrated in brief excerpts from speech samples that yield Percent Consonant Correct scores of 65, 85, and 92 for the pre-treatment, post-treatment, and follow-up assessments respectively.

Pre-treatment Speech Sample Excerpt
'Karl's putting her in there where is all fishes.'
[ɡɑɪz pʊɡɪŋ hə ɪn ɡɛʌ wɛ ɪz ɑ fɪsəz]
Post-treatment Speech Sample Excerpt
'He is putting the baby in there. In … tank. There's fishies.'
[hi ɪz pʊrɪŋ ə bebi ɪn dɛʌ … ɪn … tæŋk … dɛɹz fɪʃiz]
Follow-up Speech Sample Excerpt
'And then he takes the baby to the fish tank and the baby swimming in the fish tank.'
[æn ðɛn hi teks ə bebi tu ðə fɪʃtæŋk æn ðə bebi swɪmɪn ɪn ðə fɪʃtæŋk]

Further Information, and an Invitation

More information about the application of perceptually based approaches to speech therapy can be found in Rvachew (Rvachew, 2005b), Rvachew (Rvachew, 2005a), and (Rvachew, 2007a). Please contact the author at susan.rvachew@mcgill.ca if you wish to create new stimuli appropriate to a different dialect or language group.

The Principles Underpinning Phonological Intervention

Like Grunwell (1975, 1985b) and Ingram (1976), Fey (1992) observed that three principles underlie phonology-based approaches to treatment such as conventional minimal pairs therapy (Weiner, 1981a) that use meaningful ('real') word contrasts.

1. **Modifying groups of sounds, or syllable structures**
   The first principle concerned the modification of *groups* of sounds targeted according to an organizing feature or systematic rule (of the child's), rather than focusing on 'correcting' or 'perfecting'

the articulation of individual phones. Levelling intervention at *groups* of sounds indicated two things, first, recognition of the systematic nature of phonology, and second, acknowledgement that enhancing part of the system increased the possibility of generalization of new learning across the child's speech sound system.

The speech production errors that the systematic rules represented fell into two main categories: **substitution processes** (also called *systemic processes*, *systemic patterns*, and *substitution patterns*) where one sound or sound class is substituted for another; and **structural processes** (also called *syllable structure processes*, *structural errors*, *structural patterns*, and *syllable structure patterns*), where the structure of the syllable or word changes. The phonological processes/patterns listing in Tables 2.1 and 4.3 is not exhaustive. Those marked with asterisks in Table 4.3 regularly occur in children with SSD but are uncommon in typical development (TD) in English.

2. Establishing feature contrasts

The second phonological principle was around establishing feature contrasts as opposed to perfecting articulatory execution sound-by-sound and word-position-by-word-position. Phonetic placement techniques, such as *hunting* (Van Riper & Irwin, 1958), the 'trail blazing' (*sic*) *progressive approximations* method (Van Riper, 1963), the *successive approximation* procedure (Kaufman, 2005; McCurry & Irwin, 1953), and *shaping* (Bernthal & Bankson, 2004; Shriberg, 1975) are goal attack strategies used as intermediary steps towards adult-like phonetic execution of a target. Fostering such articulatory precision, clinicians may verbally encourage children to produce 'a good crisp /s/', 'a clear /tʃ/', 'a perfect /k/', 'a sharp /t/', 'a nice /ŋ/', or 'a lovely /l/'.

By contrast, in phonological therapy, the child is rewarded for creating *contrast* by using a sound in the target sound class, or a reasonable approximation to the target. For instance, with a child working

Table 4.3 Examples of phonological processes / phonological patterns.

Substitution Processes / Substitution Patterns	
(systemic processes / systemic patterns)	
Abbreviations: **TD** Typical Development, **SIWI** Syllable Initial Word Initial, **SIWW** Syllable Initial Within Word, **SFWF** Syllable Final Word Final, **SFWW** Syllable Final Within Word	
*Alveolarization / Apicalization	An alveolar consonant replaces a dental (labiodental /f, v/ or interdental /θ, ð/) consonant. For example, [ˈsʌˌni] for *funny*, [ˈzɪki] for *Vicky*, [sɪŋ] for *thing*, and [zæt] for *that*.
Assimilation: Velar assimilation	A non-velar consonant changes to a velar due to the presence of a neighbouring velar, for example, [gʌk] for *duck*; [kɪk] for *tick*.
*Assimilations that are unusual in TD	Nasal assimilation: a non-nasal consonant changes to a nasal due to the presence of a neighbouring nasal, for example, [ˈnæˌni˙] for *Danny*, [nəˈnaˌnə] or [məˈmaˌmə] for *banana*, [bəˈgɪŋˌɪŋ] for *beginning*. Alveolar assimilation, for example, [deɪd] for *paid*, [tʊt] for *put*. Palatal assimilation, for example, [ʃʌʃ] for *rush*. Liquid assimilation, for example, [ˈlouˈlou] for *yoyo*. An exception is [ˈlɛˌlou] for *yellow* which is common in TD.
Backing	A velar ('back consonant') replaces an alveolar ('front consonant'), for example, [kiː] for *tea*, [geɪk] for *date*.
Cluster simplification	A glide replaces a liquid in a consonant cluster, for example, [bwuː] or [bjuː] for *blue*, [fwɪp] for *flip*, or simplifies a fricative, for example, [fɹiː] or [fwiː] for *three*, [θtwɪŋ] for *string*, [ˈɛnˌtwəns] for *entrance*.
Deaffrication	A fricative replaces an affricate, for example, [ʒʌmp] for *jump*, [ʃɪn] for *chin*, [peɪʒ] for *page*, [wɪs] for *wish*.

(Continued)

Table 4.3 (*Continued*)

Fricative simplificationThis term, Fricative simplification, rather than Labialization, is reserved for substitutions of [f] for /θ/ and [v] for /ð/, commonly heard in TD.	Considered to be Labialization in some classifications (Edwards & Shriberg, 1983), [f] replaces /θ/ and [v] replaces /ð/, for example, [fɪŋk] for *think*, [vɛm] for them, ['bɹʌvə] for *brother*, [baf] for *bath*. Because Labialization is uncommon in TD, 'fricative simplification' is preferable. Fricative simplification may be dialectal, but it is also common in English TD, cross dialectally. Speakers who replace /θ/ and /ð/ with [t] and [v] may be pigeonholed or stereotyped, by some listeners who do not, as low in social status or 'uneducated'.
Fronting of Palatals / Palatal fronting / Depalatalization	An alveolar consonant replaces a postalveolar consonant, for example, [suː] for *shoe*, ['mɛzə] for *measure*, ['æl'seɪ,sən] for *Alsatian*, [wɒs] for *wash*, [beɪz] for *beige*.
Fronting of velars / Velar fronting	An alveolar ('front consonant') replaces a velar ('back consonant'), for example, [tiː] for *key*, [daɪ] for *guy*, [ɹɒn] for *wrong*.
Gliding of affricates	A glide replaces an affricate, for example, [wouk] for *choke, joke*; [jouk] for *choke, joke*.
Gliding of fricatives	A glide replaces a fricative, for example, [wɛd] for *fed, head, said, shed, zed*; [juː] for *shoe, sue, who, zoo*, ['wɛwi] or ['wɛɹi] for *very*.
Gliding of liquids	A glide replaces a liquid, for example, [ji] for *Lee*, [wɛd] for *red*.
*Labialization	A labial (bilabial or labiodental) consonant replaces a non-labial consonant, for example, ['fɪkŋ] for *chicken*, [fil] for *seal*, ['faɪni] for *shiny*. See Fricative simplification, above, re [f] for /θ/ and [v] for /ð/ substitutions (called fricative simplifications).
Post-vocalic devoicing (an Assimilation of voice)	A voiced consonant that follows a vowel is replaced with its voiceless cognate, for example, [wɪk] for *wig*, [ɹʌp] for *rub*, [ɛtʃ] for *edge*, [keɪf] for *cave*, ['ælə,keɪtə] for *alligator*.
Pre-vocalic voicing (an Assimilation of voice)	A voiceless consonant that precedes a vowel is replaced with its voiced cognate, for example, [bɔl] for *Paul*, /gʌp/ for *cup*.
Stopping of affricates Stopping of fricatives	A stop replaces an affricate or fricative, for example, [diː] for *fee, see, she, he*; [deɪn] for *chain, Jane, Shane*, ['bʌniː] for *funny*.
*Stopping of liquids	A stop (usually a voiced stop) replaces a liquid, for example, [dɛt] for *let*, [daɪn] for *line*, [beɪt] for *late*, ['fɒ,dou] for *follow*.
Systematic sound preference (Weiner, 1981b), can create widespread homophony, greatly reducing intelligibility, and provoking both speaker and listener frustration.	A sound class, or many members of a sound class, particularly fricatives and affricates, is replaced by a 'favourite sound' (often, but not necessarily a voiced stop), for example, [d] or [b] replace SIWI and SFWF fricatives in *chew, chews, fee, fees, jay, jays, sew, sews, show, shows, zoo, zoos*, so they are realized, highly unintelligibly, as [duː, duːd, diː, diːd, deɪ, deɪd, dou, doud, dou, doud, duː, duːd] respectively, or [buː, buːb, biː, biːb, beɪ, beɪb, bou, boub, bou, boub, buː, buːb] respectively.
*Vocalization / Vowelization	A vowel replaces a syllabic consonant, for example, ['lɪtʊ] for *little*, ['tækʊ] for *tackle*, ['gɹæpʊ] for *grapple*, ['fʌnʊ] for *funnel*, and ['tʌnʊʷ]for *tunnel* (alternatively, [lɪtʊʷ], [tækʊʷ], [gɹæpʊʷ], [fʌnʊʷ], [tʌnʊʷ]). Edwards and Shriberg (1983) posited that vocalization can occur with syllabic nasals (e.g., [bʌtʊ] for *button*), while Grunwell (1982) proposed that this was best characterized as final consonant deletion.

Structural Processes / Structural Patterns
(syllable structure processes / syllable structure patterns)

Cluster reduction	A consonant within a cluster (usually a marked consonant) is deleted, for example, [bu] for *blue*, [neɪk] for *snake*, [stɪŋ] for *string*.
*Coalescence	Features of two adjacent phones (usually in a consonant cluster) are replaced by a different phone, for example, ['faɪ,də] for *spider*, [doun] for *stone*. In ['faɪ,də] for *spider*, the [+ continuant] manner feature of /s/ coalesces with the [LABIAL] place feature of /p/, to make [f] – which is [LABIAL] and [+ continuant]. In [doun] for *stone*, the [ALVEOLAR] place feature of /s/ coalesces with the [-continuant] manner feature of /t/ making [d] – which is alveolar.

Table 4.3 *(Continued)*

*Diminutization	The vowel /iː/ is appended to a word, for example, [ˈhɔˌsi] for horse, [ˈʃiːpi] for sheep. Some diminutization may be 'taught' when parents use child directed speech, for example, 'Time for beddy-byes' (bed), 'Nighty night'(goodnight), 'Where's froggy?' (frog), or euphemisms, for example, /ˈbɒˌti/ (*bottom*: a euphemism for *buttocks*),
*Epenthesis This is sometimes called schwa insertion when the epenthetic segment is the neutral vowel, /ə/.	A segment is inserted after a SIWI or SIWW consonant or within a cluster, for example, [pəˈleɪn] for *plain*, [kɜˈliːn] for *clean*, [təˈɹiː] for *tree*, [ˈhɛnˌəˈɹi] or [ˈhɛnˌɜˈɹi] for *Henry*, [spəˈɹeɪd] for *sprayed*, [ˈæθˌʌˈlɪt] for *athlete*, [ˈbæˈɹɪzˌbn̩] or [ˈbʌˈɹɪzˌbn̩] for *Brisbane*, [ˈæd ˌvəˈkɑːˌdou] *avocado*, [ˈæˌtəˈlɪs] for *atlas*.
Final consonant deletion	A final consonant (SFWF or SFWW) is deleted, for example, [pɛ] for *peck*, [pɛˈɪŋ] for *pecking*.
*Initial consonant deletion	An initial consonant (SIWI or SIWW) is deleted, for example, [uːz] for *shoes*, [ˈuːˈɒp] for *shoe shop*, [ˈuːˈeɪs] for *shoelace*.
*Metathesis	The sequence of two adjacent or nonadjacent consonants is reversed, for example, [ˈɛˌfəˈlənt] for *elephant*, [mɑːks] for *mask*, [touts] for *toast*, [ˈhɒsˌtəˈpʊl] for *hospital*, [ˈbɪsˌtɪk] for *biscuit*, [ˈvæsˌkɪnˈeɪʃn̩] for *vaccination*, [ˈvæˈskiːn] for *vaccine*.
*Migration	A sound in a word position, or word combination, relocates to a different position, for example, [ˈpeɪtˌstɹiː] for *pastry*, [aɪ ˈpaɪs] for *I spy*.
Reduplication / Doubling	A syllable is repeated twice, for example, [ˈdɪˈdɪ] or [ˈdɪnˈdɪn] for *dinner*, [ˈnaˈna] for *banana*, [ˈwɔˈwɔ] or [ˈwaˈwa] for *water*. Doubling is sometimes 'taught' when parents use child directed speech, for example, 'Pat your tum-tum' (tummy), or euphemisms, for example, 'Let's wipe your bot-bot' (bottom/buttocks).
Weak syllable deletion / Unstressed syllable deletion	A weak, or unstressed syllable is deleted, for example, [ˈæˌmul] for *animal*, [ˈstɹeɪˌjə] for *Australia*, [ˈtɛˌvɪʒn̩] for *television*, [ˈkæˌpɪˌlə] for *caterpillar*.

at the systemic (substitution process) level to eliminate stopping of fricatives, a production like /ʃʌn/ for *sun* rather than /dʌn/ for *sun* would be rewarded, because /ʃ/ and /s/ are in the same (fricative) sound class, and both are voiceless. With a child working at the structural level, learning final consonant inclusion, a production such as /biːm/ for *bean* rather than /biː/ for *bean* would be rewarded, because a final consonant was included, and furthermore the /m/ is a nasal consonant (like /n/).

The clinician's acceptance of phonemic contrast and the lack of emphasis on fine tuning of phonetic form, particularly in the early stages of therapy, can be hard to explain or 'sell' to parents and caregivers (and even some SLPs/SLTs), especially if they are anxious, and impatient to see progress. Their expectation of a clinician's role may be that we are 'supposed to be' encouraging perfection, and they can find it difficult to understand that, if a goal in therapy is to eliminate stopping of fricatives, then /fɪp/ for *ship* is 'more correct' than /dɪp/ for *ship* and /sɪp/ for *ship* is even better!

3. Working at word level and above – to make meaning

> *The function of the phonological system of a language is to signal the meaning differences required by the grammatical and lexical systems.*
>
> Grunwell, 1985a, p. 93

The third principle related to the goal of making *meaning*, with the implication that the therapy must, perforce, be constructed around listening to, discriminating between, decoding, and saying 'real' words. Indeed, it is a truism that phonological therapy *must* be at word level or above (i.e., employing, as stimuli, words, phrases, sentences, or conversation) to signal to the child that the function of phonology is to communicate (or to make meaning). This emphasis on meaning begins in the assessment phase, with the clinician gathering single word and connected speech data for phonological analysis, or to identify systemic phoneme collapses. Then, intervention is designed so that the child recognizes that homophony must be avoided, and meaningful contrasts established. If *bum, come, crumb, drum, dumb, gum, hum, plum, some,* and *thumb* are 'collapsed' and realized homonymously as [dʌm], the child is led to discover that something (phonological) *must* change (see Storkel, 2022 for helpful discussion).

Applying the Phonological Principles in Intervention

When implementing the phonological principle of **targeting groups of sounds or groups of syllable structures**, a clinician selects either a substitution process, or a syllable structure process, or both, as a therapy target or targets, with the goal of eliminating the process or processes. This 'elimination' is achieved via the second principle of **establishing feature contrasts**.

To recap, the function of feature contrasts is to signal meaning differences between words, or **to make meaning**, necessitating the third phonological principle of **working at word level and above**. With some children who have phonological impairment, it may *also* be necessary to work at a phonetic or articulatory level using the phonetic placement techniques described early in this chapter: auditory discrimination activities, imitation, shaping, phonetic-placement cues, motor-kinaesthetic cues, and touch cues. Some children will require the stimulability approach (Miccio, A17), and some – considerably more that was once thought (Rvachew, 1994) – may also require speech perception intervention (Rvachew, A18). Recall that intervention for *any* SSD includes metalinguistic cues (see Table 4.1).

Minimal/Near Minimal Pairs; Minimal/Maximal Oppositions

Minimal pairs, near minimal pairs, minimal oppositions and maximal oppositions are discussed detail in Chapter 2. For convenience, more examples follow.

Minimal pairs are two words that contrast by one phoneme, causing them to have different meanings. For example, *ship-sip, cap-gap, word-bird,*

safe-save, supper-sucker, berry-belly, tip-tap, and *bungle-bangle* are all minimal pairs.

Near minimal pairs are word pairs that differ because the syllable structure changes, as in

- Singleton vs. cluster contrasts, for example, lie-fly, pay-play (CV vs. CCV), *call-crawl, back-black* (CVC vs. CCVC), and *sash-splash, wrong-strong, catch-scratch,* (CVC vs. CCCVC), and boat-boast, Tess-test (CVC vs. CVCC).
- Cluster vs. cluster contrasts, for example, *fly-fry* (CCV vs. CCV), *spin-skin,* (CCVC vs. CCVC), *spring-string* (CCCVC vs. CCCVC), and *slinky-Blinky* (CCVCCV vs. CCVCCV). For the uninitiated, a slinky is a 'tumbling' spring-like toy, and Blinky is the eponymous koala from the children's classic Blinky Bill by Dorothy Wall (1894–1942). Today, Blinky Bill is monetized as toys, games, figurines, cartoons, comic books, movies, at least one App, and TV shows.
- Via the inclusion or exclusion of a consonant such as *bee-bean, chew-choose, weigh-wait* (CV vs. CVC), *eel-feel, up-cup, ice-rice, out-shout* (VC vs. CVC).
- Via the inclusion or exclusion of a (usually weak) syllable, for example, *tar-guitar, leave-believe, cross-across, cos-because, Nana-banana, Tsar-bazaar, la-galah.* It is difficult to find suitable, picturable near minimal pairs for weak syllable deletion (unstressed syllable deletion) but it can be done with a little ingenuity. In the preceding list, a cos /kɒz/ is a type of lettuce, Nana /ˈnaˌna/ is a girls' name, la [la] is a musical note, and a galah /gəˈla/ is a parrot-like bird.

Minimal oppositions, for example, *buy-pie, cab-cap, cab-cub, caber-caper,* and *blot-plot,* are *minimal pairs* in that one sound changes, that are *minimally opposed.* In a minimal opposition, there only one feature change. In the preceding list, in *buy-pie* voicing, but not place and manner of articulation change, while in *cab-cub* only the vowels change, and the consonants remain the same.

Maximal oppositions occur in minimal pairs where there are two or more feature differences. In *bun-sun, mob-moss, Bobby-bossy,* we see that the voiced labial stop /b/ is maximally opposed to the voiceless alveolar fricative /s/. While they are still minimal pairs, they form maximal oppositions with their three maximally opposing features: voiced vs. voiceless, labial vs. alveolar, stop vs. fricative (continuant). In *sea-me, seal-meal, send-mend, silk-milk,* and *sign-mine*; and *weed-feed, wig-fig, one-fun, walk-fork,* and *wire-fire,* there are three feature differences (in voice, place, and manner) and an additional class feature, contrast: obstruent /s/ or /f/ vs. sonorant /m/ or /w/ respectively.

Minimal and Near Minimal Pairs in Phonological Therapy

The minimal pair approach is based on minimal word pairs that a child realizes (says) homonymously. Generally, they form minimal oppositions (*nail-mail*) or are near minimal pairs (*nail-snail; ale-nail*). For instance, for a child who exhibits stopping of affricates (e.g., pronouncing *chain* /tʃeɪn/ as [teɪn] and *Jane* /dʒeɪn/ as [deɪn]), rhyming word-pairs containing /tʃ/ and /t/, or /dʒ/ and /d/, would make up the treatment sets for minimal pair intervention. The SLP/SLT constructs meaningful pairs because the thrust of minimal pair therapy is to teach the child to avoid homonymy and make meaning. Suitable pairs in this example would be a selection – say, three to five pairs or more – from a choice of *cheat-teat, cheese-Ts, chin-tin, cheer-tear, chip-tip, chick-tick, chess-Tess, chop-top, chew-two,* or *chalk-talk*; a choice of *jeep-deep, G/D, jig-dig, Jill-dill, J-day, jam-dam, jog-dog,* or *junk-dunk, juice-deuce,* or *jive-dive.*

Before initiating a minimal pairs approach, it is important to determine that

- assessment data show that the substitution error production is consistent: for example, *chin* is pronounced *tin* [tɪn] every time, and not variably and variously with two or more of these: *tin, din, gin, shin,* tsin [tsɪn] and *zhin* [ʒɪn].
- the error does not vary in terms of syllable structure, for example, *chin* is realized consistently as [tɪn], and not inconsistently as two or more of these: [tɪn], [tə͜ɪn], [tsɪn], [tɪ], and [tɪʔ].
- errors to be remediated have a phonological (linguistic) basis and not a phonetic (articulatory) explanation.
- word pair sets demonstrate, to the child, lost contrast and ultimately, their own homonymy.

- the chosen minimal pair approach suits the child in terms of factors such as their phonology, age, temperament, and availability to attend sessions.

The Meaningful Minimal Pairs Approach

Trevor, 2;11 engaged in a meaningful minimal pair approach, and his intervention is described Box 4.1. Meaningful minimal pairs therapy occurs in three general steps:

Step 1. Familiarization with treatment words (errors and targets) and picture stimuli.

Step 2. Listening and pointing to or picking up, requested pictured words.

Step 3. Production of error-target pairs, and then target words in longer utterances.

It is helpful to know that in her openly accessible tutorial, Storkel (2022) advised that using the conventional minimal pair approach should be restricted to children with a small number of errors, older children, or children with mild SSD.

Box 4.1   Case Illustration: meaningful minimal pairs intervention

Trevor, 2;11

Trevor, who was coming up to his third birthday, exhibited prevalent final consonant deletion, with open syllables dominating his syllable structures. He was monolingual, learning a non-rhotic variety of English, and was stimulable for the phones he omitted in CVs, and in vowel plus fricative VCs. His parents, Liane and Wenchang were second generation Chinese Australians who had 'lost' most of their Cantonese which they had both spoken with people in their grandparents' generation in early childhood. When Dave, Trevor's SLP asked Wenchang, how intelligible Trevor was to him, he replied, '*I feel terrible about this, but I guess I only "get" about 25% of what he's trying to say. Liane does a lot better, but she and Trev get super frustrated with each other at times.*' Dave had anticipated a response along these lines, knowing that Wenchang mainly saw him at weekends due to long work hours, and given Trevor's extensive homophony. He put the same question to Liane who said, '*I get around 95%, but only if I know what he's talking about. I get uptight when he tells me about something at preschool and I don't know the other children's names.*' Dave, who was attuned to children with SSD estimated that for him, Trevor's intelligibility was around 80%.

Phonological analysis revealed for his VC, CVC and CVCC words alone, Trevor's homonymous productions included [kɪ] for *kid, kick, kill, kiss, Kim,* and *king;* [bʌ] for *bub, budge, bug, bum, bun, bunch, bus, but,* and *buzz;* [pɛ] for *peck, peg, pen, pest,* and *pet;* [ɛ] for *edge, eff, egg, ell, end, ess,* and '*X*', and [ʌ] for *Ugg, up,* and *us.* Despite this, Dave reasoned that Trevor's SSD was in the mild range in that only one phonological process, Final Consonant Deletion (FCD), was evident (Storkel, 2022).

Following the phonological principle of targeting errors as a group, Trevor's parents and therapist encouraged, in general conversation, final consonant inclusion across his disordered system. This was preferable to laboriously treating word-final /p/, /b/, /t/, /d/, /k/, /g/, /m/, /n/, /ŋ/, /f/, /v/, /θ/, /ð/, /s/, /z/, /ʃ/, /ʒ/, /tʃ/, /dʒ/, /ɹ/, and /l/ individually and serially as syllable-final-word-final (SFWF) singleton omissions.

Dave carefully selected meaningful near minimal pair exemplars, optimistic that there would be generalization to non-targeted contrasts. Trevor started with 5 pairs, from a choice of 18: *bay-Babe, row-road, cow-couch, sir-surf, key-quiche, bay- beige, pay-page, buy-bike, E-eel, lie-lime, tray-train, bee-beep, K-cage, hoe-hose, buy-bite, lay-lathe, two-tooth,* and *high-hive.* Trevor chose *bay-Babe, sir-surf, buy-bike, K-cage,* and *high-hive* (representing the final consonants /b, f, k, dʒ,* and v/) and they were used in the first session for **Step 1: familiarization.** Only *K, sir* and *hive* were absent from his lexicon at the outset of therapy. Still in the first session, he quickly moved to **Step 2: listening and pointing to or listening and picking-up** words spoken by Dave. Again, he caught on quickly and Dave was able to introduce **Step 3: production** practice comprised of drill and a small palette of drill-play. This progression, from Step 1 to Step 3 in the first session is reasonably typical, even for children as young as Trevor.

At 2.11, Trevor did not need a wide variety of drill-play (production) activities. He willingly engaged in uncomplicated 'card posting' games, especially if they involved a *Smart Chute,* and would put the pairs through the chute saying the

words as he put them in, and again when they emerged at the foot of the chute, in exchange for praise, stars, stickers and smiley stamps for final consonant inclusion, at the end of a set. He would also enthusiastically pick up and say the word pairs in simple turn-taking games and engage in 'say these (pairs) after me' with a model, or 'tell me what these are' production drill without a model. He particularly enjoyed crossing a river on stepping-stones, climbing a ladder, or climbing stairs with the pictures and printed words on the stepping-stones, rungs, or steps. He also required very little metalinguistic cueing for final consonant inclusion, but when he did, Dave used a magnetic steam train to convey the metaphor that the locomotive was the beginning of a word, and the tender (coal car) was the final consonant. Both Liane and Wenchang were pleased with his persistence, and cooperation telling him often that he had 'a great work ethic'!

Trevor attended with either Liane or Wenchang, twice weekly for 8 weeks, for 40-minute sessions, with 30 minutes devoted to a combination of drill and drill-play activities, and structured play. He was uninterested in child-led semi-structured play, preferring to have Dave take the lead. He consistently produced 100 trials within 30 minutes. Dave engineered the semi structured play bursts and would have prominently on view an appealing (to Trevor) book, game or toy that reflected one of the target words, for example, a vintage **Babe** and *Friends Mini Farm Collection* (plush figures) from the 1998 feature film *Pig in The City* which Dave bought on eBay, Dave's vintage Super **Surf** Smurf collection also from eBay, the book *Bear on a **Bike*** by Hannah Shaw, the Dr. Seuss book *If I Ran the Zoo* (for **cage**), and a Clamp Bee to **Hive** matching game.

Once he was mostly adding a final consonant in the right sound class (not necessarily the correct consonant) to *Babe, surf, bike, cage,* and *hive,* Trevor chose another 5 pairs from the remaining thirteen: *cow-couch, row-road, E-eel, key-quiche,* and *hoe-hose* (representing 5 different final consonants /tʃ, d, l, ʃ,* and z/). He progressed well with those too, with the same combination of therapy activities. Because Trevor liked all the pictures and requested them, Dave combined the two sets (10 pairs). They worked with them until he could produce the VC (*eel*) and the nine CVCs accurately.

Dave then assessed progress with a single-word probe set of unpractised pairs that Trevor had not seen before, representing the 10 *targeted* final consonants /b, f, k, dʒ, v, tʃ, d, l, ʃ,* and z/. He achieved

90-to-100% accuracy with all but the affricates /ʧ, and dʒ/ which stood at 40%. In a second single word probe, he also included the *untreated* consonants /g, m, n, ŋ, s, and l/ with 70% accuracy word finally.

At this juncture Dave did two things. First, he introduced a 6 near minimal pair set for the final consonants /ʧ, dʒ, and θ/: *ow-ouch, E-each, for-forge, sea-siege, sow-south, tea-teeth*. True to form, Trevor was quickly familiarized with the 'new words' (for him) *forge, south*, and *siege*, and progressed through the first two steps to Step 3 production in the first session. Second, he used the structured play materials to develop production practice activities beyond a single-word level, for example, a card game with pictures of large and small items where Trevor and an adult would take turns requesting a big or small one (a big bike vs. a little bike, a big quiche vs. a little quiche, a big road vs. a little road, a big hose vs. a little hose). Dave would praise correct productions (*That's right, a little **quiche***) or challenge incorrect ones (*I heard you say key, but there's no key there. Did you mean quiche? Try again, give me the little **quiche**.*) He loved the phrase and sentence activities, progressing steadily.

Gains with the newly introduced /ʧ, dʒ, and θ/ targets were slow in coming, and frustrating for Trevor, and his parents and therapist agreed to move on to minimal pairs intervention for SFWW targets, using the phonemes he was successful with in the SFWF positions, and return to the SFWF /ʧ, dʒ, and θ/ targets after a three-week break.

After the short break, Trevor now almost 3;3, had a series of 40-minute sessions with 30 minutes of drill and drill play, and 10 minutes structured play, twice weekly for two weeks and once weekly for four (eight sessions). By the eighth session, final consonant inclusion SFWF and SFWF had generalized across Trevor's system, and he was self-correcting errors without prompting, and enjoying praise for self-correcting. All that was required at this point was for his parents to provide occasional reminders, models, and labelled praise.

Overall, Trevor had one initial assessment session and 27 × 40-minute treatments, spread over 19 weeks from the ages of 2;11 to 3;6, with brief probe assessments integrated into the eighth and 27th intervention session. He was an obliging, sociable preschooler who happily produced 100 trials within 30 minutes in each session. He returned for a follow-up assessment at age 3;9 when his speech sound system was within normal limits.

Meaningful vs. Perception-production Minimal Pairs

*Children who have one particularly pervasive process or only a few age-inappropriate phonological processes seem to be better candidates for the **perception-production minimal pairs procedure** because it involves concentration on one process at a time.*

Tyler et al., 1987, p. 405

Trevor, whose intervention is described in Box 4.1, participated in a meaningful minimal pairs approach. An alternative approach is perception-production minimal pairs intervention (described by Baker, 2010, 2021). Casey received the perception-production option, and this is illustrated in Box 4.2. The approach comes from Crosbie et al. (2005), Elbert et al. (1990, 1991), and Tyler et al. (1987, 1990). In a perception-production minimal pairs approach just one phonological process is targeted at a time. The therapist first teaches a child to produce their target words using imitation strategies and does not introduce minimal pair words until the child produces the target words relatively accurately.

The use of minimal pairs was not incorporated until the child displayed some ability to correctly produce the target sound in single words. (Based on previous clinical experience, this was believed necessary… for the child to experience success.) At the minimal pairs level, the child was required to independently produce the target sound in five words during a variety of activities designed to take advantage of the semantic confusion created by an error production.

Tyler et al., 1987

The rationale for ensuring production that matches, or almost matches the adult target is to ensure the child's production success (Tyler et al., 1987, p. 396). Although Tyler et al. do not say so explicitly, reasonable target word production may render it easier for the child to repair communication breakdowns when a clarification request is issued by the clinician. It may also minimize the child's frustration when asked by an adult to revise production, when semantic confusion due to homonymy, is made overt. The 'production success' rationale differs from the meaningful minimal pair approach, where semantic confusion or listeners' misunderstandings – whether feigned or authentic – are thought to raise a child's awareness that an aspect of their speech *must* change.

Recall that the meaningful minimal pairs approach (Blache, 1982; Blache et al., 1981; Weiner, 1981a) as for Trevor in Box 4.1 has three steps: (1) Familiarization. (2) Listening and pointing or picking up. (3) Production. By contrast, the perception-production approach is in four general steps:

Step 1. Familiarization and perception training
Step 2. Production via word-imitation of 10 words comprising five target words vs. five error words. For example, for a child with prevocalic voicing, replacing /k/ with [g], the target words might be *coat, cap, card, curl,* and *cold,* paired with the minimal pair words *goat, gap, guard, girl,* and *gold.* Similarly, for a child backing alveolar stops, and replacing /d/ with [g], suitable, picturable, child-friendly, SIWI error-target contrast would be *go-dough, gull-dull, gust-dust, gash-dash,* and *gown-down,* or SFWF *sag-sad, beg-bed, bug-bud, thug-thud,* and *bag-bad.*
Step 3. Production via independent naming
Step 4. Production of minimal pair words (as in step three of the meaningful minimal pairs approach).

Perception-production Minimal Pairs

Step 1: Familiarization and Perception Training

Step 1 begins with the clinician sitting at a small table facing the child and spreading three to five picture-pairs on the table, the right way up for the child. The clinician teaches the child, in a listening-and-pointing procedure, to identify the two treatment sounds in isolation, and then in words.

For the sake of the example, let's say there are five pairs of words (on 10 cards), the phonological process is gliding of fricatives (see Table 4.3), and the words and pictures are *well-shell, wall-shawl,*

whip-ship, wake-shake, and *wave-shave* to represent a glide vs. fricative error-target contrast. The therapist says to the child, something to the effect of, '*I want you to pick up the one I say*' and then says: '*This is well*', '*This is shell*', '*This is wall*', '*This is shawl*', '*This is whip*'…etc.

This task, with the instruction to '*pick up—*', '*point to—*' or '*show me—*' continues until the child's matching of the pictures with the therapist's spoken word is 90% accurate.

Crosbie et al. (2005) added a sorting-into-pairs activity after the pick-up/point-to/show-me procedure, where the child matched *well* with *shell,* etc. The therapist praises listening ('*Super listening, yes, that's the shell*', '*That's right, this is shawl – great listening*' etc.) and provides feedback cues for incorrect responses ('*Oops. You chose whip with a [w] at the start. Listen again and pick up ship with a [ʃ]*).'

Step 2: Production via Word Imitation

In Step 2, the child is given auditory and production cues, as required, and imitates five to 10 target words. In our example there are five: *shell, shawl, ship, shake,* and *shave.* The SLP/SLT praises correct production (e.g., '*Excellent [ʃ] in ship*'; '*I'm loving your beautiful [ʃ] in ship!*') and instructional feedback for errors (e.g., '*Try it again. Listen and watch my pouty lips: ship. It's ship*'; '*Uh-oh. Listening? Watching? Try again, ship. Say ship*' and the like).

Step 2 continues until the child imitates the five target words with 90% accuracy or greater, in 50 or more trials.

Step 3: Production via Independent Naming

The child progresses in Step 3 to producing the same pictured words: *shell, shawl, ship, shake,* and *shave* in a picture-naming task with no model. Praise and instructional input (if necessary) continue, as in Step 2.

Step 3 lasts until the child imitates the five ʃ-words with 90% accuracy or greater in at least 50 trials.

Step 4: Production of Minimal Pair Words

Step 4 is the same as in Step 3 of the meaningful minimal pairs approach (as in Trevor's therapy in Box 4.1) in which the child requests a target (a ʃ-word in this example) or its pair (a w-word in this example). The child is free to choose whether to say *well* or *shell*, *wall* or *shawl*, *whip* or *ship*, *wake* or *shake*, or *wave* or *shave*. Tyler et al. (1987), proposed that the inclusion of imitated models and independent naming of the word targets words prior to the child naming the minimal pairs in Step 2 and Step 3 helped to expedite successful production in Step 4, averting any frustration on the child's part arising from realizing that they made a production error, or in response homonymy confrontation by the SLP/SLT.

Box 4.2   Case illustration: perception-production minimal pairs

Casey, 4;9

Casey had a history of otitis media with effusion between six and 36 months. The infections stopped when he had ventilation tubes inserted at 3;0. He had two episodes of mild stuttering as a three-year-old and was referred to his SLP, Melissa at that time. His dysfluency resolved with parent management advice and six visits for intervention. Melissa noted velar fronting and that he was non-stimulable for /k, g and ŋ/ and proposed to his parents that they might have his speech assessed. For financial reasons, Gough, and Jan elected not to proceed with an assessment and they did not return to Melissa's practice for nine months.

At 4;9 Casey presented as an anxious, reactive boy who had difficulty leaving Jan's side to sit at a small table with she and Melissa, and who protested quietly with 'Not today', 'It makes my tummy sore' and 'My tummy's sore'. Jan appeared to be anxious in the situation too and to have some difficulty separating from him, wanting him to sit on her lap at the table. She explained that Casey was frequently reluctant to attend preschool, saying his tummy was sore, and that on those mornings she would 'give him a day off' and 'make sure he had a lovely day at home'. She said he probably associated the speech room with preschool and thought that if he used the same tactic the adults would back off.

After a shaky start he sat in a chair by himself and Melissa gained his hesitant cooperation, observing that he had a low frustration threshold and avoided ('*Maybe later*') or abandoned tasks ('*Too hard for boys*') readily. Jan hovered anxiously, unwittingly reinforcing his responses by directing comments such as '*I think that's a bit too tricky for boys, isn't it Case?*' and '*That's a hard one, isn't it Case?*' to him.

Standardized assessment showed that his receptive and expressive language skills were well advanced with a high score on vocabulary particularly, and that he was a competent 'beginning reader' with well advanced phonological awareness.

He had 100% velar fronting, for example, [tuːl] for *cool*, [baɪt] for *bike*, ['lʌti] for *lucky*, [dou] for *go*, [bɪd] for *big*, ['daɪdə] for *tiger*, [win] for *wing*, ['hænə] for *hanger*, ['jʌndə] for *younger*, [təˈlʌb] for *club*, [dəˈlaːs] for *glass*; [təˈræb] for *crab*, [dəˈɹiːn] for *green* and [stəˈɹiːn] for *screen*, [stəˈwɪd] for *squid*.

Curiously, although velar fronting *and* epenthesis (see Syllable Structure Processes in Table 4.3) were evident when Casey attempted words like *club, glass, crab, green,* and *screen*, and other words with /kl, gl, kɹ, gɹ, and skɹ/ clusters, his other clusters, including /tɹ/, /stɹ/ and /dɹ/ in obligatory contexts (e.g., in *astronaut, dry, stray, try, undress*) matched the adult target. Intrigued, Melissa made a small probe with picture-and-word cards for *train-drain-crane-grain*, and *true-drew-crew-grew* to find that *train, drain, true,* and *drew* were produced correctly, and *crane, crew, grain,* and *grew* were invariably realized, with epenthesis, as [təˈɹeɪn], [təˈɹuː], [dəˈɹeɪn], and [dəˈɹuː]. He was still non-stimulable for velars, saying '*I can't*' when asked to imitate, displaying frequent communicative frustration.

In deciding which intervention approach to apply, Melissa took account of Casey's reactive temperament, retiring personality, and anxious, clingy behaviour, as well as his speech characteristics. Further down the line, it emerged that Gough and Jan considered Casey to be 'highly-strung and sensitive', harbouring concerns, based on discussion with well-meaning but misinformed family members, that speech intervention might trigger another episode of stuttering. Melissa settled on the perception-production minimal pairs approach because it might be more acceptable to, and less threatening for Casey and his family than the meaningful minimal pairs alternative.

Melissa decided to introduce word-final [t] (error) vs. /k/ (target) contrasts as Casey's first treatment set, as voiceless velar stops often emerge first word-finally in typical development. Indeed, most SLPs/SLTs who have been around for a while know children who can say *peek, back, neck, buck, pack,* and *shack* with every final /k/ correct, but not the other way around, *keep, cab, cap, Ken, cub,* and *cash* with /k/ in the initial position

For his first intervention session, she chose the error-target pairs *beat-beak, pet-peck, net-neck, pit-pick,* and *sit-sick.* She set aside two more sets of five pairs, *pat-pack, fort-fork, rat-rack, fete-fake, dart-dark;* and *bite-bike, light-like, bat-back, mat-mac, eight-ache* for possible future use. She also prepared two sets of [t] vs. /k/ SIWI picture cards for later sessions. They were *tea-key, tap-cap, tub-cub, tool-cool* and *tape-cape;* and *tease-keys, tail-kale, top-cop, two-coo,* and *tough-cuff.*

Step 1. Familiarization and perception training (introduced in Session 1)

Using picture cards, Melissa familiarized Casey with /t/ and /k/ in isolation. The /t/ was represented as a dripping tap picture and given the imagery name 'tippy' associated with the verbal prompt in Step 1 '*Hear that tippy?*'. In Step 2 this was modified to become production prompts, '*Remember your tippy*', '*You forgot your tippy*', '*Great, you remembered your tippy*' associated with the verbal prompt 'Tongue up' (see Table 4.1). The /k/ was represented with coughing cow picture from Miccio's stimulus cards (see Table A17.1 and Figure A17.1) associated with a gesture cue in which the SLP placed her hand near the top of her throat and the imagery name 'throaty': '*Hear the throaty sound?*', '*Remember your throaty sound*', '*Terrific! I heard your throaty sound*'.

Using a listening-and-pointing routine, Casey was taught to identify /t/ and /k/ in isolation, and then in the 10 words: *beat-beak, pet-peck, net-neck, pit-pick,* and *sit-sick.* Melissa said to him, '*I want you to pick up the one I say*' and then: '*This is beat*', [followed by feedback for a correct of incorrect selection] '*This is beak*', [feedback again, and after each move] '*This is pet*', [feedback] '*This is peck*', [feedback] '*This is net*' [feedback]...etc. Feedback for a correct selection was for Melissa simply to say the correctly picked-up word to Casey, with a smile, or '*Yes, that's right. This is neck*', or '*Good choice! Net*'. Feedback for an incorrect choice comprised responses like, '*Listen again, and give me neck*', or '*That one's net, but I asked for neck with a throaty*' said with a gesture cue. This task, with the instruction to '*pick up*', '*point to*' or '*show me*' continued until Casey matched the pictures with Melissa's spoken

word with 90% accuracy. Casey and Jan beamed when Melissa told the preschooler, '*You got 90 out of 100, that's pretty good*' and '*Do you know why you got 90 out of 100? Because you tried hard*'.

Noticing that Casey was warming to the situation, Melissa followed the suggestion of Crosbie et al. (2005) by introducing a sorting-into-pairs activity after the pick-up/point-to/show-me procedure in which Casey matched *beat* with *beak,* etc. Melissa praised listening ('*Terrific listening, yes, that's the beak*', '*Correct! This is sick – nice listening*' etc.) and provided feedback cues for incorrect responses ('*Uh-oh. That's* neck *with a [k] at the end. Listen again and pick up* neck *with a [k]*).' She also told him, '*You're going for 90 out of 100 again; we know you can do it!*' At intervals Casey would ask '*Is it 90 yet?*' and tolerated it when Melissa replied, '*Not yet, but you're getting there by trying hard*'. Jan took the hint, saying things like '*What a good tryer, Case*' and '*Keep trying like a big boy*'. He achieved 90% accuracy within the session, but instead of moving along onto Step 2, Melissa repeated the same activities in the second session, so that he could experience high levels of success before she 'graduated' him. At the end of the session, she told him, '*We're going for something a bit harder next time*' to which he replied '*OK*', while Jan looked a little uneasy.

Step 2: Production via word imitation (introduced in Session 3)

In Step 2, Casey was given production cues (imagery names, verbal and gesture cues, phonetic placement cues, shaping/successive approximations, and models, see Table 4.1), as required, to help him imitate five of the target words. He could have had up to 10 words, but Melissa was still negotiating a fine balance between shaping sound production and maintaining minimal pair recognition on one hand and circumventing a return of Casey's unwilling, apprehensive behaviour. Pushing him too hard was to be avoided.

When he arrived for his third session, he claimed that his tummy was sore. Melissa made a sympathetic face and said '*Let's see if we can take your mind off it*'; he replied breezily, '*OK. Are we going for 90?*'

His five words were *beak, peck, neck, pick,* and *sick.* Melissa praised correct production (e.g., '*Love your [k] at the end of neck*'; '*Wow your throaty [k] at the end of pick sounded great!*') and instructional feedback for errors (e.g., '*Have another try. Beak needs your throaty* [touching her neck with thumb and fingers in a "U" shape]. *Watch and listen,* beak *say* beak', '*Uh-oh. Listening? Watching? Beak*'). Aiming for at least 90% accuracy in 50 or more trials, Casey said the five words correctly in 2 × 70 trials.

Step 3: Production via independent naming (introduced in Session 4)

Casey progressed to producing the same pictured words: *beak, peck, neck, pick,* and *sick* without a model. Praise and instructional input (when necessary) continue, as in Step 2. The aim was for 90% or greater *independent* production, for the five final-k words, in at least 50 trials, a goal Casey achieved within the session in 2 × 65 trials.

Step 4: Production of minimal pair words (introduced in Session 5).

Step 4 of the perception-production minimal pairs approach is the same as Step 3 of the meaningful minimal pairs approach. In it, Casey asked for either a target word (with final-k) or its pair (with final-t). He could request *beak,* or *beat, peck,* or *pet, neck,* or *net, pick,* or *pit, sick, or* sit. He accomplished the task unerringly.

Sessions 5 to 8

At the beginning of Session 5, Melissa showed Casey the 10 pictured pairs she had set aside at the outset: *pat-pack, fort-fork, rat-rack, fete-fake, dart-dark, bite-bike, light-like, bat-back, mat-mac, eight-ache.* After brief familiarization he was able to point to them, and then say them accurately.

Melissa surprised him with an award certificate and a large smiley badge before introducing Step 1 again, with /k/ vs. [t] word initially. This time however, he had 10 pairs, not five: *tea-key, tap-cap, tub-cub, tool-cool* and *tape-cape;* and *tease-keys, tail-kale, top-cop, two-coo,* and *tough-cuff.* Following the perception-production approach's guideline of working on one sound at a time, they did the four steps for initial /k/ in only three weeks, while doing structured play activities for final /k/ in phrases and short sentence in sessions six and seven.

Melissa was pleased to see that final /k/ had generalized to several final /g/ words by session seven, for example, [bɪk] for *big,* [fɹɒk] for *frog,* [ɛk] for *egg,* and [mʌk] for *mug.* She pointed it out to Jan (as progress) and suggested that she and Gough model and recast such words when they came up, for example, if Casey said [bɪk] for *big,* they would repeat the word correctly as /bɪg/ two-to-four times, conversationally, without pressing Casey repeat it.

The following week (Week 8) Casey arrived with the news that he could say his own name. He demonstrated proudly. Jan said, '*Tell Melissa what*

else you can say, Case', to which he responded, *I can say my Daddy's name: [gɒf, gɒf, gɒf, gɒf, gɒf,]!*

Beyond Session 8

Progress from then on was rapid. The velar stops generalized to conversational speech, and the velar nasal /ŋ/ normalized with two weeks of perception-production minimal pairs with *fan-fang, pin-Ping, run-rung, pin-ping, thin-thing, Ron-wrong, bin-Bing,* and *gone-gong.* During those two weeks Melissa noticed that his epenthesis had resolved without intervention, and without anyone, including the SLP, even noticing. His sessions complete, he (rather sadly) said goodbye to Melissa with a promise to visit in three months' time. At his follow-up assessment, his speech was age typical.

Auditory Input

Several intervention approaches include the delivery of intense auditory input as key components. The rationale is the same for each, but the way input is provided to children differs somewhat. The approaches are: CPPA with amplified auditory stimulation and focused auditory stimulation (Prezas, Magnus, & Hodson, A5); PACT with listening lists and alliterative input delivered without amplification (Bowen, 2010); and Auditory Input Therapy (Flynn & Lancaster, 1996; Lancaster et al., 2010; Lancaster & Pope, 1989) described in Chapter 5. Finally, there is Naturalistic Recast Intervention (Camarata, 2021) which is also described in Chapter 5. In Camarata's intervention, multiple exemplars of target words are delivered as 'broad target recasts' to facilitate both increased sentence length and speech intelligibility.

Amplified Auditory Stimulation in CPPA[1]

Hodson and Paden (1983) incorporated amplified 'auditory bombardment' (AB), at the beginning and end of intervention sessions using the *Cycles Phonological Remediation Approach* (Prezas & Hodson, 2010). 'Cycles' has more recently become known as the *Cycles Phonological Patterns Approach (CPPA)* (Prezas, Magnus, & Hodson, A5). Children listen, through headphones, to the clinician reading

20 slightly amplified words representing the week's target pattern. From the session described in Hodson and Paden (1991, pp. 107–109) AB is but one important component, and '*it is stressed that each intervention session is devoted to production-practice* [within] *motivational activities...The child must produce the target pattern appropriately before they can take a turn*' (Hodson, personal correspondence, 2013).

In the current Cycles protocol, the small auditory input component involves children listening to the 15–20 amplified words, spoken by an adult, for <30 seconds, at the beginning and end of each session, and once daily at home with no amplification. Professor Hodson now prefers the terms 'amplified auditory stimulation' and 'focused auditory input' over 'auditory bombardment (AB)' because of criticisms from some caregivers and audiologists that the word 'bombardment' suggests that the procedure might damage the ears (it does not!). The term 'focused auditory stimulation' only relates to a technique used for one cycle, in intervention with toddlers (see below).

Hodson and Paden (1983) proposed that AB helped develop 'auditory images', that helped the child learn to monitor incorrect productions, while production practice helped them to develop accurate kinaesthetic images, which also assisted in error monitoring. Commenting on their proposal, Ingram (1989), citing Pye et al. (1987) posited that a promising explanation for the apparent usefulness of AB might lie in preliminary data from cross-linguistic phonetic acquisition studies of phonological acquisition. The 1987 study by Pye et al. suggested that the acquisition of first sounds is influenced more by their linguistic prominence than by their assumed articulatory difficulty. For instance, /v/ is acquired early by monolingual French-speaking and late by monolingual English-speaking children. The incidence of /v/ in French is higher than in English. Accordingly, Ingram (1989) suggested that AB might aid phonological change by increasing the frequency, in input, of some targets.

Focused Auditory Stimulation for Toddlers

Professor Hodson describes a second procedure, focused auditory stimulation (also known as focused auditory input). It is for very young children who are unwilling or unable to do regular production practice activities when SLPs/SLTs first see them. In this case *no* production is requested. The clinician designs the environment to offer many opportunities for the child to hear the target sound or pattern. The clinician essentially does language stimulation activities (following child's lead, talking about what the child is doing, etc.) so that the child is exposed to many examples of the target. Focused auditory input is only used for one cycle.

Auditory Input in Parents and Children Together (PACT)

In PACT intervention (Bowen & Cupples, 1999), described in Chapter 5, a variation of Hodson and Paden's (1983) 'original' AB is a constituent of the Multiple Exemplar Training component. Hodson and Paden used headphones *and* amplified AB, but in PACT neither is employed. Auditory input, or AB, without amplification, is used in PACT on the basis that phonological progress is sensitive to phonological input (Ingram, 1989). In practice AB, and the minimal pair games listed in Chapter 5, overlap. AB in the context of PACT sees the child:

- Listening to words with common phonetic features (e.g., all starting with /ʃ/).
- Listening to minimally, or near-minimally contrasted words that exemplify a phonological process (e.g., minimal pairs *ship–sip, shell–sell*, etc., for palatal fronting; near minimal pairs *two–toot, tie–tight*, etc., for final consonant deletion; near minimal pairs *nip–snip, nail – snail*, etc., for cluster reduction).
- Hearing alliterative input within games and stories (Bowen & Rippon, 2013).
- Engaging in Auditory Input Therapy (Lancaster & Pope, 1989), naturalistic intervention (Camarata, 2010), which has been rebadged Naturalistic Recast Intervention (Camarata, 2021).

Auditory Input Therapy (AIT)

Not to be confused with auditory integration training (also abbreviated AIT) (ASHA, 2004), Auditory Input Therapy (Flynn & Lancaster, 1996; Lancaster

& Pope, 1989) has the advantage of being suitable for younger children and children with cognitive and/or behavioural challenges, *and* it encourages the active participation of their caregivers (Lancaster, 1991). Camarata (2010) and co-workers use the term 'Naturalistic Intervention' to refer to similar 'whole word' procedures to improve the overall intelligibility and sentence length of children with severe SSD, including children with Down syndrome, children with autism and children who stutter. The essence of both AIT and naturalistic intervention is in devising attractive activities, called 'thematic play' in some literature, in which the client is exposed to multiple 'repetitions' of sound or word targets, spoken by the adult, with no requirement for them to practice saying sounds or words. AIT incorporates Conventional Minimal Pair therapy and metalinguistic activities.

Feature Contrasts in English

Phonemes are not 'contrastive' but their features are. Featural distinctions serve to create 'opposition' between phonemes. The non-major class distinctions are in *place*: differentiating labial, coronal, and dorsal consonants; *manner*: differentiating stops, fricatives, affricates, nasals, liquids, glides; and voice: differentiating the voiced–voiceless cognate pairs, /p b, t d, k g, f v, s z, ʃ ʒ, tʃ dʒ, θ ð/. Major class features distinguish between the main groupings of sounds in a language, namely, consonants versus vowels, glides versus consonants and obstruents (stops, fricatives, affricates) versus sonorants (nasals, liquids, glides, vowels).

Bake vs. Make, Make vs. Wake, and Silly vs. Billy

The minimal pair *bake–make* illustrates a major class distinction between obstruents and sonorants; *make–wake* illustrates the major class distinction between consonants and glides. In the minimal pair *silly* versus *Billy*, the contrast is not *quite* maximal, but it is 'maximal enough' to be highly salient for a child receiving intervention. In *silly* versus *Billy* is labial /b/ versus coronal /s/, stop /b/ versus fricative /s/ and voiced /b/ versus voiceless /s/. It cuts across

many featural dimensions, but as /s/ and /b/ are both obstruents there is no obstruent versus sonorant opposition (i.e., no major class feature distinction).

Highly Salient Non-homonymous Contrasts

Maximal Oppositions (Gierut, 1990) and a variation of it, treatment of the Empty Set (Gierut, 1992) are minimal pair intervention approaches built on the principles of language learnability, perceptual saliency, and complexity. Their originators and main proponents are Judith Gierut and colleagues from the University of Indiana.

The same implementation procedures are used for Maximal Oppositions and Empty Set. The difference between them resides in whether one new target sound is paired, in a non-homonymous contrast, with a sound the child 'knows' (can say), or whether two new 'unknown' sounds are paired, in a non-homonymous contrast. In other words, a Maximal Opposition sees an unknown and a known sound paired, and an Empty Set sees two unknown sounds paired. Whatever the pairing, known-unknown or unknown-unknown, there is a maximal feature distinction between the sounds, so that they are highly perceptually salient (different) from each other.

Minimal Pair Approaches: Maximal Oppositions

Maximal Oppositions (Gierut, 1989, 1992) is not based on homophony. Rather, the premise is that heightened *saliency* of contrasts increases *learnability*, thereby facilitating phonemic change. The word pairs are *minimal pairs* with one sound change, but the feature contrasts are *maximal* or *near-maximal* (as in *silly* vs. *Billy* exampled above). Gierut applies feature geometry to create contrastive pairs that are high and low on the feature tree called *nonproportional pairs*. Because non-proportional pairs share few features in common with other minimal pairs, they are highly perceptually salient, and, according to Gierut's findings, more learnable. In Maximal Oppositions and Empty Set, the clinician aims to present a target and contrasting word that differ by many features: in place, manner, and voice; and major class. The contrasting sound in Maximal Oppositions is (1) independent of the target, (2) produced correctly by the child and (3) maximally distinct. In Empty Set the child produces both sounds incorrectly and the two are maximally distinct.

As in the Conventional Minimal Pairs approach, only one contrast is presented at a time. For example, Xing-Fu, 4;5 was a monolingual Australian English speaker with a severe SSD. He replaced /k/ with [t] in all contexts, whereas /n/ was one of only eight consonants he produced correctly in all obligatory contexts. So, /k/ was unknown, and /n/ was known. The voiced, velar nasal /n/ differs from the voiceless, alveolar stop /k/ in place, manner, voice, major class (and markedness, for that matter), so when it came to contrasting a sound that he knew with a sound he needed to learn, /n/ vs. /k/ was one obvious choice within the Maximal Oppositions paradigm.

Gierut advocated the use of eight '*novel word*' pairs in a treatment set. In the literature, novel words are also called *non-words*, *nonce words*, and *nonsense words*. Xing-Fu's clinician had seen the video demonstrations of *modified* versions of Gierut's interventions, using real words, in the SCIP Software (Williams, 2006a, 2016) but had not read Gierut's original work in detail. Accordingly, the maximally opposed minimal pairs used in Xing-Fu's therapy included five real-word pairs: *key–knee, cat–gnat, coat–note, cow–now*, and *cot–knot*.

Had his therapist followed Gierut's suggestion, a novel word pair set might have been: /kif-nif, kæs-næs, koub-noub, kɒm-nɒm, kɜʃ-nɜʃ, kɛz-nɛz, kag-nag, kʊt-nʊt/. The novel words are assigned lexical meanings – the names of actions, objects, or characters (Gierut, 2008) – and children are familiarized with them through stories. The child receives intervention in two phases: imitation, then spontaneous production.

Phase 1 Imitation

The child is prompted to repeat the SLP's/SLT's spoken model of each of the words. Positive verbal feedback, on a continuous schedule, greets each correct response, and incorrect responses are met with cues. These cues might be for the therapist to repeat the model, to provide instructional cues about

place, manner, or voicing; tactile cues, manual positioning of the child's articulators, successive approximations (shaping), metaphoric cues, and orthographic cues (written sounds or words), in any combination as needed. Phase 1 continues until the child achieves 75% production accuracy, in the imitative condition, over two consecutive sessions, or until completion of the child's seventh session (Gierut, 1992).

Phase 2 Spontaneous Production

The child is encouraged to produce the novel words with no model. Phase 2 continues until the child has 90% production accuracy over three consecutive sessions, or until 12 sessions have occurred (Gierut, 2008). In Phase 2, verbal praise is provided by the SLP/SLT, intermittently (not continuously as in Phase 1).

For both phases, Gierut (1992) suggests activities such as sorting and matching word pairs, storytelling, and 'disambiguation of word pairs' (p. 1053). To achieve a high response rate of approximately 100 trials per session, Gierut (1999) suggests using drill-play (Shriberg & Kwiatkowski, 1982) to support attention and motivation and to keep the child interested. Production practice homework is encouraged with parents helping their child work though personalized homework sheets, and complete specially selected colouring-in pictures. Also at home, between sessions the child listens to audio recordings of the target words.

With Phase 2 complete, the SLP/SLT evaluates the child's performance on a phonological generalization probe of the targeted sound(s) in untreated words. Ideally, a child would achieve about 70% conversational accuracy before intervention on that target ceased and work on a new target started, or before ending intervention. The 70% criterion is a guide drawn from Tyler (1995), Tyler et al. (1993), and Williams (1991). The SLP/SLT would also consistently probe other implicationally related phonemes (see below) that might also have improved in response to the intervention.

Implicational Relationship

The concept of implicational relationships in phonology dictates that the presence of a **marked** feature in a phonological system implies the necessary presence of its **unmarked** counterpart, and that the relationship is unidirectional (from marked to unmarked). **Marked features** are the features of phonological systems that are

- phonetically more complex,
- universally less common across the languages of the world, and
- later developing in typical acquisition.

The following list of implicational relationships is adapted from Gierut (2001, 2007); and Gierut and Hulse (2010).

- Consonants imply vowels (e.g., Robb et al., 1999)
- Fricatives imply stops (plosives) (e.g., Elbert et al., 1984)
- Voiced obstruents imply voiceless obstruents (e.g., McReynolds & Jetzke, 1986)
- Liquids imply nasals (e.g., Gierut et al., 1994)
- Velars imply coronals (e.g., Bernhardt & Stoel-Gammon, 1996)
- Affricates imply fricatives (e.g., Schmidt & Meyers, 1995)
- Clusters imply singletons (e.g., Gierut & O'Connor, 2002)
- True clusters with small sonority difference scores imply true clusters with large sonority difference scores (e.g., Gierut, 1999) where 'true clusters' exclude the adjuncts /st, sp/, and /sk/

The Maximal Oppositions approach is reported to be suitable for children aged three to eight years, like Xing-Fu with severe phonological impairment, as is Empty Set. Note, however, that despite their longevity over more than three decades, any supporting evidence remains preliminary or emerging. For Multiple Oppositions there is a between-group study (Mota et al., 2007), four single-case experimental studies (Gierut, 1989, 1992; Topbaş & Ünal, 2010), and case studies (Donicht et al., 2011; Mota et al., 2005). Studies of Empty Set include a between-groups study (Pagliarin et al., 2009), three single-case experimental studies (Gierut, 1991, 1992; Gierut & Neumann, 1992), and case studies (Mota et al., 2005). As well, *modified versions* of maximal oppositions intervention were positively reported by Dodd et al. (2008) and Williams (1993). Intervention delivery, duration, and target selection differed between these two, and from the original,

so making meaningful comparisons is problematic. Nevertheless, it is noteworthy that Dodd et al. (2008) found no between group difference in children receiving conventional minimal pairs intervention and those receiving modified maximal oppositions.

Minimal Pair Approaches: Empty Set (Unknown Set)

Empty Set (Gierut, 1992) is a variation of Maximal Oppositions that also uses non-proportional pairs and does not rely on homophony motivating phonemic change. Again, the principle is that enhanced perceptual saliency of contrasts improves learnability, facilitating phonological restructuring. In it, two targets are addressed concurrently. An *error* the child has (the first target) is contrasted with *another* erred sound (the second target), and the two targets are maximally distinct.

Probably the better name for this is 'Unknown Set' as it signals that the child does not 'know' either of the sounds and therefore must learn two *new* sounds. So, error is contrasted with error – but not *any* error pair! For example, my colleague's client Vaughan, 5;8 was from a monolingual South African English background, and was a recent migrant, with his family, to Australia. He had a severe SSD, and a PCC of 41%. Vaughan replaced /f/ with [b] (stopping) and /ɹ/ with [w] (gliding), and both /f/ and /ɹ/ were absent from his repertoire. Recognizing the severity of his impairment, and wanting to use the Unknown Set approach, his SLP needed to find a contrasting sound for his minimal-pair–maximally-opposed treatment set that was maximally distinct from /f/, remembering that the sound had not only to be maximally distinct but also *absent* from Vaughan's repertoire (representing least phonological knowledge: see Table 9.4). His non-stimulable /ɹ/ was a perfect choice. His clinician, also influenced by the Williams (2006a) videos, and not Gierut's publications, elected to use real words. Accordingly, Vaughan's (non-proportional and maximally contrasting) minimal word pairs set included *rind–find*, *reel–feel*, *red–fed*, and *rocks–fox*, which he produced at the outset of therapy as: [waɪnd-baɪnd, wil-bil, wɛd-bɛd, wɒks-bɒks]. As it happened, Vaughan's error productions were also maximally distinct (non-proportional), but not homonymous. Had the SLP followed Gierut's advice, a suitable eight-pair novel word (non-word) treatment set might have been: /ɹaɪk-faɪk, ɹun-fun, ɹɛs-fɛs, ɹɪv-fɪv, ɹɔb-fɔb, ɹaud-faud, ɹʌp-fʌp/, and /ɹig-fig/.

The schedule (Phase 1 and Phase 2) and procedures used in Empty Set are the same as for Maximal Oppositions, and may include phonemic place and manner cues, suggestions and 'instructions' to the child, and metaphors.

Drawing on the results of several experiments, Gierut (1992) determined that therapy was most effective, with the greatest generalization, if two new maximally opposed phonemes representing a major class feature difference were targeted, as in Vaughan's case using Empty Set. By contrast, targeting one new maximally opposed phoneme representing a non-major class distinction was effective, but less effective than the preceding option. Between these two were two further equally effective Maximal Opposition alternatives. The first was to target two new maximally opposed phonemes representing a nonmajor class distinction; and the second was to target one new maximally opposed phoneme representing a major class feature difference.

Minimal Pair Approaches: Multiple Oppositions

The use of larger treatment sets in multiple oppositions may lead to several new phonemic contrasts being added to a child's system. Thus, multiple oppositions has a potential advantage over singular contrastive models of phonological intervention in terms of shortened length of treatment, improved intelligibility, and more efficient intervention.

Williams, 2000a

Unlike the Conventional Minimal Pairs approach, in Multiple Oppositions Therapy it is not assumed that minimal or maximal *feature* contrasts will be formed. This is because the child's phoneme collapses (homonymous productions), with several targets realized the same way, determine which

contrastive oppositions will be used. In an intervention session, several targets are presented to the child, all contrasting with the error-sound the child produces as a substitute. For example, if a child collapsed the voiceless velar stop /k/, the voiceless affricate /tʃ/, the voiceless alveolar fricative /s/, and the consonant cluster /tɹ/to [t] so that *cap*, *chap*, *sap*, and *trap* were all realized homophonously as [tæp], the treatment sets (in the first two columns below), and a corresponding untreated set to use as a generalization probe (shown in the third column), might look like this:

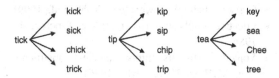

Any non-words would be made meaningful by using it as the name for a person, pet, or fantasy creature or object, so you might have a picture of a character called *Chee* included in the probe set I column 3 above, as shown in Figure 4.1.

Multiple Oppositions

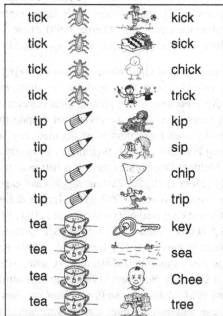

Figure 4.1   Multiple Opposition word pairs. Drawings by Helen Rippon, Speech and Language Therapist, www.blacksheeppress.co.uk.

Two further examples of 'phoneme collapses', the term Williams uses to denote the simplified one-to-many correspondence between the child's error production and targets, are: *lick, wick, rick,* and *flick* realized as [jɪk]; and *beat, been, beak,* and *beach* all produced as a CV [bi]. The collapse to /jɪk/ is not amenable to description in terms of phonological processes or phonological patterns, although it *could* be termed a systematic sound preference for /j/, while the collapse to [bi] *could* be described as deletion of coda or final consonant deletion.

In the Multiple Oppositions approach, it is neither assumed, nor important in target selection, that either minimal or maximal feature contrasts will be formed. The characteristics of the sounds are immaterial – it is irrelevant whether they are early, or later developing, stimulable or non-stimulable, known, or unknown, most deleterious to intelligibility; socially important to the child or family; marked, or unmarked. This is because the contrasts are based on a child's errors relative to adult targets. As well, the Multiple Oppositions paradigm is not based on the idea that a child's developing sound system can be adequately described in phonological processes (phonological patterns) terms, which Williams says fragments description of the child's sound system into pre-determined categories, using sound-to-sound comparisons.

The phoneme collapse perspective allows clinicians to describe a child's phonological organization more broadly than the phonological processes approach permits. Using it provides an account of the child's unique phonology that is both *child-based* and *systemic*. In practice, a phoneme collapse is considered as one rule, rather than several separate phonological processes (phonological rules). Accordingly, Multiple Oppositions intervention is distinct from other minimal pair approaches in (1) having *more targets in training*, and (2) the way the *targets relate to each other as components of one rule set*. In essence, Multiple Oppositions represents a paradigm shift to view SSD from a *systemic* standpoint as opposed to an *error* standpoint. Up to four treatment targets are selected from one rule set (phoneme collapse). They are chosen relative to the child's system rather than the characteristics of the sounds.

Using the *distance metric* in target selection, sounds are chosen from across the phoneme collapse that represent different *manners* and *places* of articulation, different *voicing* characteristics, and different *phonetic sequences* (i.e., whether they are singletons or clusters). Thus, there is phonetic distance across the targets that reflects the learning the child must achieve. With targets that have utmost phonetic distance from each other, and represent the different parameters in the rule set, the frame of learning the child must achieve is expanded.

To treat multiple targets concurrently across a child's rule set, they are contrasted one at a time with the child's customary substitute, making the multiple oppositions word sets. The activities used are the same as for Conventional Minimal Pairs (see Boxes 4.1 and 4.2) and intervention is in four phases (Williams, 2000b).

Phase 1: Familiarization + Production.
Phase 2: Contrasts + Naturalistic Play: This begins with imitative production moving to spontaneous production by the child when the first training criterion of 70% accuracy is achieved.
Phase 3: Contrasts within Communicative Contexts.
Phase 4: Conversational Recasts.

Regarding production accuracy in connected speech, Williams uses a structured and systematic treatment paradigm to program for generalization in all phases of intervention. She aims for high response rate per treatment session (about 60–80 trials in a 30-minute session). In the early phases, she begins a session with focused production practice of the contrasts and ends it with a conversation-based naturalistic activity. She believes that the conversation-based activity provides a bridge to the focused practice and allows children to hear and practice their sound(s) in a more naturalistic activity (in Phase 2). These brief naturalistic activities include sound-loaded conversational activities (cf., Bowen, 2010; Camarata, 2010, 2021; Prezas et al., A5) in which the child hears, and has opportunities to produce, a large proportional frequency of their target sounds. The approach is geared to children with severe phonological disorders and those at the more severe end of the moderate range.

Sound Contrasts in Phonology: SCIP

From the 1970s, clinically useful developments arose from Generative and Natural Phonology as Linguists focused, for the first time, on the plight of children with speech impairment. Their significant work held recognizable clinical potential (see Grunwell's guidelines in Chapter 5) but moulding it into ecologically valid treatment that was practical, efficient, effective, and acceptable to practitioners and clients was difficult. It needed adequately funded, time consuming research effort from the SLP/SLT side, but this was in a milieu of often overstretched services with most clinicians only dimly aware of how the new knowledge from linguistics could inform practice. Lynn Williams, who had developed, and demonstrated the efficacy of Multiple Oppositions intervention, knew that it is likely for important clinical research to be published widely in the peer-reviewed literature (which it has) while remaining almost undiscovered by most clinicians. She acted creatively, and innovatively for 2006, by delivering her own and *other* evidenced phonological treatments (Conventional Minimal Pairs, Maximal Oppositions, and Empty Set) to the world's workplace in the form of computer software. The first iteration of the *Sound Contrasts in Phonology (SCIP)* assessment and intervention software was on disc (Williams, 2006a) and was eventually succeeded by an iPad App (Williams, 2016).

Implementing Multiple Oppositions using *SCIP* is not simply a question of client plus clinician plus app with a dash of homework! Whether it is done with the aid of the app or not, effective intervention rests on understanding the organization of the child's sound system relative to the adult, or ambient, sound system, and this requires meticulous assessment. Although Williams used a (lengthy) 245-item protocol for her clinical research, a clinician can base the analysis on a standardized test,

such as the *GFTA*-3 or the *DEAP*, completing the analysis faster. Detailed assessment allows the clinician to map the child's sound system onto the adult system determining the extent to which the child's system aligns with the adult system and what remains for the child to learn. By applying a systemic assessment, the SLP/SLT can establish a treatment plan, with highly specified goals, aimed at expeditious restructuring of the child's disordered system so that it matches age-expectations.

Dr. Lynn Williams is Associate Dean in the College of Clinical & Rehabilitative Health Sciences and Professor in the Department of Audiology and Speech-Language Pathology at East Tennessee State University (ETSU) in Johnson City, Tennessee, United States. She was the 2021 President, is a Fellow of the American Speech-Language-Hearing Association (ASHA), and she has served as an Associate Editor of *Language Speech and Hearing Services in the Schools* (2004–2007) and *American Journal of Speech-Language Pathology* (2009–2017). Lynn is the author of *Speech Disorders Resource Guide for Preschool Children* (Williams, 2003), co-editor of *Interventions for Speech Sound Disorders in Children* 2nd ed. (Williams et al., 2021), and she has published and presented extensively, nationally, and internationally, on her research with children who have speech sound disorders. Lynn has received several grants from the National Institutes of Health in support of her translational research, resulting in the development of *Sound Contrasts in Phonology (SCIP)* (Williams, 2006a, 2016). Embedded in *SCIP* is her own approach to speech therapy, *Multiple Oppositions*.

Q19. A. Lynn Williams: The Multiple Oppositions Approach

The *SCIP* app includes clinical training videos that show, with helpful commentaries, snippets of four contrastive therapies in action, namely: Conventional Minimal Pairs, Multiple Oppositions, Maximal Oppositions, and 'Empty' or Unknown Set. What assessment process is typical for a suitable candidate for Multiple Oppositions therapy? And in terms of the intervention itself, can you give us a case example that demonstrates the aspects of the therapy not shown in the available videos (Williams, 2016; Williams et al., 2021)? For example, how long are the treatment sessions, how frequent are they, are families involved in sessions or in homework, what procedures and activities are incorporated, and at what stages of the child's progress are they introduced?

A19.   Lynn Williams: A Systemic Approach to Phonological Re-Organization: Multiple Oppositions

Nature of the Assessment

To implement the systemic treatment approach of multiple oppositions, it is important to describe the child's speech disorder *systemically*. A systemic approach is a *system-based* approach in which the SLP/SLT compares the child's system to the adult system by mapping the two sound systems to each other using phoneme collapses. For example, a child might produce [t] for several sounds (e.g., /s ʃ k tʃ st/) that occur in the adult, or target system. This is viewed as one rule involving a phoneme collapse of voiceless obstruents and cluster (adult system) to the voiceless obstruent, [t] (child system).

This broader system-to-system comparison provides a more holistic description of the child's speech than is possible with a sound-based approach that utilizes a narrower sound-to-sound comparison of the child's production relative to an adult target. Using this example, a sound-to-sound comparison using phonological (processes) patterns would describe the phoneme collapse as four separate and independent error patterns (i.e., stopping, fronting, deaffrication, and cluster reduction).

Additionally, a systemic analysis is *child-based* rather than adult-based, as is common in many traditional assessment approaches that are founded on a pre-determined and finite number of rules (or processes/patterns) to describe the child's error patterns. Consequently, the broader system-to-system comparison and child-based aspects of a systemic analysis allow the clinician to: 1) describe idiosyncratic errors that are common in unintelligible speech, and 2) gain insight into the organizational structure the child has developed to compensate for a smaller sound system relative to the adult sound system. As Grunwell (1997) stated, we can discover the 'order in the disorder'.

Implementing the Assessment

To execute a systemic description of a child's speech, I complete the *Systemic Phonological Analysis of Child Speech (SPACS)* that provides information on the child's phonetic inventory (Word Initial and Word Final), distribution of English consonants relative to the ambient sound system, and mapping of child-to-adult sound systems using phoneme collapses. For a more detailed description of the *SPACS* approach, readers can refer to Williams (2001, 2003, 2006b, 2010, 2019; Williams & Sugden, 2021).

In my clinical research, I use a 245-item single-word elicitation probe (*Systemic Phonological Protocol*, Williams, 2003) and a 15–20-minute conversational sample. Clinically, however, this sample is likely to be too time consuming for SLPs/SLTs who have large caseloads and severe time constraints. Clinicians can complete a *SPACS* on smaller databases, such as the *Goldman-Fristoe Test of Articulation-2 (GFTA-3;* Goldman & Fristoe, 2015), or other sound inventory tests, that are commonly used. Phoneme collapses can be constructed *by initial and final word position* by mapping the adult sound targets that are replaced by the error production in the child's system. Using the *GFTA-3*, the clinician can look down the word-initial column on the response matrix to diagram phoneme collapses of frequently occurring error productions.

Case Study

Adam aged 4;6 produced [g] for adult targets /b, d, f, v, ð, s, z, ʃ, tʃ, dʒ, dɹ, fɹ, gl, gɹ, kw, st, tɹ/ in word-initial position on the *GFTA-2*. This represents a 1:17 (1-to-17) phoneme collapse between Adam's sound system and the adult sound system. A closer examination of the adult targets revealed that they were obstruents and clusters. Thus, Adam collapsed obstruents and clusters to the obstruent [g].

This *SPACS* was completed easily and quickly, and it represented Adam's logical and systemic organization more clearly than if a phonological process/pattern analysis were completed on his *GFTA-2* responses.

Applying the Distance Metric to Treatment Target Selection

After the child's system has been described, a systemic approach called the *distance metric* (Williams, 2005, 2017) is used to select up to 4 targets from one phoneme collapse or rule set. With this approach, target sounds are selected based on phonetic distance between the child's error and the target sounds (maximal distinction) and across the selected targets (maximal classification). By increasing the phonetic distance along these two parameters (distinction and classification) clinicians achieve two objectives. First, they increase the saliency of the sound(s) to be learned, and second, they increase the frame of learning that the child must achieve.

Returning to Adam, four targets were selected from the 1:17 phoneme collapse to [g]; namely, /d, f, tʃ, st/. In this way, targets are selected based on each individual child's unique sound system and not on the characteristics of the sounds themselves, such as developmental norms, stimulability, or consistency of knowledge. The distance metric assumes the importance of the target sound's *function* in a child's system is greater than the characteristics of an individual sound. It also reflects Adam's need to learn more than a single aspect of sound production, such as manner, or place, or voicing.

Streamlined Intervention

Aligned with the systemic analysis and target selection, a systemic intervention approach using multiple oppositions is implemented to facilitate phonological restructuring with the greatest amount of change occurring in the least amount of time. I structure intervention using a treatment paradigm described in detail elsewhere (Williams, 2000b, 2003, 2005, 2010; Williams & Sugden, 2021). There are four phases: All are data-based except for Phase 1, which is time-based. Basically, **Phase 1** involves Familiarization (of the rule, the sounds, and the vocabulary) + Production of the contrasts. This initial phase creates a meaningful context that lays a foundation for the feedback and work that will be carried out in the following treatment phases. **Phase 2** encompasses focused practice of the contrasts at an imitative level with a dense response rate (about 60–80 responses in a 30-minute individual session or 20–40 responses in a 30-minute small group session).

Although the Multiple Oppositions paradigm has larger treatment sets of target sounds, the contrasts are practiced one at a time. For example, *tip-sip; tip-ship; tip-Kip; tip-trip*. The focused practice is followed by a short (5 minute) naturalistic play activity. These are brief, sound-loaded activities that bridge the focused practice that occurs on a narrow training set with the communicative use of the contrast within meaningful play activities. An example might be *I Spy* using objects or pictures of items that have the target sound in untrained words. The clinician and child take turns giving hints for the other to guess the item. I typically use the naturalistic activity for one sound per session and generally choose the sound with which the child is having greatest difficulty. The focused practice continues at an imitative level until the child achieves training criterion (70% accuracy across two consecutive treatment sets where 1 treatment set = 20 responses). Once the criterion is met, **Phase 2 continues** with focused practice + naturalistic play, but at a spontaneous level of production. Intervention continues at the spontaneous level of Phase 2 until the second training criterion is met (90% accuracy across two consecutive treatment sets). At that point, treatment moves to **Phase 3**: contrasts within naturalistic communicative contexts. This treatment phase integrates the focused practice and play so that the child plays games with the contrasts (such as, *Go Fish*). Although most children achieve the generalization criterion (50% accuracy in conversational speech) in Phase 3, some children need additional intervention at a conversational level to attain generalization (see Williams, 2000b for longitudinal data from an intervention study with 10 children). For those children who are doing well in Phase 3 at a spontaneous response level in communicative contexts, but not reaching generalization, movement to Phase 4 occurs. **Phase 4** involves conversational recasts that encompass Stephen Camarata's *Naturalistic Speech Intelligibility Training* (cf., Camarata, 2010, 2021). In this phase, treatment switches from the contrasts in games to using the contrasts communicatively in conversational scenarios, such as ordering food at a restaurant that includes food items containing the target sounds. For example, for Adam with his 1:17 collapse to /g/, described above, words might include *dinner, doughnut, fish, fudge, stew,* and *steak*.

The treatment paradigm provides structure, or a blueprint, for intervention and the child's progression through the treatment phases. As noted earlier, the child is in the driver's seat, so to speak, and matriculation through the treatment phases is based on the child's performance data. The paradigm structures intervention to address two important aspects of phonological intervention: (1) the duality of sound learning: phonetic and phonemic aspects; and (2) programming for generalization. In the early phases of treatment, greater emphasis and support are placed on helping the child learn the production aspects of the new contrast (the imitative response level, plus the focused practice with dense response rates). The early phases also control for extraneous distractors, such as playing board games, for the child to achieve the focused practice and dense response rates. Yet, I program for generalization from the outset by pairing the focused practice with the bridging activities of naturalistic play involving the new contrast in sound-loaded activities. I want to quickly bring in the phonemic aspects of sound learning (moving from imitation to spontaneous with a lower training criterion level) and gradually and systematically re-introduce the distractors (playing games with the contrasts in Phase 3 or conversational recasts in Phase 4).

A summary of the treatment phases and activities is provided in Table A19.1. As you look at the treatment phases, activities, and response levels, you will notice the systematic and gradual programming for generalization, as well as the shift in intervention focus from phonetic learning to phonemic learning.

Table A19.1 Summary of treatment phases and activities in Multiple Oppositions intervention.

Treatment Phase	Intervention Focus	Response Rate	Response Level	Example of ActVowel Interventioivities	Criterion
Phase 1: Familiarization + Production EXAMPLE:	Create a meaningful context that lays a foundation for the work the child will do	1 treatment set = 20 responses (5 contrastive word pairs of 4 target sounds = 20 responses)	Imitative	Familiarization of: • Rules (long versus short [t~ s, ʃ]; front versus back [t ~ k]; buddy sounds [t ~ tɹ]) • Sound (ticking clock sound versus flat tire sound and quiet lady sound; coughing man sound; sounds that go together) • Vocabulary	First treatment session

Table A19.1 *(Continued)*

Treatment Phase	Intervention Focus	Response Rate	Response Level	Example of ActVowel Interventioivities	Criterion
Phase 2: Contrasts + Naturalistic Play	Initial focus is on the phonetic aspects of sound learning (imitative) and then moves to phonemic aspects (spontaneous)	60–80 responses (individual session); 20–40 responses (group session)	Imitative then Spontaneous	Produce contrasts [5 contrastive word pairs] with imitative model (control distractors and get high response rate); give tokens for each response regardless of accuracy – when child gets 20 tokens, s/he has completed one treatment set and s/he gets a sticker; switch order of presentation of contrasts to prevent child developing articulatory set. Naturalistic Play (e.g., *I Spy*)	70% accuracy across two consecutive treatment sets (move to Spontaneous); 90% accuracy across two consecutive treatment sets (move to Phase 3)
Phase 3: Contrasts within Communicative Contexts	Rule Learning (phonemic)	60–80 responses (20–40 responses for group session)	Spontaneous	*Go Fish*; *Concentration*; *Memory*; *Teacher*	90% accuracy across two consecutive treatment sets (if generalization criterion of 50% accuracy in conversation speech not met, move to Phase 4)
Phase 4: Conversational Recasts	Incorporate new contrast into conversational rule	60–80 responses (20–40 responses for group session)	Spontaneous	Communicative Scenarios, such as a family restaurant	50% accuracy in conversational speech

Intervention Frequency and Intensity

Regarding the intervention 'dosage' an analysis of practice trials using multiple oppositions related to treatment outcomes (Williams, 2012) revealed the following:

- A minimum dose of ≥ 50 trials for a duration of 30 sessions twice weekly is required for intervention to be effective
- Greater intensity (70 trials for about 40 sessions) is required for children with more severe SSD.
- Quantitative changes in dose occur over the course of intervention with greater intensity at the beginning that decreases by about 20% during the second half of intervention on a specific goal.
- Qualitatively, focused practice and naturalistic play activities are implemented with a 2:1 ratio throughout intervention as the bridging activities are used to program for generalization.

The Role of Families

Engaging families in the intervention process is an important component of treatment and can take many different forms from active to passive involvement. The way that I involve families reflects my philosophy that (1) learning a sound system is like learning language – it involves communication; and (2) parents are not trained therapists. Consequently, I ask parents to leave the focused practice of facilitating new sound contrasts to me as the trained professional, *and* I ask them to extend the work the child and I are doing in the clinic at home through fun, play-based, sound-loaded activities that involve models and recasts.

I interview the parent(s) to find typical routines they share with their child through the week and then I develop naturalistic activities that they can implement within those routines. I know that many families live full and hectic lives with dual careers and a heavy load of after school activities, so the naturalistic activities I send home have a greater chance of being completed (and enjoyed!) if I can ask them to do them within their normal routines. For example, at the grocery store, play a game to see who can identify the most items with the /k/ sound (*coffee, candy, cauliflower, carrots,* etc.). I teach the parents how to use set-ups, protests, models, and recasts in the activity, such as identifying *beans* so the child can say a word that doesn't have their coughing man sound; or saying *torn* for *corn* to see if the child can correct them.

I give the parents two to three activities each week, along with a questionnaire they complete about the number of times they used the activities, how well the activities worked, what questions they had, and so on. The questionnaire structures the home activities and communicates to the parents an expectation that they will carry out these activities regularly. Occasionally, I give the parents a tape recorder to take home and record an activity that we will review together. In a 2020 study by Sugden et al., parents were taught to implement multiple oppositions as part of a parent- and clinician-delivered intervention over an 8-week period. One 60-minute session per week was delivered by an SLP in a university clinic, and two sessions of modified-for-parents Multiple Oppositions intervention were delivered in the same week by a trained parent at home Measures of treatment fidelity indicated that parents can be trained to deliver multiple oppositions competently and confidently.

Minimal Pairs Intervention with Added Elements

The value, in phonological intervention, of drawing on techniques and procedures that may be more closely associated with articulation, stimulability, and perceptual therapy, when appropriate is shown in a case illustration from Isla, 5;2 (Box 4.3). Isla's intervention was primarily a meaningful minimal pair approach, with elements of speech perception training for /ɹ/ vs. /w/, followed by traditional articulation therapy for /ɹ/, /ð/ and /θ/ towards the end of her treatment sessions.

Box 4.3 Case illustration: meaningful minimal pairs, plus

Isla, 5;2

Isla aged 5;2 had a systematic sound preference for /b/ and /d/ (see Table 4.3; Weiner, 1981b). She stopped the affricates /tʃ/ and /dʒ/, and eight of the nine English fricatives, /f, v, s, z, θ, ð, ʃ/, and /ʒ/, but not /h/. Like typically developing three- and four-year-old children who tend to stop affricates and fricatives, she stopped *and* voiced the voiceless affricate /tʃ/ and the voiceless fricatives /f, s, θ/, and /ʃ/ (see Table 2.1). A rough guide to the elimination of stopping is that: stopping of /f, s/ usually disappears by 3;0, /v, z/ by 3;6, /ʃ, tʃ, dʒ/ by 4;6, and /θ, ð/ by 5;0. Interestingly, Isla used the singleton stops /p, b, t, d, k, g/ correctly (contrastively). She also reduced many clusters, but not /pj, bj, tj, dj, kj, mj, nj, and hj/ as in *pure, bugle, tune, duet, cute, mute, new,* and *Hugh* respectively; /bl, kl and gl/ as in *blue, clue,* and *glue* respectively; and /tw, dw, kw and gw/ as in *twin, dwarf, quick* and *guava* respectively. Less obviously, she exhibited weak syllable deletion inconsistently in a small selection of multisyllabic words (e.g., *Australia, computer, Samantha,* and *tomato*), and in a few frequently used word combinations (e.g., *Auntie Veronica, Mira Royal Detective,* and unsurprisingly, *Pinkalicious and Peterrific*).

Isla had extensive homonymy, due to realizing fricatives and affricates as the voiced stops with her 'favourite sounds', the voiced stops /b/ or /d/. For example she produced, systematically: *fan*, *than*, and *van* as [bæn], *sum*, and *thumb* as [dʌm], *safer* and *saver* as ['seɪbə], *do*, *Sue*, *shoe*, and *zoo* as [du], *seven* as ['dɛbən], *session* as ['dɛdən], *sushi* and *Suzie* as ['dudiː], *duffle*, *shovel*, and *shuffle* as ['dʌbl], *lead*, *leave*, *leash* and *leech* as [liːd], and *jeep*, *sheep*, and *cheap* as [diːp]. Affected clusters were reduced to singletons: as [d] in words like *swim*, *slide*, *three*, and *healthy*, and as [b] in words like *flower*, *freezer*, *fresh*, *elf*, *Kelvin*, and *solve*. She was stimulable in isolation, but not in syllables, for both affricates and all fricatives except /θ, ð/, and /ʒ/.

Deciding to address Isla's substitution process of stopping of fricatives as a treatment priority, Therese, her therapist used a meaningful minimal pairs approach (i.e., a conventional minimal pairs approach as reported by Weiner, 1981a). Therese's plan was to target fricatives as a sound class, rather than treating /f/, /v/, /s/, /z/, /ʃ/, and ʒ/ individually as articulatory targets.

Because Isla collapsed all fricatives except /h/, and many clusters, to either [d] or [b] an alternative might have been to analyse her phonology in terms of phoneme collapses (Williams, 2003) and use a multiple oppositions approach to intervention (Williams, A19).

Therese based her choice of intervention on several factors. First, in terms of phonological processes, Isla only evidenced stopping, cluster reduction with voicing of voiceless fricative clusters, and to a considerably lesser extent, weak syllable deletion. Second, she already used one fricative /h/: a hopeful sign in Therese's view. Third, she included all four stops /p, b, t, d, k, and g/ accurately in obligatory singleton contexts; and showed strong signs of consonant cluster acquisition. In Therese's opinion, looking at Isla's output in phonological pattern terms, this amounted to a small number of errors.

Taking advantage of Isla's stimulability, albeit only in isolation, for /f, v, s, z, and /ʃ/, Therese created a set of five minimal pair picture cards: *fog-bog*, *V-bee*, *sock-dock*, *zip-dip*, and *show-dough*. Dock (wharf) was the only word absent from Isla's lexicon at the outset, and familiarization with the captioned pictures was accomplished rapidly. A willing, interested little girl who received strong support for her learning at home, Isla was soon able to play, with enjoyment, a 'point to the one

I say' drill-play game with Therese and then with her mother, Julie, who observed and participated in all treatment sessions. Over eight sessions (twice weekly for four weeks), Isla engaged in drill and drill-play aimed at eliciting at least 100 production practice trials ('repeats') of words with her stimulable fricatives in onset. This involved 'best production' of the first set of pictured minimal pairs (*fog-bog*, etc.) and comparable sets of five (e.g., *fin-bin*, *van-ban*, *suck-duck*, *zoo-do*, and *ship-dip*), and pictured, captioned words representing the targets (e.g., *fog*, *V* (vee), *sock*, *zip*, *show*, *fin*, *van*, *suck*, *zoo*, *ship*) to perform:

- **Cloze tasks with short sentences,** for example, The rabbit's not skinny, it's———(*fat*); Grapes grow on a———(*vine*); Whales live in the———(*sea*); My jeans have a———(*zip*); Little Bo-Peep has lost her———(*sheep*); Mr. Whippy drives a———(*van*). When Isla stopped any of these SIWI fricatives, Therese would gently challenge her production with **homophony confrontation**, saying both target and error: for example, '*I showed you a* **fat** *bunny, but I think you said* **bat***; did you mean* **fat** *with a quiet, long sound for the* **fat** *bunny?' 'It's not* **dee***, is it? You meant to say* **sea***. Try* **sea** *again with a long snake sound?* **Sea***.' 'Did I hear* **dine** *or* **shine***? Try* **shine** *again with your lovely sh-be-quiet sound.* **Shine***.'* Maintaining a light touch, homophony confrontation was integrated consistently into the following tasks and activities too, alongside reinforcement, that included modelling the correctly produced word, when Isla produced the right fricative (e.g., '*That's right* **vine***.' 'You remembered your sh-be-quiet sound;* **shine***.'*) or any fricative (e.g., when Isla produced [ʃiː] for *sea* Therese said, '*Great, you remembered there's a quiet blowy sound in* **sea***. Put your pouty lips away and try* **sea** *with your long snake sound? Watch, teeth shut, little smile,* **sea***.'*). Similarly, when Isla produced vine as [βaɪn], with the voiced bilabial fricative /β/ replacing /v/ and reflecting her customary [b] for /v/ error, Therese praised her voicing and frication: '*Super, you did a buzzy long sound, for* **vine***, but you forgot to show us your teeth for the vacuum cleaner sound, vv…, so it came out as* [βaɪn]*. Have another go. Bite your lip like a bunny rabbit and say* **vine***'.*
- **Cloze tasks** in rebus stories made by Therese, with help from Isla and Julie.
- **Cloze tasks** in shared book reading, with a familiar story, for example, 'The———(*sun*) did

not—(*shine*), it was too wet to play, so we—(*sat*) in the house all that cold, cold wet day. I—(*sat*) there with—(*Sally*). We—(*sat*) here we two and we—(*said*) 'How we wish we had—(*something*) to do.'

- **Rhyme completion activities contrasting error and target in input**: for example, dine rhymes with———(*shine*); bat rhymes with———(*sat*); dead rhymes with———(*said*); dally rhymes with———(*Sally*); bun rhymes with———(*sun*).
- **Word-pair imitation activities**, for example, 'Say these words after me' (with and without pictures): *sun-done, shine-dine, fun-bun, vet-bet, thin-din*.
- **I spy**, for example, 'I spy with my little eye something beginning with [f...].'.
- **Confrontation naming activities**, for example, 'Tell me what's in these pictures.'
- **Reading activities**, for example, 'Read these words to me' (with, and without pictures).

Isla worked on the voiceless fricatives /f/, /s/, and /ʃ/ for four weeks, maintaining the high production rate ('session dose') of 100 trials per half hour, with all sessions comprising 30 minutes drill and drill-play, plus 10 minutes free play at the ends of sessions. Free play was Isla's preferred 'reward' and she sometimes wanted Therese and/or Julie to participate. She attended twice weekly (accumulating at least 800 productions over 8 sessions, or 240 minutes). At this time (Week 5), Therese and Jenny observed that /s/ and /ʃ/ were generalizing spontaneously to the SIWW, SFWF, and SFWW positions, and in many SIWI contexts (remembering that SIWI had been addressed in intervention).

As Therese anticipated, in a probe comprising 10-minute client-clinician conversation, Isla's single-word accuracy met the 70% accuracy rubric, operationalized by Baker and McLeod (2004) that signalled generalization of a therapy target. Therese watched, waited, and encouraged Isla while her production accuracy of /s/ and /ʃ/ across word positions in conversation crept up over ensuing weeks.

Although Isla displayed better than 90% single word accuracy without a model for /f/ SIWI after 5 weeks of intervention, generalization to conversation was only evident in words that were 'special' to her: *Fozzie*, the family dog, *Aoife* /ˈiːˌfə/ her best friend, *five* [faɪb] her age, and *farm*, *farmer*, *foal*, and *filly* because her grandparents were farmers and they had a new filly.

Production practice of minimal pairs beyond a single-word level. In the first of two sessions in Week 6, Therese introduced production trials of /f/ vs. /b/ SIWI in phrases and sentences, with high levels of homophony confrontation, at the same dose rate per session. Isla caught on quickly and 'graduated' to producing contrasting, semantically congruent sentences for /f/ vs. /b/ (e.g., *Don't bite me kittycat.* vs. *Don't fight me kittycat. The dog saw the bone.* vs. *The dog saw the phone.*) SIWI in the following session. By now, Therese was confident that /θ, ð, and ʒ/ could be added to Isla's phonetic repertoire easily, thinking that they might even emerge spontaneously.

/f/ vs. /b/ sentences

She moved on to a sentence imitation task with incongruent vs. congruent, /b/ vs. /f/ minimal pair sentences, for example, Dad put his *bone/phone* in his pocket; Beauty and the Prince ate the delicious *Beast/feast* (Isla laughed every time this came up); and We crossed the harbour by *berry/ferry*. Alternatively, Isla, Julie and Therese joined in structured-play such as a picture lotto game (played like bingo with pictures instead of numbers) taking turns requesting pictures on cards to superimpose on identical pictures on a board until the board was covered: I need *filly/billy*, give me the *fox/box*, I want the *ferry/berry*, hand me the *phone/bone*, may I have the *foal/bowl*, I need the *fin/bin*, let me have the *farm/balm*. Therese would take Isla's requests literally, and give her, for example, the bone even when she knew Isla needed the phone. Isla would have one chance to revise her production without a model, and if successful could put the card in its spot on the board. *Farm, filly*, and *foal* were included to ensure success for Isla. When Therese made a 'mistake' it would often be billy for *filly*, bowl for *foal*, or balm for *farm*. Once Isla was achieving close to 100% success with the meaningful sentence contrasts she moved on to 'good sentences' vs. 'silly sentences', for example, when she attempted 'When we leave him behind, Fozzie makes a fuss' and said 'bus' for 'fuss' Therese or Julie would feign confusion or give her an enquiring look. If neither prompt elicited a revised production, they would say something like, 'Bus?' or 'Fozzie makes a bus? I think you mean "fuss"' and ask her to try again: 'Can you say that again? Bite your lip and blow for [f]. "Fozzie makes a fuss"'.

By Week 8 Isla was achieving over 70% accuracy conversationally with /f/ SIWI without a model, while /f/ emerging within words and word-finally.

Isla started the second session of Week 9 by announcing 'I can say treasure'. She could, with a perfect [tɹ] and [ʒ]. Julie explained that Aoife had stayed for a sleepover and she and Isla had been to a Saturday pirate-themed birthday party together and spent the rest of the weekend devising treasure hunts. When the weather deteriorated on the Sunday afternoon the girls came inside to find that Julie had made picture cards for *treasure, television, tape measure, Persian cat, Eurovision*, and *explosion* in readiness for a game of 'Speech Therapy'! When the girls tired of taking turns being the SLP/SLT and the client, Julie produced treasure chest colouring pages, downloaded from the internet.

Delighted with Isla's response to the treatment program, and Julie's part in it, in Week 12 Therese reassessed her phonology to find an improvement in overall intelligibility and clinically significant change and generalization across the child's speech sound system. In terms of her fricatives, Isla now rarely misarticulated /f, v, s, z, ʃ, or ʒ/. Her /θ and ð/ were no longer subject to stopping, but rather Fricative Simplification: /θ/→[f] and /ð/→[v] in the correct sound class. She was stimulable in VCs for /tʃ/ and /dʒ/ and replacing them with [ʃ] and [ʒ] respectively, rather than /b/ and /d/. The adjuncts /st, sp, and sk/ were now evident, as were the clusters /kw, tw, dw, sm, sn/. She simplified the liquid clusters: e.g., brave→[bweɪv], drum→[dwʌm], claws→[kwɔz], slow→[swou], and was using singleton /l/ consistently in conversation. The /ɹ/, /ð/, /θ/ remained non-stimulable. Weak Syllable Deletion occurred rarely, and she could even say *Pinkalicious and Peterrific*. When she produced an error Isla usually noticed, and self-corrected readily.

Isla and her family were away for the summer school holiday. Isla contracted bacterial pneumonia soon after their return, requiring brief hospitalization and missing the first two weeks of the new school term. Because of this, Therese did not see her for a review until she was 6;1 when her speech was within normal limits, although /ɹ/, /ð/ and /θ/ remained non-stimulable. Her parents were anxious for her to work on these three phonemes, and she returned at 6;4 for 40 minute once-weekly sessions for 12 weeks. The intervention comprised a combined program of minimal pairs intervention: /ð/ vs. /v/ and /θ/ vs. /f/, and speech perception training for /ɹ/ vs. /w/, followed by traditional articulation therapy for /ɹ/, /ð/ and /θ/— successfully accomplished by 6;7 with maintenance confirmed at a follow-up review at 6;10.

Mistaken Ideas about Vowels

Describing vowels as the 'poor relation' in the child phonology *research* literature and venturing that the vowels might be neglected because they are acquired easily and are of little theoretical interest, Davis and MacNeilage (1990) dismissed both speculations as mistaken. They held that much could be learned about children's speech acquisition if researchers were to turn the spotlight on vowels to a similar degree as the customary focus on consonants.

Over two decades later, Speake et al. (2011) noted that the study of vowels in children's speech had received much less attention than consonants; while Speake et al. (2012) surveyed the *intervention* literature, pointing out that compared to the treatment of consonants, the treatment of vowels was described infrequently; and in their timely, one-of-a-kind book Ball and Gibbon (2013) devoted a single chapter to intervention. Fast forward eight or so years, to discover a flurry of enthusiasm for vowel development and disorders (e.g., Ingram et al., 2019; Kent & Rountrey, 2020; Roepke & Brosseau-Lapré, 2021); and many helpful chapters in Ball 2021, e.g., Titterington and Bates (2021). There is even the odd article on the perils of vowel transcription (e.g., Sloos et al., 2019). Amid all this activity, scant attention is given to the assessment and treatment, by SLP/SLT clinicians, of children with difficulties with vowel discrimination, perception, and production.

Dr. Karen Pollock is a SLP and Professor in the Department of Communication Sciences and Disorders at the University of Alberta in Edmonton, Canada, where she served as Chair of the program for over 15 years. Her research and clinical interests include the production of vowels in children with and without SSDs, including children who speak different dialects of North American English. She has co-edited 3 books, published over 40 articles/chapters, and supervised countless graduate students. Her work on vowels was funded by the National Institute on Deafness and Communication Disorders (NIDCD). Her current research explores speech development (yes, including vowels!) in Canadian children learning Chinese as a heritage language or second language in bilingual schools and is funded by the Social Sciences and Humanities Research Council (SSHRC).

Q20.   Karen Pollock: Achieving a Better Understanding of Vowel Errors

In Pollock (2013, pp. 285–286) you commented on the pervasive and idiosyncratic vowel-error patterns that some children with SSD may display, noting that the consequent neutralization of phonemic contrasts highlights the potentially devastating effect of vowel errors on intelligibility. You went on to say, 'A better understanding of the nature and significance of vowel errors in phonological disorder is needed to plan effective remediation strategies for such children'. Are we any closer to this important goal, and how would you guide information-hungry clinicians?

A20.   Karen E. Pollock Characteristics, Assessment, and Treatment of Vowel Errors in Children with SSD

As a speech-language pathologist trained in the 1980s, I never gave much thought to vowels – until I ran across a client who presented with moderate to severe vowel errors. Vowels were known to be challenging for children who are deaf (e.g., Angelocci et al., 1964; Monsen, 1976) or have dysarthria due to cerebral palsy (Byrne, 1959; Levy et al., 2016; and see Pennington, A30), with centralized vowels significantly impacting intelligibility. But until the early 80s, the literature suggested that in the absence of hearing loss, velopharyngeal incompetence, or cerebral palsy, vowels were acquired by two or three years of age and were rarely misarticulated. Hence, vowels were not generally addressed in tests of speech sound development and treatment methods were practically non-existent.

In 1982, Pat Hargrove published a case study of a child with SSD who exhibited vowel errors and suggested that perhaps these cases are more common that we were led to believe, but that clinicians are generally insensitive to them because our clinical training and assessment tools are overwhelmingly focused on consonants. Over the years, several other authors have provided detailed descriptions of individual or small groups of children with vowel errors (e.g., Gibbon et al., 1992; Penney et al., 1994; Reynolds, 2013; Speake, 2013; Speake et al., 2012; Stoel-Gammon & Herrington, 1990), confirming that although less frequent than consonant errors, some children with SSD also produce vowel errors. However, larger group studies were needed to determine just how common vowel errors are among children with SSD.

Pollock and Berni (2003) sought to determine the incidence of non-rhotic vowel errors in a relatively large group of children with SSD (n = 149; 30 to 82 months of age) compared to a group with typical speech development (n=165; 18 to 81 months of age) learning a southern variety of American English. Overall, the children with SSD had lower accuracy (percent of non-rhotic vowels correct or PVC-nr) and greater variability in vowel production (M = 94.76, SD = 6.95) than age-matched peers with typical speech (M = 98.30, SD = 2.03). Consonant and vowel accuracy were strongly correlated for children with typical development and moderately correlated for those with SSD. Using different cut-offs for determining the presence of vowel errors (PVC-nr <95%, <90%, <85%), we found that vowel errors were rare in children with typical speech development beyond 3 years of age (0–4%), but higher in those under 3 (24–65%) and those with SSD (11–32%). For children with SSD, the likelihood of vowel errors increased dramatically with the severity of SSD (as determined by PCC): 4–23% of children with mild-moderate SSD, 8–41% of children with moderate-severe SSD, and 42–70% of children with severe SSD exhibited some vowel errors.

More recently, Roepke and Brosseau-Lapré (2021) found similar results with a group of 84 children (48 to 71 months of age) learning a mid-western variety of American English, including 45 children with SSD and 39 with typical speech development. Using a measure that excluded not only rhotic vowels but also syllabic /l/ (Percent Vowels Correct – Non-Liquid or PVC-NL), those with typical speech development had higher vowel accuracy (M = 97.7, SD = 1.7) than those with SSD (M = 93.7, SD = 4.0). The number of vowel errors was moderately but significantly correlated with severity of SSD (as measured by their standard score on the GFTA-3) in both studies. The authors concluded that children with more severe SSD are at risk of having vowel errors as well as consonant errors.

There is a growing body of literature on typical and atypical vowel development, including an edited book (Ball & Gibbon, 2013) devoted to vowels and vowel disorders. Errors on vowels are frequently included as a potential marker of Childhood Apraxia of Speech (CAS), along with prosodic errors and sequencing difficulties (ASHA, 2007). More recently, studies have found that children with Developmental Language Disorder (DLD) have difficulty with vowel perception & vowel accuracy in non-word repetition (NWR) tasks (Roepke et al., 2020; Vuolo & Goffman, 2020). Recent publications on vowel development in typically developing children and those with SSD (e.g., Kent & Rountrey's 2020 review which emphasized acoustic studies) also draw attention to the importance of vowels in both typical and disordered speech development. This work has important implications for vowel assessment and intervention and has the potential for translation into clinically applicable tools and strategies for addressing vowel errors.

Importance of Vowel Errors in Children with SSD

Vowels have been routinely ignored when working with children with SSDs. Stoel-Gammon (1990) and others have discussed possible reasons for this neglect, positing that vowels are less discrete than consonants, making them more difficult to perceive and to transcribe reliably *and* more difficult to teach. In addition, listeners may be accustomed to hearing differences in vowel production across different dialects, making them more tolerant of vowel variations in children's speech, especially if they involve relatively minor shifts in height, centrality, or rounding.

Vowel errors that result in a loss of phonemic contrast (or multiple phoneme collapses), however, can have a significant impact on intelligibility, especially when they occur in combination with consonant errors, which is most often the case for children with SSD. For example, a child reported in Pollock (2002), whose PCC and PVC-nr on a single word elicitation task were both 75, frequently produced the vowels /ɛ/ and /æ/ as [ɑ], replaced /ɔɪ/ and sometimes /eɪ/ with [aɪ], and used [ɔ] for /aʊ/ and all rhotic vowels and diphthongs. Another child, reported in Pollock (1991), had an idiosyncratic substitution of [eɪ] for all lax vowels (although it applied inconsistently), the rhotic monophthong [ɝ/ɚ], and to rhotic diphthongs with front vowels ([ɪɚ] and [ɛɚ]). The resulting loss of phonemic vowel contrasts for these children resulted very poor intelligibility.

Vowel errors have been shown to have a detrimental effect on intelligibility for speakers who are deaf or dysarthric (e.g., Levy et al., 2016; Markides, 1970), but there is little direct evidence of the impact of vowel errors on intelligibility for children with an SSD other than childhood dysarthria. An intriguing finding reported by Speake et al. (2012) was that intelligibility increased for two 10-year-old children with persisting speech difficulties and normal hearing following intervention directly targeting vowel production. Pre-treatment intelligibility was quite low (8 and 32%) but increased (to 52 and 47%, respectively) along with improvements in PVC but no or limited changes in PCC. Although additional research with more children with vowel errors is needed, this finding supports a direct link between vowel errors and intelligibility for children with SSD as well as positive outcomes for vowel intervention.

In an experimental study using a synthesized child voice, Vaughn and Pollock (1997) controlled the number and type of vowel and consonant errors in an unpredictable word at the end of a sentence. Consonant and vowel errors had similar effects on the listeners' ability to identify the target word. Furthermore, it appeared that some types of errors (e.g., laxing, diphthong reduction) affected intelligibility to different extents. A partial replication by Mackie (2015) using live voice and single word stimuli controlled for frequency and neighborhood density reported a similar finding that vowel errors and consonant errors affected intelligibility equally, but failed to find a significant difference between different types of vowel errors. In both studies, words containing a consonant error and a vowel error had the biggest impact on intelligibility, suggesting that children who have vowel errors in addition to consonant errors will have a difficult time being understood.

Assessment of Vowels

Common assessment tools for SSD focus heavily (if not exclusively) on consonants. Although there is growing recognition that the inclusion of vowels is important for a full assessment of a child's speech sound development, constructing a test that assesses vowels is complicated.

Widespread variation exists in the English– or 'Englishes'–spoken in different parts of the world (e.g., British varieties of English vs. Australian varieties of English vs. North American varieties of English) and most of this variation is in the vowel system (e.g., see review in Watt, 2013). Within these major varieties, regional variations in vowel production also exist (e.g., see Jacewicz et al., 2011, for American English; Cox & Palethorpe, 2007, for Australian English). As a result, any vowel assessment must be adapted to the ambient language and dialect of the child being assessed. Recognizing this need, Bowen's (2010) *Quick Vowel Screener* offers different versions for Australian and New Zealand English vowels, as well as a form without symbols on which the examiner can write the phonetic symbols of the client's variety of English. Similarly, the transcription of target words on response form for the *Hodson Assessment of Phonological Patterns – 3rd Edition* (HAPP-3; Hodson, 2004) includes blank spaces for vowels and vocalic liquids; clinicians can write in the phonetic symbols appropriate to the child's dialect if their child does not speak Standard American English (SAE).

Another issue that complicates vowel assessment is the transcription of vowels. Linguists regularly disagree on the most appropriate system for transcribing the vowels of a given language, particularly when it comes to diphthongs and rhotic vowels. For example, the diphthong in the word 'sky' is transcribed by some as two vowel symbols, often with a tie bar ([aɪ̯]) but by others as a vowel followed by a glide ([aj]). There is even less agreement on the transcription of rhotic vowels, as in 'b<u>ir</u>d', 'butt<u>er</u>', which may be transcribed as rhotic vowel symbols ([ɝ, ɚ]), syllabic consonants ([ɹ̩]) or neutral vowels followed by /ɹ/ ([ʌɹ, əɹ]). Similarly, postvocalic rhotics as in '<u>ear</u>' and 'd<u>oor</u>' may be transcribed as rhotic diphthongs ([ɪɚ] and [ɔɚ]) or as a vowel followed by /ɹ/ ([ɪɹ] and [ɔɹ]). These differences in transcription of vocalic and postvocalic rhotics impact whether they are analyzed as vowels or consonants. Other transcription-related challenges include selecting the appropriate level of transcription (/phonemic/ or [phonetic]) when transcribing target vowels (Cox, 2008) and determining the level of phonetic detail (narrow transcription) required for clinical purposes (e.g., Müller & Damico, 2002; Titterington & Bates, 2021). Research has also shown that the speaker's accent and the transcriber's knowledge of that accent can bias phonetic transcription (Sloos et al., 2019).

Not surprisingly, vowels are difficult to transcribe (e.g., Howard & Heselwood, 2013, and many clinicians express a lack of familiarity with IPA vowel symbols, causing a circular problem. Because vowels are not a focus in assessment tools, clinicians have less practice transcribing them, therefore lacking experience and confidence. Tutorials addressing vowel transcription are available for clinicians wishing to improve their skills (e.g., Ball et al., 2010; Pollock & Berni, 2001), but clearly more attention should be paid to vowels when learning and maintaining phonetic transcription skills.

Acoustic-aided transcription may help clinicians who are familiar and comfortable with acoustic analysis. Fortunately, acoustic-aided transcription is becoming more feasible with freely downloadable software like Phon (Hedlund & Rose, 2020), which provides a platform for transcribing and analyzing children's speech samples and incorporates functions for acoustic analysis from Praat (Boersma & Weenink, 2022). Acoustic analysis can enhance knowledge by offering more objective acoustic measurements and is especially useful for uncovering covert contrasts (subtle differences between sounds that are not perceptually salient), which can indicate an intermediate stage in the development of phonemic contrasts (Munson et al., 2010).

Standardized tests are commonly used to identify SSD in children, but none were designed to assess vowels. Those that purport to assess vowels often provide only one opportunity to produce each vowel target. Although some tests include an option to record an inventory of the vowels that were produced incorrectly by the child on the test form, and the *Khan-Lewis Phonological Analysis – 3rd edition* (KLPA-3; Khan & Lewis, 2015) devotes a full page to a supplemental analysis of vowels, most tests do not incorporate vowel errors in the calculation of scores. Accordingly, a child with vowel errors as well as consonant errors could score the same as a child with consonant errors only – underestimating the additional impact of the vowel errors on intelligibility and severity. One notable exception is the *Diagnostic Evaluation of Articulation and Phonology* (DEAP; Dodd et al., 2002) which includes vowel errors in the calculation of the Articulation Score, a norm-referenced scaled score. The DEAP also includes a modified vowel accuracy (PVC) calculation, based on the vowels in test target words.

Over the past 3 decades, several authors have suggested that standardized tests of articulation and phonology may provide a starting point for vowel assessment and have examined the distribution of vowels in the test stimuli to determine whether they provide an adequate sample of vowels to complete a non-standardized analysis (Pollock, 1991; Eisenberg & Hitchcock, 2010; Roepke & Brosseau-Lapré, 2021). Each set different criteria for an acceptable sample for vowel assessment. For example, Pollock (1991) looked across 5 tests for the number of opportunities for each non-rhotic and rhotic vowel and diphthong in open and closed syllables in monosyllabic words and in stressed and unstressed syllables of disyllabic and multisyllabic words. Eisenberg and Hitchcock (2010) surveyed the stimulus words of 11 tests for at least two opportunities to produce each of 15 stressed vowels in monosyllabic or disyllabic words when not followed by a liquid. In their assessment of the vowel targets in the GFTA-3, Roepke and Brosseau-Lapré (2021) used the same criteria as Eisenberg and Hitchcock but added a requirement that the vowel be elicited in two of three different post-vocalic consonantal contexts (labial, coronal, or dorsal). The authors of the three studies concluded that such tests do not provide an adequate representation of vowel targets (understandable, as that was never their intent) and suggested that supplemental words be added to obtain a sufficient sample for assessment. Clinicians may look to these articles to find suggestions for additional words to supplement the sample obtained from their preferred test(s) for children with vowel errors. Post-vocalic liquids are known to influence preceding vowels and should be avoided (or systematically controlled).

Several researchers have developed their own vowel assessment tools for use in research, but these tools have not been normed or validated psychometrically. Pollock's *Vowel-Consonant Assessment Protocol* (VCAP; Pollock, 2002, 2013) includes 140 words elicited from photographs. The word list includes 6 to 9 opportunities of each of the 14 non-rhotic vowels of American English (11 monophthongs /i ɪ e ɛ æ u ʊ o ɔ ɑ ʌ(ə)/ and 3 diphthongs /aɪ aʊ ɔɪ/) and 5 rhotic vowels (1 monophthong /ɝ(ɚ)/ and four diphthongs /ɪɚ ɛɚ ɔɚ ɑɚ/). Each vowel is targeted in open syllables (if permissible) and closed syllables of monosyllabic words with a variety of following consonants (excluding /ɫ/) and in and disyllabic or multisyllabic words with and without primary stress. Some words are elicited more than once, to assess consistency. A story-retelling task containing each non-rhotic and rhotic vowel provides the opportunity to assess vowels in connected speech. The full list of words and the story script are included in the appendix of Pollock (2002) illustrating the scores that can be obtained: percent correct for each vowel/diphthong target, PVC-non-rhotic and PVC-rhotic, and a weighted score for PVC-non-rhotic vowels that considers frequency of occurrence of target vowels in conversational speech. Speake et al. (2012) created an assessment of Southern British English vowels containing 12 CV words beginning with a plosive, fricative, or nasal, 12 VC words ending in a plosive, fricative, or nasal, 52 CVC words with a variety of initial consonants and a final plosive, fricative, nasal, or continuant (including /ɫ/). Eight imitated sentences containing a range of vowels are also included to assess vowels in connected speech. For Australian and New Zealand English, Bowen's online *Quick Vowel*

Screener (Bowen, 2010) offers target words (with copyright free colour clipart) for each vowel. A longer version with 4 words and pictures per vowel is also available.

The importance of assessing vowels in more complex words has been highlighted through studies finding lower accuracy in multisyllabic words as compared to monosyllabic words. In a study of children with typical speech development, James et al. (2001) found that PVC was lower in longer words. Likewise, Masso et al. (2016) assessed 93 children with SSD and found significantly more vowel errors on the *Polysyllable Preschool Test* (POP; Baker, 2013), which consists of 30 three- to five-syllable words, more than on the DEAP, which includes only 5 (out of 50) words greater than two syllables. Interestingly, consonant accuracy was not different across the two assessments. These findings suggest that vowel accuracy may be overestimated when using assessments that include mostly monosyllables and disyllables and demonstrate the importance of including polysyllable sampling tasks (that tax the child's system) when assessing vowels.

Phonetic context must also be considered when assessing vowels, rather than assuming vowels have been learned as independent units. Failure to assess vowels in a variety of phonetic environments could lead to faulty assumptions about a child's abilities. For example, if a child produces a vowel incorrectly in one context, it does not mean that they may not be able to produce it correctly in other contexts. At the same time, just because a child produces a vowel correctly in one context it does not mean they can do so in all contexts. Bates et al. (2013) summarize literature on consonant-vowel (C-V) interactions and provide examples of both vowel-conditioned consonant errors and consonant-conditioned vowel errors. The most common C-V interaction pattern is the co-occurrence of alveolar stops with front vowels, velar stops with back vowels, and labial stops with back rounded vowels, and the pattern may be extended to different manner classes (e.g., nasals, fricatives) in children with SSD. Bates et al. (2013) provide a summary of C-V sequences that are most likely to be problematic as well as more facilitative contexts that could be used to select target words for intervention.

Treatment of Vowel Errors

In some, but certainly not all, cases vowel errors may resolve spontaneously or following treatment for consonant errors (e.g., Robb et al., 1999; Watson et al., 1994). Pollock (1994) described a boy with severe vowel errors (PVC 33%) who had previously received treatment for multiple consonant errors; the consonant errors had been mostly remediated, but numerous vowel errors remained. In a larger group study, 8 children with SSD including vowel errors were followed longitudinally, during which time they received direct intervention for consonant errors only; although most showed improvements in vowel accuracy, several continued to exhibit vowel errors following up to 18 months of intervention (Pollock, 2002). In a more recent study on the effectiveness of direct vowel-targeted intervention for two children, Speake et al. (2012) found significant improvements in PVC as well as intelligibility as judged by peers. Both Pollock (1994) and Speake et al. (2012) found greater improvement during interventions for vowels that were stimulable pre-treatment.

Information regarding clinical strategies for direct treatment of vowel errors comes primarily from a dozen or so case studies (see Gibbon & Beck, 2002 for a summary of early case reports) and an overview of general principles and approaches to speech sound intervention that can be applied to vowels as well as consonants (Gibbon, 2013). Indeed, vowel-targeted intervention has been shown to be effective with children with who are deaf as well as children with SSD. Strategies reported include auditory-perceptual approaches such as structured listening or auditory bombardment, linguistic/phonological approaches such as minimal pair contrasts or *Metaphon*, motor/articulatory approaches including intensive repetitive drill practice, facilitative contexts, and gestures or hand cues representing (see Gibbon & Beck, 2002 for a review).

When providing intervention for consonant errors, clinicians often utilize placement cues for tongue position, jaw opening, and lip rounding. For vowel intervention, jaw opening and lip rounding cues may be helpful, but tongue position is much more difficult to describe and/or demonstrate. Visual biofeedback technology (e.g., electropalatography: EPG, ultrasound imaging) may help fill that need by providing information about relative tongue position within the oral cavity. Such approaches have been successfully used to target vowels with adolescents and adults who are deaf or who have dysarthria (e.g., Fletcher & Hasegawa, 1983; Levy et al., 2016) and have also been proposed for children with SSD (Bernhardt et al., 2010). Cleland and Preston (2021) suggest that ultrasound and visual acoustic biofeedback are more appropriate for vowel intervention than EPG, which may also be used for intervention with high front vowels such as /i/ that involve some linguapalatal contact, but not for mid or low vowels. Cleland and Preston also advise that biofeedback is most effective with school-age children and adolescents with residual speech errors, given the cognitive skills needed 'to integrate the visual feedback with their feedforward speech production systems' (p. 576).

Intervention using acoustic biofeedback has also been used with vowel intervention, primarily for children who are deaf but also with children with persistent residual speech errors, including rhotic vowels (e.g., Ertmer et al., 1996; Shuster et al., 1995). Such acoustic feedback is typically in the form of a real-time spectrogram or linear predictive coding (LPC) spectrogram. More recent acoustic biofeedback methods have emerged as low-cost, accessible, user-friendly apps. For example, the Complete Speech VowelViz app offers real-time acoustic feedback in the form of a cursor showing the speaker's attempts to hit vowel targets on a screen displaying the non-rhotic English vowel monophthongs in a classic vowel quadrilateral. However, the vowel formant data used to map the vowels to the quadrilateral are approximations and do not represent all speakers of American English, nor are they adjusted for speaker age or gender. Difficulties may be encountered in targeting the high front vowels /i/ and /ɪ/. Diphthongs can be visualized by adjusting the length of the tail that follows the cursor from one vowel position to another. VowelViz Pro includes feedback for rhotic as well as non-rhotic vowels. Research on the effectiveness of VowelViz is not available, but its existence confirms the interest in and market for technology targeting vowels.

Another iOS app for residual rhotic errors currently in development at New York University, *Speech Therapist's App for /r/ Treatment* (staRt) uses a real-time LPC spectrum (presented as a beach-themed wave) with an adjustable target line for F3 (McAllister Byun et al., 2017). As the client speaks, the clinician cues them to make articulatory adjustments until their F3 peak reaches the target line. The LPC filter order can be adjusted for speaker age, gender, and height. Users can practice or test their production of selected rhotic vowels and diphthongs (as well as pre-vocalic /ɹ/) at the syllable or word level. McAllister Byun et al. (2017) presented a case study of a 13-year-old girl with residual rhotic errors who had not shown long-term improvement following other forms of treatment. Her accuracy increased from 1 to 73% correct in 10 sessions and maintained 65% accuracy after clinician cues and biofeedback were systematically withdrawn. The staRt app has also been successfully used in telepractice (Peterson et al., 2022). Thus far, the app shows great potential but further research on a larger group of children is needed to determine its effectiveness.

Recent attention to the nature, assessment, and treatment of vowel errors in children points to the significance of vowels in understanding children's complete phonological systems. Furthermore, the documented impact of vowel errors on intelligibility suggests that vowels be considered as intervention targets. Clinicians who are hesitant to address vowels in intervention may take comfort in the knowledge that the same principles and strategies used for treating consonants may also be used with vowels. Meanwhile, further development of assessment tools and documentation of treatment efficacy are needed to ensure that children with vowel errors are identified and supported.

More Intervention Approaches

This chapter includes accounts of Phonetic Intervention (Articulation Therapy), Stimulability Intervention, Perceptual Intervention, and Minimal Pair Approaches to Phonological Intervention: Conventional Minimal Pairs (Meaningful Minimal Pairs and Perception-Production Minimal Pairs), and three approaches based upon complexity principles (Maximal Oppositions, Empty Set, and Multiple Oppositions interventions), and Vowel Intervention. Another evidenced approach to intervention with children with phonological disorder, the Cycles Phonological Patterns Approach (CPPA) appears in Chapter 1. Coming up in Chapter 5, are details of Naturalistic Recast Intervention, Grunwell's guidelines for phonological intervention, *Metaphon*, Parents and Children Together (PACT), Core Vocabulary Intervention, the Psycholinguistic Framework (Schäfer & Fricke, A21), and Phonological Awareness intervention (McNeill, A22). Looking further ahead, in Chapter 7, there are details of Phonotactic Therapy (Velleman, 2002) which has wide applicability to children with motor speech disorders (MSD) and those with phonological disorder. Then, the principles of motor learning: PML (Schmidt et al., 2019) for children with MSD are laid out in Chapter 8 where research, assessment, and treatments for MSD are presented by Megan Overby (A27), Amy Skinder-Meredith (A28), Kristen Allison (A29), Lindsay Pennington (A30), Edythe Strand (A31), Patricia McCabe (A32 and A34), and Pam Williams (A33).

Note

1. This sections on the Amplified Auditory Stimulation and Focused Auditory Stimulation (Focused Auditory Input) within the *Cycles Phonological Remediation Approach* was written in November 2013 with invaluable editorial input from Barbara Williams Hodson. It was updated for the 3rd edition of this book to reflect more recent developments, and the name-change to the *Cycles Phonological Patterns Approach (CPPA)*.

References

Adams, M. J., Treiman, R., & Pressley, M. (1998). Reading, writing and literacy. In I. Sigel & A. Renninger (Eds.), *Handbook of child psychology, Volume 4: Child psychology in practice* (pp. 275–355). Wiley.

Angelocci, A., Kopp, G., & Holbrook, A. (1964). The vowel formants of deaf and normal-hearing eleven- to fourteen-year-old boys. *Journal of Speech and Hearing Disorders*, 29(2), 156–170. https://doi.org/10.1044/jshd.2902.156

ASHA. (2004). *Auditory integration training* [Technical Report]. https://www.asha.org/policy

ASHA. (2007). *Childhood apraxia of speech* [Position Statement]. https://doi.org/10.1044/jshd.2902.156

Bain, B. (1994). A framework for dynamic assessment in phonology: Stimulability revisited. *Clinics in Communication Disorders*, 4(1), 12–22. PMID: 8019548.

Baker, E. (2010). Minimal pair intervention. In A. L. Williams, S. McLeod, & R. J. McCauley (Eds.), *Interventions for speech sound disorders in children* (1st ed., pp. 41–72). Paul H. Brookes.

Baker, E. (2013). *Polysyllable preschool test*. Author.

Baker, E. (2021). Minimal pair intervention. In A. L. Williams, S. McLeod, & R. J. McCauley (Eds.), *Interventions for speech sound disorders in children* (2nd ed., pp. 33–60). Paul H. Brookes.

Baker, E., & McLeod, S. (2004). Evidence-based management of phonological impairment in children. *Child Language Teaching and Therapy*, 20(3), 261–285. https://doi.org/10.1191%2F0265659004ct275oa

Baldwin, D. A., & Markham, E. M. (1989). Establishing word-object relations: A first step. *Child Development*, 60(2), 381–398. https://doi.org/10.2307/1130984

Ball, M. J. (Ed.). (2021). *Manual of clinical phonetics*. Routledge. https://doi.org/10.4324/9780429320903

Ball, M. J., & Gibbon, F. E. (Eds.). (2013). *Handbook of vowels and vowel disorders* (2nd ed.). Psychology Press. https://doi.org/10.4324/9780203103890

Ball, M. J., Muller, N., Klopfenstein, M., & Rutter, B. (2010). My client is using non-English sounds! A tutorial in advanced phonetic transcription. Part II: Vowels and diacritics. *Contemporary Issues in Communication Science and Disorders*, 37(Fall), 103–110. https://doi.org/10.1044/cicsd_36_f_103

Bates, S., Watson, J., & Scobbie, J. (2013) Context conditioned error patterns in disordered systems. In M. J. Ball & F. E. Gibbon (Eds.), *Handbook of vowels and vowel disorders* (2nd ed., pp. 288–325). Psychology Press. https://doi.org/10.4324/9780203 103890.ch11

Bernhardt, B., & Stemberger, J. P. (2000). *Workbook in nonlinear phonology for clinical application*. Pro-Ed.

Bernhardt, B., & Stoel-Gammon, C. (1996). Under-specification and markedness in normal and disordered phonological development. In C. E. Johnson & J. H. V. Gilbert (Eds.), *Children's language* (Vol. 9, pp. 33–54). Lawrence Erlbaum Associates.

Bernhardt, B. M., Stemberger, J., & Bacsfalvi, P. (2010). Vowel intervention. In L. Williams, S. McLeod, & R. McCauley (Eds.), *Interventions for speech sound disorders in children* (pp. 41–72). Brookes.

Bernthal, J. E., & Bankson, N. W. (2004). *Articulation and phonological disorders* (5th ed.). Allyn & Bacon.

Blache, S. E. (1982). Minimal word pairs and distinctive feature training. In M. Crary (Ed.), *Phonological intervention: Concepts and procedures* (pp. 61–96). College-Hill Press Inc.

Blache, S. E., Parsons, C. L., & Humphreys, J. M. (1981). A minimal-word-pair model for teaching the linguistic significant difference of distinctive feature properties. *Journal of Speech and Hearing Disorders*, *46*(3), 291–296. https://doi.org/10.1044/jshd.4603.291

Boersma, P., & Weenink, D. (2022). *Praat: Doing phonetics by computer* (Version 6. 2.23)[computer software]. http://www.praat.org

Bowen, C. (1996). Evaluation of a phonological therapy with treated and untreated groups of young children (Unpublished doctoral dissertation). Macquarie University. http://hdl.handle.net/1959.14/304812

Bowen, C. (2010a). Parents and children together (PACT) intervention for children with speech sound disorders. In A. L. Williams, S. McLeod, & R. J. McCauley (Eds.), *Interventions for speech sound disorders in children* (pp. 407–426). Brookes Publishing Co.

Bowen, C. (2010b). *The quick vowel screener*. www.speech-language-therapy.com

Bowen, C. (2019). Articulation therapy (phonetic intervention) In J. S. Damico & M. J. Ball (Eds.), *The SAGE encyclopedia of human communication sciences and disorders* (pp. 168-174). Sage Publications.

Bowen, C., & Cupples, L. (1999). Parents and children together (PACT): A collaborative approach to phonological therapy. *International Journal of Language and Communication Disorders*, *34*(1), 35–55. https://doi.org/10.1080/136828299247603

Bowen, C., & Rippon, H. (2013). *Consonant clusters: Alliterative stories and activities for phonological intervention*. Black Sheep Press.

Byers, B. A., Bellon-Harn, M. L., Allen, M., Whisenhunt Saar, K., Manchaiah, V., & Hanspani, R. (2021). A comparison of intervention intensity and service delivery models with school-age children with speech sound disorders in a school setting. *Language, Speech, and Hearing Services in Schools*, *52*(2), 529–541. https://doi.org/10.1044/2020_lshss-20-00057

Byrne, M. (1959). Speech and language development of athetoid and spastic children. *Journal of Speech and Hearing Disorders*, *24*(3), 231–240. https://doi.org/10.1044/jshd.2403.231

Camarata, S. M. (2010). Naturalistic intervention for speech intelligibility and speech accuracy. In A. L. Williams, S. McLeod, & R. J. McCauley (Eds.), *Interventions for speech sound disorders in children* (pp. 381–405). Brookes Publishing Co.

Camarata, S. M. (2021). Naturalistic recast intervention. In A. L. Williams, S. McLeod, & R. J. McCauley (Eds.). *Interventions for speech sound disorders in children* (2nd ed., pp. 227–361). Brookes Publishing Co.

Carter, E. T., & Buck, M. W. (1958). Prognostic testing for functional articulation disorders among children in the first grade. *Journal of Speech and Hearing Disorders*, *23*(2), 124–133. https://doi.org/10.1044/jshd.2302.124

Cleland, J., & Preston, J. (2021). Biofeedback interventions. In A. L. Williams, S. McLeod, & R. J. McCauley (Eds.), *Interventions for speech sound disorders in children* (2nd ed., pp. 573–600). Paul H. Brookes Publishing.

Cohen, J. H., & Diehl, C. F. (1963). Relation of speech sound discrimination ability to articulation-type speech defects. *Journal of Speech and Hearing Disorders*, *28*(2), 187–190. https://doi.org/10.1044/jshd.2802.187

Cox, F. (2008). Vowel transcription systems: An Australian perspective. *International Journal of Speech-Language Pathology*, *10*(5), 327–333. https://doi.org/10.1080/17549500701855133

Cox, F., & Palethorpe, S. (2007). Australian English. *Journal of the International Phonetic Association*, *37*(3), 341–350. https://doi.org/10.1017/S0025100307003192

Crosbie, S., Holm, A., & Dodd, B. (2005). Intervention for children with severe speech disorder: A comparison of two approaches. *International Journal of Language and Communication Disorders*, *40*(4), 467–491. https://doi.org/10.1080/13682820500126049

Davies, K. E., Marshall, J., Brown, L. J., & Goldbart, J. (2017). Co-working: Parents' conception of roles in supporting their children's speech and language development. *Child Language Teaching & Therapy*, *33*(2), 171–185. https://doi.org/10.1177%2F0265659016671169

Davis, B. L., & MacNeilage, P. F. (1990). Acquisition of correct vowel production: A quantitative case study. *Journal of Speech and Hearing Research*, *33*(1), 16–27. https://doi.org/10.1044/jshr.3301.16

DeVeney, S. L., Cabbage, K. L., & Mourey, T. (2020). Target selection considerations for speech sound disorder intervention in schools. *Perspectives of the ASHA Special Interest Groups*, *5*(6), 1722–1734. https://doi.org/10.1044/2020_PERSP-20-00138

Dodd, B., Crosbie, S., McIntosh, B., Holm, A., Harvey, C., Liddy, M., Fontyne, K., Pinchin, B., & Rigby, H. (2008). The impact of selecting different contrasts in phonological therapy. *International Journal of Speech-Language Pathology*, *10*(5), 334–345. https://doi.org/10.1080/14417040701732590

Dodd, B., Crosbie, S., Zhu, H., Holm, A., & Ozanne, A. (2002). *Diagnostic evaluation of articulation and phonology (DEAP)*. Psychological Corporation.

Donicht, G., Pagliarin, K. C., Mota, H. B., & Keske-Soares, M. (2011). The treatment with rothics and generalization obtained in two models of phonological therapy. *Jornal da Sociedade Brasileira de Fonoaudiologia*, *23*(1), 71–76. https://doi.org/10.1590/s2179-64912011000100015

Edwards, J., Fox, R. A., & Rogers, C. L. (2002). Final consonant discrimination in children: Effects of phonological disorder, vocabulary size, and articulatory accuracy. *Journal of Speech, Language, and Hearing Research*, *45*(2), 231–242. https://doi.org/10.1044/1092-4388(2002/018)

Edwards, M. L. (1983). Selection criteria for developing therapy goals. *Journal of Childhood Communication Disorders*, *7*(1), 36–45. https://doi.org/10.1177%2F152574018300700105

Edwards, M. L., & Shriberg, L. D. (1983). *Phonology: Applications in communicative disorders*. College-Hill.

Eisenberg, S., & Hitchcock, E. (2010). Using standardized tests to inventory consonant and vowel production: A comparison of 11 tests of articulation and phonology. *Language, Speech and Hearing Services in Schools*, *41*(4), 488–503. https://doi.org/10.1044/0161-1461(2009/08-0125)

Elbert, M., Dinnsen, D., & Powell, T. (1984). On the prediction of phonological generalization learning pattern. *Journal of Speech and Hearing Disorders*, *49*(3), 309–317. https://doi.org/10.1044/jshd.4903.309

Elbert, M., Dinnsen, D. A., Swartzlander, P., & Chin, S. B. (1990). Generalization to conversational speech. *Journal of Speech and Hearing Research*, *55*(4), 694–699. https://doi.org/10.1044/jshd.5504.694

Elbert, M., & Gierut, J. (1986). *Handbook of clinical phonology: Approaches to assessment and treatment*. College-Hill Press.

Elbert, M., Powell, T. W., & Swartzlander, P. (1991). Toward a technology of generalization: How many exemplars are sufficient? *Journal of Speech and Hearing Research*, *34*(1), 81–87. https://doi.org/10.1044/jshr.3401.81

Ertmer, D., Stark, R., & Karlan, G. (1996). Real-time spectrographic displays in vowel production training with children who have profound hearing loss. *American Journal of Speech-Language Pathology*, *5*(4), 4–16. https://doi.org/10.1044/1058-0360.0504.04

Fazio, B. B. (1997). Learning a new poem: Memory for connected speech and phonological awareness in low-income children with and without specific language impairment. *Journal of Speech, Language, and Hearing Research*, *40*(6), 1285–1297. https://doi.org/10.1044/jslhr.4006.1285

Fey, M. E. (1985). Clinical forum: Phonological assessment and treatment. Articulation and phonology: Inextricable constructs in speech pathology. *Human Communication Canada*, *9*(1), 7–16. Reprinted as Fey (1992). https://cjslpa.ca/files/1985_HumComm_Vol_09/No_01_1-50/Fey_HumComm_1985.pdf

Fey, M. E. (1986). *Language intervention with young children*. College-Hill Press.

Fey, M. E. (1992). Clinical forum: Phonological assessment and treatment. Articulation and phonology: Inextricable constructs in speech pathology. *Language, Speech, and Hearing Services in Schools*, *23*(3), 225–232. https://doi.org/10.1044/0161-1461.2303.225

Fey, M. E., & Stalker, C. (1986). A hypothesis testing approach to treatment of a child with an idiosyncratic (morpho)phonological system. *Journal of Speech and Hearing Disorders*, *51*(4), 324–336. https://doi.org/10.1044/jshd.5104.324

Fletcher, P., & Hasegawa, A. (1983). Speech modification by a deaf child through dynamic orometric modeling and feedback. *Journal of Speech and Hearing Disorders*, *48*(2), 178–185. https://doi.org/10.1044/jshd.4802.178

Flynn, L., & Lancaster, G. (1996). *Children's phonology sourcebook*. Winslow Press.

Gibbon, F. (2013). Therapy for abnormal vowels in children with speech disorders. In M. J. Ball & F. E. Gibbon (Eds.), *Handbook of vowels and vowel disorders* (2nd ed., pp. 429–446). Psychology Press. https://doi.org/10.4324/9780203103890.ch17

Gibbon, F., & Beck, M. (2002). Therapy for abnormal vowels in children with phonological impairment. In M. J. Ball & F. E. Gibbon (Eds.), *Vowel disorders* (pp. 217–248). Butterworth-Heinemann.

Gibbon, F., Shockey, L., & Reid, J. (1992). Description and treatment of abnormal vowels. *Child Language Teaching and Therapy, 8*(1), 30–59. https://doi.org/10.1177/026565909200800103

Gierut, J. (1989). Maximal opposition approach to phonological treatment. *Journal of Speech and Hearing Disorders, 54*(1), 9–19. https://doi.org/10.1044/jshd.5401.09

Gierut, J. (2001). Complexity in phonological treatment: Clinical factors. *Language, Speech, and Hearing Services in Schools, 32*(4), 229–241. https://doi.org/10.1044/0161-1461(2001/021)

Gierut, J. (2007). Phonological complexity and language learnability. *American Journal of Speech-Language Pathology, 16*(1), 6–17. https://doi.org/10.1044/1058-0360(2007/003)

Gierut, J. A. (1990). Differential learning of phonological oppositions. *Journal of Speech and Hearing Research, 33*(3), 540–549. https://doi.org/10.1044/jshr.3303.540

Gierut, J. A. (1991). Homonymy in phonological change. *Clinical Linguistics & Phonetics, 5*(2), 119–137. https://doi.org/10.3109/02699209108985509

Gierut, J. A. (1992). The conditions and course of clinically induced phonological change. *Journal of Speech and Hearing Research, 35*(5), 1049–1063. https://doi.org/10.1044/jshr.3505.1049

Gierut, J. A. (1999). Syllable onsets: Clusters and adjuncts in acquisition. *Journal of Speech, Language, and Hearing Research, 42*(3), 708–726. https://doi.org/10.1044/jslhr.4203.708

Gierut, J. A. (2008). Fundamentals of experimental design and treatment. In D. A. Dinnsen & J. A. Gierut (Eds.), *Optimality theory, phonological acquisition and disorders* (pp. 93–118). Equinox.

Gierut, J. A., & Hulse, L. E. (2010). Evidence-based practice: A matrix for predicting phonological generalization. *Clinical Linguistics & Phonetics, 24*(4–5), 323–334. https://doi.org/10.3109/02699200903532490

Gierut, J. A., & Neumann, H. J. (1992). Teaching and learning /θ/: A non-confound. *Clinical Linguistics & Phonetics, 6*(3), 191–200. https://doi.org/10.3109/02699209208985530

Gierut, J. A., & O'Connor, K. M. (2002). Precursors to onset clusters in acquisition. *Journal of Child Language, 29*(3), 495–517. https://doi.org/10.1017/S0305000902005238

Gierut, J. A., Simmerman, C. L., & Neumann, H. J. (1994). Phonemic structures of delayed phonological systems. *Journal of Child Language, 21*(2), 291–316. https://doi.org/10.1017/S0305000900009284

Gillam, S. L., & Gillam, R. B. (2014). Improving clinical services: Be aware of fuzzy connections between principles and strategies. *Language, Speech, and Hearing Services in Schools, 45*(2), 137–144. https://doi.org/10.1044/2014_LSHSS-14-0024

Glaspey, A. M., & Stoel-Gammon, C. (2005). Dynamic assessment in phonological disorders: The scaffolding scale of stimulability. *Topics in Language Disorders: Clinical Perspectives on Speech Sound Disorders, 25*(3), 220–230. https://doi.org/10.1097/00011363-200507000-00005

Glaspey, A., & Stoel-Gammon, C. (2007). A dynamic approach to phonological assessment. *Advances in Speech Language Pathology, 9*(4), 286–296. https://doi.org/10.1080/14417040701435418

Goldman, R., & Fristoe, M. (2000). *Goldman-Fristoe test of articulation* (2nd ed.). American Guidance Service.

Goldman, R., & Fristoe, M. (2015). *Goldman-Fristoe test of articulation 3*. Pearson.

Grunwell, P. (1982). *Clinical phonology*. Croom Helm.

Grunwell, P. (1975). The phonological analysis of articulation disorders. *British Journal of Disorders of Communication, 10*(1), 31–42. https://doi.org/10.3109/13682827509011272

Grunwell, P. (1985a). *Phonological assessment of child speech (PACS)*. NFER–Nelson.

Grunwell, P. (1985b). Developing phonological skills. *Child Language Teaching and Therapy, 1*(1), 65–72. https://doi.org/10.1177%2F026565908500100108

Grunwell, P. (1992). Process of phonological change in developmental speech disorders. *Clinical Linguistics & Phonetics, 6*(1–2), 101–122. https://doi.org/10.3109/02699209208985522

Grunwell, P. (1997). Developmental phonological disability: Order in disorder. In B. W. Hodson & M. L. Edwards (Eds.), *Perspectives in applied phonology* (pp. 157–196). Aspen Publications.

Hargrove, P. (1982). Misarticulated vowels: A case study. *Language, Speech, and Hearing Services in Schools, 13*(2), 86–95. https://doi.org/10.1044/0161-1461.1302.86

Hearnshaw, S., Baker, E., & Munro, N. (2018). The speech perception skills of children with and without speech sound disorder. *Journal of Communication Disorders, 71*(Jan-Feb), 61–71. https://doi.org/10.1016/j.jcomdis.2017.12.004

Hearnshaw, S., Baker, E., & Munro, N. (2019). Speech perception skills of children with speech sound disorders: A systematic review and meta-analysis. *Journal of Speech and Hearing Research*, *62*(10), 3771–3789. https://doi.org/10.1044/2019_JSLHR-S-18-0519

Hedlund, G., & Rose, Y. (2020). *Phon 3.1* [Computer Software]. https://phon.ca.

Hodson, B. (2004). *Hodson assessment of phonological patterns* (3rd ed.). Pro-Ed.

Hodson, B. W., & Paden, E. P. (1983). *Targeting intelligible speech: A phonological approach to remediation*. College-Hill Press.

Hodson, B. W., & Paden, E. P. (1991). *Targeting intelligible speech: A phonological approach to remediation* (2nd ed.). Pro-Ed.

Hoffman, P. R., Daniloff, R. G., Bengoa, D., & Schuckers, G. (1985). Misarticulating and normally articulating children's identification and discrimination of synthetic [r] and [w]. *Journal of Speech and Hearing Disorders*, *50*(1), 46–53. https://doi.org/10.1044/jshd.5001.46

Hoffman, P. R., Stager, S., & Daniloff, R. G. (1983). Perception and production of misarticulated /r/. *Journal of Speech and Hearing Disorders*, *48*(2), 210–215. https://doi.org/10.1044/jshd.4802.210

Howard, S., & Heselwood, B. (2013). The contribution of phonetics to the study of vowel development and disorders. In M. J. Ball & F. E. Gibbon (Eds.), *Handbook of vowels and vowel disorders* (2nd ed., pp. 61–112). Psychology Press. https://doi.org/10.1080/02699200210135893

Ingram, D. (1976). *Phonological disability in children*. Edward Arnold.

Ingram, D. (1981). *Procedures for the phonological analysis of children's language*. University Park Press.

Ingram, D. (1989). *Phonological disability in children* (2nd ed.). Cole & Whurr Publishers.

Ingram, S. D., Reed, V. A., & Powell, T. W. (2019). Vowel duration discrimination of children with childhood apraxia of speech: A preliminary study. *American Journal of Speech-Language Pathology*, *28*(S), 857–874. https://doi.org/10.1044/2019_AJSLP-MSC18-18-0113

Jacewicz, E., Fox, R. A., & Salmons, J. (2011). Regional dialect variation in the vowel systems of typically developing children. *Journal of Speech, Language, and Hearing Research*, *54*(2), 448–470. https://doi.org/10.1044/1092-4388(2010/10-0161)

James, D., van Doorn, J. A., & McLeod, S. (2001). Vowel production in mono-, di- and polysyllabic words in children aged 3;0 to 7;11 years. In L. Wilson & S. Hewat (Eds.), *Evidence and innovation: Proceedings of the 2001 speech pathology australia national conference* (pp. 127–135). Speech Pathology Australia.

Jamieson, D. G., & Rvachew, S. (1992). Remediation of speech production errors with sound identification training. *Journal of Speech-Language Pathology and Audiology*, *16*(3), 201–210. https://cjslpa.ca/files/1992_JSLPA_Vol_16/No_03_177-250/Jamieson_Rvachew_JSLPA_1992.pdf

Kaufman, N. (2005). *Kaufman speech praxis workout book*. Northern Speech Services.

Kent, R. D., & Rountrey, C. (2020). What acoustic studies tell us about vowels in developing and disordered speech. *American Journal of Speech-Language Pathology*, *29*(3), 1749–1778. https://doi.org/10.1044/2020_AJSLP-19-00178

Khan, L. M. L., & Lewis, N. P. (2015). *Khan-Lewis. Phonological analysis* (3rd ed.). Pearson.

Lancaster, G. (1991). The effectiveness of parent administered input training for children with phonological disorders. Unpublished Master's thesis, City University, London.

Lancaster, G., Levin, A., Pring, T., & Martin, S. (2010). Treating children with phonological prob-problems: Does an eclectic approach to therapy work? *International Journal of Language and Communication Disorders*, *45*(2), 174–181. https://doi.org/10.3109/13682820902818888

Lancaster, G., & Pope, L. (1989). *Working with children's phonology*. Winslow Press.

Levy, E., Leone, D., Moya-Gale, G., Hsu, S., Chen, W., & Ramig, L. (2016). Vowel intelligibility in children with and without dysarthria: An exploratory study. *Communication Disorders Quarterly*, *37*(3), 171–179. https://doi.org/10.1177/1525740115618917

Lof, G. L. (1996). Factors associated with speech-sound stimulability. *Journal of Communication Disorders*, *29*(4), 255–278. https://doi.org/10.1016/0021-9924(96)00013-5

Mackie, K. M. (2015). *Vowels and consonants: The relative effect of speech sound errors on intelligibility* (Unpublished master's thesis). University of Alberta. https://doi.org/10.7939/R3WM14024

Markides, A. (1970). The speech of deaf and partially-hearing children with special reference to factors affecting intelligibility. *International Journal of Language & Communication Disorders*, *5*(2), 126–139. https://doi.org/10.3109/13682827009011511

Masso, S., McLeod, S., Baker, E., & McCormack, J. (2016). Polysyllable productions in preschool children with speech sound disorders: Error categories and the framework of polysyllable maturity. *International Journal of Speech-Language Pathology*, *18*(3), 272–287. https://doi.org/10.3109/17549507.2016.1168483

McAllister Byun, T., Campbell, H., Carey, H., Liang, W., Park, T. H., & Svirsky, M. (2017). Enhancing intervention for residual rhotic errors via app-delivered biofeedback: A case study. *Journal of Speech-Language-Hearing Research*, *60*(6S), 1810–1817. https://doi.org/10.1044/2017_JSLHR-S-16-0248

McCurry, W. H., & Irwin, O. C. (1953). A study of word approximations in the spontaneous speech of infants. *Journal of Speech and Hearing Disorders*, *18*(2), 133–139. https://doi.org/10.1044/jshd.1802.133

McReynolds, L., & Jetzke, E. (1986). Articulation generalization of voiced-voiceless sounds in hearing-impaired children. *Journal of Speech and Hearing Disorders*, *51*(4), 348–355. https://doi.org/10.1044/jshd.5104.348

Miccio, A. W. (2002). Clinical problem solving: Assessment of phonological disorders. *American Journal of Speech-Language Pathology*, *11*(3), 221–229. https://doi.org/10.1044/1058-0360(2002/023)

Miccio, A. W. (2005). A treatment program for enhancing stimulability. In A. G. Kamhi & K. E. Pollock (Eds.), *Phonological disorders in children: Clinical decision making in assessment and intervention* (pp. 163–173). Paul H. Brookes Publishing Co.

Miccio, A. W., & Elbert, M. (1996). Enhancing stimulability: A treatment program. *Journal of Communication Disorders*, *29*(4), 335–352. https://doi.org/10.1016/0021-9924(96)00016-0

Miccio, A. W., Elbert, M., & Forrest, K. (1999). The relationship between stimulability and phonological acquisition in children with normally developing and disordered phonologies. *American Journal of Speech-Language Pathology*, *8*(4), 347–363. https://doi.org/10.1044/1058-0360.0804.347

Milisen, R. (1954). A rationale for articulation disorders. *Journal of Speech and Hearing Disorders*. (Monograph supplement), *4*, 6–17, ASHA.

Monsen, R. (1976). Normal and reduced phonological space: The production of English vowels by deaf adolescents. *Journal of Phonetics*, *4*(3), 189–198. https://doi.org/10.1016/s0095-4470(19)31243-4

Mota, H. B., Bagetti, T., Keske-Soares, M., & Pereira, L. F. (2005). Generalizatio n based on implicational relationships in subjects treated with phonological therapy. *Pro-Fono Revista de Atualizacao Cientifica, Barucri (SP)*, *17*(1), 99–110. PMID: 15835574

Mota, H. B., Keske-Soares, M., Bagetti, T., Ceron, M. I., & Melo Filha, M. G. C. (2007). Comparative analyses of the effectiveness of three different phonological therapy models. *Pro-Fono Revista de Atualizacao Cientifica, Barucri (SP)*, *19*(1), 67–74. https://doi.org/10.1590/S0104-56872007000100008

Müller, N., & Damico, J. (2002). A transcription toolkit: Theoretical and clinical considerations. *Clinical Linguistics & Phonetics*, *16*(5), 299–316. https://doi.org/10.1080/02699200210135901

Munson, B., Baylis, A., Krause, M., & Yim, D.-S. (2006). Representation and access in phonological impairment. *Paper presented at the 10th Conference on Laboratory Phonology*, Paris, France, June 30-July 2.

Munson, B., Edwards, J., & Beckman, M. E. (2005). Relationships between nonword repetition accuracy and other measures of linguistic development in children with phonological disorders. *Journal of Speech, Language, and Hearing Research*, *48*(1), 61–78. https://doi.org/10.1044/1092-4388(2005/006)

Munson, B., Edwards, J., Schellinger, S., Beckman, M., & Meyer, M. (2010). Deconstructing phonetic transcription: Covert contrast, perceptual bias, and an extraterrestrial view of *Vox Humana*. *Clinical Linguistics & Phonetics*, *24*(4–5), 245–260. https://doi.org/10.3109/02699200903532524

Namasivayam, A. K., Huynh, A., Granata, F., Law, V., & van Lieshout, P. (2021). PROMPT intervention for children with severe speech motor delay: A randomized control trial. *Pediatric Research*, *89*(3), 613–621. https://doi.org/10.1038/s41390-020-0924-4

Pagliarin, K. C., Mota, H. B., & Keske-Soares, M. (2009). Therapeutic efficacy analysis of three contrastive approach phonological models. *Pró-Fono Revista de Atualização Científica*, *21*(4), 297–302. https://doi.org/10.1590/s0104-56872009000400006

Penney, G., Fee, E. J., & Dowdle, C. (1994). Vowel assessment and remediation: A case study. *Child Language Teaching & Therapy*, *10*(1), 47–66. https://doi.org/10.1177/026565909401000103

Peterson, L., Savarese, C., Campbell, T., Ma, Z., Simpson, K. O., & McAllister, T. (2022). Telepractice treatment of residual rhotic errors using app-based biofeedback: A pilot study. *Language, Speech, and Hearing Services in Schools*, *53*(2), 256–274. https://doi.org/10.1044/2021_LSHSS-21-00084

Pollock, K. E. (1991). Identification of vowel errors using traditional articulation or phonological process test stimuli. *Language, Speech, & Hearing Services in Schools, 22,* 39–50. https://doi.org/10.1044/0161-1461.2202.39

Pollock, K. E. (1994). Assessment and remediation of vowel misarticulations. *Clinics in Communication Disorders, 4*(1), 23–37. PMID: 8019549.

Pollock, K. E. (2002). Identification of vowel errors: Methodological issues and preliminary data from the Memphis Vowel Project. In M. J. Ball & F. E. Gibbon (Eds.), *Vowel disorders* (pp. 83–113). Butterworth-Heinemann.

Pollock, K. E. (2013). The Memphis Vowel Project: Vowel errors in children with and without phonological disorders. In M. J. Ball & F. E. Gibbon (Eds). (2013). *Handbook of vowels and vowel disorders* (2nd ed., pp. 260–287). Psychology Press. https://doi.org/10.4324/9780203103890.ch10

Pollock, K. E., & Berni, M. (2001). Transcription of vowels. *Topics in Language Disorders, 21*(4), 22–40. https://doi.org/10.1097/00011363-200121040-00005

Pollock, K. E., & Berni, M. C. (2003). Incidence of non-rhotic vowel errors in children: Data from the Memphis Vowel Project. *Clinical Linguistics & Phonetics, 17*(4–5), 393–401. https://doi.org/10.1080/0269920031000079949

Powell, T. W., Elbert, M., & Dinnsen, D. A. (1991). Stimulability as a factor in the phonological generalization of misarticulating preschool children. *Journal of Speech and Hearing Research, 34*(6), 1318–1328. https://doi.org/10.1044/jshr.3406.1318

Powell, T. W., Elbert, M., Miccio, A. W., Strike-Roussos, C., & Brasseur, J. (1998). Facilitating [s] production in young children: An experimental evaluation of motoric and conceptual treatment approaches. *Clinical Linguistics and Phonetics, 12*(2), 127–146. https://doi.org/10.3109/02699209808985217

Powell, T. W., & Miccio, A. W. (1996). Stimulability: A useful clinical tool. *Journal of Communication Disorders, 29*(4), 237–253. https://doi.org/10.1016/0021-9924(96)00012-3

Prezas, R. F., & Hodson, B.W. (2010). The cycles phonological remediation approach. In A. L. Williams, S. McLeod, & R. J. McCauley (Eds.), *Interventions for speech sound disorders in children.* Paul H. Brookes.

Pye, C., Ingram, D., & List, H. (1987). A comparison of initial consonant acquisition in English and Quiche. In K. E. Nelson & A. Van Kleek (Eds.), *Children's language,* Chapter 8 Erlbaum. http://dx.doi.org/10.4324/9781315792668-8

Rauscher, F. B., Krauss, R. M., & Chen, Y. (1996). Gesture, speech, and lexical access: The role of lexical movements in speech production. *Psychological Science, 7*(4), 226–231. https://doi.org/10.1111%2Fj.1467-9280.1996.tb00364.x

Rescorla, L., & Bernstein Ratner, N. (1996). Phonetic profiles of typically developing and language delayed toddlers. *Journal of Speech and Hearing Research, 39*(1), 153–165. https://doi.org/10.1044/jshr.3901.153

Reynolds, J. (2013). Recurring patterns and idiosyncratic systems in some English children with vowel disorders. In M. J. Ball & F. E. Gibbon (Eds.), *Handbook of vowels and vowel disorders* (2nd ed., pp. 229–259). Psychology Press. https://doi.org/10.4324/9780203103890.ch9

Robb, M. P., Bleile, K. M., & Yee, S. S. L. (1999). A phonetic analysis of vowel errors during the course of treatment. *Clinical Linguistics and Phonetics, 13*(4), 309–321. https://doi.org/10.1080/026992099299103

Roepke, E., Bower, K., Miller, C., & Brosseau-Lapré, F. (2020). The speech "bamana": Using the syllable repetition task to identify underlying phonological deficits in children with speech and language impairments. *Journal of Speech, Language, and Hearing Research, 63*(7), 2229–2244. https://doi.org/10.1044/2020_jslhr-20-00027

Roepke, E., & Brosseau-Lapré, F. (2021). Vowel errors produced by preschool-age children on a single-word test of articulation. *Clinical Linguistics & Phonetics, 35*(12), 1161–1183. https://doi.org/10.1080/02699206.2020.1869834

Rvachew, S. (1994). Speech perception training can facilitate sound production learning. *Journal of Speech and Hearing Research, 37*(2), 347–357. https://doi.org/10.1044/jshr.3702.347

Rvachew, S. (2005a). Phonetic factors in phonology intervention. In A. G. Kamhi & K. E. Pollock (Eds.), *Phonological disorders in children: Assessment and intervention* (pp. 175–188). Paul Brookes Publishers.

Rvachew, S. (2005b). Stimulability and treatment success. *Topics in Language Disorders, 25*(3), 207–219.

Rvachew, S. (2007a). Perceptual foundations of speech acquisition. In S. McLeod (Ed.), *International guide to speech acquisition* (pp. 26–30). Thomson Delmar Learning.

Rvachew, S. (2007b). Phonological processing and reading in children with speech sound disorders. *American*

Journal of Speech-Language Pathology, 16(3), 260–270. https://doi.org/10.1044/1058-0360(2007/030)

Rvachew, S., & Brosseau-Lapré, F. (2015). A randomized trial of 12-week interventions for the treatment of developmental phonological disorder in francophone children. *American Journal of Speech-Language Pathology, 24*(4), 637–658. https://doi.org/10.1044/2015_AJSLP-14-0056

Rvachew, S., & Nowak, M. (2001). The effect of target-selection strategy of phonological learning. *Journal of Speech, Language and Hearing Research, 44*(3), 610–623. https://doi.org/10.1044/1092-4388(2001/050)

Rvachew, S., Nowak, M., & Cloutier, G. (2004). Effect of phonemic perception training on the speech production and phonological awareness skills of children with expressive phonological delay. *American Journal of Speech-Language Pathology, 13*(3), 250–263. https://doi.org/10.1044/1058-0360(2004/026)

Rvachew, S., Rafaat, S., & Martin, M. (1999). Stimulability, speech perception and the treatment of phonological disorders. *American Journal of Speech-Language Pathology, 8*(1), 33–43. https://doi.org/10.1044/1058-0360.0801.33

Saben, C. B., & Ingham, J. C. (1991). The effects of minimal pairs treatment on the speech-sound production of two children with phonologic disorders. *Journal of Speech and Hearing Research, 34*(5), 1023–1040. https://doi.org/10.1044/jshr.3405.1023

Schmidt, A. M., & Meyers, K. A. (1995). Traditional and phonological treatment for teaching English fricatives and affricates to Koreans. *Journal of Speech and Hearing Research, 38*(4), 828–838. https://doi.org/10.1044/jshr.3804.828

Schmidt, R. A., Lee, T. D., Winstein, C. J., Wulf, G., & Zelaznik, H. N. (2019). *Motor control and learning: A behavioral emphasis* (6th ed.). Human Kinetics Europe Ltd.

Sherman, D., & Geith, A. (1967). Speech sound discrimination and articulation skill. *Journal of Speech and Hearing Research, 10*(2), 277–280. https://doi.org/10.1044/jshr.1002.277

Shriberg, L. D. (1975). A response evocation program for /ɚ/. *Journal of Speech and Hearing Disorders, 40*(1), 92–105. https://doi.org/10.1044/jshd.4001.92

Shriberg, L. D., & Kwiatkowski, J. (1980). *Natural process analysis*. Academic Press.

Shriberg, L. D., & Kwiatkowski, J. (1982). Phonological disorders II: A conceptual framework for management. *Journal of Speech and Hearing Disorders, 47*(3), 242–256. https://doi.org/10.1044/jshd.4703.242

Shuster, L., Ruscello, D., & Toth, A. (1995). The use of visual feedback to elicit correct /r/. *American Journal of Speech-Language Pathology, 4*(2), 37–44. https://doi.org/10.1044/1058-0360.0402.37

Shuster, L. I. (1998). The perception of correctly and incorrectly produced /r/. *Journal of Speech, Language, and Hearing Research, 41*(4), 941–950. https://doi.org/10.1044/jslhr.4104.941

Sloos, M., García, A. A., Andersson, A., & Neijmeijer, M. (2019). Accent-induced bias in linguistic transcriptions. *Language Sciences, 76*, 101176. https://doi.org/10.1016/j.langsci.2018.06.002

Sommers, R. K., Leiss, R. H., Delp, M., Gerber, A., Fundrella, D., Smith, R., Revucky, M., Ellis, D., & Haley, V. (1967). Factors related to the effectiveness of articulation therapy for kindergarten, first and second grade children. *Journal of Speech and Hearing Research, 10*(3), 428–437. https://doi.org/10.1044/jshr.1003.428

Speake, J. (2013). *Children with persisting speech difficulties: Exploring speech production and intelligibility across different contexts* (Publication No. 10660775) [Doctoral dissertation, University of Sheffield]. ProQuest Dissertations & Theses Global. https://etheses.whiterose.ac.uk/21867

Speake, J., Howard, S., & Vance, M. (2011). Intelligibility in children with persisting speech disorders: A case study. *Journal of Interactional Research in Communication Disorders, 2*(1), 131–151. https://doi.org/10.1558/jircd.v2i1.131

Speake, J., Stackhouse, J., & Pascoe, M. (2012). Vowel targeted intervention for children with persisting speech difficulties: Impact on intelligibility. *Child Language Teaching and Therapy, 28*(3), 277–295. http://doi.org/10.1177/0265659012453463

Stoel-Gammon, C. (1990). Issues in phonological development and disorders. In J. Miller (Ed.), *Progress in research on child language disorders*. Pro-Ed.

Stoel-Gammon, C., & Herrington, P. (1990). Vowel systems of normally developing and phonologically disordered children. *Clinical Linguistics & Phonetics, 4*(2), 145–160. https://doi.org/10.3109/02699209008985478

Storkel, H. L. (2022). Minimal, maximal, or multiple: Which contrastive intervention approach to use with children with speech sound disorders? *Language, Speech, and Hearing Services in Schools, 53*(3), 632–645. https://doi.org/10.1044/2021_LSHSS-21-00105

Sugden, E., Baker, E., Munro, N., Williams, A. L., & Trivette, C. M. (2018). An Australian survey of parent involvement in intervention for childhood speech sound disorders. *International Journal of Speech-Language Pathology*, *20*(7), 766–778. https://doi.org/10.1080/17549507.2017.1356936

Sugden, E., Baker, E., Williams, A. L., Munro, N., & Trivette, C. M. (2020). Evaluation of parent and speech-language pathologist delivered multiple oppositions intervention for children with phonological impairment: A multiple-baseline design. *American Journal of Speech-Language Pathology*, *29*(1), 111–126. https://doi.org/10.1044/2019_AJSLP-18-0248

Sugden, E., Munro, N., Trivette, C. M., Baker, E., & Williams, A. L. (2019). Parents' experiences of completing home practice for speech sound disorders. *Journal of Early Intervention*, *41*(2), 159–181. https://doi.org/10.1177%2F105381511982 8409

Sutherland, D., & Gillon, G. T. (2007). The development of phonological representations and phonological awareness in children with speech impairment. *International Journal of Language and Communication Disorders*, *14*(2), 229–250. https://doi.org/10.1080/13682820600806672

Titterington, J., & Bates, S. (2021). Teaching and learning clinical phonetic transcription. In M. J. Ball (Ed.), *Manual of clinical phonetics* (pp. 175–186). Routledge.

Topbaş, S., & Ünal, Ö. (2010). An alternating treatment comparison of minimal and maximal opposition sound selection in Turkish phonological disorders. *Clinical Linguistics and Phonetics*, *24*(8), 646–668. https://doi.org/10.3109/02699206.2010.486464

Travis, L. E. (1931). *Speech pathology: A dynamic neurological treatment of normal speech and speech deviations*. D. Appleton Co.

Tyler, A. A. (1995). Durational analysis of stridency errors in children with phonological impairment. *Clinical Linguistics and Phonetics*, *9*(3), 211–228. https://doi.org/10.3109/02699209508985333

Tyler, A. A., Edwards, M. L., & Saxman, J. H. (1987). Clinical application of two phonologically based treatment procedures. *Journal of Speech and Hearing Disorders*, *52*(4), 393–409. https://doi.org/10.1044/jshd.5204.393

Tyler, A. A., Edwards, M. L., & Saxman, J. H. (1990). Acoustic validation of phonological knowledge and its relationship to treatment. *Journal of Speech and Hearing Disorders*, *55*(2), 251–261. https://doi.org/10.1044/jshd.5502.251

Tyler, A. A., & Figurski, G. R. (1994). Phonetic inventory changes after treating distinctions along an implicational hierarchy. *Clinical Linguistics & Phonetics*, *8*(2), 91–107. https://doi.org/10.3109/02699209408985299

Tyler, A. A., Figurski, G. R., & Langsdale, T. (1993). Relationships between acoustically determined knowledge of stop place and voicing contrasts and phonological treatment progress. *Journal of Speech and Hearing Research*, *36*(4), 746–759. https://doi.org/10.1044/jshr.3604.746

Van Riper, C. (1963). *Speech correction: Principles and methods*. Prentice Hall.

Van Riper, C. (1978). *Speech correction: Principles and methods* (6th ed.). Prentice-Hall.

Van Riper, C., & Irwin, J. V. (1958). *Voice and articulation*. Prentice Hall.

Vaughn, A., & Pollock, K. E. (1997, November). The relative contribution of vowel and consonant errors to intelligibility. *Presentation at the Annual Convention of the American Speech-Language-Hearing Association*, Boston, MA, United States.

Velleman, S. (2002). Phonotactic therapy. *Seminars in Speech and Language*, *23*(1), 43–57. https://doi.org/10.1055/s-2002-23510

Vuolo, J., & Goffman, L. (2020). Vowel accuracy and segmental variability differentiate children with developmental language disorder in nonword repetition. *Journal of Speech, Language, and Hearing Research*, *63*(12), 3945–3960. https://doi.org/10.1044/2020_jslhr-20-00166

Watson, M., Martineau, D., & Hughes, D. (1994). Vowel use of phonologically disordered identical twin boys: A case study. *Perceptual and Motor Sills*, *79*(3S), 1587–1597. https://doi.org/10.2466/pms.1994.79.3f.1587

Watt, D. (2013). Sociolinguistic variation in vowels. In M. J. Ball & F. E. Gibbon (Eds.), *Handbook of vowels and vowel disorders* (2nd ed., pp. 207–228). Psychology Press. https://doi.org/10.4324/9780203103890.ch8

Weiner, F. (1981a). Treatment of phonological disability using the method of meaningful contrast: Two case studies. *Journal of Speech and Hearing Disorders*, *46*(1), 97–103. https://doi.org/10.1044/jshd.4601.97

Weiner, F. (1981b). Systematic sound preference as a characteristic of phonological disability. *Journal of Speech and Hearing Disorders*, *46*(3), 281–286. https://doi.org/10.1044/jshd.4603.281

Williams, A. L. (1991). Generalization patterns associated with least knowledge. *Journal of Speech and Hearing Research*, *34*, 722–733. https://doi.org/10.1044/jshr.3404.733

Williams, A. L. (2000a). Multiple oppositions: Theoretical foundations for an alternative contrastive intervention approach. *American Journal of Speech-Language Pathology*, *9*(4), 282–288. https://doi.org/10.1044/1058-0360.0904.282

Williams, A. L. (2000b). Multiple oppositions: Case studies of variables in Phonological intervention. *American Journal of Speech-Language Pathology*, *9*(4), 289–299. https://doi.org/10.1044/1058-0360.0904.289

Williams, A. L. (2001). Phonological assessment of child speech. In D. M. Ruscello (Ed.), *Tests and measurements in speech-language pathology* (pp. 31–76). Butterworth-Heinemann.

Williams, A. L. (2003). *Speech disorders: Resource guide for preschool children*. Thomson Delmar Learning.

Williams, A. L. (2005). Assessment, target selection, and intervention: Dynamic interactions within a systemic perspective. *Topics in Language Disorders*, *25*(3), 231–242. https://doi.org/10.1097/00011363-200507000-00006

Williams, A. L. (2006a). *Sound contrasts in phonology (SCIP)*. Super Duper.

Williams, A. L. (2006b). A systemic perspective for assessment and intervention: A case study. *Advances in Speech-Language Pathology*, *8*(3), 245–256. https://doi.org/10.1080/14417040600823292

Williams, A. L. (2010). Multiple oppositions intervention. In A. L. Williams, S. McLeod, & R. J. McCauley (Eds.), *Interventions for speech sound disorders in children* (pp. 73–94). Paul H. Brookes Publishing Co.

Williams, A. L. (2012). Intensity in phonological intervention: Is there a prescribed amount? *International Journal of Speech-Language Pathology*, *14*(5), 456–461. https://doi.org/10.3109/17549507.2012.688866

Williams, A. L. (2016). SCIP 2: Sound contrasts in phonology 2 (1.0) [Mobile application software]. https://itunes.apple.com

Williams, A. L. (2017, May 1). Sound proof: What's the evidence on target selection for speech sound disorders? Medbridge Blog. https://www.medbridgeeducation.com/blog/2017/05/sound-proof-whats-evidence-target-selection-speech-sound-disorders

Williams, A. L. (2019, February 1). Linguistic detectives: Systemic phonological analysis of child speech. Medbridge blog. https://www.medbridgeeducation.com/blog/2019/02/linguistic-detectives-systemic-honological-analysis-of-child-speech

Williams, A. L., McLeod, S., & McCauley, R. J. (Eds.). (2021). *Interventions for speech sound disorders in children* (2nd ed.). Paul H. Brookes Publishing Co.

Williams, A. L. & Sugden, E. (2021). Multiple oppositions intervention. In A. L. Williams, S. McLeod, & R. J. McCauley (Eds.). *Interventions for speech sound disorders in children* (2nd ed., pp. 1689–361). Brookes Publishing Co.

Chapter 5
More Intervention Approaches

Expose the child systematically to the dimensions of the target system absent from his or her speech in a way in which both their form and communicative functions are made evident.

Grunwell, 1989

Chapter 5 contains Grunwell's guidelines for phonological therapy, and accounts of Auditory Input Therapy, Naturalistic Recast Intervention, Metaphon, Imagery Therapy, Whole Language Therapy, Parents and Children Together (PACT), Core Vocabulary Therapy, Psycholinguistic Intervention (Schäfer & Fricke A21), and Phonological Awareness Intervention for Children with SSD (McNeill, A22).

Grunwell's Guidelines for Phonological Therapy

British Linguist Pamela Grunwell drew on David Stampe's natural phonology theory (Stampe, 1969, 1973, 1979) identifying phonological processes as *the* key aspect of speech assessment (Grunwell, 1975, 1985a, 1987). In influential work, she proposed treatment based on the principle that homophony

motivates phonemic change, describing four main types of change that might become a clinician's focus in target selection and intervention:

1. **Stabilization**: the resolution of a variable pronunciation pattern into a stable one.
2. **Destabilization**: the disruption of a stable pattern, resulting in variability.
3. **Innovation**: the introduction of a new pattern.
4. **Generalization**: the transfer of a pronunciation pattern across four possible contexts: phonological, lexical, syntactic, and socioenvironmental.

In selecting targets, Grunwell advised working in developmental sequence where possible, prioritizing patterns most deviant from normal phonology and/or prioritizing those most destructive of communicative adequacy. There was no attempt to increase the saliency of contrasts. Systemic feature contrasts were minimal (e.g., *fan* vs. *van*; *comb* vs. *cone*) and structural contrasts near minimal (e.g., *top* vs. *stop*; *Ben* vs. *bend*). The (unexplained) grounds for this was that with small feature difference between the target and the error, '*there was nothing else to get in the way*'. Clinicians tended to accept, unquestioningly, the notion that

Children's Speech Sound Disorders, Third Edition. Caroline Bowen.
© 2023 John Wiley & Sons Ltd. Published 2023 by John Wiley & Sons Ltd.

something *might* 'get in the way' if there were more than one feature difference within a word pair. I am still thinking about that idea.

In Grunwell's intervention approach, the procedures used are systemic, or what Grunwell called **system-based** (metalinguistic) or word based (**manipulative**). Meaningful minimal pair therapy was conceptualized as a metalinguistic method that showed a child that sound differences signal meaning differences; so in practice, it involved metaphonological procedures. A manipulative procedure might involve listening to, and eventually saying in context, words with common phonetic or phonotactic features (e.g., all with fricatives SIWI, or all with stops SFWF). Grunwell advised incorporating into intervention a variety of tasks and games that involved auditory discrimination, meaningful minimal pairs, and near-minimal pair games, homophony confrontation, phoneme–grapheme correspondences, and metaphonological processes.

Grunwell (1981) considered the therapy suitable for children with mild through to severe 'phonological disability' but see Storkel (2022) who advises that conventional minimal pairs should be confined to children with few errors. Typically, these are children with mild SSD and older children with a few persistent (or 'residual') errors.

The sweeping influence of Grunwell's innovative research, pedagogy, and her so-called phonological principles is apparent in Auditory Input Therapy (Flynn & Lancaster, 1996), Multiple Oppositions Intervention (Williams, A19), Phoneme Awareness Therapy (Hesketh, 2004, 2010; Hesketh et al., 2000, 2007; McNeill, A22; McNeill & Hesketh, 2010); contrastive Vowel Intervention (e.g., Gibbon & Mackenzie Beck, 2002; Gibbon et al., 1992; Gibbon, 2013; Pollock, A20; Speake et al., 2012), PACT (Bowen & Cupples, 1999a, 1999b), and *Metaphon* (e.g., Dean et al., 1995).

Auditory Input, and Naturalistic Recast Intervention

Auditory Input Therapy: AIT (Flynn & Lancaster, 1996; Lancaster et al., 2010; Lancaster & Pope, 1989), and Naturalistic Recast Intervention (Camarata, 2021) formerly called Naturalistic Intervention for Speech Intelligibility and Speech Accuracy (Camarata, 2010) are broadly similar. Both involve devising attractive games and tasks, often called 'thematic play', during which the client is exposed, *in input*, to multiple 'repetitions' of sound or word targets, spoken by the adult. The child is not required to say the sounds or words (e.g., no production drill) but spontaneous production attempts are reinforced by the SLP/SLT.

Usually administered as a component of an 'eclectic therapy' approach (Lancaster et al., 2010) AIT is not a total 'therapy package' (Lancaster, 2015). In practice, AIT incorporates both Conventional Minimal Pair therapy and metalinguistic activities. I am indebted to Gwen Lancaster, who contributed to the first and second editions of this book, for the information in the following section.

Auditory Input Therapy (AIT)

Evolving from clinical practice with three-to-six-year-olds with speech impairment, AIT was developed in the mid-1980s in the UK.

Assessment and Target Selection

Assessment involves independent and relational analysis (Stoel-Gammon, A8; Stoel-Gammon & Dunn, 1985), including contrastive assessment (Grunwell, 1985a). Target selection is based on the assessment findings and is largely founded on developmental norms (e.g., those proposed by Dodd et al., 2002), so that for English-learning children /p/, /b/, and the nasals, are selected before sounds and structures that are later in typical acquisition. Appropriate normative expectations are considered for speakers of languages other than English (Lancaster, 2015).

Theoretical Rationale

AIT was inspired in part by the 'AB' ('auditory bombardment') component of the Cycles Phonological Pattern Approach (Prezas et al., A5) as described by Hodson and Paden (1983), and later dubbed 'focused auditory input' (Hodson, 2007). AIT centres on the child listening to rather than producing speech, helping to increase the information the child has (and needs) about the speech sound system via repeated, intense auditory models delivered naturalistically.

Lancaster (2015) felt that the Velleman and Vihman (2002) account of typical language learners unconsciously registering, and implicitly acquiring, the features of their language or languages, by listening, provided a solid theoretical rationale for the effects of AIT. She pointed out that at least some children with SSD gain from intense exposure to wisely selected targets that are germane for them. This facilitates acquisition of new syllable structures, phones, and contrasts (Lancaster et al., 2010).

Implementation with Individuals or Groups of up to Six Three-to-six-year-olds

In implementing AIT, Lancaster followed Grunwell's guidelines (1985a, 1985b; and see above) and Hodson and Paden (1991). Lancaster (2015) recommended that the AIT activities be carried out daily at home or in educational settings for 5 or 10 minutes, at least once daily. Different people could play the games with the child, and siblings, friends and peers could join in. Treatment dose – the number of teaching episodes in one session – was unspecified. The AIT activities, delivered individually or in groups of up to six three-to-six-year-olds, are based around:

- **Topics**, for example, things found outside such as *stick*, *rock*, and *bike* to target final /k/.
- **Semantic groups**, for example, foods, such as *bean*, *burger*, and *bun* to target initial /b/.
- **Stories**, for example, a story about a 'sad seal' in the 'sea' to target initial /s/.

Such activities may be used to target language and/or speech goals (Ellis Weismer et al., 2017).

Regarding *speech* activities, materials for most consonants are provided in Flynn and Lancaster (1996), and there is ample scope for SLPs/SLTs and caregivers to devise novel activities to target consonants, vowels, and syllable shapes according to individual children's intervention needs, and their interests. Indeed, AIT can be incorporated into *any* appealing pastime, which means that adults *can* – and in the case of 'reluctant candidates' for intervention, *must* – follow the child's lead in the choice of materials and activities (Girolametto & Weitzman, 2006).

Research Support

In her MSc research (Lancaster, 1991; Lancaster et al., 2010), Lancaster compared the speech progress of (1) a group receiving once-weekly parent delivered AIT, (2) a deferred-treatment control group, and (3) a group receiving 15 half-hour therapy sessions of clinician-delivered eclectic intervention with full parental participation, over six months. The setting was a National Health Service (NHS) centre, and the participants were 15 three-and-four-year-olds with moderately to severely impaired speech (Hodson & Paden, 1983), referred to the service by health or education professionals, and randomly assigned to the three groups. Intervention extended for six months, followed by reassessment.

The parents assigned to Group 1 were provided two hours of group training using materials later published in Flynn and Lancaster (1996). They were then supplied with materials to carry out AIT activities once weekly for six weeks. The activities addressed each child's speech targets determined via contrastive assessment (Grunwell, 1985a). At the end of each 6-week period, Lancaster met with each child's parent(s) to discuss progress and set new targets. To evaluate the effectiveness of parental intervention only, the child was not included in these meetings but was seen for reassessment after the 6-month treatment phase. The children in Groups 1 and 3 improved significantly more than those in Group 2, in terms of their percentage of occurrence of speech error patterns in a citation naming test of 55 words: 41 from the *Edinburgh Articulation Test* (Anthony et al., 1971) and 14 additional words. The results of this and other studies indicate that therapy directly involving both clinicians and parents or caregivers is the most effective (Lancaster et al., 2010). Lancaster (2015, p. 187) commented, '*Although intervention by caregivers alone may not be the most **effective** therapy, it can be used **efficiently**. My small study (*Lancaster, 1991*) demonstrated that the children who received AIT made significantly more progress than children who received no therapy, suggesting that AIT may provide a partial solution in situations where **long waiting lists**, unmanageable caseloads or gaps in provision exist.*' See McGill et al. (2020) for insights into parents' views on waiting times for services, where '*many wasted months*' in the title speaks volumes.

Naturalistic Recast Intervention

Like Auditory Input Therapy, described above, Naturalistic Recast Intervention for speech intelligibility and speech accuracy is an input-oriented, or focused stimulation procedure. It was developed by Stephen Camarata (Camarata, 1993), for children who have difficulty engaging in imitation-based and drill-based approaches by virtue of their ages, primary diagnosis, or both (Camarata, 2010). There are three intended populations for the approach:

1. **Primary:** Any individual with a severe SSD; and very young children – toddlers and some pre-schoolers – who are not amenable to direct instruction (Camarata, 2021).
2. **Secondary:** Children with complex communication needs, such as those with Down syndrome (Camarata et al., 2006; Yoder et al., 2016), and those with autism (Smith & Camarata, 1999).
3. **Tertiary:** Children who stutter, noting that imitation and drill might aggravate their dysfluency (Louko et al., 1999; Unicomb et al., 2013) or distress them.

The fundamental goal of Naturalistic Recast Intervention is to improve children's comprehensibility and speech intelligibility rather than the usual goal of speech treatments which is to improve speech accuracy. Its aim is to raise the number of utterances that the child's listeners can understand. The intervention occurs within naturalistic, child-directed contexts where children's verbal initiations are met with conversational recasts, or 'broad target recasts' containing words with the child's target speech sound or sounds. Importantly, while the activities used are child-directed, the therapist 'influences' the activities to facilitate frequent opportunities for the child to hear the target(s), and this takes considerable skill.

Meet Hamish, 6;0 who has Down syndrome, and who consistently stops /ʃ/, replacing it with [d], calling himself ['heɪˌnɪd]. He enters the therapy room for his session and immediately spots a temptingly positioned row of 10 sheep figurines that his SLP/SLT has 'harvested' from farm animal sets. They are out of his reach atop a cabinet. Alongside the sheep he can see clip-together plastic fences and gates, a small bowl of water, a sponge, and a shoebox labelled 'sheep shed'. The clinician knows Hamish loves sheep and waits for him to initiate an unprompted utterance.

Hamish: *Sheep* [diːp] (Points to the line-up of sheep) *sheep me?*

SLP/SLT: You do like *sheep, Hamish!*

Hamish: *Sheep* me. Sheep *Hamish* (['diːp 'heɪˌnɪd]).

SLP/SLT: You want a *sheep, Hamish.* Here you go! One *sheep* for *Hamish!*

Hamish: (takes it and points to the remaining nine) *Sheep* me?

SLP/SLT: Another *sheep* for you? (Hands one to him) Now your *sheep* has a friend.

Hamish (bouncing on his bottom, pointing at the sheep): *Sheep-sheep-sheep, Hamish!*

SLP/SLT: I think you want ALL the *sheep, Hamish*? *Shall* I get them down?

Hamish: *Sheep, sheep, sheep, Hamish. Yes please!*

SLP/SLT: *Sure.* Do the *sheep* need a *sheep shed*?

Hamish: *Sheep shed* [diːp dɛd]

SLP/SLT: (hands him the 'shed', fences and gates, sponge, and water) Here.

Hamish: *Wash sheep?* [wɒdiːp] *Wash sheep* me?

SLP/SLT: (had planned for the water to be sheep-dip but followed his lead) *Sure.*

Hamish: *Wash sheep* me. ['wɒtʃˌip 'mi] (the SLP/SLT makes a note)

SLP/SLT: Where *should* we put the *sheep* when they've had a *wash*? In the *shed*?

Hamish: *Shed. Sheep shed.* Clean *sheep* go in *shed.* Dirty *sheep* NOT go in.

SLP/SLT: Let's *shut* them in the *sheep* pen to wait for their *wash.*

(The clinician and Hamish set about assembling a fence to encircle the waiting sheep)

SLP/SLT: Which *sheep should* have the first *wash*?

Hamish: *Wash sheep* me. This *sheep* now. ['wɒtʃˌip 'mi ‖ dɪʔ'diːp ˌnau]

SLP/SLT: This *sheep* first? (The clinician mimes washing a sheep). *Wash* the sheep!

Hamish: *Wash* the *sheep, wash* the *sheep.* Come here *sheep*, you got so dirty face.

(Hamish spits on his finger and rubs the sheep's face, then puts his hand in the water)

(The clinician shows him how to dampen the sponge)

Hamish (scrubs a sheep with the sponge):   Good boy *sheep*. Clean face. Go *shed* now.

[Long pause while Hamish admires the sheep in the shed]

Hamish: This *sheep* cleanie beanie boy now!

SLP/SLT   Can he stay in the *sheep shed* now?

Hamish: Yes, he in *sheep shed*.

SLP/SLP: He needs friends in the *sheep shed*. Is it a boy *sheep* or girl *sheep* next?

Hamish: Them's all boy *sheeps*.

SLP/SLT: No *she-sheep*? Is their mummy here?

Hamish: Her at work. Her goed on the train. Them's ALL boy *sheeps*.

SLP/SLT: There's a lot of boy *sheep* waiting for a *wash*.

Hamish: Wait for *wash*. Wash, wash, wash. Then put in *shed*. Shh, my *sheep* in bed.

SLP/SLT: Did you say *shh*, Hamish?

Hamish: Yes. *Shh* ([ʃ]). I say *shh* ([ʃ]) for my *sheep* ([diːp])

SLP/SLT: Your *sheep* go to bed in the *sheep* shed?

Hamish: Yes. Where bed? Where *sheep* bed?

SLP/SLT: (Improvises quickly) They sleep on soft *tissues*. *Shh*, sleep tight, *sheep*.

Hamish: (Puts the sheep on a tissue covering it with another) *Shh*, cleanie boy *sheep*.

The SLP/SLT must be responsive to the child's output and nimble in deciding, on an utterance-by-utterance basis, whether to recast the phonetic content of what the child has just said, or to recast the grammar, or to provide an expansion. For example, when Hamish said, '*Him no like him lunch*' [ˈhɪˌnou ˈwaɪ ˌhɪn ˈwʌts] the clinician decided on the spot whether to recast:

1. '*He doesn't **like** his **lunch. Lunch**.*' or '*He doesn't **like** it. What do you **like** for **lunch**?*', (attending to whole-word phonetic production of *like* and *lunch*), or

2. '**He** doesn't like **his** lunch', (attending to grammar), or

3. '*Yes. He doesn't like it. He wants a different lunch*' (expanding the meaning).

In the process, care is taken not to combine speech recasts with sentence recasts, or speech recasts with expansions (Camarata et al., 2006; Yoder et al., 2016). This is because, speculatively, working on more than one domain simultaneously might be overwhelming for the child. Typically, the clinician would reserve expansions for the child's more intelligible utterances. So, for example, the relatively more comprehensible [ˌhɪm ˈheɪʔ ˌhɪmd ˈwʌts] with discrete word boundaries ('*Him hate him's lunch*') would be more likely to receive an expansion-response than the same comment pronounced [ˌhɪˈheɪʔ ˌhɪəˈwʌts] ('*He hate his lunch*').

Metaphon

Metaphon (Dean et al., 1990, 1995; Dean & Howell, 1986) is also based on the principle that homophony motivates phonemic change. Its theoretical base was greatly influenced by Grunwell (1981, 1982, 1985b, 1989, 1992) who was especially active in publishing her theoretical and research works while *Metaphon* was in development.

Using the assessment materials in the *Metaphon Resource Pack* (Dean et al., 1990), now out of print, the SLP/SLT performs a phonological analysis of the child's single-word production in a picture-naming task. Errors, treatment targets, and goals are specified in terms of phonological processes. Meaningful minimal pair picture-cards are constructed with the target contrasted with the child's customary production, as in Conventional Minimal Pair intervention (Weiner, 1981a). For example, to eliminate palatal fronting, the target /ʃ/ might be contrasted with its substitute, [s], in word pairs such as *ship–sip*, *shine–sign*, *show–sew*, *shell–sell*, *shower–sour*, *push–puss*, *mesh–mess*, *gash–gas* and *ash–ass*. Feature contrasts are usually, but not necessarily, minimal or near minimal.

Metaphon encompasses two overlapping treatment phases followed by a discrete final phase. Metaphonetic and metaphonological skills are trained to improve a child's 'cognitive awareness' of the properties of the sound system, and metalinguistic tasks are implemented to increase the child's communicative effectiveness through more successful use of repair strategies.

Metaphon Phase 1

In Phase 1, the child is taught that language is used to communicate and that language which is normally opaque can be made transparent. Phase 1 comprises four Levels: Concept, Sound, Phoneme, and Word. Phase 1 is considered by its developers to be the most important phase of *Metaphon*, and the one that distinguishes the approach from other published phonological therapies (Howell & Dean, 1994). The aim is to capture the child's interest in the phonology of the target language, to

1. Alert the child to the place, voice, and manner (PVM) properties of sounds, and their contrastive potential.
2. Show that contrasts between sounds convey meaning (e.g., that *'The bee is on the vine'* means something different from *'The bean is on the vine'*).
3. Help the child know that these properties can be manipulated to increase the probability of being understood.

Concept Level

At Concept Level, individual speech sounds are *not* contrasted, and the child learns a conceptual vocabulary to use later for PVM awareness tasks. Metaphors associated with voicing features are used: for example, Mr. Noisy or Mr. Growly to denote voiced consonants and Mr. Whisper or Mr. Quiet for voiceless ones. Other concepts, such as long sound vs. short sound (denoting fricative vs. stop) and back sound vs. front sound (velar vs. alveolar) are introduced, with the aim of having children identify sounds by their properties with 100% accuracy. The *Metaphon* team reported that it might not take long for children to achieve 100% accuracy.

The next step, Sound Level, is different depending on whether the targets are substitution processes (e.g., fronting, stopping, or gliding, where one sound replaces another) or syllable structure processes (e.g., cluster reduction, or final consonant deletion, where the structure of the syllable changes).

Substitution Processes

For substitution processes at **Sound Level**, the vocabulary the child has learned (Mr. Growly, Short Sound,

Long Sound etc.) is transferred to describing non-speech sounds: castanets, whistles, the therapist's vocalizations and animal and vehicle noises. The aim is to show the child that those environmental sounds and vocalizations can be classified as long–short, front–back and noisy–whisper (growly–quiet). Then, at **Phoneme Level**, entire sound classes are contrasted, using visual cues. For example, all fricatives vs. all stops are presented to the child, still referring to the sound properties (long–short, etc.). Next, the child enters **Word Level**, and minimally contrasted word pairs are introduced for *listening* (not production). The child judges whether a word has a long–short, front–back or noisy–whisper sound in it. Again, visual support is provided in the form of gesture cues and pictures. For example, the 'long sound' like the fricative /f/ might be accompanied by a picture of a can of aerosol hair spray, to represent the ff... sound it makes in use, or a l-o-n-g hand gesture, or both; and a 'short sound' like the stop /b/ with a stop sign picture or object, or an abrupt (short) hand gesture, or both.

Syllable Structure Processes

For syllable structure processes at **Sound Level**, concepts such as 'beginning', as a preparation for working on initial consonant deletion (ICD), and 'end', in preparation for addressing final consonant deletion (FCD), are introduced, as well as imagery and concrete demonstrations. For example, for cluster reduction SIWI, imagery coupled with a concrete demonstration might involve a train with one locomotive representing /ɹ/ vs. a train with two locomotives representing /tɹ/, in preparation for a near minimal pair such as *rip–trip* or *rap–trap*. At **Syllable Level** and **Word Level**, nonsense syllables vs. real words are contrasted (e.g., *hot* has an engine, *ot* does not).

Metaphon Phase 2

In Phase 2, metaphonological tasks involving minimal pairs (introduced in Phase 1) and homonymy confrontation are emphasized. Now, the focus shifts to developing communicative effectiveness, with the SLP/SLT providing feedback about success or failure to convey meaning, through behavioural responses, prompting the child to review output. Dean and Howell (1986) postulated that, in the short term, such feedback would improve production by triggering the use of repair strategies based on the new knowledge of sound contrasts learned in Phase 1, and that the long-term effect would be a change in central phonological processing. Phase 2 is concerned with developing phonological and communicative awareness, and the link between Phases 1 and 2 is achieved by merging Phase 1 activities into Phase 2. Phonological awareness and awareness speech sounds' PVM properties must be well developed before the core activity of Phase 2 can be successful.

Core Activity

In the *Metaphon* core activity, the clinician and child take turns to *produce* and *select* meaningful minimal pair words (e.g., *fin* vs. *bin*, *fall* vs. *ball*, *fun* vs. *bun*, *fight* vs. *bite*, *foal* vs. *bowl*) pictured on cards or worksheets. If the child says a target word, such as *fin*, correctly: (1) The therapist selects the correct word; (2) feedback is given; and (3) guided discussion occurs; for example, '*Yes. That was a long sound. I guess you know lots of other long sounds.*' If the child says the target word *incorrectly* (e.g., *bin* for *fin*): (1) The therapist selects the incorrect word (the one the child said); and (2) no feedback is given directly to the child, but attention is drawn to the sound property, for example, '*That was a short sound. Should it have been a long sound?*' The aim of the core activity is to have the child revise incorrect productions 'spontaneously'.

Metaphon Final Phase

In the final phase of *Metaphon*, minimal pair **sentences** are introduced. The therapist and child take turns, each instructing the other to, for example, 'Draw a *bin/fin* on the fish'; 'Draw a *bog/fog* on the farm'; 'Draw a *bone/phone* in the fridge'; 'Give the *bead/feed* to the foal'. Emphasis is still on guided discussion of sound properties ('Shouldn't *fin* have a long sound?') to facilitate the spontaneous use of repair.

Imagery Therapy

In Imagery Therapy (Klein, 1996a, 1996b), error and target are contrasted, and feature differences are usually minimal or near-minimal, so oppositions like *Sue–zoo*, *Sue–shoe*, or *Sue–soon*, *Sue–soup* are typical. Imagery terms (or imagery labels) for, and images (pictures) of phonetic characteristics are used to aid the child's learning of new phonological rules, and the rational for the approach is that homonymy motivates phonemic change. According to Klein (1996a) it is suitable for 'children with one or many phonological processes' with mild to severe SSD. The intervention proceeds in three steps.

Step 1: Identification and Production of the Contrast in Nonsense Syllables

Imagery terms or imagery labels are assigned to the 'intruder' (Klein's term for error) and sound class (target). For example, if the child stops fricatives, the stops (intruders) may be called poppies and fricatives (the sound class) may be called windys, and it must be conceded that participating parents can find this hilarious. The target and error (sound class and intruder) are combined with vowels to make CVs, representing the intruders (e.g., *pah*, *pee*, *paw*; *tah*, *tee*, *taw*) and target sound classes (e.g., *fah*, *fee*, *faw*; *sah*, *see*, *saw*; *shah*, *she*, *shaw*). The therapist produces a syllable (e.g., *paw*), and the child indicates (points to) the associated imagery term on a poppy's poster or a windy's poster (if the therapist says *paw*, the child should choose the poppy's poster). The child is then asked to produce a syllable containing a sound from each imagery class (e.g., '*Give me a poppy sound*' or '*Give me a windy sound*'). If the child is confused, the therapist provides a choice, usually with the target produced first: 'which one is windy, *faw* or *paw*?' Printed captions accompany all picture-and-object stimuli to support literacy acquisition. Note that the child is required to produce CVs and not isolated phones.

Step 2: Identification, Classification, and Production of Single-word Contrasts

Next, the therapist *shows* a picture or an object representing a real word containing either the intruder or the target, *says* the word and asks the child to indicate the imagery term associated with the word. For instance, the therapist says 'sail', and the child should respond correctly by placing the picture on the poster for 'windys' because the child knows that /s/ is 'windy'.

Then, the therapist *silently* shows a picture or object with either the intruder or target, and the child indicates the associated imagery term on one of the posters. By now, the clinician's production has been eliminated. The child draws on their internal representation to make the classification. Each treatment word is classified thus.

Following classification of a word, the child is asked to *produce* the word, keeping in mind the classification. For example, the child is shown a picture of *sail* and classifies it as 'a windy'. The clinician responds, 'That's right. Now make it with a windy sound'. Here, the child is told to say the target word, but *no model* is provided. The clinician responds to any errors in production by referring to the classification the child provided. For example, if the child said *tail* for *sail*, the therapist might say, '*Tail? You said it was a windy word, but you made it with a poppy sound. Can you try it again and put in the windy sound that you said it should have?*' Conventional Minimal Pair activities (Weiner, 1981a) with communicative consequences for using either the intruder or the target are *also* used at this level.

Throughout Step 1 and Step 2, isolated sounds are not elicited, and the clinician does not overtly model how to say the treatment words. For example, when eliciting g-words, the therapist might say, proffering a picture, '*Can you say this one with your throaty?*' Natural feedback is given if the child errs, perhaps by producing /d/ in place of /g/: '*But you said it was a throaty and you said it with a tippy. Try it again with your throaty?*'

Step 3: Production in Narratives and Conversational Speech

The procedures from this point onwards are quite 'traditional' and include activities such as storytelling, games incorporating the child's target sound classes and what Klein called controlled conversation tasks (like 'guided discussion' in *Metaphon*).

Whole Language Intervention

Whole Language Therapy (Hoffman, 1992; Hoffman & Norris, 2010; Tyler, 2002) is intended for children experiencing moderate to severe phonological issues and expressive language impairment concomitantly (McCauley, A15).

In a typical treatment session, targets might include question forms, personal pronouns and /h/ SIWI. The clinician reads to the child a book such as '*Are you my Mother?*' by Stan and Jan Berenstain, modelling the question form, pronouns and /h/ SIWI, especially in *he*, *his* and *her* that occur frequently in the story. Then, the therapist re-tells the story, starting with short utterances and progressively increasing their length. As the story is re-told, the child repeats each brief utterance and then, if able, tells the story again (perhaps to a puppet or doll).

Intervention takes place via conversational interactions and story contexts, incorporating cues, cloze sentences, rebus stories, story reading (to the child) and storytelling, to the child and by the child, with no picture- or object-naming as such.

Core Vocabulary Therapy[1]

The Core Vocabulary Approach (Crosbie et al., 2005, 2006) is intended for children with inconsistent speech disorder (Broomfield & Dodd, 2004a; Dodd, 2005), a category of phonological disorder in Dodd's *Differential Diagnostic Classification System; DDCS* (Dodd, 2005), described in Chapter 2. The origins of Dodd's DDCS can be found in Leahy and Dodd (1987) and Dodd and Iacono (1989), and the early foundations of Core Vocabulary Therapy (CVT) in Dodd and Iacono (1989).

Hypothetically, the underlying deficit of inconsistent speech disorder is a phonological planning deficit, not a cognitive–linguistic deficit, with most affected children in the severe SSD range. The rationale for the approach is that different parts of the speech-processing chain respond differently to therapy targeting different processing skills, and that treatment that specifically targets the speech-processing deficit underlying the child's speech disorder will result in system-wide change.

Assessment

Dodd advises that to differentially diagnose children with speech disorder it is important to collect, via independent and relational analysis (Stoel-Gammon, A7), information on the child's:

- Phonetic inventory: the ability to produce individual sounds
- Phonological system: the ability to use sounds in context
- Consistency of production: the ability to produce words the same way
- Phonotactics: syllable structures, constraints that limit where phones can occur
- Oromotor skill: the ability to perform volitional lip, tongue, and jaw movements

Following Independent and Relational Analysis, an Inconsistency Assessment, a component of the *DEAP* (Dodd et al., 2002) is administered.

Inconsistency Assessment

Twenty-five pictures are named on 3 separate occasions within one session, ensuring that the same lexical items are elicited within an identical context. The child will need a break between citation naming each 25-word series, so a workable format might be to (1) name 25 words then read a story or play a game, (2) name the 25 words again then do a puzzle or converse on a topic of interest to the child, (3) name the 25 pictures for a final time then colour or draw a picture. Importantly, the inconsistency assessment trials should not be interspersed with assessment tasks, or intervention activities, if the child is to do his or her best.

As the child names the pictures, using a form like the one displayed in Table 5.1, in the Trial 1 column enter an '=' symbol if the child says the word correctly and transcribe the word phonetically if they say the word incorrectly. Do the same in the Trial 2 and Trial 3 columns. Compare the three to calculate a score and express it as a %-inconsistency.

Consistent Production

In the 'score' column, give the child a score of 0 (zero) if they say a word the same way all three times. For example, if for the word *five* they say [faɪv, faɪv, faɪv] or [faɪb, faɪb, faɪb] or [faɪz, faɪz, faɪz] or [ɸaɪv,ɸaɪv, ɸaɪv] with a voiceless bilabial fricative, consistently on each trial they achieve a score of 0 (zero) for that word, because there is no inconsistency. Don't worry about how they say the word; the only concern is consistency vs. inconsistency.

Inconsistent Production

If the child says the word inconsistently (e.g., [faɪv, faɪb, faɪ] or [faɪb, faɪb, faɪz] or [faɪv, faɪv, faɪʔ] or [faɪd, faɪf, faɪv] for *five*) put a score of 1 (one) in the 'score' column, because it is one example of inconsistent production.

In terms of the DDCS, children are judged to have Inconsistent Speech Disorder if test words are produced with 40% variability or greater, and to have Consistent Speech Disorder if they have two or more atypical patterns and inconsistency is below 40%.

Diagnostic Features of Inconsistent Speech Disorder

Dodd cautions that Inconsistent Speech Disorder may be mistaken for CAS and stresses the following diagnostic features that distinguish the two, emphasizing the need for careful differential diagnosis. A child with Inconsistent Speech Disorder has:

- A high degree of inconsistent productions of the same lexical item in the same context. That is, 40% or more of words are produced differently in single-word confrontation naming across three trials on the same occasion of testing (e.g., within one 30-, 40-, or 60-minute session).
- Age appropriate oromotor ability.
- Better accuracy in imitating words compared with word production accuracy in spontaneous production.
- The ability to produce most sounds in isolation.
- Fluent speech with normal intonation.

Table 5.1 Inconsistency assessment: data collection form (https://speech-language-therapy.com/images/inconsistencyform.pdf).

NAME	AGE	DATE	%INCONSISTENT

0 all responses the same 1 any response is different FC forced choice IM imitation

	Trial 1	Trial 2	Trial 3	SCORE
1. shark				
2. boat				
3. rain				
4. zebra				
5. birthday cake				
6. parrot				
7. jump				
8. vacuum cleaner				
9. bridge				
10. teeth				
11. elephant				
12. slippery slide				
13. tongue				
14. umbrella				
15. five				
16. kangaroo				
17. chips				
18. fish				
19. thank you				
20. witch				
21. girl				
22. helicopter				
23. dinosaur				
24. ladybird				
25. scissors				

Total Score /25×4 = %

Core Vocabulary Intervention

The Core Vocabulary Therapy procedure begins with the child, parents and teacher selecting, with the therapist's help if required, 50 words from a pool of 70 words, that are functionally 'powerful' (make things happen) for the child and 'mean something', or are 'important' to him or her, such as names of family, friends, teacher, pets; places, for example, school, library, park, pool, McDonalds; functional words like please, thank you, toilet; and favourite things like a sport, programs, superheroes, games,

and characters. Children are seen twice-weekly (Sessions 1 and 2) for 30–45 minutes. The research team conducted 2 × 30 to 45-minute 'paired' sessions per week. Dodd notes that once weekly, and four times weekly, have also been successful.

Session 1

Ten words (picture cards or written-word cards) are randomly selected, by the child, from the list of 50. Typically, the words, with pictures and captions on cards, or just the written words on cards, are kept in a cloth bag with a drawstring, or a hat, or other container and the child selects them without looking or even wearing a blindfold. Having selected the words, 'best production' – not necessarily perfect production – is established using traditional articulation intervention techniques. For example, the best

production Alice 9;4 (see Figure 5.1) had for *bridesmaids* was [ˈbɹaɪzˌmeɪdz] and for her sisters' names [ˈdʒetˌsɪˌkə] for *Jessica* and [ˌfəˈlɪtˌsəˈti] for *Felicity*.

These were 'accepted' during drill and drill-play, but as soon as Alice improved production of any of the words, the new pronunciation became the new best-production. When modelling *bridesmaids*,

Alice 9 Core Vocabulary

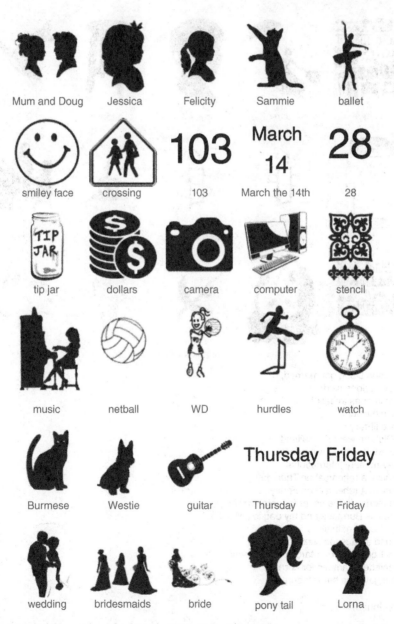

Figure 5.1 Core Vocabulary words and selected sentences for Alice, 9;4.

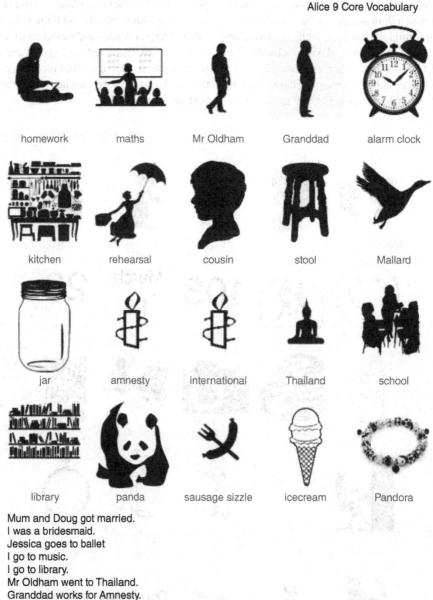

Alice 9 Core Vocabulary

homework   maths   Mr Oldham   Granddad   alarm clock

kitchen   rehearsal   cousin   stool   Mallard

jar   amnesty   international   Thailand   school

library   panda   sausage sizzle   icecream   Pandora

Mum and Doug got married.
I was a bridesmaid.
Jessica goes to ballet
I go to music.
I go to library.
Mr Oldham went to Thailand.
Granddad works for Amnesty.
I like Amnesty International.
We have a rehearsal on Thursday.
We have a rehearsal on Friday.
I get money in the tip jar for doing my homework.
Our cat is Burmese and my dog is a Westie.
I am WD for netball.
We had a sausage sizzle at school.
Mary Poppins is on March the fourteenth.
We minded Sammie for Lorna.
Lorna gave me her Pandora.

Figure 5.1 (Continued)

Jessica, and *Felicity* the SLP used correct production (*not* Alice's [ˈbɹaɪzˌmeɪdz], [ˈʤɛtˌsɪˌkə] and [ˌfəˈlɪtˌsəˈti]). Once best production is established, drill and drill-play can begin.

Shaping Best Production

Alice chose *Pandora* as one of her words. To teach *Pandora*, the clinician might say: '*Pandora has three syllables – [pæn] and [dɔ] and [ɹə]. The first syllable [pæn] has three sounds: /p/, /æ/, /n/. Start with your lips shut for /p/; you try it [p]*'. Give feedback. Build the word and then have the child blend the parts. If it is helpful, link sounds to letters. Children with Inconsistent Speech Disorder can usually imitate all sounds. If it is not possible to elicit correct production then best production may include developmental errors (e.g., *Pandora* pronounced as [ˈpænˈdɔˌwə]). Emphasize that you want the word said the same way each time, ensuring parents understand you are not bent on achieving error-free production.

Session 2

Best production is confirmed, or re-established if necessary, and drilled for 30–45 minutes. Motivating games are used to elicit a high number of productions, aiming for 150 or more productions in 30 minutes. At the end of the week, the child produces the 10 words three times. Words produced consistently are removed from the list of 50 words. Words that are inconsistently produced remain on the list, from which the next week's 10 words are randomly chosen.

Duration

According to Dodd, six to eight weeks (or 6–8 hours), should be sufficient for most children to establish consistency of production.

Providing Feedback

When the child makes an error, the feedback should be explicit, stating what went wrong and what to do to fix it. Simply asking the child to imitate the target word is avoided since imitation

provides a phonological plan that 'inconsistent children' can use without generating their own plan for the word.

Generalization

Core Vocabulary Therapy aims to stabilize a child's system resulting in consistent productions. The therapy would not be beneficial if its effect were limited to the treated words. To monitor generalization a set of untreated items (10 words) is provided (see Figure 5.2). The most words, so far, taken to achieve generalization of consistency, is 70.

Therapy Agent(s): The SLP/SLT is the primary agent of therapy. Parents play an important role in administering practice at home (2× 10-minutes daily). It is helpful if teachers are aware of the target words so they can reinforce correct productions.

Number of target words: Typically, pre-school and school children have 10 words per week (range 5–15). Younger children, or those with special needs have fewer. Single words are taught first, and towards the end of the second session children put them into carrier sentences (e.g., *I see a…*; *Here is the…*), and finally in formulated sentences containing two of the words per sentence.

Goal of Intervention

Intelligible speech.

Long-term Goal

The child will produce at least 50 target words consistently.

Target-Specific Short-term Goals

The child will achieve an appropriate productive realization of each target based on their phonological system and phonetic inventory (i.e., 'best production', and consistently use the established 'best production').

Figure 5.1 above, shows the 50 words, and some of the sentences used in Core Vocabulary Therapy for Alice aged 9;4. Alice's words and sentences were:

Efficacy monitoring sheet

Name: **Date:**

Target	Transcription	Trial 1	Trial 2	Trial 3	Score
ice-cream	aɪskrim				
octopus	oktəpus				
rocket	rokət				
motorbike	moutəbaɪk				
pencil	pɛnsəl				
butterfly	bʌtəflaɪ				
snail	sneɪl				
fish	fɪʃ				
caterpillar	kætəpɪlə				
helicopter	hɛlikoptə				
				Total:	

Ask the child to name the pictures 3x and separate each trial with a therapy activity
- Compare the 3 productions for each word.
- If the 3 productions are the same, assign the word a score of 0.
- If the 3 productions differ, assign the word a score of 1.
- Calculate the percentage of inconsistency by dividing the number of words that received a score of 1 by the number of words produced 3 times x 100

Figure 5.2 Core Vocabulary efficacy (progress) monitoring sheet.

- Mum and Doug, Jessica, Felicity, Sammie, ballet, 103, March 14, 28, smiley face, crossing, tip jar, dollars, camera, computer, stencil, music, netball, WD, hurdles, watch, Thursday, Friday, Burmese, Westie, guitar, wedding, bridesmaids, bride, pony tail, Lorna, homework, maths, Mr. Oldham, Granddad, alarm clock, kitchen, rehearsal, cousin, stool, Mallard, jar, amnesty, international, Thailand, school, library, panda, sausage sizzle, ice-cream, Pandora.
- Mum and Doug got married. I was a bridesmaid. Jessica goes to ballet. I go to music. I go to the library. Mr. Oldham went to Thailand. Grandad works for Amnesty. I like Amnesty International. We have a rehearsal on Thursday. We have a rehearsal on Friday. I get money in a tip jar for doing my homework. Our cat is Burmese, and my dog is a Westie. I am WD for netball. We had a sausage sizzle at school. *Mary Poppins* is on March the fourteenth. We minded Sammie for Lorna. Lorna gave me her Pandora.

Effects of Core Vocabulary Intervention

Crosbie et al. (2005) reported that children with inconsistent speech disorder benefit most from Core Vocabulary Therapy in terms of increased consistency and PCC, whereas children with consistent speech disorder make the most change in PCC when error patterns are targeted. These results, for children aged 4;8 to 6;5, provided support for the hypothesis that the underlying deficit of inconsistent speech disorder is phonological planning and not a cognitive-linguistic deficit. By improving the child's ability to form or access phonological plans, the phonological system self-corrected and operated successfully. Further research support comes from Rvachew and Matthews (2019).

Efficacy Monitoring

The form in Figure 5.2 is reproduced three times on an A4 or US Letter page and the SLP/SLT uses it to 'probe', once every two weeks, as intervention proceeds.

What is to Be Done When the Child's Speech is Consistent?

The effect Core Vocabulary Therapy has on a child's speech sound system can vary. Some children need more than one intervention approach to achieve age-appropriate speech. For example, Dodd and

Bradford (2000) report a case study of a boy with inconsistent speech production. Once consistency was established, he benefited from minimal pair intervention via 'a standard *Metaphon* programme' (p. 195) described by Dean et al. (1995) that targeted his remaining developmental error patterns.

The Psycholinguistic Framework

The Psycholinguistic Framework developed by Stackhouse and Wells (1997) offers a processing-based means of explaining and profiling – but not describing – specific areas of difficulty with speech and literacy that children with SSD experience. The product of the explanation or profile is not a diagnosis of this or that disorder; that is, it does not tell the investigator that the child 'has phonological disorder' or 'has CAS', for example. Rather, once an individual child's difficulties are explained, the SLP/SLT is guided towards the skills areas that require intervention.

In its conceptualization and implementation, the framework draws on psycholinguistic accounts of children's speech perception and production, described and illustrated since the 1970s with box-and-arrow models (see, Baker et al., 2001, for a comprehensive review). The basic version of the Psycholinguistic Framework sees a sound or word travelling between speaker and listener on a pathway that goes, **input** → **storage** → **output**. When the input is **speech**, sound is transmitted from the **ear** → **brain** → **mouth**, and when the input is **writing** (or **signing**), **words** (or **signs**) are relayed from the **eye** → **brain** → **hand**. Stackhouse and Wells (1997) developed this basic framework into the Speech Processing Model In the model, an acoustic signal is heard as a sound (peripheral auditory processing), recognized as speech or not speech (speech/non-speech discrimination), and perceived as a word (phonological recognition).

Stackhouse and Wells (1997) posited a single underlying representation (which they called a **lexical representation**) that incorporated phonological and semantic representations. Speech is produced via a pathway that runs from motor programming to motor planning, to motor execution to speech input. Over many years, Stackhouse,

Wells, and co-workers have generated test tools and intervention resources to complement the model (Pascoe et al., 2006; Stackhouse & Wells, 2001). Crosses A-K on the simple speech processing model displayed in Figure 5.3 indicate the levels at which tests cluster.

Dr. Blanca Schäfer is a German Speech and Language Therapist (SLT). Since completing her degree in Teaching and Research Logopedics (RWTH Aachen University, Germany) she has had a special interest in the acquisition of speech. Her PhD project at the University of Sheffield included the development of a phonological awareness test battery based on psycholinguistic principles (in collaboration with Silke Fricke). Having worked as a post-doctoral research associate on two projects in the UK (Newcastle University, University of Sheffield), as a professor in Germany (Hochschule Fresenius, University of Applied Sciences) and a lecturer at the University of Sheffield, she is now a freelance SLT in Germany. Her clinical work and research interests focus on child speech, language, and literacy acquisition in mono- and multilingual children, including appropriate assessment and intervention tools.

Dr. Silke Fricke is a Speech and Language Therapist (SLT) and a Senior Lecturer in the Division of Human Communication Sciences, University of Sheffield. Having qualified and practised as an SLT with a specialization in children with speech and literacy difficulties in Germany, she completed an MSc followed by a PhD in Human Communication Sciences in the UK. In her longitudinal PhD project, she investigated the influence of speech and language processing skills on early literacy development in monolingual and bilingual German-speaking children. From 2009 to 2011, she was a Post-Doctoral Research Fellow on the Nuffield Early Language Intervention project (an oral language intervention RCT) at the Department of Psychology, University of York. She joined the Division of Human Communication Sciences in January 2011 as a Lecturer. In her research, Dr. Fricke focuses on understanding speech, language, and literacy development, difficulties and their interrelationships in monolingual and multilingual children, and the evaluation of early support and intervention approaches for children's speech, language, and literacy development.

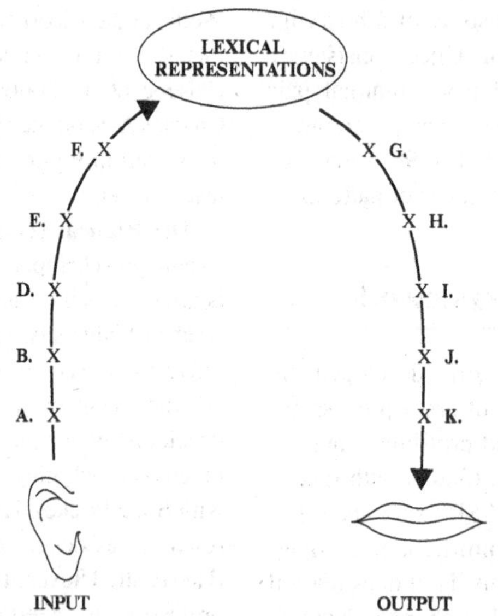

Figure 5.3 Crosses A–K on the simple speech processing model mark levels at which tests cluster. Adapted from Stackhouse and Wells (1997). Text adapted from Gardner, 2015.

Input

A. Tasks may require the child to discriminate between two speech sounds spoken in isolation, for example, pointing pictures representing /k/ and /t/. Because they are not in word or word-like contexts, simple perception or 'bottom-up processing', with no reference to lexical representations, is the skill tested.

B. The child's task is asked to discriminate between a series of non-words or listen for syllables that rhyme, without needing to access word knowledge (i.e., lexical representations) per se.

D. This is higher up the processing pathway and the child now must access the lexicon (engaging in top-down processing). At this 'height' we can ask whether the child can discriminate between real spoken words. Does the child recognize a segmental change, for example, from *kidding* to *skidding* as producing different meanings? Would the child point to the correct picture or respond at 'chance' (guess) because no meaningful contrast is established?

E. A child must detect whether the adult is saying a word correctly and spot any errors. Children with unclear storage of phonological information may respond to errors, for example, *fum* vs. *thumb* vs. *pum*, as if the words were interchangeable.

F. At this, the highest level, children can manipulate sound segments in patterns that change the word and the meaning by generating the information required for themselves, for example, sorting pictures according to their phonological similarity, without hearing the words spoken by another person.

Output

G. At this level the child should be able to access accurate motor programs from the lexical store and name pictures spontaneously, without hearing another speaker provide a model. The child may be able to say sounds in nonsense words accurately but cannot overcome habitual patterns to produce the correct version of a real word when accessing strongly established (incorrect) lexical representations.

H. and I. Here, the child can manipulate or play with sound segments. These levels relate to phonological output where the child has some ability to create novel rhymes or omit final consonants from a recently heard word (consonant deletion). The child can imitate and articulate (or repeat parrot-fashion) real words accurately, with no motor difficulty, without thinking about what the words mean.

J. At this level, output tasks involve non-words, building or repeating syllables modelled by another person. Because they are non-words there is no recourse to the lexical store.

K. Physical or articulatory difficulties that prevent accurate production of the target are at this, the lowest level of processing.

Q21. Blanca Schäfer and Silke Fricke: Psycholinguistic Profiling and Intervention

Readers in the UK are familiar with the application and principles of the psycholinguistic framework's underlying theory, assessment, goal setting and intervention for children with speech and literacy difficulties (Pascoe & Stackhouse, 2021; Stackhouse & Wells, 1997) and its empirical basis. In other parts of the world, it is not as well known. Can you provide, for SLPs/SLTs and Education professionals who are new to it, and who are interested to include it in their treatment repertoire, an account of its origins, practical application, and ongoing development? How do Stackhouse, Wells and co-workers conceptualize and explain the roots of SSD, making links between speech production skills including intonation, phonological awareness, and literacy acquisition, working from a child's speech processing strengths and addressing their areas of weakness: all without framing assessment and treatment within a diagnostic category?

A21. Blanca Schäfer and Silke Fricke: The Psycholinguistic Framework – Five Reasons Why it can Benefit Clinical or Education Practice

The basic premise of a psycholinguistic approach is that children's speech difficulties arise from one or more points in their underlying speech processing system and that, unless this is identified, the intervention delivered may not be effective. The Psycholinguistic Framework, originally developed by Stackhouse and Wells (1997), aims to provide practitioners with the tools to question results of auditory, speech, phonological awareness, literacy, and prosodic assessments, thus providing them with a stronger foundation on which to build intervention programmes.

Here is a familiar scenario: We sit with a child who shows speech sound errors. We have gathered medical notes, information on their education and psychosocial situation. Now they are trying to tell us about their day or favourite toy, but their speech is unintelligible. A linguistic analysis of their speech reveals a range of phonetic difficulties and phonological patterns. Now what? Where do we start? Our detective work is about to begin. Questions that go through our minds are: *Why does the child have speech sound errors? What are this child's specific difficulties? How do they impact communication?* We ask ourselves these questions because we know that despite similar speech sound errors, some children respond well to certain intervention approaches while others do not. Some children go on to learn to read and write successfully whereas others struggle to acquire literacy because their underlying difficulties in processing and producing speech interfere with their ability to develop skills such as phonological awareness. This then triggers the question: *What assessments do we need to profile the underlying strengths and weaknesses of this child's speech processing system?* Once we have chosen and administered the assessments, we ask: *How can we use the test results to inform our intervention planning and management of the child's speech sound disorder (SSD)?* Finally, we want to know: *How can we ensure that what we are doing is effective?*

Wouldn't it be great to have a roadmap that helped us to answer these questions? By adopting a psycholinguistic way of thinking, and using the tools provided by the Psycholinguistic Framework, we can address such questions and:

- Systematically gather and document our clinical observations,
- Build hypotheses about the underlying deficits of SSD and,
- Support our decision making for what to target in an intervention.

In the following sections, we use the expressions clinical practice, education practice, clinical professionals, and educational professionals. Because these terms may be unclear to some readers, we explain them here. **Educational practice** refers to support provided within the education system, for example, in nursery, kindergarten, preschool or school context. **Educational professionals** who may be involved in the assessment and support of children (directly or in a consultative/supervisory role) may include teachers or other educational staff (e.g., teaching assistants or Special Educational Needs Coordinators: SENCOs). These roles in education settings and their responsibilities differ across countries and education systems. **Clinical practice** refers to direct or consultative support provided within healthcare system(s) by **clinical professionals** such as SLPs/SLTs or SLP/SLT Assistants.

Here are five reasons why using the psycholinguistic framework can benefit professionals involved in educational and clinical practice.

Reason 1: Find the Source! Use the Framework to Search for Underlying Difficulties

The Psycholinguistic Framework allows clinicians and educators to explore beneath the surface of a child's speech productions and find out which parts of the speech processing system are impaired. When we have a toothache, as a first step, we might treat the symptom and take an analgesic to numb the pain but to alleviate this pain in the longer term we really need to get to the source of the problem and target treatment there. It is the same with SSD.

For some children with SSD a medical diagnosis informs appropriate treatment, for example repair of a cleft palate. However, many children with SSD do not present with a diagnosed medical condition. Because the psycholinguistic approach helps us to consider where the speech processing system itself is breaking down, this is not a problem. It can be used with any child with SSD, with the SLP/SLT/Educator bearing in mind associated medical conditions when planning intervention. Those implementing the psycholinguistic approach adopt a linguistic

perspective such as systematic phonetic and phonological descriptions of a child's speech output errors, which is necessary for considering hypotheses about the level(s) of speech processing breakdown. Thus, a psycholinguistic approach is not an alternative to the medical and linguistic approaches: the three are complementary and mutually informing.

But how do we identify where the child's speech processing is breaking down? The framework includes a speech processing profile and a box-and-arrow-model of speech processing. Both allow us to describe and compare three key components:

1. Speech input skills, i.e., how a child perceives speech (e.g., speech discrimination skills tested by questions such as: 'do /kʌf/ and /nʌf/ sound the same?').
2. Speech output skills, i.e., how a child produces speech (e.g., articulation skills tested by asking the child to repeat pseudowords such as *kalepo* /kalɛpəʊ/).
3. Stored information (also called lexical representations), i.e., how phonological information is retained in lexical entries (tested by showing a picture, for example of a bus, and asking the child: 'is this a /bʌs/? Is this a /bʌf/? Is this a /bʌp/?').

The profile comprises a range of diagnostic questions, such as: *Can the child discriminate between real words? Can the child access accurate motor programs?* They help clinicians and educators to pick the right assessment tools, for example, a real word auditory discrimination task to find out if the child struggles with speech perception at word level.

The psycholinguistic box-and-arrow model helps clinical and educational professionals to conceptualize speech processing. It illuminates how speech and language are processed and produced, while helping to interpret a child's assessment data.

Once the location of the speech processing impairment has been explored and identified, the framework can help practitioners to decide if or what further assessments are suitable for evaluating the child's input and output skills and stored lexical information.

Reason 2: Put It to the test! The Framework Allows a Critical Evaluation of Familiar and Unfamiliar Assessments

Our cupboards or digital folders often house a large range of test kits or assessment tools. The challenge can be to categorize them according to their focus, for example **input tests** (i.e., that only require the child to complete receptive tasks) or **output tests** (i.e., tasks that require a spoken answer). We must also decide whether a task targets bottom-up or top-down skills. **Bottom-up tasks** assess basic auditory processing or speech production skills which do not include the involvement of lexical knowledge (e.g., listening to different sounds and deciding whether they sound the same, repeating nonsense or new words not yet stored in the lexicon). By contrast, **top-down tasks** test whether a child can successfully use lexical knowledge to complete an activity, for example, when seeing a picture of a bus and asked the question: is this a /bʌf/? Is this a /bʌs/? Is this a /bʌt/?, a child may accept 'buf' or 'but' as a form of 'bus' if their stored representation of the word 'bus' is not precise. Some assessments mix these different task demands (e.g., including real and pseudowords in the same subtest), making it difficult to establish the areas of difficulty and strength for an individual child.

Using the dichotomies of input vs. output and bottom-up vs. top-down, the Psycholinguistic Framework allows practitioners to critically review existing tests and categorize them according to what they do and do not test. Key questions include:

1. Is it an output or input task? For example, does the child have to provide a verbal answer by producing a rhyming word or is it enough to just indicate 'yes' or 'no'?
2. Can children use their lexical knowledge to complete the task?
3. If yes, *must* they use their lexical knowledge to complete the test? In other words, can children complete the test without using their lexical representations or is some lexical knowledge necessary for successful completion?

Expanding on the three questions above, if a child is asked to decide whether two real words rhyme (e.g., cat/hat), they have two options:

first, to complete the task by accessing their lexicon or second, to compare the word forms based on their word structure. If the same task were done with obscure- or non-words (e.g., /dæt/ vs. /gæt/), the child would have no entry in their lexicon for these items and the task would be completed without lexical support.

Assessment tasks can therefore be sorted according to whether they entail input vs. output, bottom-up vs. top-down, or both. If it is not clear what a task is testing, a different assessment tool may need to be considered. Alternatively, assessors can use those components to systematically design new tasks. By applying the questions and selecting a range of input vs. output tasks and bottom-up vs. top-down assessments a comprehensive (psycholinguistic) profile of a child is established and can be used to plan intervention.

While it might seem like hard work at first to get your head around these principles, in our experience studying the psycholinguistic framework is time well spent as, once the principles are internalized, it is easier to choose appropriate assessment tools for clients and to interpret the results.

Reason 3: Have a plan! The framework Helps to Systematically Set Intervention Goals by Revealing a Child's Strengths and Weaknesses in Speech Processing

Following a critical review of assessments, available therapy materials can also be sorted according to the principles outlined above, in the form of activities that target input vs. output or bottom-up vs. top-down skills. In a second step, after considering the strengths and weaknesses of a child, the Psycholinguistic Framework can be used to design or pick intervention materials that are tailored to a child's needs (see Stackhouse & Wells, 2001 and Pascoe et al., 2006 for more information and intervention examples). The framework has demonstrated that children with the same speech sound errors (based on a phonetic and phonological analyses of their speech) can have different underlying difficulties. For example, fronting of velar stops (e.g., /t/for /k/) may arise from input or output difficulties or both. Individual tailoring circumvents the pitfall of choosing an intervention approach/procedure, or activity based on surface errors alone. This does not mean, however, that all children with SSD need to be seen individually for therapy. Group therapy sessions with a focus on speech skills can be a suitable choice if the SLP/SLT/Educator is aware of how to pitch an activity to benefit individuals within the group. In sum, by incorporating psycholinguistic principles into assessment, a deeper understanding of a child's SSD and identification of any risk for literacy issues is ensured. It also simplifies and structures clinicians' and/or educators' workflow, allowing easier progress monitoring.

Reason 4: Let it Grow! The Framework Offers a Developmental Perspective by Defining Key Developmental Stages

Another aim of an assessment of SSD might be to determine a child's developmental stage and then monitor further development. Therefore, the Psycholinguistic Framework offers a third component in the form of a Developmental Phase Model which allows a developmental perspective. Its purpose is to describe how children progress through five stages of speech development while acknowledging the struggle some children with SSD have. They are:

1. *The Prelexical Phase.* This is the pre- /first words period up to about 12 months of age and is characterized by nonverbal skills such as speech discrimination and early expressive skills such as babbling.
2. *The Whole Word Phase.* Here, children up to 24 months of age show stronger receptive capabilities in comparison to their more limited expressive speech and language skills. Lexical entries are still imprecise and stored as whole units, which is considered to result in inconsistent word production.
3. *The Systematic Simplification Phase.* Now, children between 2;6 and 4;0 have more

consistent sound systems, simplifying the adult word forms in their speech output with patterns such as fronting or cluster reduction. They also store more information about the word form, allowing more refined phonological representations.
4. *The Assembly Phase.* In this phase, which extends from about ages 3;0 to 4;0, there is more focus on connected speech. This requires a child to learn how to produce sentences with greater complexity, and some of them may become non-fluent in the process.
5. *The Metaphonological Phase.* Finally, by about the fifth birthday, children learn to reflect on their speech. Children with difficulties in one or more of the earlier phases may struggle to employ phonological awareness skills. This in turn may adversely affect the development of their written language skills (Gillon, 2017, p. 45; Stackhouse, 2006, p. 28).

Alongside this developmental perspective, a child's cultural and linguistic background needs to be considered, and any 'at risk' factors, such as social disadvantage, identified.

Reason 5: For the Many! The Framework can Used with Children from Diverse Linguistic Backgrounds

At its core, the Psycholinguistic Framework is a way of thinking (Pascoe & Stackhouse, 2021). Once its key principles are incorporated into an SLP's/SLT's/Educator's thinking, they can be applied to a wide variety of children and families with diverse family structures and parenting styles, assessments, or intervention approaches. Therefore, it can be used to support children from different linguistic and cultural backgrounds.

For example, Geronikou and Rees (2016) applied psycholinguistic profiling to a group of Greek children with SSD. Paralleling studies of English-speaking children (e.g., Ebbels, 2000; Pascoe et al., 2005), the researchers could identify a range of individual underlying speech processing difficulties, resulting in different intervention goals for the children. The

Psycholinguistic Framework principles have also been successfully applied in the design of assessment tools for cohorts with different language backgrounds (e.g., *Arabic*: Alkheraiji, 2018; *French*: Wells et al., 1999; *German*: Fricke & Schäfer, 2021; *Greek*: Geronikou et al., 2018; *isiXhosa*: Pascoe et al., 2016; *Mandarin*: Yeh et al., 2015; and *Portuguese*: Vance, 1996).

Where to from Here? Speaking Practitioner to Practitioner

The Psycholinguistic Framework has three main components: A speech processing profile, a speech processing model, and a developmental phase model. These derive from a hypothesis-testing approach to children's speech and literacy difficulties that complements medical and linguistic approaches.

So, time to put it to the test! Our advice is to have a look at what your resources are tapping in terms of input/output and bottom-up and bottom-down. In a second step, see how you can incorporate your material into the Psycholinguistic Framework. Follow up reading will help you familiarize yourself with core elements of the approach. A good overview is provided by Pascoe and Stackhouse (2021). For more in-depth reading, we suggest Stackhouse and Wells (1997), the first book of their series, which introduces the reader to the whole Psycholinguistic Framework, including a multitude of examples and practical activities. Books 2 (Stackhouse & Wells, 2001) and 3 (Pascoe et al., 2006) of the series provide more information and examples of intervention. Book 4, the Stackhouse et al. (2007) *Compendium of Auditory and Speech Tasks* provides a valuable collection of assessments which can be used or adapted to profile children's speech processing skills. For those who want guidance on how to include intonation in the intervention process, book 5 (Wells & Stackhouse, 2016) is an accessible and practical resource.

We hope that we have presented a convincing case for the Psycholinguistic Framework as a useful tool for examining children's speech

systematically and a comprehensive methodology for planning intervention for children with SSD and tracking their progress.

Acknowledgement

The authors thank Joy Stackhouse and Bill Wells for reviewing an early version of their manuscript and are appreciative of their input.

Facilitating Phonological Awareness Development

There are many reports in the literature of diverse, evidence-based therapies for SSD in children that incorporate metalinguistic techniques in general, and phonetic awareness and/or phonemic awareness in particular (e.g., Blache, 1982; Bowen & Cupples, 1999a; Dean & Howell, 1986; Dean et al., 1995; Dodd et al., 2006; Flynn & Lancaster, 1996; Gillon, 2006; Grunwell, 1985b, 1992; Hesketh et al., 2000, 2007; Klein, 1996a, 1996b; Moriarty & Gillon, 2006; Weiner, 1981a; Williams, 2000a). To varying extents, these approaches specifically target and use *phoneme* awareness in therapy with pre-literate children, sometimes with the aim of improving the child's intelligibility, sometimes with the aim of enhancing literacy acquisition or pre-empting reading and spelling difficulties in at-risk populations, and sometimes with both aims paramount.

Dr. Brigid McNeill is a SLP, Professor and Associate Dean (Research) in the Faculty of Education at the University of Canterbury, New Zealand. Brigid is also the successful learning theme leader for A Better Start National Science Challenge, a 10-year programme of research designed to uplift children's wellbeing in Aotearoa, New Zealand. Her research interests include enhancing the literacy outcomes of children with speech sound difficulties, including children with childhood apraxia of speech; initial teacher education and implementation research to embed evidence-based literacy approaches. Brigid is an Associate Editor for the journal, *Early Childhood Research Quarterly*. She currently holds three externally funded research projects that examine the implementation of culturally responsive and structured approaches to early literacy learning in New Zealand schools, supporting older students with literacy and/or communication difficulties in the upper school and connecting effective literacy teaching across the curriculum.

Q22.　Brigid McNeill: The Speech-Language-Literacy Link

Can you walk readers who are unfamiliar with Integrated Phonological Awareness Intervention for speech sound disorders through its theoretical underpinning, evidence-base and the nuts and bolts of target selection, and implementation? Which research articles are important for SLPs/SLTs and students to read before embarking on this therapy?

A22.　Brigid McNeill: Integrated Phonological Awareness Intervention

Integrated Phonological Awareness intervention is a therapeutic approach for children with speech sound disorder (SSD) that simultaneously targets their speech production, phonological awareness, and letter-sound knowledge skills. The development of this intervention was driven by the need to enhance literacy outcomes of children with SSD (e.g., Tambyraja et al., 2020) and theoretical models of speech production which identify the importance of precise phonological representations from which to drive accurate speech production (e.g., Dodd, 2005). My aim here is to provide a brief outline of the rationale for the development of the approach, summarizes its efficacy and then offer a practice checklist to help direct clinicians to implement the approach with fidelity.

Rationale

Children with SSD (or a history of SSD) are at heightened risk for literacy difficulties (e.g., Brosseau-Lapré & Roepke, 2022; Hayiou-Thomas et al., 2017; Lewis et al., 2018;

McNeill et al., 2017; Rvachew et al., 2003; Tambyraja et al., 2020). Children who have a language impairment in addition to their speech difficulty are more likely to experience low phonological awareness and literacy difficulties than children who only have a speech sound production difficulty (Nathan et al., 2004; Peterson et al., 2009) Additionally, the types of speech errors present contribute to the likelihood that a child with SSD will also need intervention for phonological awareness and literacy development.

Risk and Protective Factors

There is a large body of research showing that the presence of atypical speech sound errors or error patterns (i.e., speech substitutions and/ or omissions that are unusual in the speech of younger children with typical language development) increases a child's risk for phonological awareness difficulties and thus literacy difficulties (e.g., Brosseau-Lapré & Roepke, 2022; Dodd, 2005; Hayiou-Thomas et al., 2017; Pennington & Bishop, 2009; Preston & Edwards, 2010; Preston et al., 2013).

Other risk and protective factors will also play a role in determining whether a child with SSD will also need a focus on metalinguistic and literacy skills within their therapy plan. Factors such as non-verbal intelligence, classroom instructional quality and genetic risk of dyslexia will also contribute to the literacy outcomes of a child with SSD (Hayiou-Thomas et al., 2017; Peterson et al., 2009). Integrated phonological awareness intervention is more suitable for children who exhibit atypical speech error errors (alongside other speech error patterns) and/ or demonstrate a weakness in phonological processing in addition to the speech production difficulties in their assessment profile.

Quality of Phonological Representations

Another key rationale underpinning the development of integrated phonological awareness intervention is the role that phonological representations play in speech sound production. Good quality phonological representations are hypothesized to have a positive influence on both speech accuracy and phonological awareness development (e.g., Pennington & Bishop, 2009). Several studies have shown relatively poor development of phonological representations in children with SSD as measured by mispronunciation detection tasks (e.g., Rvachew, 2006; Sutherland & Gillon, 2005). Further, there is an association between phonological awareness, speech production accuracy and the quality of phonological representations. This association indicates there is a connection across these factors that can be exploited in therapy. Integrated phonological awareness intervention focuses on enhancing the specificity of children's phonological representations and their ability to access those representations, both of which are important for speech production *and* phonological awareness.

Evidence for Integrated Phonological Awareness Intervention

Gillon (2000, 2002) first described and evaluated the effectiveness of integrated phonological awareness for children with SSD in a controlled study and longer-term follow-up that compared the integrated intervention to traditional therapy focused on speech sound production alone. These studies showed that although there was no difference in speech production outcomes between intervention groups, children who experienced the integrated phonological awareness condition had enhanced phonological awareness, letter-sound knowledge, reading and spelling outcomes that were maintained at long term follow-up. Since that seminal work, various studies have demonstrated the effectiveness of adapted versions of the integrated phonological awareness approach for three or more purposes including

1. the prevention of later literacy difficulties in pre-schoolers with speech sound disorder (Gillon, 2005);

2. as an approach to support the speech and literacy development of children with childhood apraxia of speech (e.g., Hume et al., 2018; McNeill et al., 2009); and
3. for children with Down Syndrome (van Bysterveldt et al., 2010).

Dosage and Treatment Intensity Matter

Other evaluations of approaches designed to integrate phonological awareness and speech production goals have highlighted key components of this intervention that contribute to its efficacy. Hesketh et al. (2000) compared 'metaphonological therapy' and traditional articulation therapy. Although metaphonological therapy also has the dual goal of supporting children's phonological awareness and speech production skills, there are key differences in the approach compared to the integrated approaches trialled by Gillon and colleagues highlighted above. For example, in the metaphonological therapy, phonological awareness activities only took place in the first four weeks of the intervention, and the stimuli used in those activities were not based on children's speech production goals. There was some focus on perceptual training for children to recognize the difference between their error form and the correct form, but speech production was limited to the last two weeks of the 10-week intervention. Results showed no difference in speech or phonological awareness outcomes across conditions suggesting that the intensity of both speech production and phonological awareness aspects of the intervention may have been inadequate.

Denne et al. (2005) evaluated the impact of 12 hours of integrated phonological awareness intervention on the phonological awareness and early literacy outcomes of children with SSD. Again, this treatment intensity is lower than the 18 to 20 hours of intervention reported in the earlier integrated phonological awareness intervention trials. Children in the integrated phonological awareness intervention had better phonological awareness outcomes than the comparison group, but this did not transfer to superior literacy outcomes. Together, these studies highlight the importance of speech production practice and treatment intensity in ensuring optimal shifts in children's speech production and phonological awareness skills.

Research Need

Although there is empirical evidence to support the use of integrated phonological awareness intervention, more research is necessary. Further information regarding the efficacy of the approach is needed through replication studies, implementation of randomized controlled trials, long term follow-up of therapy outcomes, and investigation of the utility of the approach for other types of speech production errors.

Principles of Intervention

The following list includes key components of integrated phonological awareness intervention that are important to ensure that the approach is implemented with fidelity (Baker, A26).

1. The phonological awareness activities should be primarily focused on phonemes (rather than syllables and/or rhymes) within phonological awareness. Activities focused on phonemes will have the best impact on children's reading and spelling skills (see Gillon, 2018, for review). Further, focusing on phonemes enables speech production practice to be more easily integrated in the activities. Finally, to aid generalization of the phonological awareness gains to a child's reading and spelling progress, graphemes should be included in all phonological awareness activities (Gillon, 2018).
2. It is important that the intervention is delivered at the appropriate intervention and intensity as described in the literature (i.e., 2 to 3 times per week over 18 to 20 hours) (Gillon, 2000, 2005; McNeill et al., 2009).
3. There is evidence for the effectiveness of the approach in individual (e.g., Gillon, 2000; McNeill et al., 2009) and small-group settings (e.g., Gillon, 2005).

4. The stimuli used in the phonological awareness activities should be matched to the child's current speech production goals. For example, if the target is the elimination of velar fronting, then the phonological awareness activity should include many words with /k/ in onset. In addition, each activity must ensure a minimum number of trials of the speech production target and provide feedback regarding that production attempt. An integrated phonological awareness approach will have the desired impact on children's speech production accuracy *only* if targeted speech production practice is included.
5. To capitalize on the connection between strengthened phonological representations, phonological awareness and speech production, phonological structure (phonotactics) and graphemes should be used explicitly as prompts to support speech production. For example, if a child said 'tar' for 'star', the clinician might point to the grapheme 's' and say 'when you say tar, I don't hear /s/ at the start. Try saying "star" again with the /s/ sound at the start'.
6. Integrated phonological awareness intervention is easiest to implement with stimulable sounds. If there are no stimulable sounds from which to commence therapy, it is recommended that time is spent eliciting the sound in isolation (while introducing the grapheme associated with the sound) before beginning the integrated phonological awareness therapy block.
7. It is critical that SLPs/SLTs collaborate with teachers regarding integrated phonological awareness intervention to ensure the best educational outcomes (Neilson, A49, A50). With more classrooms moving to a structured approach to literacy instruction, there may be opportunities to have alignment between classroom and therapy contexts in assessment and teaching/therapy targets.
8. As with any intervention, it is important to engage the child's family in goal setting and generalization.

Resources

Integrated phonological awareness intervention activity examples and therapy resources can be accessed from Gillon and McNeill

(2007). The resources include a manual and method to track the effectiveness of the approach within a clinical context. This is a great place to learn more about this approach to enhance both the spoken and written language development of children with speech sound disorder.

Parents and Children Together (PACT)

'PACT' is an acronym for a family-centred phonological assessment and intervention approach to speech sound disorders called *Parents and Children Together* (Bowen, 2010; Bowen & Cupples, 2006). Conceivably, PACT could stand for 'parents and child, and therapist' since all are actively involved in PACT. Delivered in planned blocks of therapy attendance, and breaks from therapy, PACT is termed 'broad-based' because it prioritizes the phonemic (phonological or cognitive–linguistic) level, *and* takes in phonetic and auditory perceptual aspects, as the difficulties children who have phonological disorder experience may not be exclusively 'phonological'. PACT directly targets speech perception and production, and hence intelligibility, in children with phonological disorder. It may also indirectly impact morphosyntax and phonological awareness (especially phonemic awareness) and hence literacy acquisition.

In the two previous editions of this book (Bowen, 2009, 2015) PACT appeared in Chapter 9. For the third edition, the description has been reduced in length and moved to Chapter 5. Chapter 9 from the second edition, including a case study of Josie, and a contribution by Dr. Deb James (James, 2015) is available at https://www.speech-language-therapy.com/images/cssd2ech9.pdf

For more about PACT, go to the header of any page at www.speech-language-therapy.com → Click on ARTICLES → Intervention to see four PACT-related pages: *Implementation, Publications, Theory and Evidence* and *Therapy for Josie*. On the *Therapy for Josie* page is a slide show (see https://www.speech-language-therapy.com/pdf/josie.ppsx) about her intervention, in 2010, from ages 6;5 to 7;6, for a severe phonological disorder with a mix of phonemic,

perceptual, and phonetic issues. There are also links to activities and picture-and-word resources we used.

Primary Population

PACT was designed for 3- to 6-year-olds and validated as an effective treatment for children in this age range diagnosed with mild, moderate, and severe phonological disorders (Bowen, 1996a; Bowen & Cupples, 1999a, 1999b). The children in the efficacy study were typical of children with intelligibility difficulties in that they did not necessarily have 'pure' phonological disorder. Children with developmental language disorder (DLD) were excluded from the study, and each child's SSD had a phonological basis, plus or minus phonetic execution and auditory perceptual difficulties. Some participants were treated for stuttering.

We had a twofold rationale for developing a therapy for pre-schoolers and younger school children. First, intelligibility difficulties may be obvious in 2- and 3-year-olds (Dodd, 2015; McIntosh & Dodd, 2011), but diagnosis of SSD is usually elusive until a child's fourth year. Withholding intervention, however, until diagnosis is 'definite' can prove counterproductive in the longer term. Second, we wanted to develop an intervention that families could access before their children started formal schooling, potentially 'catching' many of them before they were too busy (and probably too tired) and inaccessible – in the sense of not wanting to miss school – to attend speech therapy, and pre-empting or minimizing literacy acquisition difficulties.

Secondary Populations

Clinicians report acceptable outcomes with PACT with other populations, but such implementation has not been tested experimentally. The 'others' included children

- Aged 3;0- to 6;11 with language processing and production issues *and* SSD.
- With low intelligibility aged ≤10 years with Developmental Language Disorder.

- Aged ≤10 years with pragmatic issues.
- Growing up multilingual (Goldstein, A41; McLeod & Crowe, A42; Prezas et al., A5; Zajdó, A43).
- With developmental delay, for example, related to Fragile X, and Williams syndromes.
- With clefts (Peterson-Falzone et al., 2017; Ruscello, A38).
- With autism (Broome et al., 2021).
- With Down syndrome (Camarata et al., 2006; De Thorne et al., 2009; Yoder et al., 2016)
- With cochlear implants (Asad et al., A12).

Although not designed for children with CAS, it has been coupled with Dynamic Temporal and Tactile Cueing (DTTC) which is a form of integral stimulation (Strand, 2020; Strand et al., 2006), and compatible techniques that follow the principles of motor learning (McCabe et al., 2020; Schmidt et al., 2019), to help treat children diagnosed with CAS.

Theoretical Basis

PACT is based on the assumptions that phonemic change is

1. Gradual, and motivated by homophony (Grunwell, 1987).
2. Enhanced through metalinguistic awareness of phones (the phonetic level) and the phonemic system (the phonological level).
3. Facilitated by heightening the perceptual saliency of contrasts because it increases their learnability.

In common with all minimal pair approaches (Fey, 1992) PACT systematically

- Modifies groups of sounds produced in error in a patterned way.
- Emphasizes the elimination of homophony.
- Establishes feature contrasts to mark meaning distinctions, rather than putting the spotlight on accurate sound production.
- Makes it explicit to children that the function of phonology is communication.

These ends are achieved in PACT by working at word level and above, using naturalistic parent–child communicative contexts, increasing the child's (and parents') metaphonological awareness, and

targeting, as required, phonological, phonetic, phonotactic and perceptual goals.

Empirical Support

In the efficacy study, a longitudinal matched groups design was employed, with assessment, treatment, and reassessment (probe) phases. Fourteen children were treated under typical clinical conditions, and treatment was withheld from eight matched children on waiting lists. At probe, the treated children showed accelerated and highly selective improvement in their productive phonology [$F(1,20) = 19.36$, $P < 0.01$], whereas the untreated eight did not. No such selective improvement was observed in the treated children in either receptive vocabulary or Mean Length of Utterance in Morphemes, attesting to the specific effect of the therapy. PACT is practicable (Robey & Schultz, 1998) under conditions of everyday practice in terms of the in-clinic component (Bowen & Cupples, 1998, 1999a), and it is feasible and often enjoyable for families who implement homework, as well as skills they have learned in the parent education component of PACT (Bowen & Cupples, 2004).

Assessment

A 200-utterance conversational speech (CS) sample, or a 200-word CS sample, *and* single words (SWs) elicited using the *Quick Screener* (Bowen, 1996b, after Dean et al., 1990) usually provide enough data to allow independent and relational analyses (Stoel-Gammon, A7) and diagnosis, or provisional diagnosis, of phonological impairment. Additional testing may be needed, especially for children with moderate or severe SSD. This might entail administering the DEAP (Dodd et al., 2002) or the HAPP-3 (Hodson, 2004), the Locke Speech Perception Task (Locke, 1980; see Tables 9.6a and 9.6b), and an imitative PCC (Johnson et al., 2004).

Speech assessment within the PACT approach, whether initial or ongoing, is integral to intervention. As parents play a central role in management, it is highly desirable for them to be aware – through observation, participation, and explanation – of the speech-language assessment process. Essential components of data gathering are the case history interview; an audiological evaluation by an Audiologist (Asad et al., A 12); screening for language, pragmatics, voice and fluency strengths and difficulties; an oral musculature examination (see https://www.speech-language-therapy.com/images/omesf2pp.pdf); and, as noted above, a CS sample of 200 utterances, if possible, remembering that, for some children, single word tokens may predominate. Within the case history interview, parents are asked to provide an intelligibility rating using a scale of 1–5: (1) completely intelligible; (2) mostly intelligible; (3) somewhat intelligible; (4) mostly unintelligible; and (5) completely unintelligible. This is recorded at the top of the *Quick Screener* data collection form displayed in Figure 5.4.

If the child's output is so poorly intelligible that the clinician cannot discern the content, or if time is short, or the child's cooperation difficult to establish, an imitative PCC procedure is used rather than the conversational PCC procedure (Flipsen Jr., A8). Johnson et al. (2004) found that PCCs derived from conversational samples did not differ significantly from PCCs drawn from sentence imitation, using age-appropriate vocabulary, syntax, and representative distribution of speech sounds in children aged 4–6. They concluded that 'the sentence imitation procedure offers a valid and efficient alternative to conversational sampling'. In their experiment, an almost wordless picture book, *Carl Goes to Daycare* (Day, 1993), provided visual stimuli for the task, and the 36 short sentences, tapping 273 consonants, that the children repeated after the examiner included, 'Watch them dance', 'He got cold', and 'Time to go home'.

Quick Screener

Speech assessment begins with the administration of the *Quick Screener*, while parents observe, using the data collection form shown in Figure 5.4. The SLP/SLT phonetically transcribes in full, with necessary diacritics, the child's production of the first word 'cup' and immediately enters a score in the CC (consonants correct) column. For example, if the child says [kʌp] the score is 2; for [kʌ], [ʌp], [tʌp] or [gʌp] the score is 1; and for [ʌ] or [tʌ] the score is zero. Each word is scored for consonant production in this way.

There are about 100 consonants in the sample, depending on the variety of English, so a *tentative* single-word PCC can be estimated quickly, with parents watching, by adding the scores in the CC columns and calling the sum a percentage. For example, if the child scores 55 CC, the tentative PCC, or screening PCC, is 55%.

There is provision on the form to record vowel errors. The vowel and diphthong targets reflect non-rhotic Australian English. Therapists working with children speaking other varieties of English can change the vowel symbols, and 'vowelless' forms are available at www.speech-language-therapy.com (e.g., https://www.speech-language-therapy.com/pdf/QS-data-collection-SLPs-nv.pdf). If the child mispronounces the vowel or diphthong in a word, it is circled by the therapist. Vowels correct are later tallied to calculate a screening, single-word, percentage of vowels correct (PVC) with the formula VOWELS CORRECT $\div\ 47 \times 100 = $ PVC (again, while parents observe).

The PCC and the PVC derived from the screener are *screening* (tentative) measures, although it has been observed clinically that there is little variation in PCC and PVC scores between data gathered via the *Quick Screener* and larger data sets.

Several versions of the Quick Vowel Screener pictures and record forms, with and without symbols are available. Locate these and other resources by going to the header of any page at www.speech-language-therapy.com → Click RESOURCES → Index → Child Speech Assessment Resources.

Using the *Quick Screener* analysis form displayed in Figure 5.5 the clinician summarizes the child's phonological processes as percentages of occurrence, if this is considered useful, and records pertinent observations, including the therapist's own intelligibility rating. These outcomes are discussed in the child's hearing. It is explained to parents that the child's continued presence during discussion provides a demonstration to the child that his or her parents are important partners in the therapy process. It also helps to acknowledge parents, up front, as the homework experts and experts where their own child is concerned.

The word in the *Quick Screener* is based on the *Metaphon Resource Pack Screening Test* developed by Dean et al. (1990) with the word and picture for 'gun' changed to 'gone'. The stimulus pictures, data collection forms and analysis form are freely available at

Quick Screener

SINGLE-WORD SCREENING SAMPLE USING THE METAPHON STIMULUS VOCABULARY

Dean, E., Howell, J., Hill, A., & Waters, D. (1990). Metaphon Resource Pack. Windsor, Berks: NFER Nelson

Date of Birth	Observer(s)
Today's date	Examiner

① completely intelligible ② mostly intelligible ③ somewhat intelligible ④ mostly unintelligible ⑤ completely unintelligible

#	TARGET	TRANSCRIPTION	CC	#	TARGET	TRANSCRIPTION	CC
1	cup	ʌ		23	jam	æ	
2	gone	ɒ		24	house	aʊ	
3	knife	aɪ		25	path	a	
4	sharp	a		26	door	ɔ	
5	fish	ɪ		27	smoke	oʊ	
6	kiss	ɪ		28	bridge	ɪ	
7	sock	ɒ		29	train	eɪ	
8	glass	a		30	chair	ɛə	
9	watch	ɒ		31	red	ɛ	
10	nose	oʊ		32	spoon	u	
11	mouth	aʊ		33	plane	eɪ	
12	yawn	ɔ		34	fly	aɪ	
13	leaf	i		35	sky	aɪ	
14	thumb	ʌ		36	sun	ʌ	
15	foot	ʊ		37	wing	ɪ	
16	toe	oʊ		38	splash	æ	
17	snake	eɪ		39	tent	ɛ	
18	van	æ		40	salt	ɒ	
19	fast	a		41	crab	æ	
20	girl	ɜ		42	sweet	i	
21	stairs	ɛə		43	sleeve	i	
22	big	ɪ		44	zipper	ɪ ə	

Check ɔɪ boy ɪə ear   **SUBTOTAL CC:**   **TOTAL CC:**

TENTATIVE single word phonetic inventory (≈100 consonants in sample) and PVC (47 vowels/diphthongs in sample)

Vowels	i	ɪ	ɛ	æ	a	ʌ	ə	ɜ	ɒ	ɔ	ʊ	u	Vowels correct (47) %
Obstruents	p	b	t	d	k	g	f	v					Consonants % correct (≈ 100)
Obstruents	θ	ð	s	z	ʃ	ʒ	tʃ	dʒ	STIMULABILITY				MARKED p t k f v
Sonorants	m	n	ŋ	l	r	w	j	h					θ ð s z ʃ ʒ tʃ dʒ

List phonological processes/record observations

Figure 5.4 The Quick Screener data collection form, Bowen (1996b), stimulus words after Dean et al. (1990).

www.speech-language-therapy.com. Word productions can be elicited using the *Metaphon Resource Pack Screening Test* easel book (now out of print), or the *Quick Screener* pictures on cards, or presented on pdf slides (e.g., in a pdf https://www.speech-language-therapy.com/pdf/qs2007.pdf or a PowerPoint show https://www.speech-language-therapy.com/pdf/qs 2007.ppsx) on a laptop, or tablet such as an iPad.

Velar fronting

#	Target SI	0/1	#	Target SF	0/1
1	cup		7	sock	
6	kiss		17	snake	
2	gone		22	big	
20	girl		37	wing	
	TOTAL	/4		TOTAL	/4

Palato-alveolar fronting

#	Target SI	0/1	#	Target SF	0/1
4	sharp		5	fish	
30	chair		9	watch	
23	jam		28	bridge	
	TOTAL	/3		TOTAL	/3

Word-final devoicing

#	Target	0/1	#	Target	0/1
41	crab		43	sleeve	
31	red		10	nose	
22	big		28	bridge	
				TOTAL	/6

Backing

#	Target SI	0/1	#	Target SF	0/1
16	toe		15	foot	
39	tent		42	sweet	
26	door		31	red	
	TOTAL	/3		TOTAL	/3

Stopping of fricatives

#	Target SI	0/1	#	Target SF	0/1
5	fish		13	leaf	
15	foot		11	mouth	
14	thumb		6	kiss	
7	sock		38	splash	
36	sun		43	sleeve	
4	sharp		10	nose	
18	van				
44	zip(per)				
	TOTAL	/8		TOTAL	/6

Stopping of affricates

#	Target SI	0/1	#	Target SF	0/1
30	chair		9	watch	
23	jam		28	bridge	
	TOTAL	/2		TOTAL	/2

Pre-vocalic voicing

#	Target	0/1	#	Target	0/1
25	path		5	fish	
16	toe		14	thumb	
6	kiss		36	sun	
			4	sharp	
				TOTAL	/7

Liquid/glide simplification

#	Target	0/1	#	Target	0/1
9	watch		12	yawn	
13	leaf		31	red	
				TOTAL	/4

Initial consonant deletion

#	Target	0/1	#	Target	0/1
3	knife		7	sock	
22	big		30	chair	
18	van		12	yawn	
				TOTAL	/6

Final consonant deletion

#	Target SI	0/1	#	Target SF	0/1
23	jam		10	nose	
44	zip		5	fish	
31	red		28	bridge	
				TOTAL	/6

Initial cluster reduction

#	Target SI	0/1	#	Target SI	0/1
33	plane		43	sleeve	
8	glass		27	smoke	
28	bridge		17	snake	
29	train		32	spoon	
41	crab		21	stairs	
34	fly		35	sky	
42	sweet		38	splash	
				TOTAL	/14

Final cluster reduction

#	Target	0/1	#	Target	0/1
19	fast		40	salt	
39	tent				
				TOTAL	/3

Figure 5.5 Quick Screener analysis form.

I prefer the slide show option, not least because children usually find it interesting and fun, *and* quite remarkably, frequently ask to do the test 'again'!

The data collection form has space for recording stimulability data and the child's inventory of marked consonants. In stimulability testing, the child is asked to directly imitate vowels in isolation and CVs, usually [ba bi bu] etc. focusing on vowels and diphthongs already circled on the form; and consonants of interest in CV or VC contexts, or both, but not usually in isolation. Marked consonants in the child's inventory are circled, from a choice of /p t k f v θ ð s z ʃ ʒ tʃ dʒ/. The stimulability and markedness data are later used in selecting treatment targets, as outlined in Chapter 9.

Assessing Progress

It is usual to administer the *Quick Screener*, with parent observation, at the initial assessment and thereafter at the beginning of each intervention block (after a break from intervention), allowing parents to observe and discuss any changes.

Additional testing may be required; for example, the DEAP, HAPP-3 or the Locke Task might be repeated. Any decision to terminate or continue therapy is made jointly with parents (see Baker, 2010 for insightful discussion).

Goals and Goal Attack

Table 1.4 provides a schema within which to view three levels of intervention goal. **Basic Goal:** The basic goal of PACT is to work at word level or above to encourage phonological reorganization, thus facilitating the emergence of clear speech. This basic goal is achieved by increasing a child's consonant, vowel, syllable-shape, syllable-stress, phonotactic and suprasegmental repertoires and accuracy; and by promoting generalization of new segments, structures, and prosodic features to increasingly challenging contexts and situations.

Intermediate Goal: The intermediate goal is to target groups of sounds related by an organizing principle (phonological processes, rules, or patterns), addressing phonetic and perceptual levels as required.

Specific Goals: Specific intervention goals are to target a sound, sounds or syllable structures, using horizontal strategies: targeting several sounds within a sound class or manner of production, or syllable structure category, and/or targeting more than one process or deviation or structure simultaneously. Goal selection and attack strategies are primarily therapist-driven and explained to parents. Multiple goals are addressed in and across treatment sessions and in homework, sequentially and simultaneously, and rarely cyclically.

For example, Emeline, 5;1, in Session 4 of her second therapy block, had three concurrent goals. First, a phonetic goal to produce /dʒ/ and /tʃ/ in onset and coda in six paired practice words for each (cheese-Gs, chain-Jane, cheep-jeep and H-age, rich-ridge, lunch-lunge), aiming for 70 trials in a 50-minute session; second, a phonological goal to recognize distinctions in input, and to mark distinctions in output in short phrases between the cognate pairs /p b/, /t d/ and /k g/ (e.g., with Emeline instructing and adult to 'Touch the *pea/bee*', 'Touch the *toe/doe*', 'Touch the *cap/gap*'; and then switching roles) aiming for 50 trials within the same 50-minutes; and a generalization goal to use the voiceless fricatives /f/, /s/ and /ʃ/ in conversational speech in untrained words in the therapy session and during an agreed daily period at home. Emeline's parents, who were dedicated 'homework parents' who shared the task, opted for 5–7 minutes of homework twice daily, or three times daily when possible. The practice periods at home could be separated by as little as 10 minutes.

Materials and Equipment

The materials and equipment required are toys, vowel and consonant pictures and worksheets (presented on cards, as hard copies, or digitally); a 'speech book' (exercise book, ring binder or scrapbook); drawing and 'making' materials and equipment (craft supplies such as paper, card, glue, adhesive tape, stencils and craft pens); rewards such as stamps and stickers; a desktop, laptop, or tablet computer for slide shows; and an audio recorder to record therapy snippets. It is helpful but not essential for the family to have a computer or smart phone and audio recorder. Pictures usually include captions to clarify what the target words are meant to be. Captions are printed consistently with the way in which early literacy instruction is commonly delivered, with all words printed in lower case, and capital letters used only for the beginnings of proper nouns. Suitable pictures are available to clinicians and families, at no cost, at www.speech-language-therapy.com.

Intervention

Therapy Sessions

The clinician sees the child for 50–60 minutes (usually 50 minutes) once weekly in therapy blocks. Depending on the severity of the phonological disorder and the child's capacity for drill, dose rate ranges from at least 50 production per in-clinic session, through 70, and up to100 trials for more severely involved (and cooperative) children.

The minimum parent participation involves the parent joining the therapist and child for 20 minutes at the end of a session, or 10 minutes at the beginning and end. Maximum parent participation sees parents staying 50–60 minutes. A parent assumes the role of dynamic collaborator in a treatment triad with child and therapist. Episodes of parent participation always require the child's continued involvement, to properly demonstrate what should happen at home.

The following is an outline of a 50-minute session for Iain, 5;7, with his father Gordon and a therapist, towards the end of his second treatment block (of three) in which one target was addressed. Then, there is a brief comment about the activities employed in Iain's subsequent session.

Iain had a persistent [n] for /l/ sound replacement SIWI, and over the previous two weeks had *finally* become stimulable for /l/ in CVs by dint of every phonetic placement technique the therapist knew – or at least it felt that way! The breakthrough came when they tried: https://www.speech-language-therapy.com/pdf/llama.pdf Gordon left Iain with the therapist for 15 minutes while he dropped his wife Lucinda at a train station and took 7-year-old Bruce to school, returning for the final 35 minutes of the session with Iain's brother Fergus, 18 months, who played happily alone. Iain had already engaged in items 1–3 with the therapist.

Example: Outline of One of Iain's 50-Minute Sessions

1. Rhyming auditory bombardment using five pictured, captioned (in lower case printing), minimal pairs: *snip-slip, snap-slap, snow-slow, snug-slug, sneak-sleek*, was presented. The pairs were spoken to Iain at a comfortable conversational loudness level, and then he played a quick game of 'Point to the one I say', with the therapist saying the words and Iain pointing.
2. Next was auditory input cloze with the same captioned pictures, with Iain saying the /sn/-words that he was already able to pronounce correctly: Adult: *Slow* rhymes with … Iain: *snow* Adult: *Slap* rhymes with … Iain: *snap*, etc.
3. Then came a 'silent sorting' task. Four cards (*name, night, knots* and *nine*) were placed before Iain who was instructed to 'think the words' as he

placed a rhyming word (from a choice of *lame, light, lots*, and *line*) beside each (see Figure 5.6).
4. Gordon began participating in the session at this point. Iain was shown a page of pictures of *late, lei, lap, let, light, lock, lick, lame, lead, lit* and *lice*, and told, 'This time, Iain, you be the teacher and tell me if I say these words the right way or the wrong way'. Taking the role of 'student', Gordon made deliberate random errors, emulating Iain's sound replacement (e.g., 'Nate' for 'late', 'neigh' for 'lei', 'nap' for 'lap' as single word inputs or in short utterances, for example, 'He is *late* for school' vs. 'He is *Nate* for school'). Iain had to tell the 'student' whether he was right or wrong without modelling correct pronunciation.
5. The therapist, and then Gordon, presented a 'fixed-up-one routine' for /n/ vs. /l/.
6. The clinician presented a homophony confrontation task with *lei-neigh, lap-nap, lame-name* and *low-no*, and this was the one task not included in homework.
7. All three rehearsed a Knock-Knock joke (Knock, knock. *Who's there? Lettuce. Lettuce who? Lettuce in!*). This was then recorded several times on the same recording, with Iain saying '*Lettuce*' and '*Lettuce in*' and his father saying, '*Who's there*' and '*Lettuce who*?' Ian said the /l/ in 'lettuce' (which he produced as [ˈlʌˌtəs]) correctly several times during this activity. He could also say 'llama' [ˈlamə], and 'line' pronounced as [laːn].
8. The auditory bombardment was delivered again and recorded, so that it followed the 'lettuce' humour. It consisted of *snip-slip, snap-slap, snow-slow, snug-slug, sneak-sleek*, as in item one above, followed by 15 words in sequence: *leaf, lamb, lock, label, lead, lie, lake, lion, lip, letter, lunch, llama, lamp, lettuce.*
9. Homework, comprising activities 2–4 and 6–8, was explained by the clinician, demonstrated by the clinician and Iain, and then rehearsed by Iain and Gordon. Iain tried the Knock-Knock joke out on his father several more times, and the recording with the joke and bombardment sequences, with a running time of 2.5 minutes, was played.

10. In the context of putting 'children' on a toy school bus, Gordon, therapist, and Iain sang '*Lettuce-in, lettuce-in, lettuce-in*', '*Lettuce-go, lettuce-go, lettuce-go*', and '*Lettuce-out, lettuce-out, lettuce-out*' to the tune of 'Here we go, here we go, here we go' on the recording to take home, increasing the running time to 4 minutes.

11. Reinforcing /l/ via frequent recasting was discussed with Gordon (parent education), and suggestions for thematic play offered around 'llama' and 'line' and making up more words for the 'lettuce song' ('*Lettuce stop*', '*Lettuce start*', '*Lettuce see*', '*Lettuce stay*', '*Lettuce sing*', etc.). They were to do all the activities except number 6 at home, and instructions and pictures were included in Iain's speech book for Lucinda, who shared over half the homework-load with Gordon.

Because Iain had only recently become stimulable for /l/ and that he could only say the three words, *lettuce, llama,* and *line* with his target sound correct, no production drill was included in his session. When he, Lucinda and Fergus arrived the following week, Iain was able to say, imitatively, with approximately 30% accuracy *lake, lamb, letter, lettuce, lie, light, lion, lip, line, llama,* and *lunch.* In the session, he did production drill and drill play for: *lock-knock, lap-nap, low-no, lei-neigh, let-net,* and *lip-nip*; and with the word-pairs pictured in Figure 5.6 (*lame-name, light-night, lots-knots,* and *line-nine*) with a dose rate of 100 trials in 50 minutes.

Intervention Scheduling

A unique feature of PACT is its administration in planned blocks and breaks (Bowen & Cupples, 2004) that are intended to

- accommodate the gradualness of speech acquisition, mimicking typical development,
- allow for spurts and plateaus in development,
- make 'space' for consolidation of new speech skills,
- make 'space' for phonological generalization,
- make 'space' for untrained spontaneous gains, and
- provide periodic respite, allowing families to refresh and regroup.

Dose Frequency

In PACT, the dose frequency (i.e., the occasions of treatment sessions per time unit) is one 50–60-minute session a week, on the same day each week, with the SLP/SLT and a parent (or parents), and 5- to 7-minute homework (home practice) sessions, with an adult (preferably a parent), once, twice, or three times daily. The 5- to 7-minute sessions can be separated by as little as 10 minutes (e.g., practice → read a story → practice → play a game → practice → reward). The 'reward' might be a stamp, sticker, a favourite activity, or a token that builds to a more substantial reward or prize. For instance, Iain was motivated to receive one token for doing one practice, two tokens for two, and three tokens for three in a day, in the expectation of winning a Hot Wheels Diecast 1:64 Car for his collection for each 60 tokens he achieved. The cars were purchased by his grandfather who was very forthcoming with praise too.

The initial block and break are usually about 10 weeks each, and then the number of therapy sessions per block tends to reduce while the period between blocks remains constant at 10 weeks. A typical schedule is 10 weeks on, 10 weeks off, 8 weeks on, 10 weeks off, 4–6 weeks on. It is suggested to parents that, during the breaks, they do no formal practice for up to 8 weeks. In the 2 weeks prior to the next block, they are asked to enjoy looking through the speech book with the child a few times and to do any activities the child wants to do. Although they do no homework or revision in the breaks, parents continue providing continual modelling corrections, reinforcement of revisions and repairs and metalinguistic activities, as opportunities arise, applying strategies learned in 'parent education' in the therapy block(s).

Typically, those children with phonological disorder *only* have needed a mean of 21 consultations for their output phonology to fall within age-expectations, meaning that many are ready for discharge at the end of their second block (about 30 weeks after initial assessment) or immediately after their second break (about 40 weeks after initial assessment). A small number of children engaged in PACT have required a third block; fewer have needed four; and there is no record of a child needing more than four. Children with phonological disorder *and* mild language or fluency difficulties have needed about the same volume of therapy for speech, but most have had intervention for longer to address their other, non-speech goals.

Target Selection

Like goal selection and goal attack, target selection (with exceptions like Shaun's wanting to work on /ʃ/ to pronounce his own name correctly) is therapist-driven, and the reasons certain targets are given preferential treatment are explained to parents. As part of a stopping pattern, Shaun, 4;9, mentioned in Chapter 9, called himself 'Dawn'. Dawn, an adult neighbour, apparently oblivious to the misery it evoked and angry appeals from Shaun to 'Stop it', teased him endlessly to the point where *all* he and his mother were interested in doing in therapy was to work on /ʃ/ in just one word – *Shaun* (which we did, successfully).

In selecting treatment targets, the clinician uses linguistic criteria, considering motivational factors and attributes of the child and parents; is flexible regarding feature contrasts which can be minimally, maximally, or multiply opposed depending on the child's intervention needs and disposition; and applies research evidence and clinical judgement. Traditional and newer criteria (see Table 9.1) may be applied to isolating optimal targets.

Sometimes it is necessary to fall back on other, more traditional criteria. Take Tessa for example (Bowen, 2010). Superficially, Tessa 5;10, was a perfect candidate for a least knowledge approach using high-frequency lexical targets because she had a phonetic inventory of only 13 consonants, a PCC of 38%, and extensive homophony. Or *was* she? She was a fretful, diffident child with wary, apprehensive parents, ready to abandon therapy if the clinician attempted anything 'too hard'. These three were unsuited to complex maximal oppositions or empty set feature contrasts, for which Tessa had least knowledge. Instead, they needed to ease into intervention via a gentler, albeit less potent, approach using unmarked, stimulable, inconsistently erred, early developing sounds; low-frequency words with low neighbourhood density; and minimal feature contrasts. Once they were all ready to trust the clinician's target choices and to confront more difficult tasks, Tessa took more risks, handling the challenges of multiply opposed word sets within the Multiple Exemplar Training component of PACT.

PACT Components

PACT has five dynamic and interacting components: Parent Education (Family Education), Metalinguistic Training, Phonetic Production Training, Multiple

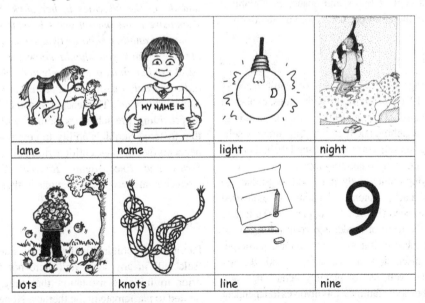

Figure 5.6 /l/ versus /n/ minimal word pairs. Drawings by Helen Rippon, Speech and Language Therapist www.blacksheeppress.co.uk.

Exemplar Training (Auditory Input and Minimal Contrasts Therapy), and Homework. The therapy involves the child, primary caregiver(s) and therapist; and sometimes older siblings, grandparents and teachers, become involved in homework.

Parent Education (Family Education)

Rationale

Recognizing that PACT will not suit every child or every family, we hypothesized that arming interested parents with techniques (e.g., modelling, recasting, fostering repair strategies, performing metaphonological tasks, and providing alliterative input in thematic play contexts) related to their own child's intervention needs, and by working with them collaboratively, we would tap a unique and powerful 'therapeutic resource'. Unique because a child (usually) only has one set of parents, and powerful because (usually) parents likely spend the most time with their child and are the people who are most motivated to help. Through supportive parent education, they would be guided to use 'speech time' optimally in homework and incidentally in real (natural and not contrived) communicative contexts as opportunities arose. This might lead to the need for fewer consultations and fewer child–clinician-parent contact hours and ensure that planned breaks from therapy were used more productively.

Methods

Incorporating simple principles of adult learning (Knowles, 1970), parents learn techniques, explained in plain-English (Bowen, 1998a, 1998b), including: delivering modelling and recasting, encouraging self-monitoring and self-correction, using labelled praise, and providing focused auditory input.

Employing clinical judgement and responding to parent feedback, parent education is delivered according to need (Bowen & Cupples, 2004). It may happen in the form of modelling, counselling, direct instruction, observation, scripted routines, participation and discussion in assessment and therapy sessions, as well as roleplaying, 'coaching' and rehearsal. For some families, this involves independent reading of handouts and publications (Bowen, 1998a,

1998b; Flynn & Lancaster, 1996) and viewing informational slide shows that are e-mailed to them, sent via file sharing software, or downloaded from www. speech-language-therapy.com, viewed on home computers, and later discussed. Some families need more support than this and are 'talked through' informational handouts and view individualized (for them and their child) slide shows in-clinic, explained carefully by the therapist.

Written information is provided in a speech book that often becomes a prized possession of the child's, particularly if it features their artwork. It is used to facilitate communication between therapist, family and others involved (e.g., grandparents or teachers). It includes current targets and goals, a progress record, homework activities, developmental norms, and information about intervention for SSD. Parents and teachers are encouraged to contribute to the book: recording progress, commenting on homework content and performance, noting favourite activities or their own innovations and often giving important pointers to the therapist that might otherwise be unavailable.

On the latter point, Bowen and Cupples (2004) reported that Sophie, 4;3, with a moderate-to-severe SSD, talked constantly at home and was chatty in the clinic, but that her teacher surprised (and enlightened) the therapist and her parents when she wrote in the speech book: '*I enjoy working with Sophie and doing the activities in her book. She is very responsive in the one-on-one – loves it – but if I try to involve another child or two, she clams up completely. I think you should know that she never speaks to her kindy peers – only to teachers and the aide, and only one-to-one, and in a quiet voice we can hardly hear*'. The teacher's insightful note led to providing pre-school personnel with strategies that fostered Sophie's ability to communicate with her peers (see the page entitled '*Adult Communicative Styles and Encouraging Reticent Children to Converse*' at www.speech-language-therapy.com).

Discussion

Parents of the children in the efficacy study were not 'selected' in any sense and were not forewarned prior to initial consultation that they would be invited to participate in the therapy. Nonetheless, all the families rose to the task willingly, becoming actively involved in therapy sessions and in homework which they did in 5- to 7-minute bursts once, twice or three times daily, as recommended. On average, homework was done 24 times per week (4 families), 18 times per week (1 family), 12 times per week (7 families), 8 times per week (1 family) and 6 times per week (1 family) (Bowen, 2010; Bowen & Cupples, 2004).

Parents vary in the amount and style of information they need, some performing well with little explanation, learning best via observation and rehearsal. Others want a lot of 'training' before they become comfortable performing activities at home. Although it is encouraged without insisting, some parents are shy about rehearsing homework tasks in the clinic with the therapist watching. Educational levels appear to have little bearing on how readily parents comprehend and work with concepts, expressed in plain-English, such as 'sound patterns', 'sound classes', 'reinforcement', 'modelling', 'labelled praise', 'revisions and repairs', 'progressive approximations', 'shaping' and 'gradualness of acquisition'.

Subjectively, it seems some parents have an instinct, 'feel', or 'gene' for this sort of thing, and some appear to have missed out! Some are intuitive 'natural teachers', and some are not. Despite this, it is amazing what parents will *learn* to do well, with adequate support, when they perceive that their child may benefit. Parents with histories of communication difficulties like their child's may possess a special empathy, although some of them may have residual issues affecting their capacity to reflect on language function and to enjoy language play (Crystal, 1996, 1998).

In delivering parent education, it is imperative to

- Avoid overwhelming families with information at any point.
- Circumvent giving them the impression that they must become 'mini-therapists'.
- Provide parents with opportunities to rehearse new skills if appropriate, while being sensitive that some adults find it embarrassing and difficult (or culturally inappropriate) to play (Watts Pappas & Bowen, 2007).
- Create an atmosphere in which parents can feel comfortable in questioning anything not understood, share their perspectives, and exercise choice.
- Listen to their ideas respectfully and incorporate them where possible.

Metalinguistic Training

Rationale

This component was inspired by a fascinating article by Dean and Howell (1986) that proposed a role for guided discussion and meta-language in helping children reflect on the features (properties) of phonemes, and the structure of syllables, with a view to improving their awareness of when and how to apply phonological repair strategies. Dean, Howell, and colleagues went on to develop *Metaphon*, described earlier in this chapter, an approach that centres on dialogue between therapist and child with only passing references to parents. We wanted to take their recommendations in a new direction, actively engaging parents, still with the aim of increasing children's metaphonological awareness, and their capacity to reflect on their speech output.

Excited by the practical connections between Ingram's (1976) schema of underlying representation, surface form and mapping rules, and the Dean and Howell (1986) suggestions for developing linguistic awareness, we considered that, if they were only implemented in weekly therapy sessions, their effects might not be optimal. Our plan was to provide parents with training, scripts, and informational handouts (later to become Bowen, 1998a in English, and in French, Bowen, 2007). We reasoned that if *child*, and *clinician* and *parents*, and *teachers* where applicable, used a common language around sound and syllable properties, and reasons for, and communicative consequences of homophony, it would improve the accuracy of that child's knowledge of the system of phonemic contrasts and increase the likelihood of spontaneous self-corrections. This would be especially the case if *all* the adults involved (not just the SLP/SLT) knew how to reinforce them. Metalinguistic training fosters 'phonological discoveries' by the child. His or her capacity to *perceive, talk about, reflect upon* and *revise and repair* homophonous productions is enhanced via simple routines and systematic feedback delivered by parents.

Methods

Using guided discussion (Dean & Howell, 1986), child, parents and clinician talk and think about the properties of speech sounds and how they are organized to convey meaning, incorporating simple metaphonological and phonological awareness (Hesketh, 2010, 2015; McNeill, A22) tasks. In finding a common language to describe phonemic features and syllable shapes, the clinician can borrow from many sources, including Klein's (1996a, 1996b) 'imagery 'imagery labels' (e.g., *poppy, windy, throaty,* and *tippy*), discussed in Chapter 4); *Metaphon* (Dean et al., 1990) terms such as *long, short, front, back, noisy, growly, whisper* and *quiet*; and the imagery names (e.g., *2-step sound, bunny rabbit sound*) and the verbal (e.g., *Where's your buzzy bee?*) and gestural cues (e.g., 'finger walking' for 2-step sounds) in Table 4.1.

Activities, at home and in therapy, involve sound picture associations (e.g., /ɹ/ is a roaring lion sound; /tʃ/ is a choo-choo train; /f/ is a bunny rabbit sound, because it is made with teeth like a bunny); phoneme segmentation for onset matching (e.g., kangaroo starts with /k/); awareness of rhymes and sound patterns (e.g., games with minimal pairs like *tie-die*; and near minimal pairs like *tie-tight*); rudimentary knowledge of the concept of 'word'; understanding the idea of words and longer utterances 'making sense'; awareness of the use of revision and repair strategies using 'judgement of correctness' games (e.g., *The boy tore his shirt* vs. *The boy tore his cert*) and the 'fixed-up-one routine'; and playing with morphophonological structures to produce lexical and grammatical innovations (e.g., *pick* vs. *picks*).

The use of spontaneous revisions and repairs is fostered, particularly at home, by use of the fixed-up-one routine. The routine is a metalinguistic technique that allows adults to talk simply to children about self-corrections. Scripts, such as the one displayed in Figure 5.7, are provided to introduce them to the technique, and various versions of it are available, with an instructional slide show at www.speech-language-therapy.com. Also, regarding self-monitoring and making revisions and repairs, the child is encouraged to *notice* phoneme collapses or homonymy (e.g., *boo* and *blue* realized homophonously as /bu/).

Discussion

The 1986 suggestions of Dean and Howell were adopted and extended, allowing metalinguistic awareness to be targeted in naturalistic, supportive clinic *and home* settings. Expressions that crop up constantly in the context of PACT being discussed with parents are *'talking task'*, *'listening task'*, *'thinking task'*, *'fixed-up-ones'*, *'word'*, *'rhyme'*, *'making sense'*, *'make the words sound different from each other'*, *'two-step word'* and *'remember the 50:50 split'*.

The latter refers to the general recommendation that the 50:50 split between 'talking tasks' versus 'thinking and listening tasks' that is observed in therapy sessions is also observed at home.

Sometimes a family generates its own appropriate terminology. Memorable offerings have included 'Bob', 'Bobs' and 'fix-its' in relation to 'fixed-up-ones' (Bob the Builder's motto is 'Can we fix it? Yes, we can') and 'Einstein Time' in relation to listening and thinking tasks! 'Einstein Time' and 'Nice one, Einstein!' were the brainchild of Sebastian's father, who was intrigued by my framed picture of Einstein, adorned with a sticky-note 'thinks bubble' that read 'THINKING'.

The picture can be on view during 'thinking tasks', such as judgement of correctness games, silent sorting of word-pairs, 'point to the one I say' activities, and word classification games, to cue everyone that (quiet) 'thinking' is supposed to be happening! Readers wishing to experiment with this idea can download six Einstein pictures from https://www.speech-language-therapy.com/pdf/docs/ae6.pdf and 20 from https://www.speech-language-therapy.com/pdf/docs/ae20.pdf

Phonetic Production Training

Rationale

'Phonological disorders arise more in the mind than in the mouth', according to Grunwell (1987), and phonological therapy is, by definition, linguistic, meaning-based, focused on activating a child's underlying system for phoneme use, and 'in the mind'. That said, some children with phonological disorder need help at the phonemic level *and* the perceptual and phonetic levels. In other words, they must be taught to *perceive* (discriminate) sounds and *produce* the sounds and structures.

seal

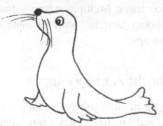

1. Say to your child, "Listen. If I said 'heel', it wouldn't sound right. I would have to fix it up and say 'seal'".

soap

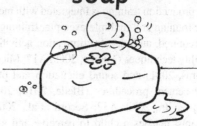

2. Say to your child, "'Hope' isn't right, is it? I need to do a fixed-up-one and say 'soap'".

soup

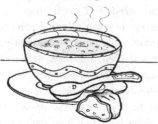

3. "Would I have to do a fixed-up-one if I said 'hoop' for this one?"

sand

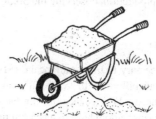

4. "What would I have to do if I accidentally said 'hand' for this one? I would have to do a ..." [fixed-up-one]

sauce

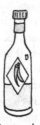

5. "If I said 'horse' instead of 'sauce' I would have to do a fixed-up-one again. I would have to think to myself not 'horse' it's 'sauce'. Did you hear that fixed-up-one?"

sun

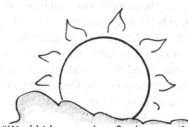

6. "Would I have to do a fixed-up-one if I said 'hun' for this one?"

Self-corrections

Adults continually make little mistakes when they speak. They barely notice these mistakes at a conscious level, and quickly correct themselves, and go on with what they are saying. This process of noticing speech mistakes and correcting them as we go is called making revisions and repairs, or self-corrections. Many children with speech sound difficulties are not very good at self-correcting. They find it difficult to monitor their speech (i.e., listen to it critically) and make corrections.

Fixed-up-ones

At home this week, introduce the idea of a "fixed-up-one", or the process of noticing speech mistakes and then saying the word(s) again more clearly, specifically in relation to the consonants at the beginnings of the six words featured on this page. Go through the following routine two or three times, and talk about fixed-up-ones. Have some fun making up other "mistakes" with words, that need correcting.

Figure 5.7 An example of a fixed-up-one routine. Drawing by Helen Rippon, Speech and Language Therapist www.blacksheeppress.co.uk.

Methods

Phonetic production training is integrated with meta-linguistic training and multiple exemplar training. It uses, as required, auditory discrimination activities, stimulability techniques (Miccio, 2005, A17; Miccio & Williams, 2021) and sound elicitation and phonemic placement procedures (Bleile, 2018, 2019, A36; Flipsen Jr., 2022; A37; Secord et al., 2007). The therapist teaches a child to perceive and generate absent phones *beyond* isolated sound level, or failing that, to produce approximations of consonants in the same sound class in CV and VC combinations. Homework for phonetic targets includes listening and production, observing the 50:50 split.

Discussion

It is rarely necessary to train intervocalic (SIWW or SFWW) stimulability or to train all vowel and diphthong contexts. For instance, having taught /tʃu/ and /ɪtʃ/, clinicians seldom have to teach /tʃu tʃi tʃɔ tʃaɪ tʃoʊ tʃeɪ tʃa/ and /utʃ itʃ ɔtʃ aɪtʃ oʊtʃ eɪtʃ atʃ/, etc. Children usually proceed from syllable to word level, having demonstrated the capacity to produce the phone in CV and/or VC contexts. Introductory stimulability or pre-practice tasks may be at individual sound (segment) and 'nonsense syllable' level, even involving 'syllable drill', but not for long. Once a child is stimulable for a target, or is producing a passable approximation, or a phone in the same sound class, in syllables or words, therapy moves onto the phonemic level and all activities are 'meaning-based' at word level and beyond (Bowen & Cupples, 2006).

The child does production practice of a few target words, usually no more than six, depending on their temperament. If the child tends to become bored with few stimuli, this can be increased to maintain their interest and cooperation. It is important to know that 'phonetic production training' does not imply hierarchical, traditional articulation therapy (Van Riper, 1978) or adaptations of it.

Multiple Exemplar Training

Rationale

Focused auditory input and the heightened perceptual saliency of phones, structures, and contrasts, provided by the therapy activities, increases the learnability of new sounds, syllable structures and word contrasts. Multiple exemplar training has two overlapping aspects: auditory input and minimal pair therapy.

Methods: Auditory Input

Auditory input involves listening-lists, alliterative input, and thematic play; and minimal contrast therapy uses minimal, maximal, or multiple oppositions between words. Listening lists comprise word lists of up to 15 words with a common phonetic feature (e.g., /s/ SIWI: *sail, seat, sigh, sew, seed, sum, sack, sun, sand, sea, sock, soup, silly, seal, saw, soap*) or up to seven minimal pairs (e.g., minimal oppositions: *sock-shock, sour-shower; sack-shack, sip-ship, sell-shell, Sue-shoe, save-shave*) or triplets (e.g., *seat-sheet-cheat, sigh-shy-chai, sip-ship-chip, sore-shore-chore, Sue-shoe-chew*) or target, error, and 'foil' (e.g., *pie-bye-boo, pig-big-boo, Paul-ball-boo, pin-bin-boo, pug-bug-boo, pat-bat-boo, poi-boy-boo*) to the child.

Foils are introduced to make some sequences more rhythmical and fun, and more enticing for the child to dance, jog, march, rap, or bop to. Sometimes the input words are pictured and sometimes not. Alliterative input can be provided via stories, songs, rhymes, games, and worksheets, such as one for /k/ SIWI from Black Sheep Press (https://www.blacksheeppress.co.uk) which depicts a *cat*: in a *cupboard*, with a *kite*, in a *coat*, in a *corner*, in a *kennel*, being *carried*, behind a *curtain* and in a *cap*.

Auditory input also involves games and books selected for their potential to allow the child to hear frequent repetitions of targets. Bowen (2010) describes an activity for 'Bruno', 4;2, who was learning /f/ SFWF. In one session, and for a week in homework, he listened to the story of Jeff, Steph, and the scarf (shown in Figure 7.6). For related homework, Bruno listened to and sorted into 'rhymes' the pairs *laugh-scarf, off-cough, Jeff-Steph*, etc.; listened to and pointed to the minimal pairs *cough-cop, Steph-step, wife-wipe*, etc.; and listened to and pointed to the near minimal pairs *la-laugh, Y-wife, Lee-leaf*, etc. work illustrated in Figure 5.8.

At intervals, outside of formal homework, Bruno initiated and played a game with his father where a superhero jumped off a roof. He also played self-initiated games with Smurf figurines with both parents.

Rhyming Pairs /f/ SFWF

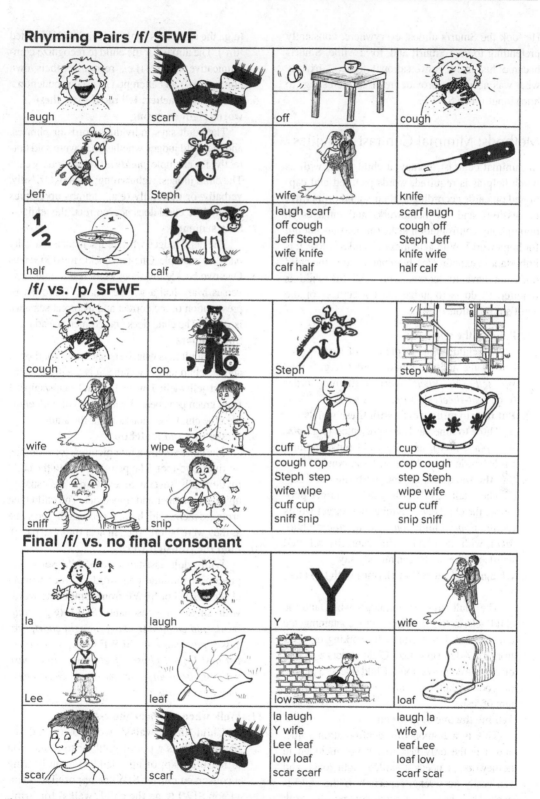

laugh	scarf	off	cough
Jeff	Steph	wife	knife
half	calf	laugh scarf / off cough / Jeff Steph / wife knife / calf half	scarf laugh / cough off / Steph Jeff / knife wife / half calf

/f/ vs. /p/ SFWF

cough	cop	Steph	step
wife	wipe	cuff	cup
sniff	snip	cough cop / Steph step / wife wipe / cuff cup / sniff snip	cop cough / step Steph / wipe wife / cup cuff / snip sniff

Final /f/ vs. no final consonant

la	laugh	Y	wife
Lee	leaf	low	loaf
scar	scarf	la laugh / Y wife / Lee leaf / low loaf / scar scarf	laugh la / wife Y / leaf Lee / loaf low / scarf scar

Figure 5.8 Minimal pair and near minimal pair sets. Drawing by Helen Rippon, Speech and Language Therapist www.blacksheeppress.co.uk.

He took the Smurfs almost everywhere, constantly pretending to be a Smurf; and, for a while, Smurfs became his main conversational topic – exactly what was needed to provide intense, interesting (to him) input for /f/ SFWF.

Methods: Minimal Contrast Activities

In minimal contrast therapy, a child sorts, with as much help as is required, words pictured and captioned on cards according to their sound properties, in sessions and for homework, and engages in homophony confrontation tasks (in sessions but not for homework). With activities 6, 7 and 8 below, it is important to explain clearly to parents that the child does not have to 'correct you'. All the child is required to do is to judge the correctness of the adult's production.

1. **Point to the one I say**

   The child points to pictures of words, spoken by the adult in random order (e.g., *sheet, sip, sell, ship, shell, seat*) or rhyming order (e.g., *seat-sheet, sip-ship, sell-shell*).

2. **Put the rhyming words with these words**

   Three to nine cards are presented (e.g., *pin, pea, pack, pole*), and the child puts rhyming cards beside them (*bin, bee, back, bowl*).

3. **Say the word that rhymes with the one I say**

   The adult says words with the target phoneme; the child says rhyming non-target words (adult: *floor*; child: *four*; adult: *flake*; child: *fake*), with the child saying carefully selected words that he or she can already say.

4. **Give me the word that rhymes with the one I say**

   The adult says the non-target word, and the child selects the rhyming word containing the target sound. For example, in working on velar fronting: Adult says 'tea'; Child selects a picture of 'key'. Adult says 'tool'; Child selects a picture of 'cool'. Adult says 'tape'; Child selects a picture of 'cape'.

5. **Tell me the one to give you**

   This is a homophony confrontation game, and it is the only task that it not included in homework. It needs a skilled, light touch and can easily go wrong, especially if the child is pushed too hard. In a game context, the adult responds to the word they heard the child say

(e.g., the child says [tɪn] for 'chin' and is handed 'tin'). The aim is for the child to recognize communicative failure (i.e., recognize their own homophony) and attempt a revised production.

6. **You be the teacher: tell me if I say these words right or wrong**

   The adult says individual words or phrases, and the child judges whether they were said correctly; for example, *puddy tat* versus 'pussy cat'. The child judges: right/wrong; yes/no; OK/silly, verbally, or gesturally (e.g., thumbs up/thumbs down). The child does not 'correct' the adult.

7. **Silly sentences**

   The child judges whether a sentence is a 'silly one'; for example, One-two buckle my doo versus One-two buckle my shoe; Mary had a little lamb versus Mary had a whittle wham. The order of presentation of the correct and incorrect sentence is varied. The child does not 'correct' the adult.

8. **Silly dinners**

   The adult says what he or she wants for dinner, and the child judges whether it is a 'silly dinner': I want jelly/deli; I want fish and chips/ships; I want green peas/bees; I want a cup of coffee/toffee. The child does not 'correct' the adult.

9. **Shake-ups and matchups**

   The child is shown four pictures, for example, tie-time, two-toot. The pairs are said to the child rhythmically several times. Cards are 'shaken up' in a container and tipped out. The child then arranges them, with help, if necessary, 'the same as they were before' (i.e., in near minimal pairs).

10. **Find the two-step-words**

    With adult assistance, the child sorts pictured near minimal pair words with consonant clusters SIWI or SFWF from contrasting words with singleton consonants SIWI (e.g., *nail-snail, nip-snip, nag-snag, nought-snort, no-snow, nap-snap*) or SFWF (e.g., *wait-waist, net-nest, goat-ghost, feet-feast, tote-toast, vet-vest, Bert-burst*; or *bus-bust, chess-chest, guess-guest, Gus-gust*).

11. **Walk when you hear the 2-steps**

    Child 'finger-walks' two steps (to a destination such as a pot of gold, or to a place on a treasure map; or up a ladder) upon hearing a consonant cluster SIWI as opposed to a singleton SIWI (e.g., the child 'walks' for 'trip', but not 'tip' or 'rip').

Discussion

Suggestions for multiple exemplar activities 1–11 above are provided to parents. For many families, the ideas trigger their creativity, and they identify novel and apt games, activities, and books, perfect for their child (and inspiring for the clinician).

Homework

Rationale

Homework administered by a parent or parents provides children with practice, reinforcement, opportunities to generalize and opportunities for discovery. It allows families to hone, generalize, and enjoy the 'teaching skills' learned in therapy sessions. By engaging in activities autonomously, families can experiment, creating new opportunities for learning in natural, functional contexts. As their knowledge, skills and confidence grow, most will innovate, making up new games and enjoyable repetitive routines, and some even instigate apposite 'next steps' in therapy. They also become more skilled in recognizing 'teaching moments' weaving them seamlessly into the child's day so that they do not feel they are 'doing speech homework all the time'. Because homework suggestions are flexible, homework is conducive to internal development and families can shape it to fit their interests, preferences, and culture. Homework can assume the family 'stamp' as well as the clinician's 'style', influencing the form, content and conduct of sessions in dynamic and striking ways, letting the adults create activities a child genuinely likes and is responsive to.

Methods

Homework comprises short bursts of home activities and the use of appropriate speech stimulation techniques (e.g., modelling corrections) when opportune. It includes activities from the most recent session, delivered in 5- to 7-minute bursts once, twice, or three times daily, one-to-one with an adult in good listening conditions. Examples of 'good' and 'poor' listening conditions are discussed.

Practices can be as little as 10 minutes apart. For example, practice-craft-practice-craft-practice-craft for children who like making things; or for booklovers, practice-story-practice-story-practice-story; or practices can be alternated with playing a game: practice-game-practice-game-practice-game or completing a puzzle: (practice-puzzle-practice-puzzle-practice-puzzle), with the 50:50 split observed between listening–thinking tasks versus talking tasks.

Parents are asked to do the homework regularly, briefly, naturalistically, encouragingly and with humour. Instructions and activities go in a homework book and are explained as often as needed. It is recommended that they *do not do homework before the child's session* on 'therapy days' (so that they start the session fresh). It is also recommended that they *always to do homework after the child's session* on 'therapy days' (to reinforce recent learning that occurred in the session).

If, for some reason, homework does not happen for a day or days, parents are asked not to 'compensate' by doing more than three practices in one day subsequently. It is suggested that they combine homework with activities the child likes, such as colouring and cutting, story reading or going to a park or favourite spot sometimes to do it.

Discussion

If one family member (e.g., the child's father) usually accompanies the child and participates in therapy sessions, other family members (e.g., the child's mother) can learn from their example during homework sessions and by watching their application of modelling, recasting and other techniques. The system fails if one parent does 'the bringing' to sessions and the other parent does *only* the formal homework without good communication between the two, as sometimes happens.

Younger children generally like the idea of doing 'homework' as something 'big kids' do. For some parents and older children, however, there may be interfering negative connotations, perhaps left over from school. A colleague in the United States commented on this, giving me pause for thought:

I use the term 'home programming' instead of 'homework'. For me homework is something that kids might hate doing, or it may be something that children are meant to complete individually. Home programming reflects effort on the parents' part and may not get the same negative response that 'homework' can sometimes get. It could also be called 'speech work' or such. It is just a preference based on my experience in providing after school services and working with parents. Many of my colleagues, I'm sure, use 'homework'.

Dr. Mark Guiberson,
personal correspondence, 2014

Implications for Service Delivery

The intervention options described in Chapters 4 and 5 carry with them serious implications for treatment fidelity, and ethical, 'common', 'best', and evidence-based practice, the themes of Chapter 6.

Note

1. Thanks to Dr. Barbara Dodd for helpful input regarding Core Vocabulary Therapy.

References

Alkheraiji, N. (2018). *Investigating speech output skills in 3–5-year-old Arabic-speaking children: A psycholinguistic approach* (Unpublished doctoral thesis). The University of Sheffield. https://etheses.whiterose.ac.uk/19483

Anthony, A., Bogle, D., Ingram, T. T. S., & McIsaac, M. W. (1971). *Edinburgh articulation test*. Churchill Livingstone.

Baker, E. (2010). The experience of discharging children from phonological intervention. *International Journal of Speech-Language Pathology*, 12(4), 325–328. https://doi.org/10.3109/17549507.2010.488326

Baker, E., Croot, K., McLeod, S., & Paul, R. (2001). Psycholinguistic models of speech development and their application to clinical practice. *Journal of Speech, Language, and Hearing Research*, 44(3), 685–702. https://doi.org/10.1044/1092-4388(2001/055)

Blache, S. E. (1982). Minimal word pairs and distinctive feature training. In M. Crary (Ed.), *Phonological intervention: Concepts and procedures*, (pp. 61–96). College-Hill Press Inc.

Bleile, K. M. (2018). *The late eight* (3rd ed.). Plural Publishing.

Bleile, K. M. (2019). *Speech sound disorders: For class and clinic* (4th ed.). Plural Publishing.

Bowen, C. (1996a). Evaluation of a phonological therapy with treated and untreated groups of young children (Unpublished doctoral dissertation). Macquarie University. http://hdl.handle.net/1959.14/304812

Bowen, C. (1996b). The quick screener. www.speech-language-therapy.com

Bowen, C. (1998a). *Developmental phonological disorders: A practical guide for families and teachers*. The Australian Council for Educational Research.

Bowen, C. (1998b). *Speech-language-therapy dot com*. www.speech-language-therapy.com

Bowen, C. (2007). *Les difficultés phonologiques chez l'enfant: guide à l'intention des familles, des enseignants et des intervenants en petite enfance*. Caroline Bowen; Rachel Fortin, traductrice et adaptatrice. Chenelière-éducation.

Bowen, C. (2009). *Children's speech sound disorders*. Wiley-Blackwell.

Bowen, C. (2010). Parents and children together (PACT) intervention for children with speech sound disorders. In A. L. Williams, S. McLeod, & R. J. McCauley (Eds.), *Interventions for speech sound disorders in children* (pp. 407–426). Paul H. Brookes Publishing Co.

Bowen, C. (2015). *Children's speech sound disorders* (2nd ed.). Wiley-Blackwell. https://doi.org/10.1002/9781119180418

Bowen, C., & Cupples, L. (1998). A tested phonological therapy in practice. *Child Language Teaching and Therapy*, 14(1), 29–50. https://doi.org/10.1177%2F026565909801400102

Bowen, C., & Cupples, L. (1999a). Parents and children together (PACT): A collaborative approach to phonological therapy. *International Journal of Language and Communication Disorders*, 34(1), 35–55. https://doi.org/10.1080/136828299247603

Bowen, C., & Cupples, L. (1999b). A phonological therapy in depth: A reply to commentaries. *International Journal of Language and Communication Disorders*, 34(1), 65–83. https://doi.org/10.1080/136828299247649

Bowen, C., & Cupples, L. (2004). The role of families in optimizing phonological therapy outcomes. *Child Language Teaching and Therapy*, 20(3), 245–260. https://doi.org/10.1191%2F0265659004ct274oa

Bowen, C., & Cupples, L. (2006). PACT: Parents and children together in phonological therapy. *Advances in Speech Language Pathology*, 8(3), 282–292. https://doi.org/10.1080/14417040600826980

Broome, K., McCabe, P., Docking, K., Doble, M., & Carrigg, B. (2021). Speech abilities in a heterogeneous group of children with autism. *Journal of Speech, Language, and Hearing Research, 64*(12), 4599–4613. https://doi.org/10.1044/2021_JSLHR-20-00651

Broomfield, J., & Dodd, B. (2004a). The nature of referred subtypes of primary speech disability. *Child Language Teaching and Therapy, 20*(2), 135–151. https://doi.org/10.1191%2F0265659004ct267oa

Brosseau-Lapré, F., & Roepke, E. (2022). Implementing speech perception and phonological awareness intervention for children with speech sound disorders. *Language, Speech, and Hearing Services in Schools, 53*(3), 646–658. https://doi.org/10.1044/2022_LSHSS-21-00117

Camarata, S. (1993). The application of naturalistic conversation training to speech production in children with speech disabilities. *Journal of Applied Behavior Analysis, 26*(2), 173–182. https://doi.org/10.1901/jaba.1993.26-173

Camarata, S., Yoder, P., & Camarata, M. (2006). Simultaneous treatment of grammatical and speech-comprehensibility deficits in children with Down syndrome. *Down Syndrome Research and Practice, 11*(1), 9–17. https://doi.org/10.3104/reports.314

Camarata, S. M. (2010). Naturalistic intervention for speech intelligibility and speech accuracy. In A. L. Williams, S. McLeod, & R. J. McCauley (Eds.), *Interventions for speech sound disorders in children* (pp. 381–405). Brookes Publishing Co.

Camarata, S. M. (2021). Naturalistic recast intervention. In A. L. Williams, S. McLeod, & R. J. McCauley (Eds.), *Interventions for speech sound disorders in children* (pp. 227–361). Brookes Publishing Co.

Crosbie, S., Holm, A., & Dodd, B. (2005). Intervention for children with severe speech disorder: A comparison of two approaches. *International Journal of Language and Communication Disorders, 40*(4), 467–491. https://doi.org/10.1080/13682820500126049

Crosbie, S., Pine, C., Holm, A., & Dodd, B. (2006). Treating Jarrod: A core vocabulary approach. *Advances in Speech Language Pathology, 8*(3), 316–321. https://doi.org/10.1080/14417040600750172

Crystal, D. (1996). Language play and linguistic intervention. *Child Language Teaching and Therapy, 12*(3), 328–344. https://doi.org/10.1177/026565909601200307

Crystal, D. (1998). *Language play.* Penguin Books.

Day, A. (1993). *Carl goes to daycare.* Farrar, Straus & Giroux.

De Thorne, L. S., Johnson, C. J., Walder, L., & Mahurin-Smith, J. (2009). When 'Simon says' doesn't work: Alternative to imitation for facilitating early speech development. *American Journal of Speech-Language Pathology, 18*(2), 133–145. https://doi.org/10.1044/1058-0360(2008/07-0090)

Dean, E., & Howell, J. (1986). Developing linguistic awareness: A theoretically based approach to phonological disorders. *British Journal of Disorders of Communication, 21*(2), 223–238. https://doi.org/10.3109/13682828609012279

Dean, E., Howell, J., Hill, A., & Waters, D. (1990). *Metaphon resource pack.* NFER Nelson.

Dean, E. C., Howell, J., Waters, D., & Reid, J. (1995). *Metaphon:* A metalinguistic approach to the treatment of phonological disorder in children. *Clinical Linguistics and Phonetics, 9*(1), 1–19. https://doi.org/10.3109/02699209508985318

Denne, M., Langdown, N., Pring, T., & Roy, P. (2005). Treating children with expressive phonological disorders: Does phonological awareness therapy work in the clinic? *International Journal of Language and Communication Disorders, 40*(4), 493–504. https://doi.org/10.1080/13682820500142582

Dodd, B. (2005). *Differential diagnosis and treatment of children with speech disorder* (2nd ed.). Whurr Publishers.

Dodd, B. (2015). Assessment and intervention for 2-year-olds at risk for phonological disorder. In C. Bowen, *Children's speech sound disorders* (2nd ed., pp. 88–94). Wiley-Blackwell.

Dodd, B., & Bradford, A. (2000). A comparison of three therapy methods for children with different types of developmental disorder. *International Journal of Language and Communication Disorders, 35*(2), 189–209. https://doi.org/10.1080/136828200247142

Dodd, B., Crosbie, S., Zhu, H., Holm, A., & Ozanne, A. (2002). *Diagnostic evaluation of articulation and phonology (DEAP).* Psychological Corporation.

Dodd, B., Holm, A., Crosbie, S., & McIntosh, B. (2006). A core vocabulary approach for management of inconsistent speech disorder. *Advances in Speech-Language Pathology, 8*(3), 220–230. https://doi.org/10.1080/14417040600738177

Dodd, B., & Iacono, T. (1989). Phonological disorders in children: Changes in phonological process use during treatment. *British Journal of Disorders of Communication, 24*(3), 333–352. https://doi.org/10.3109/13682828909019894

Ebbels, S. (2000). Psycholinguistic profiling of a hearing-impaired child. *Child Language Teaching and Therapy, 16*(1), 3–22. https://doi.org/10.1177/026565900001600102

Ellis Weismer, S., Venker, C. E., & Robertson, S. (2017). Focused stimulation approach to language intervention. In R. J. McCauley, M. E. Fey, & R. B. Gillam (Eds.), *Treatment of language disorders in children* (2nd ed., pp. 121–154). Paul H. Brookes Publishing Co.

Fey, M. E. (1992). Articulation and phonology. Inextricable constructs in speech pathology. *Language, Speech and Hearing Services in Schools*, 23(3), 225–232. https://doi.org/10.1044/0161-1461.2303.225

Flipsen, P., Jr. (2022). *Remediation of /r/ for SLPs*. Plural Publishing, Inc.

Flynn, L., & Lancaster, G. (1996). *Children's phonology sourcebook*. Winslow Press.

Fricke, S., & Schäfer, B. (2021). *Test für Phonologische Bewusstheitsfähigkeiten (TPB)* (e-edition). Schulz Kirchner Verlag.

Gardner, H. (2015). Finding the psycholinguistic model in everyday practice. In C. Bowen, *Children's speech sound disorders* (2nd ed., pp. 206–210). Wiley-Blackwell.

Geronikou, E., & Rees, R. (2016). Psycholinguistic profiling reveals underlying impairments for Greek children with speech disorders. *Child Language Teaching and Therapy*, 32(1), 95–110. https://doi.org/10.1177/0265659015583915

Geronikou, E., Vance, M., Wells, B., & Thomson, J. (2018). The case for morphophonological intervention: Evidence from a Greek-speaking child with speech difficulties. *Child Language Teaching and Therapy*, 35(1), 5–23. https://doi.org/10.1177%2F0265659018810329

Gibbon, F. (2013). Therapy for abnormal vowels in children with speech disorders. In M. J. Ball & F. E. Gibbon (Eds.), *Handbook of vowels and vowel disorders* (pp. 429–446). Psychology Press.

Gibbon, F., Shockey, L., & Reid, J. (1992). Description and treatment of abnormal vowels in a phonologically disordered child. *Child Language Teaching and Therapy*, 8(1), 30–59. https://doi.org/10.1177%2F026565909200800103

Gibbon, F. E., & Mackenzie Beck, J. (2002). Therapy for abnormal vowels in children with phonological impairment. In M. J. Ball & F. E. Gibbon (Eds.), *Vowel disorders* (pp. 217–248). Butterworth-Heinemann.

Gillon, G. T. (2000). The efficacy of phonological awareness intervention for children with spoken language impairment. *Language, Speech, and Hearing Services in Schools*, 31(2), 126–141. https://doi.org/10.1044/0161-1461.3102.126

Gillon, G. T. (2002). Follow-up study investigating the benefits of phonological awareness intervention for children with spoken language impairment. *International Journal of Language & and Communication Disorders*, 37(4), 381–400. https://doi.org/10.1080/1368282021000007776

Gillon, G. T. (2005). Facilitating phoneme awareness development in 3- and 4-year-old children with speech impairment. *Language, Speech, and Hearing Services in Schools*, 36(4), 308–324. https://doi.org/10.1044/0161-1461(2005/031)

Gillon, G. T. (2006). Phonological awareness: A preventative framework for preschool children with spoken language impairment. In R. McCauley & M. Fey (Eds.), *Treatment of language disorders in children: Conventional and controversial approaches* (pp. 279–307). Paul H. Brookes Publishing Co.

Gillon, G. T. (2017). *Phonological awareness: From research to practice* (2nd ed.). Guilford Publications.

Gillon, G. T. (2018). *Phonological awareness: From research to practice*. Guilford Publications.

Gillon, G. T., & McNeill, B. C. (2007). Integrated phonological awareness: An intervention program for preschool children with speech impairment. https://www.canterbury.ac.nz/education/research/phonological-awareness-resources/#collapse22480

Girolametto, L., & Weitzman, E. (2006). It takes two to talk – The Hanen program for parents – Early language intervention through caregiver training. In R. McCauley & M. Fey (Eds.), *Treatment of language disorders in children* (pp. 77–104). Paul H. Brookes Publishing Co.

Grunwell, P. (1975). The phonological analysis of articulation disorders. *British Journal of Disorders of Communication*, 10(1), 31–42. https://doi.org/10.3109/13682827509011272

Grunwell, P. (1981). *The nature of phonological disability on children*. Academic.

Grunwell, P. (1982). *Clinical phonology*. Croom Helm.

Grunwell, P. (1985a). *Phonological assessment of child speech (PACS)*. NFER–Nelson.

Grunwell, P. (1985b). Developing phonological skills. *Child Language Teaching and Therapy*, 1(1), 65–72. https://doi.org/10.1177%2F026565908500100108

Grunwell, P. (1987). *Clinical phonology* (2nd ed.). Williams & Wilkins.

Grunwell, P. (1989). Developmental phonological disorders and normal speech development: A review and illustration. *Child Language Teaching and Therapy*, 5(3), 304–319. https://doi.org/10.1177%2F026565908900500305

Grunwell, P. (1992). Process of phonological change in developmental speech disorders. *Clinical Linguistics & Phonetics*, *6*(1–2), 101–122. https://doi.org/10.3109/02699209208985522

Hayiou-Thomas, M. E., Carroll, J. M., Leavett, R., Hulme, C., & Snowling, M. J. (2017). When does speech sound disorder matter for literacy? The role of disordered speech errors, co-occurring language impairment and family risk of dyslexia. *Journal of Child Psychology and Psychiatry*, *58*(2), 197–205. https://doi.org/10.1111/jcpp.12648

Hesketh, A. (2004). Early literacy achievement of children with a history of speech problems. *International Journal of Language and Communication Disorders*, *39*(4), 453–468. https://doi.org/10.1080/13682820410001686013

Hesketh, A. (2010). Metaphonological intervention. In A. L. Williams, S. McLeod, & R. J. McCauley (Eds.), *Interventions for speech sound disorders in children* (pp. 247–274). Paul H. Brookes Publishing Co.

Hesketh, A. (2015). Phoneme awareness intervention for children with speech disorder: Who, when and how? In C. Bowen, *Children's speech sound disorders* (2nd ed., pp. 210–214). Wiley-Blackwell.

Hesketh, A., Adams, C., Nightingale, C., & Hall, R. (2000). Phonological awareness therapy and articulatory training approaches for children with phonological disorders: A comparative outcome study. *International Journal of Language & Communication Disorders*, *35*(3), 337–354. https://doi.org/10.1080/136828200410618

Hesketh, A., Dima, E., & Nelson, V. (2007). Teaching phoneme awareness to preliterate children with speech disorder: A randomized controlled trial. *International Journal of Language and Communication Disorders*, *42*(3), 251–271. https://doi.org/10.1080/13682820600940141

Hodson, B. W. (2004). *Hodson assessment of phonological patterns (HAPP- 3)* (3rd ed.). Pro-ed.

Hodson, B. W. (2007). *Evaluating and enhancing children's phonological systems: Research and theory to practice*. PhonoComp Publishers.

Hodson, B. W., & Paden, E. P. (1983). *Targeting intelligible speech: A phonological approach to remediation*. College-Hill Press.

Hodson, B. W., & Paden, E. P. (1991). *Targeting intelligible speech: A phonological approach to remediation* (2nd ed.). Pro-Ed.

Hoffman, P. R. (1992). Synergistic development of phonetic skill. *Language, Speech, and Hearing Services in Schools*, *23*(3), 254–260. https://doi.org/10.1044/0161-1461.2303.254

Hoffman, P. R., & Norris, J. A. (2010). Whole language (dynamical systems) phonological intervention. In A. L. Williams, S. McLeod, & R. J. McCauley (Eds.), *Interventions for speech sound disorders* (pp. 347–382). Paul H. Brookes Publishing Co.

Howell, J., & Dean, E. (1994). *Treating phonological disorders in children: Metaphon—theory to practice* (2nd ed.). Whurr.

Hume, S. B., Schwarz, I., & Hedrick, M. (2018). Preliminary investigation of the use of phonological awareness paired with production training in Childhood Apraxia of Speech. *Perspectives of the ASHA Special Interest Groups*, *3*(16), 38–52. https://doi.org/10.1044/persp3.SIG16.38

Ingram, D. (1976). *Phonological disability in children*. Edward Arnold.

James, D. G. H. (2015). The relationship between the underlying representation and surface form of multisyllabic words. In C. Bowen, *Children's speech sound disorders* (2nd ed., pp. 439–443). Wiley-Blackwell.

Johnson, C. A., Weston, A. D., & Bain, B. A. (2004). An objective and time-efficient method for determining severity of childhood speech delay. *American Journal of Speech-Language Pathology*, *13*(1), 55–65. https://doi.org/10.1044/1058-0360(2004/007)

Klein, E. S. (1996a). Phonological/traditional approaches to articulation therapy: A retrospective group comparison. *Language, Speech, and Hearing Services in Schools*, *27*(4), 314–323. https://doi.org/10.1044/0161-1461.2704.314

Klein, E. S. (1996b). *Clinical phonology: Assessment and treatment of articulation disorders in children and adults*. Singular Publishing Group, Inc.

Knowles, M. S. (1970). *The modern practise of adult education: Andragogy versus pedagogy*. Association Press.

Lancaster, G. (1991). *The effectiveness of parent administered input training for children with phonological disorders* (Unpublished Master's thesis). City University.

Lancaster, G. (2015). Auditory input therapy. In C. Bowen, *Children's speech sound disorders* (2nd ed., pp. 184–188). Wiley-Blackwell.

Lancaster, G., Levin, A., Pring, T., & Martin, S. (2010). Treating children with phonological problems: Does an eclectic approach to therapy work? *International Journal of Language and Communication Disorders*, *45*(2), 174–181. https://doi.org/10.3109/13682820902818888

Lancaster, G., & Pope, L. (1989). *Working with children's phonology*. Winslow Press.

Leahy, J., & Dodd, B. (1987). The development of disordered phonology: A case study. *Language and Cognitive Processes*, 2(2), 115–132. https://doi.org/10.1080/01690968708406353

Lewis, B. A., Freebairn, L., Tag, J., Benchek, P., Morris, N. J., Iyengar, S. K., Taylor, H. G., Stein, C. M. (2018). Heritability and longitudinal outcomes of spelling skills in individuals with histories of early speech and language disorders. *Learning and Individual Differences*, 65, 1–11. https://doi.org/10.1016/j.lindif.2018.05.001

Locke, J. L. (1980). The inference of speech perception in the phonologically disordered child. Part II: Some clinically novel procedures, their use, some findings. *Journal of Speech and Hearing Disorders*, 45(4), 445–468. https://doi.org/10.1044/jshd.4504.445

Louko, L. J., Conture, E. G., & Edwards, M. L. (1999). Treating children who exhibit co-occurring stuttering and disordered phonology. In R. F. Curlee (Ed.), *Stuttering and related disorders of fluency* (2ⁿᵈ ed., pp. 124–138). Thieme Publishers.

McCabe, P., Thomas, D. C., & Murray, E. (2020). Tutorial: Rapid Syllable Transition Treatment (ReST) – A treatment for Childhood Apraxia of Speech and other Pediatric motor speech disorders. *Perspectives of the ASHA Special Interest Groups*, 5(4), 821–830. https://doi.org/10.1044/2020_PERSP-19-00165

McGill, N., Crowe, K., & McLeod, S. (2020). "Many wasted months": Stakeholders' perspectives about waiting for speech-language pathology services. *International Journal of Speech-Language Pathology*, 22(3), 313–326. https://doi.org/10.1080/17549507.2020.1747541

McIntosh, B., & Dodd, B. (2011). *Toddler phonology.* Pearson Publishers.

McNeill, B. C., Gillon, G. T., & Dodd, B. (2009). Effectiveness of an integrated phonological awareness approach for children with childhood apraxia of speech (CAS). *Child Language Teaching and Therapy*, 25(3), 341–366. https://doi.org/10.1177/0265659009339823

McNeill, B. C., & Hesketh, A. (2010). Developmental complexity of the stimuli included in mispronunciation detection tasks. *International Journal of Language & Communication Disorders*, 45(1), 72–82. https://doi.org/10.3109/13682820902745479

McNeill, B. C., Wolter, J., & Gillon, G. T. (2017). A comparison of the metalinguistic performance and spelling development of children with inconsistent speech sound disorder and their age-matched and reading-matched peers. *American Journal of Speech-Language Pathology*, 26(2), 456–468. https://doi.org/10.1044/2016_ajslp-16-0085

Miccio, A. W. (2005). A treatment program for enhancing stimulability. In A. G. Kamhi & K. E. Pollock (Eds.), *Phonological disorders in children: Clinical decision making in assessment and intervention* (pp. 163–173). Paul H. Brookes Publishing Co.

Miccio, A. W., & Williams, A. L. (2021). Stimulability approach. In A. L. Williams, S. McLeod, & R. J. McCauley (Eds.), *Interventions for speech sound disorders in children* (pp. 279–304). Brookes Publishing Co.

Moriarty, B. C., & Gillon, G. T. (2006). Phonological awareness intervention for children with childhood apraxia of speech. *International Journal of Language and Communication Disorders*, 41(6), 713–734. https://doi.org/10.1080/13682820600623960

Nathan, L., Stackhouse, J., Goulandris, N., & Snowling, M. J. (2004). The development of early literacy skills among children with speech difficulties: A test of the critical age hypothesis. *Journal of Speech, Language, and Hearing Research*, 47(2), 377–391. https://doi.org/10.1044/1092-4388(2004/031)

Pascoe, M., Rossouw, K., Fish, L., Jansen, C., Manley, N., Powell, M., & Rosen, L. (2016). Speech processing and production in two-year-old children acquiring isiXhosa: A tale of two children. *South African Journal of Communication Disorders*, 63(2), 1–16. https://doi.org/10.4102/sajcd.v63i2.134

Pascoe, M., & Stackhouse, J. (2021). Psycholinguistic intervention. In A. L. Williams, S. McLeod, & R. J. McCauley (Eds.), *Interventions for speech sound disorders in children* (2nd ed., pp. 141–170). Brookes Publishing Company.

Pascoe, M., Stackhouse, J., & Wells, B. (2005). Phonological therapy within a psycholinguistic framework: Promoting change in a child with persisting speech difficulties. *International Journal of Language & Communication Disorders*, 40(2), 189–220. https://doi.org/10.1080/13682820412331290979

Pascoe, M., Stackhouse, J., & Wells, B. (2006). *Persisting speech difficulties in children. Children's speech and literacy difficulties (Book. 3).* John Wiley & Sons Ltd.

Pennington, B. F., & Bishop, D. V. M. (2009). Relations among speech, language, and reading disorders. *Annual Review of Psychology*, 60. https://doi.org/10.1044/1092-4388(2004/031)

Peterson, R. L., Pennington, B. F., Shriberg, L. D., & Boada, R. (2009). What influences literacy outcome in children with speech sound disorder? *Journal of Speech, Language, and Hearing Research: JSLHR*, *52*(5), 1175–1188. https://doi.org/10.1044/1092-4388(2009/08-0024)

Peterson-Falzone, S. J., Trost-Cardamone, J. E., Karnell, M., & Hardin-Jones, M. A. (2017). *The clinician's guide to treating cleft palate speech*. Mosby.

Preston, J., & Edwards, M. L. (2010). Phonological awareness and types of sound errors in preschoolers with speech sound disorders. *Journal of Speech, Language, and Hearing Research*, *53*(1), 44–60. https://doi.org/10.1044/1092-4388(2009/09-0021)

Preston, J., Hull, M., & Edwards, M. L. (2013). Preschool speech error patterns predict articulation and phonological awareness outcomes in children with histories of speech sound disorders. *American Journal of Speech-Language Pathology*, *22*(2), 173–184. https://doi.org/10.1044/1058-0360(2012/12-0022)

Robey, R. R., & Schultz, M. C. (1998). A model for conducting clinical-outcome research: An adaptation of the standard protocol for use in aphasiology. *Aphasiology*, *12*(9), 787–810. https://doi.org/10.1080/02687039808249573

Rvachew, S. (2006). Longitudinal predictors of implicit phonological awareness skills. *American Journal of Speech-Language Pathology*, *15*(2), 165–176. https://doi.org/10.1044/1058-0360(2006/016)

Rvachew, S., & Matthews, T. (2019). An N-of-1 randomized controlled trial of interventions for children with inconsistent speech sound errors. *Journal of Speech, Language, and Hearing Research*, *62*(9), 3183–3203. https://doi.org/10.1044/2019_JSLHR-S-18-0288

Rvachew, S., Ohberg, A., Grawburg, M., & Heyding, J. (2003). Phonological awareness and phonemic perception in 4-year-old children with delayed expressive phonology skills. *American Journal of Speech-Language Pathology*, *12*(4), 463–471. https://doi.org/10.1044/1058-0360(2003/092)

Schmidt, R. A., Lee, T. D., Winstein, C. J., Wulf, G., & Zelaznik, H. N. (2019). *Motor control and learning: A behavioral emphasis* (6th ed.). Human Kinetics Europe Ltd.

Secord, W., Boyce, S., Donohue, J., Fox, R., & Shine, R. (2007). *Eliciting sounds: Techniques and strategies for clinicians* (2nd ed.). Thompson Delmar Learning.

Smith, A. E., & Camarata, S. (1999). Using teacher-implemented instruction to increase language intelligibility of children with autism. *Journal of Positive Behavior Interventions*, *1*(3), 141–151. https://doi.org/10.1177%2F109830079900100302

Speake, J., Stackhouse, J., & Pascoe, M. (2012). Vowel targeted intervention for children with persisting speech difficulties: Impact on intelligibility. *Child Language Teaching and Therapy*, *28*(3), 277–295. http://doi.org/10.1177/0265659012453463

Stackhouse, J. (2006). Speech and spelling difficulties, what to look for. In M. J. Snowling & J. Stackhouse (Eds.), *Dyslexia, speech, and language: A practitioner's handbook*, (p. 28). Wiley.

Stackhouse, J., Vance, M., Pascoe, M., & Wells, B. (2007). *Compendium of auditory and speech tasks. Children's speech and literacy difficulties (Book 4)*. John Wiley & Sons, Ltd.

Stackhouse, J., & Wells, B. (1997). *Children's speech and literacy difficulties: A psycholinguistic framework (Book 1)*. Wiley.

Stackhouse, J., & Wells, B. (2001). *Children's speech and literacy difficulties (Book 2)*. Whurr Publishers.

Stampe, D. (1969). The acquisition of phonetic representation. *Papers from the 5th regional meeting of the Chicago Linguistic Society*. 443–454.

Stampe, D. (1973). *A dissertation on natural phonology* (Unpublished doctoral dissertation). University of Chicago.

Stampe, D. (1979). *A dissertation on natural phonology*. Academic Press.

Stoel-Gammon, C., & Dunn, C. (1985). *Normal and disordered phonology in children*. University Park Press.

Storkel, H. L. (2022). Minimal, maximal, or multiple: Which contrastive intervention approach to use with children with speech sound disorders? *Language, Speech, and Hearing Services in Schools*, *53*(3), 632–645. https://doi.org/10.1044/2021_LSHSS-21-00105

Strand, E. A. (2020). Dynamic temporal and tactile cueing: A treatment strategy for childhood apraxia of speech. *American Journal of Speech-Language Pathology*, *29*(1), 30–48. https://doi.org/10.1044/2019_AJSLP-19-0005

Strand, E. A., Stoeckel, R., & Baas, B. (2006). Treatment of severe childhood apraxia of speech: A treatment efficacy study. *Journal of Medical Speech-Language Pathology*, *14*(4), 297–307.

Sutherland, D., & Gillon, G. T. (2005). Assessment of phonological representations in children with speech impairment. *Language, Speech, and Hearing Services in Schools*, *36*(4), 294–307. https://doi.org/10.1044/0161-1461(2005/030)

Tambyraja, S. R., Farquharson, K., & Justice, L. (2020). Reading risk in children with speech sound disorder: Prevalence, persistence, and predictors. *Journal of Speech, Language, and Hearing Research*, *63*(11), 3714–3726. https://doi.org/10.1044/2020_jslhr-20-00108

Tyler, A. A. (2002). Language-based intervention for phonological disorders. *Seminars in speech and language*, *23*(1), 69–82. https://doi.org/10.1055/s-2002-23511

Unicomb, R., Hewat, S., Spencer, E., & Harrison, E. (2013). Clinicians' management of young children with co-occurring stuttering and speech sound disorder. *International Journal of Speech-Language Pathology*, *15*(4), 441–452. https://doi.org/10.3109/17549507.2013.783111

van Bysterveldt, A. K., Gillon, G., & Foster-Cohen, S. (2010). Integrated speech and phonological awareness intervention for pre-school children with Down syndrome. *International Journal of Language and Communication Disorders*, *45*(3), 320–335. https://doi.org/10.3109/13682820903003514

Van Riper, C. (1978). *Speech correction: Principles and methods* (6th ed.). Prentice-Hall.

Vance, M. (1996). Assessing speech processing skills in children: A task analysis. Portuguese translation. In M. Snowling & J. Stackhouse (Eds.), *Dislexia fala e linguagem: Um manual do professional* [Dyslexia, speech and language: A practicioner's handbook]. Artmet São Pablo.

Velleman, S. L., & Vihman, M. M. (2002). Whole-word phonology and templates: Trap, bootstrap, or some of each? *Language, Speech, and Hearing Services in Schools*, *33*(1), 9–23. https://doi.org/10.1044/0161-1461(2002/002)

Watts Pappas, N., & Bowen, C. (2007). Speech acquisition and the family. In S. McLeod (Ed.),

The international guide to speech acquisition, (pp. 86–90). Thomson Delmar Learning.

Weiner, F. (1981a). Treatment of phonological disability using the method of meaningful contrast: Two case studies. *Journal of Speech and Hearing Disorders*, *46*(1), 97–103. https://doi.org/10.1044/jshd.4601.97

Wells, B., & Stackhouse, J. (2016). *Children's intonation: A framework for practice and research (Book 5)*. Wiley Blackwell.

Wells, B., Stackhouse, J., & Vance, M. (1999). La conscience phonologique dans le cadre d'une evaluation psycholinguistique de l'enfant [Assessment of phonological awareness within a psycholinguistic framework]. *Re-education Orthophonique*, *197*, 3–12. https://www.researchgate.net/publication/345725962_La_Conscience_Phonologique_dans_le_cadre_d%27une_evaluation_psycholinguistique_de_l%27enfant

Williams, A. L. (2000a). Multiple oppositions: Theoretical foundations for an alternative contrastive intervention approach. *American Journal of Speech-Language Pathology*, *9*(4), 282–288. https://doi.org/10.1044/1058-0360.0904.282

Yeh, L.-L., Wells, B., Stackhouse, J., & Szczerbinski, M. (2015). The development of phonological representations in Mandarin-speaking children: Evidence from a longitudinal study of phonological awareness. *Clinical Linguistics & Phonetics*, *29*(4), 266–275. https://doi.org/10.3109/02699206.2014.1003328

Yoder, P. J., Camarata, S., & Woynaroski, T. (2016). Treating speech comprehensibility in students with Down syndrome. *Journal of Speech, Language, and Hearing Research*, *59*(3), 446–459. https://doi.org/10.1044/2015_JSLHR-S-15-0148

Chapter 6

Common, Best, and Evidence-based Practice

EBP is a valuable construct in ensuring quality of care. However, bridging between research evidence and clinical practice may require us to confront potentially difficult issues and establish thoughtful dialogue about best practices in fostering EBP itself.

Bernstein Ratner, 2006, p. 257

Addressing the theme from complementary standpoints in this chapter, Victoria Joffe, Gregory Lof, and Ruth Stoeckel reflect on aspects of common practice, evidence-based practice, and best practice. First, Joffe (A23) revisits the topic of child speech clinical work in the UK, offering helpful insights into SLTs' **common practice**, or standard care (Morgan et al., 2019). Next, Lof (A24), who has a longstanding research interest in the application of science (which fosters **evidence-based practice: EBP**) and pseudoscience (which does not foster EBP) in SLP/SLT, takes another critical look at the non-evidence-based practice – still used in the United States and beyond – of non-speech oral motor exercises: NS-OME. And third, Stoeckel (A25), who also contributed A14, considers the nexus between *critical* and *clinical* thinking, and the shifting,

evolving ideal of **best practice** in SSD management (Furlong et al., 2021; Storkel, 2022).

A key principle of evidence-based practice is that clinical decisions should be made with equal consideration of the three elements of EBP: (a) best available evidence from scientific literature (external evidence) and client data (internal evidence); (b) professional and clinical expertise; and (c) the client's values, perspectives, and circumstances. Speech-Language Pathologists face the challenge of weighting these three elements when making clinical decisions for children with speech sound disorders relating to target selection, therapy approaches, and the structural or procedural aspects of intervention.

Furlong et al., 2021, p. 581

Dr. Victoria Joffe is Professor of Speech and Language Therapy, and Dean of the School of Health and Social Care at the University of Essex. Her areas of clinical and research expertise include speech sound disorders, developmental speech, language and communication needs across the lifespan, collaborative practice and the training of teaching staff, language and literacy development, and evidence-based practice. Victoria is co-editor of the journal, *Child Language Teaching and Therapy*, and acts as a speech and language therapy partner for the Health and Care Professions Council (HCPC). She is chair of the Royal College of Speech and Language Therapist's national clinical excellence network for older children and young adults with developmental speech, language and communication needs. Victoria is currently working on three National Institute Health Research (NIHR)-funded research projects looking into new and innovative interventions for children with social communication disorder, children who stammer and children with Down syndrome.

Q23.   Victoria Joffe: Pedagogy, Research Findings and EBP in the UK

Drawing on published empirical data, and your first-hand experience as a teacher and leader in the SLP/SLT field, can you reflect and comment on the possible barriers for clinicians and administrators or 'managers', in the British context, between pedagogy, research findings, and evidence-based practice?

A23.   Victoria L. Joffe: Management of Speech Sound Disorders in the UK

We conducted two national surveys of speech and language therapy practice in the UK. One was a survey of clinical practice with children with phonological impairments (Joffe & Pring, 2008), and the second, a broader survey of the working practices and clinical experiences of paediatric speech and language therapists (SLTs) (Pring et al., 2012). Our results showed a considerable mismatch between the available research into best practice for assessment and intervention in children with speech, language and communication needs (SLCN), and current practice across the UK.

The 2008 Survey

More than 50% of the 98 SLTs who completed the first survey used a combination of what they reported to be the three most popular treatments for phonological disorder: auditory discrimination, phonological awareness, and minimal contrast therapy. Respondents appeared to use these eclectically, as a core approach, without explaining or rationalizing their inclusion in terms of the presenting nature of the speech disorder. The factors they considered in selecting the interventions were general, and included the child's age, language and cognitive abilities and parental motivation, with little reference to the type, nature or severity of the speech disorder (Joffe & Pring, 2008). This may be unsurprising, considering that the most popular test used to identify the speech disorder was reported to be the *South Tyneside Assessment of Phonology: STAP*, (Armstrong & Ainley, 1988), a relatively quick unstandardized published single-word naming test, with neither normative data nor support for in-depth data analysis to differentiate types of speech disorder and processes underlying them. For readers who are unfamiliar with STAP, the words are listed at https://clispi.com/uploads/STAP%20Test.pdf

The 2012 Survey

Our second survey, completed by 516 SLTs, with most working in the National Health Service (87.6%) and only 7.1% in private practice, showed that a large part of treatment time is consultative and indirect. It involved training other professionals, like teaching assistants and teachers (15%), and parents (13%), rather than direct therapy (23%), where the SLT works directly with the client. Nearly half of the sample (44.7%) stated that their time could be more effectively used by giving more direct therapy. This trend to train others to carry out speech and language support work perturbed some participants in this study, with several stating that they did not feel it worked, whilst others felt that although training others in the child's setting is important, it cannot replace the direct intervention given by a specialist. Another concern expressed was that not providing direct therapy could potentially deskill the professionals trained to work with this group. Furthermore, with consultative intervention continuing to be a prominent feature of interventions offered in schools in the UK, many students and newly qualified SLTs are at risk of missing the opportunity to practice working directly with the client.

Common Practice in the UK in 2016, 2018, and 2021

More recent evidence suggests that the picture of paediatric speech and language therapy practice presented in the 2008 and 2012 UK surveys, continues to reflect current practice. An online survey of 166 SLTs, by Hegarty et al. (2018) explored intervention for children with phonological impairment in the UK. The most common treatments used to remediate phonological impairments echoed the three most popular treatments identified by Joffe and Pring (2008) and were reported to be used 'always' or 'often': speech discrimination (79.5%), conventional minimal pairs (77.3%) and phonological awareness (75.6%). The 2008 and 2018 surveys also identified traditional articulation therapy (Van Riper, 1978), as a popular approach when working with children with phonological impairment, even though research has shown this is not the most effective approach to use with this client group (Lousada et al., 2013).

The two surveys, despite the 10-year gap, showed that SLTs were less likely to use the more recent complexity interventions, including maximal oppositions (Gierut, 1989) and multiple oppositions (Williams, 2000a; A19), opting for the more longstanding and familiar treatments. However, as noted by Hegarty et al. (2018), some change was apparent, with 15.9% in the 2018 study 'always' or 'often' administering the maximal opposition approach, compared with the 2008 group surveyed, where only 5.1% used it with the same frequency.

It appears that SLTs continue to use approaches and interventions with which they are most comfortable and have been using

regularly. A 2021 study conducted in the UK tapped the use of technology-assisted speech and language therapy (TASLT) with children with phonological delays in which Kuschmann et al. (2021) surveyed 158 SLTs. They found that a quarter of therapists working with this client group do not use any technology for either assessment or treatment. Interestingly, those SLTs who used technology, reported using apps that mainly focused on minimal pairs, phonological awareness and listening skills – the same three most popular approaches identified approximately 15 years before in the Joffe and Pring survey.

Despite research into child speech disorder growing in the last two decades, and more evidence becoming available around the effectiveness and efficiency of interventions with this client group, the everyday practice of SLTs in the UK does not appear to be reflecting this new evidence, with little change in how therapists work with children with speech sound disorders (SSD) in schools. There remains a gap between research and practice in the speech and language therapy profession, in the UK and internationally, and this gap has narrowed minimally over the past few decades (Froud & Randazzo, A51; McCabe, 2018).

Research and EBP

In 2016, we conducted a survey of SLTs exploring their understanding and use of research and evidence-based practice in routine clinical work in the UK, with 1020 SLTs from the UK (7.3% response rate) completing it (Pagnamenta et al., 2022 – unpublished report). Most respondents were employed in the National Health Service (64%), while 21% worked in private practice. Respondents (n = 899) were in strong agreement with statements relating to positive attitudes to Evidence-Based Practice (EBP), for example, 93% agreed that using EBP made them better clinicians, 96%, that it was their responsibility to implement EBP, and 94% agreed that applying research to clinical practice was beneficial for their clients. However, when asked about knowledge and skills in relation to EBP, responses varied, with strong agreement for understanding what it means to be an evidence-based practitioner (96%) and awareness of how to find evidence to inform their practice (86%), but lower agreement for recalling main findings and implications of research papers (45%), and only 59% reported that they had received training for EBP. Pleasingly, a greater number agreed that they would like to further develop their skills in EBP (76%). Views on opportunities and availability of training varied with only 53% of respondents stating that their managers would support them in implementing EBP, and just 44% agreeing that there were good networks and resources to support them as evidence-based practitioners.

Specific barriers to implementing EBP in the workplace included difficulty in accessing the research (42%). Having time to read the research was a barrier identified by many of the group (71%). Other obstacles to EBP that they reported included heavy caseloads, and insufficient time with clients. A further key difficulty was that the evidence available did not always reflect the realities of everyday practice. These 'clinical realities' included limited one-to-one direct service provision and the preponderance of consultative working which continues as a feature of working practice in the UK, as well as the high intensity and frequency of therapy typically included in efficacy studies, over time spans usually not available to most SLT practitioners. Despite an overall positive perspective on using EBP by therapists in the UK, there are barriers to available resources, training, and having the time to undertake any training.

Other recent national surveys reflect these findings showing a high proportion of American SLPs and their managers value the importance of EBP (Greenwell & Walsh, 2021; Thome et al., 2020), but that its implementation is difficult (e.g., Greenwell & Walsh, 2021; Thome et al., 2020). Health and Care Professions Council mandates, and the RCSLT

The limited availability of time and appropriate training and resources, that British SLTs have reported regarding EBP, is at odds with the unambiguous directive of the Health and Care Professions Council (HCPC), the professional regulator of SLTs in the UK, which sets out clear expectations for continued professional learning and development throughout an SLT career (HCPC, 2022). Regarding clinical practice in SSD, the HCPC (2013) produces standards of proficiency for SLTs and within these standards, there is explicit mention of working with this (SSD) client group and the core areas required for proficiency: – 'understand linguistics and phonetics...' and 'understand developmental...impairments of speech...' (p. 12) as well as the directive to draw on 'phonetic transcription' (p. 13).

In the curriculum guidance for the pre-registration education of SLTs, published by the Royal College of Speech and Language Therapists (RCSLT), the professional body of SLTs in the UK, there is explicit mention of speech and language therapy programmes needing support by experts in the field of linguistics and phonetics, and that all programmes must include as a clinical area, SSD, phonetics and clinical applications, and transcription (RCSLT, 2021). There is no stipulation, however, on the time that training institutions should give to these areas, and with the reduction of pre-registration training from four to three years for undergraduate study in the UK, and the increasing areas of SLT involvement (for example, respiratory and long COVID), it is challenging for Higher Education Institutions (HEIs) to incorporate the in-depth coverage of core subject areas, including for example, all available phonological interventions and their underlying evidence bases.

Variability in Training of Speech and Language Therapy Students

An example of the variability and non-standard teaching coverage of core subjects in HEIs training SLTs in the UK, is evidence from a study undertaken by Pagnamenta and Joffe (2018) exploring the pre-registration research teaching for SLT students in the UK. A survey of 14 programmes (10 undergraduate and 4 postgraduate), representing 73% and 44% of undergraduate and postgraduate courses in the UK respectively, showed substantial variability across courses in number of hours, modules and credits relating to research training. While many courses (n=7) reported that they taught research and EBP for over 30 hours, variability was high with some (n=3) teaching as few as between one to five hours. When respondents were asked to state how confident their students would be in the awareness of research, on graduation, responses were again varied with 9 rating their graduates as 'confident' or 'very confident', and 5 as 'not at all confident'. Interestingly, there was a significant positive correlation between the perceived confidence in research awareness and number of hours of research teaching in the curriculum.

The authors recommended national guidelines be developed on the quantity and content of critical areas of the curriculum, including research and EBP, and core clinical areas (including for example, SSD), to measure and maintain standards and ensure graduates have the knowledge and appropriate resources and context to follow emerging and new evidence. In the absence of such guidelines, there is the potential for new graduates to enter the workforce with variable knowledge and understanding of existing evidence-based practice, and of not having the skills or confidence to critically evaluate and advocate for the adoption of new interventions or service delivery models that are proving more effective than the status quo.

Child Speech Disorder Research Network (CSDRN)

In the UK, a group of specialist researchers and practitioners in child speech disorder became aware of and concerned about this disconnection between the research and practice in working with children with SSD, and the variable training of phonetic transcription and in-depth exploration of different profiles of SSD. Accordingly, the group came together in 2011 and formed the Child Speech Disorder Research Network (CSDRN). The aims of the network, currently comprising 14 members, is to raise the profile of SSD within the profession in the UK and internationally, to promote and support evidence-based practice with this client group, and to drive the research agenda, in close collaboration with the RCSLT and other stakeholders (Joffe & Broomfield, 2019, p. 7). The network also acts as a reference group and support for clinicians and researchers working in the field, through providing training to the RCSLT's speech clinical excellence networks (CENs).

As part of the CSDRN's work, we surveyed the research priorities for the profession at the 2014 RCSLT conference, where research questions were collated from practising clinicians on service delivery for this client group to shape the research agenda, so it more closely reflected the needs of practice. Consequently, the CSDRN has developed two sets of guidelines to support working with children with SSD: 1) *The Good Practice Guidelines for Transcription of Children's Speech Samples in Clinical Practice and Research*, and 2) *The Good Practice Guidelines for the Analysis of Child Speech*. Both guidelines serve to support critical decision making in using screening versus more in-depth sampling of single words and connected speech, as well providing an evidence-based guide to the phonetic and phonological analysis where appropriate. The CSDRN disseminates information online through its website (https://www.nbt.nhs.uk/bristol-speech-language-therapy-research-unit/bsltru-research/child-speech-disorder-research-network) and Twitter: @CSDRNetwork. The expectation is that a greater understanding of the different types of SDD, and how interventions differentially impact on each of them, as well as more availability of training post registration, and more standard and substantial coverage of this area during pre-registration training, will hopefully result in greater confidence shown by clinicians working with children with this client group, and a closer match between the evidence being produced, and the interventions implemented in practice.

With children with SSD continuing to make up a large part of the everyday caseload of the SLT in the UK and internationally, (Broomfield & Dodd, 2004; Law et al., 2000; Wren et al., 2016), sufficient time and training should be provided for this client group, both at pre-registration level, and as part of each SLT's continuing professional development, to support the change that is needed.

Appeal to Common Practice and Appeal to Novelty

Appeal to common practice is an informal logical fallacy. An informal fallacy is an unsound argument whose proposed conclusion is unsupported by its premise. For example, *'Walking across the campus for the first time today, I passed 40 or 50 people and not one said "hello". This university is far less friendly than I was led to expect'*. Appeal to common practice is also known as appeal to tradition (argumentum ad antiquitatem) and appeal to antiquity (argumentum ad antiquitam), and often expressed as 'this is what we always (or all) do', 'this is what we've always (or all) done'. When medical and other practitioners, such as SLPs/SLTs, appeal to common practice, they argue that an intervention, procedure, or activity must be correct because it is usual conduct, or conversely that a procedure, or activity must be incorrect because it is not usual conduct; or because people have done it (or avoided doing it) for a long time it must be right or good practice.

Appeal to common practice stands in contrast to **appeal to novelty** which occurs when someone asserts that something must be true or good because it's new. For example, if an SLP/SLT claims that a certain theory, assessment, or intervention is better than its predecessors, solely because it is newer, without providing credible evidence, they appeal to novelty. As clinicians and researchers, we must guard against appeal to novelty. It often crops up when developers and marketers of new intervention approaches provide little or no evidence, no scientific critique, glowing testimonials, and 'success stories' while describing them as 'proven' scientific breakthroughs, innovative or unique.

One group of interventions, strongly identified with informal logical fallacies, is Non-Speech Oral Motor Exercises (NSOME). Gregory Lof explains in A24.

Dr. Gregory Lof is Professor Emeritus in the Department of Communication Sciences and Disorders at the MGH institute of Health Professions, a graduate school founded by the Massachusetts General Hospital in Boston, Massachusetts. In his career, his research, teaching, and clinical work primarily involved children with speech sound disorders. He is also interested in professional issues, specifically the use of science and pseudoscience in speech-language pathology. Recent research, writings, and lectures have been around the lack of efficacy of using NSOME to change speech sound productions. Dr. Lof has served on many ASHA convention program committees, he was an editorial consultant for the ASHA journals, and was a member on ASHA's Center for Evidence-Based Practice in Communication Disorders that conducted evidence-based systematic reviews of oral motor exercises. He is the author of numerous articles and has presented workshops worldwide at ASHA conventions, universities, school districts, and state and international association conventions. He became a Fellow of the American Speech-Language-Hearing Association in 2012.

Q24. Gregory L. Lof NSOME: Still Under the Microscope in North America

Odd though it seems, controversy continues to surround the range of intervention activities and techniques categorized as NS-OME (non-speech oral motor exercises) or 'oral motor activities' that are implemented to address speech sound production problems. They are commonly used by SLPs in North America, often in conjunction with 'tools and toys', including bite blocks, straws and tubes, horns and other toy wind instruments, chewable objects such as 'chewy tubes', and thickened drinks.

What exercises are used and why? What is the evidence and logic against using these exercises? Is there evidence and logic in their favour? Why do clinicians continue to use them? What is the responsibility of ASHA and other continuing education providers and sponsors in ensuring that therapy techniques that are presented to CEU/CPD participants adhere to the principles of EBP?

A24.   Gregory LOF: The Persistent NS-OME Phenomenon in SLP Practice

It is puzzling to contemplate why the controversial therapy technique of nonspeech oral motor exercises (NS-OME) to change speech sound production problems is common practice internationally among SLPs/SLTs (Kamal, 2021; Lof & Watson, 2008; Pratomo & Siswanto, 2020; Rumback et al., 2017). Why 'puzzling'? Because no convincing evidence, or motor or linguistic theories support their use.

In defining nonspeech oral movements (NSOMs) Kent (2015, p. 765) proposed that they are, motor acts performed by various parts of the speech musculature to accomplish specified movement or postural goals that are not sufficient in themselves to have phonetic identity. Accordingly, one possible definition of NS-OME is, any technique that does not require the child to produce a speech sound but is used to influence the development of speaking abilities (Lof & Watson, 2008; cf., McCauley et al., 2009, Ruscello, 2008). The existence and importance of oral motor aspects of speech production is undisputed, but the use of non-speech oral motor exercises is contentious. Such exercises, aimed at directly altering the performance of the articulators for speech production, typically include activities like blowing horns, whistles, and cotton balls; tongue wags, curls, and push-ups; tongue-to-nose-to-chin and pucker-smile movements; puffing cheeks out; and blowing kisses (Lof & Watson, 2008). SLPs/SLTs who use them believe their clients' speech will benefit relative to enhanced tongue elevation and lateralization; better oral-kinaesthetic awareness; stronger tongues, lips, and sucking; and improved jaw stabilization, lip/tongue protrusion, control of drooling, and velopharyngeal competence (Lof & Watson, 2008).

Theoretical Issues

Many scholars and clinicians have questioned the use of NS-OME on theoretical grounds (Clark, 2005; Clark et al., 2003; Forrest, 2002; Lof, 2003, 2008; Lof & Watson, 2008, 2010; Ruscello, 2008; Watson & Lof, 2008), raising issues of: (1) part-whole training and transfer, (2) strengthening of the articulators, (3) task specificity/relevance, and (4) awareness.

1. Part–Whole Training and Transfer/ Relevancy

Part-whole training and transfer implies that breaking a task (in this instance, speaking) into smaller components will enhance performance of the whole task; for example, working on isolated sounds rather than linguistic units. NS-OME breaks speaking into tiny tasks when, for example, tongue tip-to-alveolar ridge isolated movement gestures are practised to teach alveolar stops, or lip puckers are elicited repeatedly in hopes of enhancing lip rounding for vowel productions. Criticizing this compartmentalization, Forrest (2002, pp. 18–19) noted, *tasks that comprise highly organized or integrated movements will not be enhanced by learning the constituent parts; rather training on parts of these organized behaviors will diminish learning.* Applying Forrest's reasoning there is inadequate theoretical justification for training disconnected, small 'component' parts of the speech gestures on the assumption that it will transfer to the whole, namely speech. They are irrelevant because isolated articulator movements do not constitute or even resemble the gestures used to articulate any English phones, rendering their value in improving production highly questionable. For instance, no speech sound requires tongue-tip elevation towards the nose, puffed-out cheeks, blowing, or tongue wagging. Oral movements that are irrelevant to speech movements are ineffective as speech therapy techniques.

2. Strengthening of the Articulators

The supposed need for strength is a frequently stated reason for conducting NS-OME (Lof & Watson, 2008), but this supposition requires examination.

- First, **how is speech strength measure?** Clinicians typically measure articulator strength subjectively, for example, by feeling the force of the tongue pushing against a tongue depressor, gloved finger, or cheek, or by simply 'observing' weakness (Solomon & Munson, 2004). But seasoned clinicians are even less accurate in their 'guesstimations' of reduced strength than are student clinicians (Clark et al., 2003). This means that SLPs/SLTs probably cannot initially verify whether strength is diminished; correspondingly, they cannot then report increases in strength following an NS-OME regimen.

- Second, **how much strength is needed for speaking?** The answer: 'not much', prompted Wenke et al. (2006, p. 15) to state, *caution should be taken when directly associating tongue strength to speech*. For example, lip muscle-force for speaking is only about 10–20% of the maximal capabilities for lip-force, and the jaws use only about 11–15% of their potential force (Bunton & Weismer, 1994; Forrest, 2002).

- Third, **do NS-OME really increase articulator strength?** Answer: 'probably not'. To strengthen any muscle, exercises must be done repeatedly, against resistance, to the point of fatigue. This standard and empirically supported muscle-strengthening paradigm, relevant to all muscle groups, is used whenever someone adheres to a weight-training program (Clark, 2008; Clark et al., 2009). So how many tongue-wag repetitions do most clinicians require clients to perform, how often, and are the wags done against resistance? If the answers are 'not many', 'not often' and 'seldom,' respectively – probably no lasting strength gains accrue from these exercises. And when strengthening does occur due to extensive exercise drills, not only are the articulator strength gains not maintained over time, but they also do not improve speech (Sjögreen et al., 2010).

- Fourth and finally, **do children with SSD have oral weakness?** Not according to Potter et al. (2019) who demonstrated objectively that preschool aged children with SSD had *stronger* articulators than their peers with age-typical speech (cf. Dworkin & Culatta, 1980).

3. Task Specificity

Addressing the topic of task specificity (H. Clark, 2012) leads to the truism: 'speech is special' (Kent, 2004; Maas, 2017). The anatomical structures used for speaking and other mouth tasks, like swallowing, sucking, and breathing, function in different ways, each mediated by different parts of the brain (Bunton, 2008; Wilson et al., 2008), although identical structures are involved, organization of movements within the nervous system is not the same for speech gestures as it is for nonspeech gestures; and the neural bases of motor control are different for speech and non-speech oral movements. This is observable in those with dysphagia, whose swallowing function (nonspeech) is compromised while the same structures function adequately for speech (Ziegler, 2003). Weismer (2006) summarizes 11 studies showing that speech and nonspeech neuromotor movements are different for numerous structures, including the facial muscles, maxilla, mandible, tongue, lips, and palate. Evidence from task specificity studies therefore indicates that working on nonspeech activities will fail to change speech (Ludlow et al., 2008; Schulz et al., 1999).

4. Awareness

Some NS-OME programs centre on a 'meta-mouth' assumption of children developing, via the exercises, metacognitive awareness of articulatory place, manner, and movement, alongside a process of 'waking up' or 'warming up' the speech musculature (Lof & Watson, 2008). Muscle warm-up may be appropriate prior to exercise routines, like distance running or weight training, designed to maximally tax the system (Pollock et al., 1998). Conversely, muscle warm-up is superfluous for less strenuous tasks that are below the maximum, like walking, handwriting, or lifting a spoon-to-mouth. Because speaking does not even approach the oral muscular maximum, warm-up is unnecessary. Besides, children up to and including seven-year-olds are probably unable to use the mouth cues provided by NS-OME to make themselves more aware of their oral structures (Klein et al., 1991). Because of this lack of 'metamouth' awareness, it is highly probable that no transfer to speech occurs from the NS-OME movements and mouth awareness cues.

Research Evidence

The theoretical underpinnings for using NS-OME to improve children's speech are weak, but might the literature hold supporting evidence for their widespread use by clinicians who want their practices to be guided by the principles of EBP? Answer: 'no'. Exhaustive systematic reviews of available published data have been conducted, only to report that no studies exist showing that NS-OME for speech are or are not beneficial (Lee & Gibbon, 2015; McCauley et al., 2009; Ruscello & Vallino, 2020). A shortage of published well-designed studies led to this unsatisfactory conclusion, pointing to a research need. Along with the few published studies (e.g., Lau & Lee, 2013), there are several unpublished research investigations that have been presented at peer-reviewed ASHA national conventions. The rare studies that suggest there is speech production improvements following a regimen of NS-OME, all have fatal methodological flaws, invalidating any results (e.g., Fields & Polmanteer, 2002; Zhang & Zhang, 2019). The available evidence overwhelming demonstrates no benefits from using NS-OME either alone or in combination with proven therapy techniques.

Research has been conducted on the popular 'horn hierarchy' (Talk Tools®) to determine its increments in blowing difficulty over a series of ten prescribed horns. Purportedly, this horn blowing strengthens targeted muscle groups in a 'measured progression' (Rosenfeld-Johnson, 2001). Jones et al. (2011) and colleagues tested the horns in this hierarchy finding that they were not at all representative of typical speech production and that the intraoral pressures required to blow them did not increase systematically from horn to horn up the supposed hierarchy. This refutes the basic premise of this blowing exercise kit. At the time of writing, similar claims for the 'straw hierarchy' have not been evaluated.

Clinicians' and Associations' Responsibilities

Given the weak theoretical underpinnings and the absence of evidence supporting the use of NS-OME, why do clinicians persist in using these techniques? Muttiah et al. (2011) conducted a qualitative study, interviewing 11 SLPs who used NS-OME and 11 researchers who do not. The main conclusion was that these two groups used different forms of 'evidence' to make clinical decisions: the researchers relied on published research and sound theoretical concepts while the clinicians relied on observations of perceived effectiveness (cf., Malamud et al., 2021).

SLPs/SLTs probably continue to use NS-OME for a range of reasons:

- the procedures offer an easy 'cookbook' approach implemented step-by-step
- the exercises give the appearance that something tangible is being 'done'
- various techniques and tools have been heavily and attractively promoted in self-published materials and workshops
- many clinicians do not read the peer-reviewed professional literature
- occupational and physical therapists on multidisciplinary teams encourage exercises; and
- clinicians often persuade colleagues to use them (Lof & Watson, 2008).

Professional organizations and universities can play a role in fostering scientific environments that enable clinicians to become more knowledgeable consumers of new, innovative, and controversial treatments (Watson & Lof, 2008).

But ultimately, the SLP/SLT must be able to critically evaluate the logic used and the evidence claimed because it is only through adherence to scientific methodologies that our field can progress (Kamhi, 2008). As Mackenzie et al. (2011) said, we must be willing to give up the 'folklore' of our profession that has been handed down by word of mouth for generations so we can move forward with the adoption of scientifically valid procedures.

Here is a cautionary statement: be aware that there are other therapeutic approaches that are essentially using NS-OME but under a different guise. Watch for promotions to use NS-OME for ankyloglossia (and tethered oral tissues, aka TOT), oral myofunctional disorders (orofacial myology), oral placement therapy (OPT), and many other topics that warrant scrutiny.

One of the reasons for EBP is not only to promote the use of proven effective treatments, but also to delay the adoption of unproven ones (American Speech-Language-Hearing Association, 2004). Currently, it seems that this delay in using NS-OME is most prudent (Kent, 2015).

Good Science is Based on Good Science

Science is a human endeavour and a process. It encompasses studies in which researchers take observations, and record them, to rigorously test hypotheses. They follow a carefully documented methodology that facilitates independent replication, by other researchers. If the hypotheses succeed, they are peer reviewed critically, by the scientific community, and considered for publication in the juried literature. Once published, studies are exposed to post-publication peer review. Concepts that work endure and those that do not fit the observed data expire. Ultimately, concepts that survive frequent, repeated scrutiny of huge quantities of observational data, via further studies, become scientific theory. The theories become as close to scientific fact as is achievable since nothing

can be proved as absolute truth. If a study conforms to this protocol, it is science; if it does not conform to this protocol, it is not science. Substantive scientific outcomes are rarely if ever achieved by one individual, or a small team working independently, who stumble fortuitously upon a 'scientific breakthrough', a 'eureka moment', an 'important new discovery', or 'find'.

Drawing on the effort of previous scientists, and the body of peer-reviewed published knowledge that those scientists created, a researcher, or research team, explains the significant concepts, models and assumptions that guide their project, showing that *their* project is grounded in reputable ('proven') knowledge.

A solid, clearly elaborated theoretical framework reveals why a researcher or team has chosen an approach to answering a research question. It also allows the reader of the research report to fully interpret and comprehend the significance of any findings. It lets researchers focus their labours on relevant data (information) for a specific line of inquiry, exclude extraneous information ('noise'), and define the exact standpoint from which the data will be analysed, interpreted, and reported in the literature.

Macro-, Meso-, and Micro-level Research

The adjectives macro (large-scale), meso (medium-scale) and micro (small-scale) refer to the levels of investigation used in social analysis research. Macro-level researchers examine the political-administrative environment, including national systems (e.g., health departments or education authorities), regulation (e.g., registration boards), and cultures (e.g., a professional associations' culture). Meso-level researchers study groups, including teams, units, and organizations. The micro-level, or 'local level' is the lowest unit of analysis in the social sciences, focusing on an individual (e.g., the parent of a child with CAS) in their social setting, or a small group of individuals (e.g., local SLPs/SLTs interested in CAS) in a social context (e.g., a local CAS special interest group).

Macro- and Meso-level Pressures on Micro-level (Practitioner) Choices

In endeavouring to understand de-implementation hesitancy and resistance, it is so vital to seek out and recognise the macro- and meso-level barriers facing, and pressures exerted on micro-level practitioners' decisions and choices, particularly when they are doing their utmost to pursue E^3BP. Only then can the profession properly address thorny issues within SSD practice such as the delivery of intervention that

- Has **too low a dose frequency** to be effective, where 'dose frequency' is the occasions of treatment sessions per time unit, e.g., 40 minutes twice per week. Note that Warren et al. (2007, p. 71) defined dose as the number of properly administered teaching episodes during a single intervention session' (and see, Baker, 2012; Hitchcock et al., 2019; Justice, 2018). Warren and colleagues considered dose to be an active ingredient of intervention – defining active ingredients as '*the procedures presumed by the interventionists to teach or enhance new learning and behaviour*'.
- Has **too low a dose rate** to be effective, where 'dose rate' is the number of trials within a session, e.g., 50, 70, or 100 production trials per in-clinic session. Farquharson et al. (2022) explored this in relation to children seen in groups in school settings, where the trials expected of each child became progressively fewer as group size increased.

Williams (2012) determined that a dose of fewer than 50 trials in 30 minutes for children with mild or moderate SSD had limited effectiveness; and that the minimum dosage requirement within a 30-minute timeframe rose to 70 trials for a child with severe SSD.

In a study of Australian SLPs, Sugden et al. (2018) found that 40% of their participants elicited between 50 and 99 production trials in a session, while 38% drew 21–49 trials per session. This differed from the contemporaneous findings of Hegarty et al. (2018) who reported that SLTs in the UK drew a dose rate of up to one trial per minute across a 30-minute session

(range 10–30 trials in single word tokens). This dose rate of 30 trials is significantly below Williams' (Williams, 2012) lower limits of at least 50 trials for mildly and moderately involved children, and at least 70 trials for those with more severe SSD.

- Tolerates **unduly short intervention session durations**, for example, fewer than 20–30 minutes once weekly for children with high-moderate to severe SSD.
- Allows **too short an intervention duration**, where intervention duration is the entire time-period an intervention runs. An example of sub-optimal intervention duration is children with high-moderate to severe SSD receiving up to 10 appointments per calendar year; or where 6-week therapy blocks are mandated.
- Occurs in the context of **inadequate intervention continuity**; that is, the scheduling of intervention sessions is at variance with the child's intervention needs in terms of the type, complexity, and severity of their SSD (with or without co-occurring conditions, see Stoeckel, A14; McCauley, A15).
- Involves **insufficient cumulative intervention intensity**, calculated as session dose expressed as trials × dose frequency per time unit × intervention duration (Cummings et al., 2019; Sugden et al., 2018).
- Uses an **intervention approach unsuited to the child's SSD**, for example, where an SLP/SLT provides traditional articulation intervention ('Van Riper therapy', described in Chapter 4) for a child with phonological disorder (see Joffe, A23).

Hegarty et al. (2018) pointed to a research-practice gap when they found that nearly half of their 166 British SLT participants (48.4%) always/often used Van Riper therapy to treat their clients with phonological impairment – an approach that is less effective than phonological intervention for this type of SSD. The effect of this gap is probably compounded by their **cumulative intervention intensity** which was markedly lower than the levels advised in the research literature. The SLT participants mostly provided once-weekly intervention (69%) for 9–12 sessions (range 5–30 sessions, 71.5%), 21–30 minutes in length (41.4%).

- Employs a **variation of an evidence-based intervention** that differs so greatly from the 'tested' intervention it is based on that it lacks fidelity (Baker, A 26; Morgan et al., 2019). This may be exacerbated when clinicians develop their own 'theories of practice' (Argyris & Schön, 1974) and 'theories of therapy' (Law et al., 2008) without considering the evidence, or when they 'cherry-pick' components of two or more intervention approaches to fashion novel eclectic therapies. Variation and individualization are in keeping with the client-patient needs-and-choices aspect of EBP (Morgan et al., 2019), but when intervention becomes 'too eclectic', so to speak, treatment efficacy will suffer.
- Employs a **less-than-optimal target selection** strategy (Storkel, 2018a, 2018b, 2022).
- Is wholly or partially **comprised of non-evidence-based NS-OME** (Lof, A24).

Macro- and meso-level pressures on micro-level practitioner decisions and choices do not only affect intervention. Rather, they impact matters including but not limited to:

- Lengthy **wait times** for assessment and/or intervention (McGill et al., 2021; Rvachew & Rafaat, 2014).
- Restricted availability of appropriate **assessment instruments**, for example, because they are shared between several clinicians at one site, or shared between sites, due to insufficient funds to purchase additional copies of tests.
- Poor access to **technology** (Williams, Thomas & Caballero, A46; Cleland & Scobbie, A47) and limited training opportunities in using it.
- Inaccessibility of **specialist consultations**.
- Limited **time allocation**, by administrators, for assessment and/or intervention.
- Unavailability of professional **interpreters** when required.

Best Practice

Best practice is the term applied to the use of procedures that arise from the best available research evidence, and/or expert opinion, where the procedures themselves are recognized – by appropriately informed practitioners – to be correct or most effective. Best practice guidelines for SLP/SLT services require clinicians to act in accordance with the evidence and ethics of their own profession while keeping a bigger picture framework of knowledge, principles, philosophies, and beliefs in mind.

Evidence-based Practice (EBP)

Evidence-based practice is the integration of (1) external scientific research evidence, (2) internal evidence drawn from clinical expertise/expert opinion, and (3) client/patient/caregiver preferences and perspectives. The purpose of EBP is to provide high-quality services that echo respectfully the interests, values, needs, preferences, and choices of the individuals served (see Leitão, A1 for informative discussion).

EBP, E^{3}BP and E^{4}BP

The bigger-picture framework grew, and is growing out of years of collective research, practice, and client-and-family experiences across disciplines, settings, and cultures. Reflecting on the big picture, Bernstein Ratner (2006) wrote the words quoted as the introduction to this chapter. She stressed that the profession must establish robust communication at all points, from laboratory to clinic. That is, between the funding bodies and researchers who develop the evidence; the academics who spread the word to students (Ellis et al., 2020) and CPD participants (Greenwell & Walsh, 2021), colleagues and the wider community; the administrators who regulate change; the employers charged with maintaining beneficial workplaces; the practitioners who implement the evidence; and the client who, in egalitarian speech intervention in everyday practice, may have the final say (Rosenzweig & Voss, 2022).

In her pithy book on Evidence-based Practice (EBP), Dollaghan (2007, p. 2) coined and defined the term E^{3}BP as a dynamic three-way arrangement, often represented as a triangle, that combines 'the conscientious, explicit, and judicious integration of best available *external* evidence from systematic research, best available evidence *internal* to clinical practice, and best available evidence concerning the preferences of a fully informed patient'. Dollaghan went on to say:

> E^3BP requires honest doubt about a clinical issue, awareness of one's own biases, a respect for other positions, a willingness to let strong evidence alter what is already known, and constant mindfulness of ethical responsibilities to patients.

Pursuing this line of reasoning and encouraging practitioners to reach for balance between unreserved acceptance of their customary practice and an open willingness to explore and accept new ideas, Kamhi (2011, p. 59) argued that '*the scientific method and evidence-based approaches can provide guidance to practitioners but will not lead to a consensus about best clinical practices*'.

In an openly accessible article, Higginbotham and Satchidanand (2019) were happy to embrace Dollaghan's three EBP *components* but pronounced the EPB triangle itself 'flawed by design'. They put a persuasive case for replacing the triangle with a diamond (cf., Hoffman et al., 2017). This, they said would better capture the critical role of internal data, based on the client's performance, in making evidence-informed choices throughout therapy. A 4-sided E^4BP diamond, with meticulous recording of these internal data, would help a clinician to answer four questions that Olswang and Bain (1994, p. 56) posed:

1. Is the client responding to the treatment program?
2. Is significant, important change occurring?
3. Is treatment responsible for the change?
4. How long should a therapy target be treated?

Ethics and Practice

The six-factor model for ethical practice displayed in Figure 6.1 was adapted from earlier work (Powell, 2007, 2013; and see, Irwin et al., 2006) in which Thomas W. Powell reviewed an international sample of codes of ethics from SLP/SLT professional associations, as well as codes from the related disciplines of linguistics, forensic phonetics, and acoustics. Dr. Powell, now retired, contributed to previous editions of this book, and the

Figure from Powell (2015) is reproduced here with his permission, as Figure 6.1.

Powell (2015, pp. 271–272) observed that 'Most ethical standards for professional and scientific associations are linked to one or more of these six principles:

Beneficence: We seek to do good by acting in the best interest in others.
Non-maleficence: We pledge to do no harm and to minimise risks to others.
Respect: We agree to respect differences, as well as the rights of others.
Integrity: We promise to be honest and to avoid conflicts of interest.
Compliance: We agree to work within established rules and laws.
Competence: We accept responsibility for ensuring a high quality of service, including appropriate delegation and referral'.

Whether you call it EBP, E^3BP or E^4BP, evidence-based practice is a process and an obligation. It is located at the juncture between clinicians' engagement with scientific theory and research and their engagement with clients and their worlds. The onus for *adopting* EBP rests with individual clinicians and cannot be imposed by professional associations, workplaces, supervisors, educators, legislators, or policy makers. But to date, most clinicians play just a small part in *constructing* the evidence component.

Academics – SLPs/SLTs, linguists, psychologists, and others – are largely responsible for developing, evaluating, adapting, synthesizing, reporting, and teaching about new SSD research evidence, theory, therapy, and best practice. They usually do so in laboratory, classroom, and CPD settings. Meanwhile, clinicians apply the outcomes of this research – aspiring to optimal fidelity (Baker, A26; Kaderavek & Justice, 2010; Schlosser, 2014) – in settings far removed from controlled laboratory conditions, in person or remotely, wherever and with whomever their clients happen to be.

So, doesn't it seem unreasonable that the burden of ensuring that speech–language pathology is an evidence-based discipline is frequently allocated to practitioners? And that it is done so without providing them with necessary

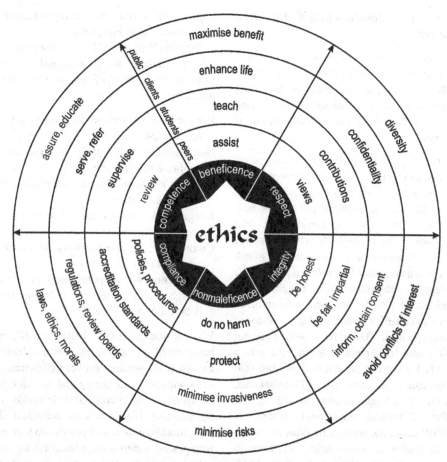

Figure 6.1 A six-factor model for ethical practice in SLP/SLT (Bowen, 2015 / Wiley-Blackwell).

team science skills (Wood et al., 2021), time, and resources to keep up with the available evidence and integrate it into practice? Might it not be fairer if the lion's share of the responsibility for the *evidence* aspect of EBP rested with the individuals who educate SLPs/SLTs, that is, the researchers and academics whose job is to address clinical and educational questions and the policy makers who channel reform?

As well as being unreasonable, it provides an environment in which gaps in communication between researchers, academics, policy makers, employers and practitioners are perpetuated and exacerbated, too often manifesting as uncertainty, antagonism, and prickly relationships. As Froud & Randazzo (A51) point out, while there has been an improvement in this unfavourable situation since the previous edition of this book, there remains ample room for further pedagogical, investigational,

translational, and practical progress to help clinicians engage meaningfully with the research literature.

Regrettably, there are still some settings where co-operation, collegiality and sharing are suboptimal, and we still hear the doubtful voices of academic researchers who are uncertain whether the product of their hard work is valued or used by clinicians. Then we find conscientious academic teachers whose students complain that they do not teach enough – or indeed *anything* – about the nitty-gritty of practice, as well as exasperated clinicians and CPD participants criticizing messages from the laboratory and the lecture hall as biased, out-of-touch, unrealistic, impractical, and impossible to implement. Such criticisms point to the importance of *modelling* and *teaching* principles of E³ BP in the academic preparation of new SLPs/SLTs by delivering higher education that is *itself* rooted in and guided by E³BP.

Social Media, Telepractice, and COVID-19

Surprising sources of improvement in SLP/SLT engagement with theoretical frameworks, research dissemination within Communication Sciences and Disorders, and vigorous knowledge-brokering (Douglas et al., 2022) have been the rise and rise of social media (Davidson et al., 2022) for professional purposes, and the gross disruption to business-as-usual arising from the COVID-19 pandemic. The pandemic also kindled a surge in telehealth/telepractice across health and education sectors (De' et al., 2020; Williams, Thomas & Caballero, A46), and these impacts are examined in Chapter 11.

Open Access

Throughout this book there are references to notable open access publications, for example, the book Bishop and Thompson (2023) and the articles Crowe and McLeod (2020), Higginbotham and Satchidanand (2019), McLeod and Crowe (2018), Nicoll et al. (2021), Storkel (2019, 2022), Verkerk et al. (2018). For scholarly works, open access is a mechanism whereby the full text of peer reviewed articles is made freely available via the internet, for users to: read, download, copy, distribute, print, search, or link to; crawl for indexing; pass between programs to share as data with software; or to use for any lawful purpose, without financial, legal or technical barriers other than those that apply to gaining internet access and capability (e.g., adequate download speeds). Articles in a repository are often referred to as being 'green' open access. These are differentiated from 'gold' open access papers where an author may have paid an article processing charge to publish the final version of record with a publisher. Research funders are increasingly mandating that publications arising from research be made openly accessible.

Clinical Decision-Making and E³BP

Three sources of information serve as the basis for decision-making within the EBP framework: client characteristics, clinician expertise, and empirical evidence. The triangulation of information garnered from these three sources is considered 'best practice'.

Kohnert, 2007

Making good clinical decisions is not easy. The existence of high-quality research can certainly help inform clinical decisions, but research is just one of several factors that influence clinical decisions. Additional factors are the two other components of EBP – client values and clinical expertise – as well as a clinician's theoretical perspective, service delivery considerations, the opinion of experts, and experimental validation with individual clients. …treatment decisions should be influenced the most by the changes that occur in client behaviors and…these changes should be empirically validated by demonstrating that the treatment provided, not some other variable, was responsible for the behavioural change.

Kamhi, 2006, pp. 277–278

Dr. Ruth Stoeckel was introduced in Chapter 3, at the top of Q25 as an academic and retired clinician with many years of experience, working with children with SSD and their families. In 2020, she and a colleague wrote an invited article on clinical decision making, for the ASHA Perspectives journal (Stoeckel & Caspari, 2020). In A25, she further explores important issues around thinking critically when making treatment decisions in (best) clinical practice, providing an illustrative case example.

Q25.   Ruth Stoeckel: Critical Thinking, Clinical Thinking and Best Practice

The fascinating evolution of clinical thinking around an individual client, from assessment through to early, and then later treatment is an interesting, and sometimes challenging process in which SLPs/SLTs strive to base their choices on evidence rather than 'belief' or their own immediate experience as a basis for choices that are made. Can you outline the process and share your thoughts on the nexus between critical thinking and clinical thinking, and their relationships with best practice?

A25. Ruth Stoeckel: Clinical Decision-Making as a Dynamic Process

Best practice that occurs at the intersection of critical thinking and clinical thinking is likely to shift over time, with the balance influenced by a combination of clinician experience and availability of empirical evidence. Clinicians in training are taught how to administer tools and tasks to obtain information that contributes to determination of whether a child has a communication disorder. Critical thinking is important for understanding the psychometric properties and other characteristics of tests. Clinicians also learn to evaluate best available evidence for developing intervention plans. Early in an SLP's/SLT's career, clinical decision-making may rely heavily on objective measures, but as a clinician gains experience, clinical thinking will likely begin to assume a larger role. Assessment may begin with the clinician developing an impression of a child based on a combination of history and brief observation, then choosing assessment tools and tasks that are expected to confirm or disprove that early impression. Once assessment has been completed, experience will likely also influence the practitioner's choice of intervention approach and how to modify intervention based on progress or lack of progress. There is an evolving balance of critical thinking about best available evidence and clinical thinking that makes use of relevant prior experiences. What follows is an account of Sarabi's assessment, intervention and discharge from therapy, and the treating clinician's engagement with her parents, and the available evidence base.

> *Sarabi is 23 months old. Her parents have brought her for evaluation because her early speech development is delayed compared to her older sibling. There are no other developmental concerns.*

Multifaceted Assessment and Intervention Planning

A plan for either assessment or intervention must take multiple factors into account. Researchers (McCormack et al., 2010; Rusiewicz et al., 2018, Thomas-Stonell et al., 2009) have surveyed parents and clinicians, basing their questions on the holistic framework provided in the World Health Organization's (WHO) International Classification of Functioning, Disability, and Health – Child and Youth Version: ICF-CY (2007). Parents tended to express concern about Participation Restrictions (social relationships and community participation) or Personal Factors (shyness, behaviour problems) as priorities, while clinicians tended to focus more on Body Structures and Function (oral structures, intelligibility). This suggests that clinicians may need to consider including parent input to develop specific goals for work on participation in play or learning tasks, and to target communication skills that support the ability to interact and socialise in different settings.

Sarabi's evaluation would first involve consideration of her language and general communication skills. Does she exhibit communicative intent and express a variety of pragmatic functions? Is there a discrepancy between receptive and expressive skills? Is speech sound development consistent with, or noticeably discrepant from, the clinician's estimate of language skills? Gathering history information from parents and caregivers is important, especially for young children, remembering the interactions among cognitive, linguistic, and motor development domains.

> *Sarabi scored within age expectations for receptive language but in the mildly delayed range for expressive language on a standardized checklist assessment. She used a combination of gestures and vocalizations to actively communicate with her parents, expressing a range of functions. She exhibited a limited speech sound inventory consisting of five differentiated vowels and two consonants*

in her spontaneous output. She did not coop-erate when standardized assessment of speech was attempted.

While Sarabi's speech sound acquisition appeared to be discrepant from the estimate of receptive language skills, further information would be needed to consider the relative contribution of linguistic skills (language, phonology) and motor speech development. Evidence towards a differential diagnosis might need to be collected over a period, based on monitoring or diagnostic therapy.

With no suspicion of other developmental disabilities and strong family support, a caregiver coaching model with periodic (monthly) monitoring was determined to be appropriate as a first step in intervention for Sarabi. AAC has been shown to facilitate development of speech and language skills in children with developmental delays (e.g., Wright et al., 2013). A goal incorporating use of simple signs and conventional gestures was included as part of the intervention and monitoring plan. Her parents were also given ideas for specific activities to facilitate engagement and to encourage verbal imitation (DeThorne et al., 2009).

Sarabi at age 27 months is producing 100 recognizable words and some 2-word combinations. She has an expanded speech sound repertoire. Her speech is understandable only to family members and familiar listeners.

A more detailed analysis of speech sound development can be attempted as a child becomes more verbal. In addition to standardized measures of articulation or phonology, important information for both speech sound inventory and language development could be obtained by analysing a sample of spontaneous verbal output. A motor speech examination might be attempted to rule a motor speech disorder in or out.

Sarabi's attention for structured testing is limited. Based on an informal picture-naming activity and spontaneous speech sample, several patterns of error were identified.

Most word approximations were produced with consistent errors. Vowels were generally accurate. Sarabi has begun to show increasing frustration when people do not understand her.

Adapting Intervention Relative to 'Child Characteristics'

Considering Sarabi's age, suspected speech disorder, communicative frustration and limited tolerance for structured tasks, speech therapy was initiated by scheduling one session per week. Goals for sessions included targeting stimulability for error patterns in play-based activities and parent education. Elements of the Parents and Children Together (PACT) approach (Bowen & Cupples, 1999) were incorporated into sessions. Her parents were taught techniques such as modelling and recasting. Sessions also included discussion between clinician and parents about speech sounds and how they are joined to make words. A variety of simple activities were taught for home practice.

At age 33 months, Sarabi is becoming more compliant for requests for direct imitation during therapy sessions. She has become much more verbal at home. She is producing 2- and 3-word utterances and occasional 4-word sequences. However, as length of utterance has increased, her intelligibility even for familiar listeners has decreased due to the number of her continuing speech errors. Parents express concern that she 'seems to be going backwards' at this point.

A Decline in Intelligibility, and a Diagnosis

It is not unexpected that Sarabi's intelligibility might be temporarily decreased with increasing length of utterance. Reduced intelligibility could be a sign that Sarabi's developing speech motor system may not be keeping up with her growing language skill. Speech therapy was increased to twice per week to work directly on speech sound production while continuing to monitor language skills. Sarabi was able to complete a standardized phonology assessment, yielding a score that confirmed skills below age expectations. An informal motor speech examination was administered to evaluate Sarabi's ability to produce syllables and syllable sequences of increasing length and phonetic complexity. Decreasing accuracy with increasing length of sequence was noted with errors that were predictable and consistent. Vowels were accurate and prosody was judged to be age-typical, with appropriate lexical stress. The overall impression was of a phonological disorder with no compelling evidence of motor speech disorder.

Sarabi's SLP/SLT made a clinical decision to adjust her therapy approach and searched the literature for information about phonological treatment approaches. A two-part series of articles on evidence-based practice (EBP) for children with speech sound disorders (Baker & McLeod, 2011a, 2011b) yielded multiple options to consider. The Cycles Phonological Patterns approach (see Hodson et al., this volume) was chosen initially due in part to a target selection protocol that allowed for addressing Sarabi's multiple error patterns in a rotating sequence, resulting in less resistance than practicing the same targets repeatedly in sequential sessions.

Using the Cycles approach, Sarabi has begun to show pride in her accomplishments as she makes progress, and she participates enthusiastically in therapy sessions. This carries over to her home practice, with her parents also pleased by her improved intelligibility and reduced frustration. Several of Sarabi's error patterns resolved after 7 months of therapy. Data from periodic probe sessions provided objective evidence of that progress. She continued to have a persistent pattern of gliding that was resistant to change.

Sarabi's SLP/SLT and parents agreed that modifying intervention appeared to be needed to address her persisting errors in a more targeted fashion. Since Sarabi was also at increased risk for reduced literacy skills relative to peers given her history. the SLP/SLT chose to address Sarabi's remaining error pattern using a conventional Minimal Pairs approach combined with the Phonological Awareness Intervention programme (e.g., Denne et al., 2005).

At 48 months of age, Sarabi's speech and language skills are much improved. She is producing sentence-length utterances with age-expected grammar and syntax that are intelligible to most listeners. She has residual inconsistent difficulty with gliding of /ɹ/ and /l/. She is stimulable for accurate production of these phonemes with effort. She has been an active participant in her preschool program. There have been no concerns about emergent literacy skills.

Deciding about Discharge and Continuing Support at Home

This can be a difficult decision point. Sarabi has made good progress and her scores on standardized assessments of language and speech sound production are in the average range for her age. Should Sarabi be released from intervention and monitored to see if there is a need, later, to 'clean up' her remaining errors? Should she remain in intervention to work on those errors? This would be an opportune time to look at language skills in detail, given research that suggests that children with an early history of language delay may be at risk for lower language skill than peers, even if they fall within the broad range of normal for age (Dale et al., 2003). This is also a time to assess phonological awareness skills more formally, based on the known connection between early history of speech-language delay and later literacy concerns (e.g., Tambyraja et al., 2020).

Sarabi's clinician made the choice to discharge her from therapy with suggestions for home practice to promote best production of remaining error sounds. Her parents were strongly advised to be proactive in seeking evaluation if concerns arose as Sarabi moves from her preschool program to formal schooling. They were provided with a list of red flags that should trigger a referral for updated speech-language assessment and/or academic testing.

The Decision-Making Process and Progress-Monitoring

Sarabi's case is an example of the kind of decisions that can occur throughout the process of assessment and intervention. Different tools for assessment will be needed depending on the developmental abilities of a child and the question(s) to be answered. Different intervention techniques may be needed over the course of intervention depending on the progress or lack of progress documented by data collected during therapy sessions. The WHO-ICF-CY model provides a framework for attention to functional outcomes.

Critical thinking and clinical thinking are interdependent processes that contribute in different ways to achieving best possible outcomes for a child with a speech sound disorder. It is unlikely that the participants in a research study will exactly reflect the characteristics of a specific child undergoing assessment or intervention. Critical thinking will be needed to consider the relevance of the approach under study for a given child, and the strength of that evidence. Clinical thinking involves combining best available evidence with practice-based evidence, such as outcome data from prior experiences with similar children. A dynamic combination of critical thinking and clinical thinking will be involved in achieving best possible outcomes for a given child.

Why Try to Overcome Barriers to Best Practice?

There are likely numerous barriers to implementing new intervention approaches, including (a) an SLP's lack of familiarity with newer approaches (Brumbaugh & Smit, 2013; Hegarty et al., 2018), (b) the dearth of effectiveness research that would provide a roadmap for delivering the approach in a typical school setting, (c) incomplete descriptions of the approach in publications (Sugden et al., 2018), and (d) the high SLP investment in

learning and adopting a new approach because of all of these factors (Furlong et al., 2021). However, newer intervention approaches may promote better outcomes for children with SSD. Consequently, it is worthwhile to try to overcome these barriers to best practice.

Storkel, 2022, pp. 632–633

References

American Speech-Language-Hearing Association. (2004). *Preferred practice patterns for the profession of speech-language pathology [Preferred Practice Patterns]*. Available from www.asha.org/policy https://doi.org:10.1044/policy.PP2004-00191

Argyris, C., & Schön, D. (1974). *Theory in practice: Increasing professional effectiveness*. Jossey-Bass.

Armstrong, S., & Ainley, M. (1988). *The South Tyneside assessment of phonology*. Stass.

Baker, E. (2012). Optimal intervention intensity in speech-language pathology: Discoveries, challenges, and unchartered territories. *International Journal of Speech-Language Pathology*, 14(5), 478–485. https://doi.org/10.3109/17549507.2012.717967

Baker, E., & McLeod, S. (2011a). Evidence-based practice for children with speech sound disorders: Part 1 narrative review. *Language, Speech, and Hearing Services in Schools*, 42(2), 102–139. https://doi.org/10.1044/0161-1461(2010/09-0075)

Baker, E., & McLeod, S. (2011b). Evidence-based practice for children with speech sound disorders: Part 2 application to clinical practice. *Language, Speech, and Hearing Service in Schools*, 42(2), 140–151. https://doi.org/10.1044/0161-1461(2010/10-0023)

Bernstein Ratner, N. (2006). Evidence-based practice: An examination of its ramifications for the practice of speech-language pathology. *Language, Speech and Hearing Services in Schools*, 37(4), 257–267. https://doi.org/10.1044/0161-1461(2006/029)

Bishop, D. V. M., & Thompson, P. A. (2023). *Evaluating What Works*. Authors. https://bookdown.org/dorothy_bishop/Evaluating_What_Works/

Bowen, C. (2015). Children's speech sound disorders, 2nd ed. Wiley-Blackwell.

Bowen, C., & Cupples, L. (1999). Parents and children together (PACT): A collaborative approach to phonological therapy. *International Journal of Language and Communication Disorders*, 34(1), 35–55. https://doi.org/10.1080/136828299247603

Broomfield, J., & Dodd, B. (2004). Children with speech and language disability: Caseload characteristic. *International Journal of Language and Communication Disorders*, 39(3), 303–324. https://doi.org/10.1080/13682820310001625589

Brumbaugh, K. M., & Smit, A. B. (2013). Treating children ages 3–6 who have speech sound disorder: A survey. *Language, Speech, and Hearing Services in Schools*, 44(3), 306–319. https://doi.org/10.1044/0161-1461(2013/12-0029)

Bunton, K. (2008). Speech versus nonspeech: Different tasks, different neural organization. *Seminars in Speech and Language*, 29(4), 267–275. https://doi.org/10.1055/s-0028-1103390

Bunton, K., & Weismer, G. (1994). Evaluation of a reiterant force impulse task in the tongue. *Journal of Speech and Hearing Research*, 37(5), 1020–1031. https://doi.org/10.1044/jshr.3705.1020

Clark, H. (2012). Specificity of training in the lingual musculature. *Journal of Speech, Language, Hearing Research*, 55(2), 657–667. https://doi.org/10.1044/1092-4388(2011/11-0045)

Clark, H. M. (2005). Clinical decision making and oral motor treatments. *The ASHA Leader*, 10(8), 34–35. https://doi.org/10.1044/leader.FTR3.10082005.8

Clark, H. M. (2008). The role of strength training in speech sound disorders. *Seminars in Speech and Language*, 29(4), 276–283. https://doi.org:10.1055/s-0028-1103391

Clark, H. M., Henson, P. A., Barber, W. D., Stierwalt, J. A. G., & Sherrill, M. (2003). Relationships among subjective and objective measures of tongue strength and oral phase swallowing impairments. *American Journal of Speech-Language Pathology*, 12(1), 40–50. https://doi.org/10.1044/1058-0360(2003/051)

Clark, H. M., O'Brien, K., Calleja, A., & Newcomb Corrie, S. (2009). Effects of directional exercise on lingual strength. *Journal of Speech, Language and Hearing Research*, 52(4), 10.3–1047. https://doi.org/10.1044/1092-4388(2009/08-0062)

Crowe, K., & McLeod, S. (2020). Children's English consonant acquisition in the United States: A review. *American Journal of Speech-Language Pathology*, 29(4), 2155–2169. https://doi.org/10.1044/2020_AJSLP-19-00168

Cummings, A., Hallgrimson, J., & Robinson, S. (2019). Speech intervention outcomes associated with word lexicality and intervention intensity. *Language, Speech, and Hearing Services in Schools*, 50(1), 83–98. https://doi.org/10.1044/2018_LSHSS-18-0026

Dale, P. S., Price, T. S., Bishop, D. V., & Plomin, R. (2003). Outcomes of early language delay: I. Predicting persistent and transient language difficulties at 3 and 4 years. *Journal of Speech, Language, and Hearing Research*, 46(3), 544–560. https://doi.org/10.1044/1092-4388(2003/044)

Davidson, M. M., Mahendra, N., & Nicholson, N. (2022). Creating clinical research impact through social media: Five easy steps to get started. *Perspectives of the ASHA Special Interest Groups*, 7(3), 669–678. https://doi.org/10.1044/2022_PERSP-21-00208

De', R., Pandey, N., & Pal, A. (2020). Impact of digital surge during Covid-19 pandemic: A viewpoint on research and practice. *International Journal of Information Management*, 55, 102171. https://doi.org/10.1016/j.ijinfomgt.2020.102171

Denne, M., Langdown, N., Pring, T., & Roy, P. (2005). Treating children with expressive phonological disorders: Does phonological awareness therapy work in the clinic? *International Journal of Language and Communication Disorders*, 40(4), 493–504. https://doi.org/10.1080/13682820500142582

DeThorne, L. S., Johnson, C. J., Walder, L., & Mahurin-Smith, J. (2009). When "Simon says" doesn't work: Alternatives to imitation for facilitating early speech development. *American Journal of Speech-Language Pathology*, 18(2), 133–145. https://doi.org/10.1044/1058-0360(2008/07-0090)

Dollaghan, C. A. (2007). *The handbook for evidence-based practice in communication disorders*. Paul H. Brookes Publishing Co.

Douglas, N., Oshita, J., Schliep, M., & Feuerstein, J. (2022). Knowledge brokering in communication sciences and disorders. *Perspectives of the ASHA Special Interest Groups*, 7(3), 663–668. https://doi.org/10.1044/2022_PERSP-21-00204

Dworkin, J., & Cullatta, R., (1980). Tongue strength: its relationship to tongue thrusting, open-bite, and artic- ulatory proficiency. *Journal of Speech and Hearing Disorders*, 45(2), 277–282. https://doi.org/10.1044/jshd.4502.277

Ellis, E., Kubalanza, M., Simon-Cereijido, G., Munger, A., & Sidle Fuligni, A. (2020). Interprofessional collaboration to promote culturally engaged and strengths-based practice. *Perspectives of the ASHA Special Interest Groups*, 6(5), 1410–1421. https://doi.org/10.1044/2020_PERSP-20-10007

Farquharson, K., McIlraith, A. L., Tambyraja, S. R., & Constantino, C. (2022). Using the experience sampling method to examine the details of dosage in school-based speech sound therapy. *Language, Speech, and Hearing Services in Schools*, 53(3), 698–712. https://doi.org/10.1044/2021_LSHSS-21-00130

Fields, D., & Polmanteer, K. (2002, November). Effectiveness of oral motor techniques in articulation and phonology therapy. *Poster presented at the Annual Meeting of the American Speech-Language-Hearing Association*, Atlanta, GA, ASHA.

Forrest, K. (2002). Are oral-motor exercises useful in treatment of phonological/articulation disorders? *Seminars in Speech and Language*, 23(1), 15–25. https://doi.org/10.1055/s-2002-23508

Furlong, L. M., Morris, M. E., Serry, T. A., & Erickson, S. (2021). Treating childhood speech sound disorders: Current approaches to management by Australian speech-language pathologists. *Language, Speech, and Hearing Services in Schools*, 52(2), 581–596. https://doi.org/10.1044/2020_LSHSS-20-00092

Gierut, J. A. (1989). Maximal opposition approach to phonological treatment. *Journal of Speech and Hearing Disorders*, 54(1), 9–19. https://doi.org/10.1044/jshd.5401.09

Greenwell, T., & Walsh, B. (2021). Evidence-based practice in speech-language pathology: Where are we now? *American Journal of Speech-Language Pathology*, 30(1), 186–198. https://doi.org/10.1044/2020_AJSLP-20-00194

Health and Care Professions Council (HCPC) (2013). Standards of proficiency. *Speech and Language Therapists*. London: HCPC. https://www.hcpc-uk.org/resources/standards/standards-of-proficiency-speech-and-language-therapists

Health and Care Professions Council (HCPC) (2022). *Standards of continuing professional development*. https://www.hcpc-uk.org/standards/standards-of-continuing-professional-development HCPC

Hegarty, N., Titterington, J., McLeod, S., & Taggart, L. (2018). Intervention for children with phonological impairment: Knowledge, practices and intervention intensity in the UK. *International Journal of Language & Communication Disorders*, 53(5), 995–1006. https://doi.org/10.1111/1460-6984.12416

Higginbotham, J., & Satchidanand, A. (2019). Triangle to diamond: Recognizing and using data to inform our evidence-based practice, *ASHA Journals Academy*. ASHA. https://academy.pubs.asha.org/2019/04/from-triangle-to-diamond-recognizing-and-using-data-to-inform-our-evidence-based-practice.

Hitchcock, E. R., Swartz, M. T., & Lopez, M. (2019). Speech sound disorder and visual biofeedback intervention: A preliminary investigation of treatment intensity. *Seminars in Speech and Language*, 40(2), 124–137. https://doi.org/10.1055/s-0039-1677763

Hoffman, T., Bennett, S., & Del Mar, C. (2017). *Evidence-based practice across the health professions* (3rd ed.). Elsevier. https://doi.org/10.1044/1058-0360(2003/086)

Irwin, D., Pannbacker, M., Powell, T. W., & Vekovius, G. T. (2006). *Ethics for speech-language pathologists and audiologists: An illustrative casebook*. Thomson Delmar Learning.

Joffe, V. L., & Broomfield, J. (2019) What is the child speech disorder research network? RCSLT Bulletin, Ask the Expert. Child speech sound disorder: special edition, (pp. 6–7).

Joffe, V., & Pring, V. (2008). Children with phonological problems: A survey of clinical practice. *International Journal of Language & Communication Disorders*, 43(2), 154–164. https://doi.org/10.1080/13682820701660259

Jones, D., Hardin-Jones, M., & Brown, C. (2011, November). Aerodynamic requirements for blowing novelty horns. *Poser presented at the Annual Convention of the American Speech-Language-Hearing Association*, San Diego, CA, ASHA.

Justice, L. M. (2018). Conceptualising "dose" in paediatric language interventions: Current findings and future directions. *International Journal of Speech-Language Pathology*, 20(3), 318–323. https://doi.org/10.1080/17549507.2018.1454985

Kaderavek, J. N., & Justice, L. M. (2010). Fidelity: An essential component of evidence-based practice in speech-language pathology. *American Journal of Speech-Language Pathology*, 19(4), 369–379. https://doi.org/10.1044/1058-0360(2010/09-0097)

Kamal, S. (2021). The use of oral motor exercises among speech language pathologists in Jordan. *Journal of Language Teaching and Research*, 12(1), 99–103. https://doi.org/10.17507/jltr.1201.10

Jones, D., Hardin-Jones, M., & Brown, C. (2011, November). Aerodynamic requirements for blowing novelty horns. *Poser presented at the annual convention of the American Speech-Language-Hearing Association*, San Diego, CA.

Kamhi, A. (2008). A meme's-eye view of nonspeech oral motor exercises. *Seminars in Speech and Language*, 29(4), 331–339. https://doi.org/10.1055/s-0028-1103397

Kamhi, A. G. (2006). Treatment decisions for children with speech-sound disorders. *Language, Speech, and Hearing Services in Schools*, 37(4), 271–279. https://doi.org/10.1044/0161-1461(2006/031)

Kamhi, A. G. (2011). Balancing certainty and uncertainty in clinical practice. *Language, Speech, and Hearing Services in Schools*, 42(1), 59–64. https://doi.org/10.1044/0161-1461(2009/09-0034)

Kent, R. D. (2004). The uniqueness of speech among motor systems. *Clinical Linguistics & Phonetics*, 18(6–8), 495–505. https://doi.org/10.1080/02699200410001703600

Kent, R. D. (2015). Nonspeech oral movements and oral motor disorders: A narrative review. *American Journal of Speech-Language Pathology*, 24(4), 763–789. https://doi.org/10.1044/2015_AJSLP-14-0179

Klein, H. B., Lederer, S. H., & Cortese, E. E. (1991). Children's knowledge of auditory/articulator correspondences: Phonologic and metaphonologic. *Journal of Speech and Hearing Research*, 34(3), 559–564. https://doi.org/10.1044/jshr.3403.559

Kohnert, K. (2007). Evidence-based practice and treatment of speech sound disorders in bilingual children. *Perspectives in Language and Learning*, 14(2), 17–20. https://doi.org/10.1044/cds14.2.17

Kuschmann, A., Nayar, R., Lowit, A., & Dunlop, M. (2021). The use of technology in the management of children with phonological delay and adults with acquired dysarthria: A UK survey of current speech-language pathology practice. *International Journal of Speech-Language Pathology*, 23(2), 145–154. https://doi.org/10.1080/17549507.2020.1750700

Lau, T. H. M., & Lee, K. Y. S. (2013). Oral motor performance in children with suspected speech sound disorders: A comparison with children with typically developing speech. *Speech, Language and Hearing*, 16(3), 139–148. https://doi.org/10.1179/2050572813Y.0000000009

Law, J., Boyle, J., Harris, F., Harkness, A., & Nye, C. (2000). Prevalence and natural history of primary speech and language delay: Findings from a systematic review of the literature. *International Journal of Language & Communication Disorders*, 35(2), 165–188. https://doi.org/10.1080/136828200247133

Law, J., Campbell, C., Roulstone, S., Adams, C., & Boyle, J. (2008). Mapping practice onto theory: The speech and language practitioner's construction of receptive language impairment. *International Journal of Language & Communication Disorders*, 43(3), 245–263. https://doi.org/10.1080/136828200247133

Lee, A. S. Y., & Gibbon, F. E. (2015). Non-speech oral motor treatment for children with developmental speech sound disorders. *Cochrane Database of Systematic Reviews*, 2015(3), CD009383. https://doi.org/10.1002/14651858.CD009383.pub2

Lof, G. L. (2003). Oral motor exercises and treatment outcomes. *Perspectives on Language, Learning and Education*, 10(1), 7–11. https://doi.org/10.1044/lle10.1.7

Lof, G. L. (2008). Controversies surrounding nonspeech oral motor exercises for childhood speech disorders. *Seminars in Speech and Language*, 29(4), 253–255. https://doi.org/10.1055/s-0028-1103388

Lof, G. L., & Watson, M. (2008). A nationwide survey of nonspeech oral motor exercise use: Implications for evidence-based practice. *Language, Speech, and Hearing Services in Schools*, 39(3), 392–407. https://doi.org/10.1044/0161-1461(2008/037)

Lof, G. L., & Watson, M. (2010). Five reasons why nonspeech oral-motor exercises do not work. *Perspectives in Language and Learning*, 11(4), 109–117. https://doi.org/10.1044/sbi11.4.109

Lousada, M., Jesus, L. M., Capelas, S., Margaça, C., Simões, D., Valente, A., Hall, A., & Joffe, V. L. (2013). Phonological and articulation treatment approaches in Portuguese children with speech and language impairments: A randomized controlled intervention study. *International Journal of Language & Communication Disorders*, 48(2), 172–187. https://doi.org/10.1111/j.1460-6984.2012.00191.x

Ludlow, C. L., Hoit, J., Kent, R., Ramig, L. O., Shrivastav, R., Strand, E., Yorkston, K., & Sapienza, C. M. (2008). Translating principles of neural plasticity into research on speech motor control recovery and rehabilitation. *Journal of Speech, Language and Hearing Research*, 51(1), S240–S258. https://doi.org/10.1044/1092-4388(2008/019)

Maas, E. (2017). Speech and nonspeech: What are we talking about? *International Journal of Speech-Language Pathology*, 3(19), 345–359. https://doi.org/10.1080/17549507.2016.1221995

Mackenzie, C., Muir, M., & Allen, C. (2011). Nonspeech oromotor exercise use in acquired dysarthria management: Regimes and rationales. *International Journal of Language & Communication Disorders*, 45(6), 617–629. https://doi.org/10.3109/13682820903470577

Malamud, H., McDaniel, J., Krimm, H., & Schuele, M. (2021, April). Understanding the research-practice gap for speech-language intervention via SLPs' endorsement of myths. *Poster presented at the Gatlinburg Conference on Research and Theory in Intellectual and Developmental Disabilities.*

McCabe, P. J. (2018). Elizabeth usher memorial lecture: How do we change our profession? Using the lens of behavioural economics to improve evidence-based practice in speech-language pathology. *International Journal of Speech-Language Pathology*, 20(3), 300–309. https://doi.org/10.1080/17549507.2018.1 460526

McCauley, R. J., Strand, E., Lof, G. L., Schooling, T., & Frymark, T. (2009). Evidence-based systematic review: Effects of nonspeech oral motor exercises on speech. *American Journal of Speech-Language Pathology*, 18(4), 343–360. https://doi.org/10.1044/ 1058-0360(2009/09-0006)

McCormack, J., McLeod, S., Harrison, L. J., & McAllister, L. (2010). The impact of speech impairment in early childhood: Investigating parents' and speech-language pathologists' perspectives using the ICF-CY. *Journal of Communication Disorders*, 43(5), 378–396. https://doi.org/10.1016/j.jcomdis. 2021.106099

McGill, N., McLeod, S., Crowe, K., Wang, C., & Hopf, S. C. (2021). Waiting lists and prioritization of children for services: Speech-language pathologists' perspectives. *Journal of Communication Disorders*, 91, 106099. https://doi.org/10.1016/j.jcomdis.2021. 106099

McLeod, S., & Crowe, K. (2018). Children's consonant acquisition in 27 languages: A cross-linguistic review. *American Journal of Speech-Language Pathology*, 27(4), 1546–1571. https://doi.org/ 10.1044/2018_AJSLP-17-0100

Morgan, L., Marshall, J., Harding, S., Powell, G., Wren, Y., Coad, J., & Roulstone, S. (2019). 'It depends': Characterizing speech and language therapy for preschool children with developmental speech and language disorders. *International Journal of Language & Communication Disorders*, 54(6), 954–970. https://doi.org/10.1111/1460-6984.12498

Muttiah, N., Georges, K., & Brackenbury, T. (2011). Clinical and research perspectives on nonspeech oral motor treatments and evidence-based practice. *American Journal of Speech-Language Pathology*, 20(1), 47–59. https://doi.org/10.1044/1058-0360(2010/09-0106)

Nicoll, A., Maxwell, M., & Williams, B. (2021). Achieving 'coherence' in routine practice: A qualitative case-based study to describe speech and language therapy interventions with implementation in mind. *Implementation Science Communications*, 2(1), 56. https://doi.org/10.1186/s43058-021-00159-0

Ogg, K., Jones, D., & Hardin-Jones, M. (2012, November). Oral pressure requirements for common blow toys. *Poster presented at the Annual Convention of the American Speech-Language-Hearing Association*, Atlanta, GA ASHA. RCSLT.

Olswang, L. B., & Bain, B. (1994). Data collection: Monitoring children's treatment progress. *American Journal of Speech-Language Pathology*, 3(3), 55–65. https://doi.org/10.1044/ 1058-0360.0303.55

Pagnamenta, E., Bangera, S., Wallinger, J., & Joffe, V. L. (2022). Speech and language therapists' understanding and use of research and evidence based practice in routine clinical work in the UK. *Unpublished Report*. RCSLT.

Pagnamenta, E., & Joffe, V. L. (2018). Preregistration research training of speech and language therapists in the United Kingdom: A nationwide audit of quantity, content and delivery. *International Journal of Evidence-Based Healthcare*, 16(4), 204–213. https://doi.org/10.1097/XEB.0000000000000143

Pollock, M. L., Gaesser, G. A., Butcher, J. D., Després, J. P., Dishman, R. K., Franklin, B. A., & Garber, C. E. (1998). The recommended quantity and quality of exercise for developing and maintaining cardiorespiratory and muscular fitness, and flexibility in healthy adults. *Medicine and science in sports and exercise*, 30(6), 975–991. https://doi.org/10.1097/ 00005768-199806000-00032

Potter, N. L., Nievergelt, Y., & VanDam, M. (2019). Tongue strength in children with and without speech sound disorders. *American Journal of speech-Language Pathology*, 28(2), 612–622. https://doi.org/10.1044/2018_AJSLP-18-0023

Powell, T. W. (2007). A model for ethical practices in clinical phonetics and linguistics. *Clinical Linguistics & Phonetics*, 21(11–12), 851–857. https://doi.org/10.1080/02699200701576777

Powell, T. W. (2013). Research ethics. In N. Müller & M. J. Ball (Eds.), *Research methods in clinical linguistics and phonetics: A practical guide* (pp. 10–27). Wiley-Blackwell.

Powell, T. W. (2015). NS-OME: An ethical challenge. In C. Bowen, *Children's speech sound disorders* (2nd ed.). Wiley-Blackwell.

Pratomo, H. G. A., & Siswanto, A. (2020). Penggunaan non speech oral motor treatment (NSOMT) Sebagai Pendekatan Intervensi Gangguan Bunyi Bicara. *Jurnal Keterapian Fisik*, 5(2), 109–121. https://doi. org/10.37341/jkf.v5i2.213

Pring, T., Flood, E., Dodd, B., & Joffe, V. (2012). The working practices and clinical experiences of paediatric speech and language therapists: A national UK survey. *International Journal of Language & Communication Disorders*, 47(6), 696–708. https:// doi.org/10.1111/j.1460-6984.2012.00177.x

Rosenfeld-Johnson, S. (2001). *Oral-motor exercises for speech clarity*. Innovative Therapists International.

Rosenzweig, E. A., & Voss, J. (2022). Their words, their world: A paradigm for culturally relevant family-centered intervention. *Perspectives of the ASHA Special Interest Groups*, 2(7), 553–559. https://doi.org/10.1044/2021_PERSP-21-00074

Royal College of Speech and Language Therapists (RCSLT). (2021). *RCSLT guidance: Curriculum guidance for the pre-registration education of speech and language therapists*.

Rumback, A. F., Rose, T. A., & Cheah, M. (2017). Exploring Australian speech-language pathologists' use and perceptions of non-speech oral motor exercises. *Disability and Rehabilitation*, 41(12), 1463–1474. https://doi.org/10.1080/09638288.2018.1431694

Ruscello, D. M. (2008). Nonspeech oral motor treatment issues related to children with developmental speech sound disorders. *Language, Speech, and Hearing Services in Schools*, 39(3), 380–391. https://doi.org/10.1044/0161-1461(2008/036)

Ruscello, D. M., & Vallino, L. D. (2020). The use of nonspeech oral motor exercises in the treatment of children with cleft palate: A re-examination of available evidence. *American Journal of Speech-Language Pathology*, 29(4), 1811–1820. https://doi.org/10.1044/2020_AJSLP-20-00087

Rusiewicz, H. L., Maize, K., & Ptakowski, T. (2018). Parental experiences and perceptions related to childhood apraxia of speech: Focus on functional implications. *International Journal of Speech-Language Pathology*, 20(5), 569–580. https://doi.org/10.1080/17549507.2017.1359333

Rvachew, S., & Rafaat, S. (2014). Report on benchmark wait times for pediatric speech sound disorders. *Canadian Journal of Speech-Language Pathology and Audiology*, 38(1), 82–96. https://www.cjslpa.ca/detail.php?ID=1145&lang=en

Schlosser, R. W. (2014). Treatment fidelity in single-subject designs. *ASHA Journals Academy CREd Library*. ASHA. https://academy.pubs.asha.org/2014/10/treatment-fidelity-in-single-subject-designs

Schulz, G. M., Dingwall, W. O., & Ludlow, C. L. (1999). Speech and oral motor learning in individuals with cerebellar atrophy. *Journal of Speech, Language and Hearing Research*, 42(5), 1157–1175. https://doi.org/10.1044/jslhr.4205.1157

Sjögreen, L., Tulinius, M., Kiliaridis, S., & Lohmander, A. (2010). The effect of lip strengthening exercises in children and adolescents with myotonic dystrophy type 1. *International Journal of Pediatric Otorhinolaryngology*, 74(10), 1126–1134. https://doi.org/10.1016/j.ijporl.2010.06.013

Solomon, N. P., & Munson, B. (2004). The effect of jaw position on measures of tongue strength and endurance. *Journal of Speech, Language, and Hearing Research*, 47(3), 584–594. https://doi.org/10.1044/1092-4388(2004/045)

Stoeckel, R., & Caspari, S. (2020). Childhood apraxia of speech: Clinical decision making from a motor-based perspective. *Perspectives of the ASHA Special Interest Groups*, 5(4), 831–842. https://doi.org/10.1044/2020_PERSP-19-00090

Storkel, H. L. (2018a). The complexity approach to phonological treatment: How to select treatment targets. *Language, Speech, and Hearing Services in Schools*, 49(3), 463–481. https://doi.org/10.1044/2017_LSHSS-17-0082

Storkel, H. L. (2018b). Implementing evidence-based practice: Selecting treatment words to boost phonological learning. *Language, Speech, and Hearing Services in Schools*, 49(3), 482–496. https://doi.org/10.1044/2017_LSHSS-17-0080

Storkel, H. L. (2019). Using developmental norms for speech sounds as a means of determining treatment eligibility in schools. *Perspectives of the ASHA Special Interest Groups*, 4(1), 67–75. https://doi.org/10.1044/2018_PERS-SIG1-2018-0014

Storkel, H. L. (2022). Minimal, maximal, or multiple: Which contrastive intervention approach to use with children with speech sound disorders? *Language, Speech, and Hearing Services in Schools*, 53(3), 632–646. https://doi.org/10.1044/2021_LSHSS-21-00105

Sugden, E., Baker, E., Munro, N., Williams, A. L., & Trivette, C. M. (2018). Service delivery and intervention intensity for phonology-based speech sound disorders. *International Journal of Language & Communication Disorders*, 53(4), 718–734. https://doi.org/10.1111/1460-6984.12399

Tambyraja, S. R., Farquharson, K., & Justice, L. M. (2020). Reading risk in children with speech sound disorder: Prevalence, Persistence, and Predictors. *Journal of Speech, Language, and Hearing Research*, 63(11), 3714–3726. https://doi:10.1044/2020

Thomas-Stonell, N., Oddson, B., Robertson, B., & Rosenbaum, P. (2009). Predicted and observed outcomes in preschool children following speech and language treatment: Parent and clinician perspectives.

Journal of Communication Disorders, 42(1), 29–42. https://doi.org/10.1016/j.jcomdis.2008.08.002

Thome, E. K., Lovell, S. J., & Henderson, D. E. (2020). A survey of speech-language pathologists' understanding and reported use of evidence-based practice. *Perspectives of the ASHA Special Interest Groups*, 5(4), 984–999. https://doi.org/10.1044/2020_PERSP-20-00008

Van Riper, C. (1978). *Speech correction: Principles and methods* (6th ed.). Prentice-Hall.

Verkerk, E. W., Tanke, M. A. C., Kool, R. B., van Dulmen, S. A., & Westert, G. P. (2018). Limit, lean or listen? A typology of low-value care that gives direction in de-implementation. *International Journal for Quality in Health Care*, 30(9), 736–739. https://doi.org/10.1093/intqhc/mzy100

Warren, S. F., Fey, M. E., & Yoder, P. J. (2007). Differential treatment intensity research: A missing link to creating optimally effective communication interventions. *Mental Retardation and Developmental Disabilities Research Reviews*, 13(1), 70–77. https://doi.org/10.1002/mrdd.20139

Watson, M., & Lof, G. L. (2008). Epilogue: What we know about nonspeech oral motor exercises. *Seminars in Speech and Language*, 29(4), 320–330. https://doi.org/10.1055/s-0028-1103398

Weismer, G. (2006). Philosophy of research in motor speech disorders. *Clinical Linguistics & Phonetics*, 20(5), 315–349. https://doi.org/10.1080/02699200400024806

Wenke, R. J., Goozee, J. V., Murdoch, B. E., & LaPointe, L. L. (2006). Dynamic assessment of articulation during lingual fatigue in myasthenia gravis. *Journal of Medical Speech-Language Pathology*, 14(1), 13–32. https://espace.library.uq.edu.au/view/UQ:79917

Williams, A. L. (2000a). Multiple oppositions: Theoretical foundations for an alternative contrastive intervention approach. *American Journal of Speech-Language Pathology*, 9(4), 282–288. https://doi.org/10.1044/1058-0360.0904.282

Williams, A. L. (2012). Intensity in phonological intervention: Is there a prescribed amount. *International Journal of Speech- Language Pathology*, 14(5), 456–461. https://doi.org/10.3109/17549507.2012.688866

Wilson, E. M., Green, J. R., Yunusova, Y., & Moore, C. A. (2008). Task specificity in early oral motor development. *Seminars in Speech and Language*, 29(4), 257–266. https://doi.org/10.1055/s-0028-1103389

Wood, C., Romano, M., Levites Strekalova, Y. A., Lugo, V. A., & McCormack, W. T. (2021). State of the practice of team science in speech-language pathology and audiology. *Journal of Speech, Language and Hearing Research*, 64(9), 3549–3563. https://doi.org/10.1044/2021_JSLHR-21-00072

World Health Organization. (2007). *International classification of functioning, disability and health: Children and youth version: ICF-CY*. World Health Organization. https://apps.who.int/iris/handle/10665/43737

Wren, Y., Miller, L. L., Peters, T. J., Emond, A., & Roulstone, S. (2016). Prevalence and predictors of persistent speech sound disorder at eight years old: Findings from a population cohort study. *Journal of Speech, Language, and Hearing Research*, 59(4), 647–673. https://doi.org/10.1044/2015_JSLHR-S-14-0282

Wright, C. A., Kaiser, A. P., Reikowsky, D. I., & Roberts, M. Y. (2013). Effects of a naturalistic sign intervention on expressive language of toddlers with Down syndrome. *Journal of Speech, Language, and Hearing Research*, 56(3), 994–1008. https://doi.org/10.1044/1092-4388(2012/12-0060)

Zhang, Y., & Zhang, J. (2019). Oral motor exercises for CSL learners to master productions of retroflex and non-retroflex consonants, *Asia-Pacific Signal and Information Processing Association Annual Summit and Conference*, 2064-2069. https://doi.org/10.1109/APSIPAASC47483.2019.9023174

Ziegler, W. (2003). Speech motor control is task-specific: Evidence from dysarthria and apraxia of speech. *Aphasiology*, 17(1), 3–36. https://doi.org/10.1080/729254892

Part II
Speech Intervention in Everyday Practice

Introduction to Part II

Building on theory and evidence presented in Part I, the emphasis in Part II is the real-world implementation of assessment and treatment of children for their speech sound disorders. As an introduction, the reader is invited to reflect on four quotations from the 'older' literature, presented chronologically, namely: Dodd (2007); DeThorne et al. (2009); Baker (2010); and Olswang and Prelock (2015), and at the end of the chapter, a more recent quotation from Fulcher-Rood et al. (2020), citing Harold (2019).

> *For some diagnostic categories, the research literature in speech language pathology does not provide any usable data concerning the best treatment approach. ...Given the lack of definitive evidence, and the heterogeneous nature of the population served by speech language pathologists, there is a need for reliance on clinical expertise and building the knowledge base by recording the outcome of intervention.*
>
> Dodd, 2007, p. 125

SLPs/SLTs do not have to look far for advice on *reading* (Greenhalgh, 2019) and *understanding* (Donohue et al., 2022) clinically applicable literature, and abundant work is available *explaining* facilitators that help, and barriers that impede clinicians' access to, and exact application of, scholarly research (Fulcher-Rood et al., 2020; Greenwell & Walsh, 2021; Harold, 2019; Ludemann et al., 2017; Thome et al., 2020; Utianski et al., 2022). But what Dodd (2007) suggested was that clinicians have an important role to play not only in *consuming* research, but also as partners in *developing* it.

Some roles that clinicians can assume within research partnerships (Roberts et al., 2020) may not be instantly recognisable. For example, some clinicians may not have considered the potential usefulness of their clinical data, derived from keeping meticulous case-by-case records of *experiences*, and intervention *outcomes* (Baker et al., 2022). **Experiences** might include the socioenvironmental, emotional, and educational impacts of SSD on an individual child and/or the child's family (e.g., Krueger, 2019; McCormack et al., 2022). **Outcomes** could embrace reasons for discharge (was the client

---

'better' or was their time allocation exhausted?), data that might be highly valued by research teams striving to improve implementation science (Davidson et al., 2022; Davidson & Morris, 2022; Douglas et al., 2022; Gallagher et al., 2022). By sharing clinical case studies (e.g., Carrigg et al., 2015; Jasso & Potratz, 2020; Schleif et al., 2021), and other accounts of our day-to-day work, with researchers, or submitting it for publication, clinicians can play several important roles (Apel, 2009; 1999), including:

- Helping close the theory–therapy, research–practice gaps (Douglas & Burshnic, 2019), potentially further improving communication and collaboration between the clinic and the academe (Froud & Randazzo, A51).
- Demonstrating the clinical utility (or not) of an intervention that looked good on paper when delivered in idealized conditions to carefully chosen participants, offering potential modifications to help it work with a general clinical population exhibiting the usual range of complicating factors, comorbidities and confounds (Apel, 1999).
- Fostering scrutiny and possible evaluation of treatments and techniques which currently lack empirical support, but which are theoretically strong and intuitively appealing. This brings us to the second quotation with its echoes of Clark (2003):

> *EBP encompasses varied forms of evidence, including theoretical grounding and clinical expertise, and does not preclude use of experimental interventions. However, EBP dictates that we be aware of what evidence does or does not exist for our practices and that we give thought to why certain strategies and techniques might be successful. Without an understanding of why something works, there is always the danger that it will be misapplied, and we will be left unable to build on the strategy to form new and potentially better ideas.*
>
> DeThorne et al., 2009, p. 134

Readers will recall from Leitão, A1 that Clark discussed two strategies SLPs/SLTs can employ when selecting an intervention. She suggested starting with the question *'Does this therapy work;*

is it evidence-based?' and seek answers by conducting a literature search (Donohue et al, 2023). If searching fails to reveal evidence for the therapy, the clinician can then ask a different question: *'Should this therapy work; is it theoretically sound?'* and seek an understanding of how the nonevidence-based intervention is *supposed* to work, developing an account of the mechanism underpinning the intervention. If that too proves unsatisfactory, then usually the treatment will be rejected. We do not wittingly action an intervention approach unless we believe it will likely work for the client, and in the best-case scenario, culminate in intelligible speech and discharge. But then, best cases, intelligibility and discharge do not always coincide, and the experience of dismissing clients from our caseloads is not necessarily upbeat or well understood, as reflected in the third quotation:

> *The experience of discharging children and their families from phonological intervention can be both rewarding and disheartening. As Hersh (2010) points out, there is a pressing need to better understand this complex yet understudied issue. Given the potential for children with a phonological impairment to be discharged with intelligible speech, it would be important that this research consider the impact of the discharge experience on SLPs, the children and the families they work in both ideal and less than ideal situations. It would also be worthwhile knowing how SLPs can be best equipped to cope with discharge dilemmas. What is more, it would be valuable to determine the ideal intensity of intervention needed to make unintelligible speech intelligible, to help SLPs navigate a course of phonological intervention for a child and his or her family towards a happy ending.*
>
> Baker, 2010, p. 328

The fourth quotation harks back to Dodd, 2007 above, and concerns the frequently discussed barriers to the clinical implementation of published research findings.

> *…an inherent problem exists in relying on journals and guidelines for dissemination: They place the responsibility on the practitioner to read, accurately interpret, and effectively apply the findings in their settings. This pushing of information into practice is compromised by*

several factors, including but not limited to the following issues: (a) relevance of the research findings to practice, (b) sufficient treatment descriptions that can be implemented with fidelity, (c) access to an organizational structure that embraces and supports the adoption of treatment innovations, (d) practitioners' motivation to change what they are currently doing, and (e) realized benefits for a targeted population sufficient to sustain application.

Olswang & Prelock, 2015. P. S1819

Implementation Science (IS)

De-implementation inquiry (Nicoll et al., 2021; Verkerk et al., 2018), discussed in Chapter 6, concerns ditching *ineffective and untested practice*, otherwise known as *entrenched practice*, *'things we do for no reason'*, and *low-value care*. Its antithesis is a fledgling area of investigation (Davidson & Morris, 2022) in health care and education, devoted to implementation science (Finestack & Betz, 2021; Finestack & Fey, 2017; Glasgow et al., 2012). Implementation Science (IS) goes beyond efficacy and effectiveness research to ascertain and evaluate likely barriers to the faithful adoption, application, and retention, as go-to standard care, of evidence-based approaches. Fixsen et al. (2019, p. 4) said that it is *the study of factors that influence the full and effective use of innovations in practice*, while Glasgow et al. (2012) described it as *the study of how evidence-based practices are adopted and implemented in real-world settings.*

Like assessment and intervention, implementation research must happen in a real-world environment, whether academic, clinical, domiciliary, educational, recreational, or virtual; with clients/students seen in a group or individually; in a publicly funded or private/independent agency; or in some combination of these, and more. It is essential to implementation success, therefore, for the setting in which an assessment or intervention may be carried out to be well understood. Evaluation of the meso-level demands, and micro-level requirements, of the local context may reveal a need to adapt an EBP (while maintaining fidelity) to optimise its application.

To date, there have been no comparative studies to reveal whether IS research in Communication Sciences and Disorder (CSD) takes place in one context or setting more than it does in others (Douglas et al., 2022). However, the scale of extant implementation studies ranges from having a micro-level focus where the goal is practice change by individual clinicians or a small team; via the meso-level that concerns practice change within larger teams, units, and organizations; to the big picture macro-level of the political-administrative environment, including national systems, organizations, regulators, and authorities.

Intervention Implemented Faithfully, as Intended

Across health and education settings, an agency or organization's culture, morale, and climate significantly influence the application of evidence-based practices (Williams & Beidas, 2019). For one thing, organizations where administrators and staff are highly proficient, nurturing a positive ambiance and workers' wellbeing, boast higher fidelity to EBP and better workplace attitudes than do organizations where administrative personnel are inflexible, and the atmosphere is tense (Williams & Beidas, 2019). Great skill is applied in implementing interventions faithfully, according to the developers' intent (*understanding* what fidelity is, and maintaining it), while adjusting the intervention, when necessary, to fit the unique needs of a particular client (*still* maintaining fidelity). The resultant balancing act requires a blend of the clinician's rich knowledge and deep understanding of what the various interventions can deliver, deciding sensibly between them, and knowing when to change tack if the 'fit' between client and intervention is found wanting. All of this is balanced against SLPs'/SLTs' ever-developing clinical experience and their capacity to apply clinical reasoning (Stoeckel, A25). Sometimes straightforward, sometimes complex, and sometimes a mixture of the two, delivering interventions for SSD with adequate fidelity is a longstanding interest of Elise Baker's.

Dr. Elise Baker is a qualified SLP/SLT and clinical researcher with expertise in the management of speech sound disorders in children. As Conjoint Associate Professor of Allied Health with Western Sydney University and South Western Sydney Local Health District, Elise enjoys conducting research with her academic and clinical colleagues finding feasible and innovative solutions to clinical challenges. She also enjoys drawing on theory to inform research into why children can say 'not *dark* [dɐːk], I mean *shark* [dɐːk]'. As a Fellow of both Speech Pathology Australia (SPA), and the American Speech-Language-Hearing Association (ASHA), and long-serving steering committee member of the NSW Speech Pathology Evidence-based Practice Network, Elise is passionate about

supporting SLPs/SLTs in their conduct of evidence-based practice and the translation of research to practice.

Q26.   Elise Baker: Treatment Fidelity

What is treatment fidelity, why does it matter, and how does it relate to E³BP? When an SLP/SLT considers adding a new (to them) intervention approach to their repertoire, what are the necessary steps they should take if their aim is to achieve acceptable fidelity?

Elise Baker: Implementing Interventions with Acceptable Fidelity

What Is Treatment Fidelity?

Treatment fidelity refers to the degree to which an intervention is implemented in accordance with the developer's prototype or gold standard implementation (Kaderavek & Justice, 2010; McCormack et al., 2017). The term is synonymous with intervention fidelity, implementation fidelity, treatment integrity, and procedural reliability (Breitenstein et al., 2010; Noell & Gansle, 2014). In research contexts, treatment fidelity is studied to determine if independent variables (interventions) are implemented by researchers exactly as planned (e.g., Topbaş & Ünal, 2010). Treatment fidelity underscores the internal validity of experiments and strengthens conclusions about the cause-effect relationship between interventions and outcomes. In clinical contexts, the goal is to implement interventions as closely to the gold standard or prototype as possible.

Why Does Treatment Fidelity Matter?

Fidelity matters because children and their families rely on SLPs/SLTs to do their job – to assess and differentially diagnose SSD in children and to provide appropriate and effective evidence-based intervention. Acceptable fidelity is crucial to success (Breitenstein et al., 2010). However, fidelity cannot be assumed, and successful outcomes cannot be guaranteed. Why? Various interventions exist for managing SSDs in children – variety means clinicians must make evidence-informed choices (Williams et al., 2021). In addition, unlike a pharmaceutical pill or vaccine where the active ingredient is manufactured to be identical in every dose, SSD interventions are complex. They comprise multiple elements to be implemented in dynamic human-to-human interactions (Baker & Williams, 2021). The nuanced tailoring or modification of interventions to suit individual children's needs further adds to the challenge of achieving acceptable fidelity and creates uncertainty about outcomes.

This idea of knowing the elements in an intervention but then attenuating fidelity by adapting the elements to the individual was highlighted by Charles Van Riper in a letter to Wayne Secord et al. (2007). In it, Van Riper – the developer of traditional articulation therapy – reflects on his own implementation of traditional articulation therapy:

Personally, in actual therapy, I constantly violated all the precepts I promulgated in the text. Unto their needs was my motto and to heck with what Van Riper or anyone else says. Rarely did I make my clients climb that staircase step-by-step.

Van Riper, 1993 as cited
in Secord et al., 2007, p. viii

To move beyond the point of uncertainty, intervention outcomes and the fidelity of implementation must be measured. Although it is possible to collect routine measures of the outcome of intervention, insight into why a particular outcome is, or is not realized must be appreciated in the context of measures of treatment fidelity. Why? Without measures of treatment fidelity, 'it is possible to assume the intervention was ineffective when in fact it was simply not implemented' or not implemented as intended (Noell & Gansle, 2014, p. 389). This situation can lead to faulty conclusions that a potentially effective intervention is ineffective (Breitenstein et al., 2010). The reverse scenario is also possible: promoting an intervention that happens to be successful, that is not actually successful when implemented with acceptable fidelity. Such faulty conclusions can have negative flow-on effects for children with SSDs. Children can 1) miss out on receiving more effective interventions; 2) receive inefficient interventions when more efficient and effective options are possible; and 3) parents/carers and colleagues can be encouraged to use an intervention that should not be used when implemented according to the prototype. How can such faulty conclusions be avoided? One way is to engage in E^{3}BP.

How Does Treatment Fidelity Relate to E^{3}BP?

Treatment fidelity is integrally related to E^{3}BP. A lock-and-key metaphor illustrates this close relationship (Gansle & Noell, 2007). The lock is the type and severity of a child's SSD. The key is the specific intervention approach required to treat or unlock the SSD. Three aspects of the lock and key relationship are central to intervention success – intervention *fit*, intervention *strength*, and intervention *implementation* (Gansle & Noell, 2007).

Intervention Fit

Just as keys have critical cuts along the shaft that fit and open a lock, interventions comprising unique combinations of elements are necessarily the best possible fit for a child and their type of SSD. The elements of interventions for SSDs can be broadly categorized into four domains: goals (e.g., what will be targeted), teaching moment (e.g., how the goals will be targeted), the context (e.g., the service delivery model, resources, and activities that will be used to provide intervention), and procedural issues (e.g., the SLP/SLT training requirements required, and how the effect of intervention will be evaluated; Baker et al., 2018). Consideration of external empirical evidence (e.g., high quality peer reviewed published research) alongside the internal evidence (e.g., findings from a comprehensive assessment with a child and their family) can help to guide evidence-based decisions. By knowing the evidence, SLPs/SLTs can identify interventions most likely to 'unlock' a child's SSD. Comparison research highlights the importance of fitting interventions to SSDs. For example, in a comparison of minimal pairs therapy and core vocabulary, Crosbie et al. (2005) reported that minimal pairs therapy was suitable for children with consistent pattern-based errors or phonological impairment, whereas core vocabulary therapy was suitable for children with inconsistent speech disorder.

Intervention Strength

The selection of a suitable intervention does not however guarantee that a child's SSD can be 'unlocked'. The material the key is made of must also be considered – it must be strong enough to operate the locking mechanism (Gansle & Noell, 2007). In this context, the strength of a key is akin to the intensity of an intervention. Inadequate dose in a session, inadequate session frequency, and/or inadequate total duration of a robust empirically supported intervention can impact success (Williams, 2012). Just as a perfectly cut key made of rubber will not release a lock, inadequate intervention intensity will not change children's speech. Reviews of external empirical evidence (e.g., Sugden et al., 2018) can help to guide SLP's/SLT's decisions and plans for realizing an acceptable intensity for managing SSD in children.

Intervention Implementation

One final important step follows, to ensure that the lock is opened – the key needs to be used in the way it was intended. Even if an appropriate intervention is selected and plans are put in place to provide an optimal intensity, plans alone cannot 'unlock' SSDs in children. Intervention plans must be implemented, and the fidelity of implementation must be measured. Measurement is crucial for tracking a child's response to intervention, knowing if intervention was implemented as planned, and avoiding faulty conclusions.

The value of measuring treatment fidelity was evident in an evaluation of a randomized controlled trial of a computerized input-based intervention for children with phonological impairment (McLeod et al., 2017). McCormack et al. (2017, p. 265) reported that treatment fidelity for dose was poor: 'less than one-third of children received the prescribed number of days of intervention, while approximately one-half participated in the prescribed number of intervention plays [dose]'. While comprehensive statistical analyses of the speech outcomes for the subgroup of children who received the intervention as planned compared to the control group did not change the null finding (McLeod et al., 2017), the findings from McCormack et al. highlight the importance of not only measuring the outcome of intervention on children's speech, but the fidelity of implementation.

Strategies for Measuring Treatment Fidelity

It is necessary for strategies for measuring treatment fidelity to find a balance between detail and practicality (Noell & Gansle, 2014). One strategy is to use a checklist of the elements comprising an intervention (e.g., Hayden et al., 2015; Schlosser, 2002; Sugden et al., 2020). When an observation checklist is used, treatment fidelity is measured by the difference between intended treatment fidelity and achieved treatment fidelity (e.g., 27/30 elements present = 90% treatment fidelity and 10% treatment infidelity) (Kaderavek & Justice, 2010).

Given that self-completion of treatment fidelity checklists can be upwardly biased (Noell & Gansle, 2014), it is important to combine a self-completed checklist with another practical strategy. For example, a peer or supervisor could observe sessions randomly and complete the observation checklist, and/or a more experienced peer or clinician could conduct a post-session coaching session with the treating SLP/SLT about whether all elements were implemented and how they could optimise treatment fidelity (e.g., Schlosser, 2002).

Implementing a New (to the SLP/SLT) Intervention Approach

When learning how to implement faithfully an intervention approach for children with SSD (whether it be new to them or new to the profession), SLPs/SLTs could consider taking five steps (Figure A26.1).

First, determine if the key fits the lock. That is, determine if the intervention is a good fit for the type of SSD observed in a child or group of children. Also consider what you already know (or believe) about the intervention approach, and how you have measured fidelity of implementation for other intervention approaches.

Step 1.
What is your goal?

e.g., Implement a named intervention for children with severe phonological impairment with 90% fidelity within 2-months.

- Identify an intervention approach you would like to learn or revise, and reflect on what you already know or believe about the approach.
- Ensure that the intervention is suitable or fits the SSD for a child or children on your caseload.
- Describe your current strategies for measuring treatment fidelity, and note your current fidelity of implementation for other SSD intervention approaches.
- Identify factors (both internal and external) that will drive your behaviour towards your goal.

Step 2. Prepare

Create a list of continuing education activities, personnel, and resources that could help you learn the approach.

- Read the evidence about the intervention approach.
- Observe another clinician implement the approach, attend continuing education events, join an evidence-based practice network, attend case discussion meetings with colleauges, and participate in online forums.
- Consider answering Baker and Williams' (2021) 20-questions to consider when learning a new intervention approach.
- Use journal articles and books, in addition to reputable websites, clinicians, and therapy resources.

Step 3. Implement

Trial implementation of the intervention approach.

- Select a client who has the type of SSD that closely fits the intervention approach.
- Develop an implementation plan and collect data on fidelity of implementation (e.g., self- and peer-completed checklist of intervention elements; interview with colleague), and collect data on the outcome of intervention.

Step 4. Evaluate

Evaluate the clinical outcomes and treatment fidelity

- Determine your % fidelity, and reflect on implementation--did you achieve your goal?
- Compare fidelity and outcome data with data on the client experience (i.e., patient-reported experience measures [PREMS])
- If fidelity is acceptable and good outcomes are achieved, move to Step 5.
- If fidelity and/or outcomes need to improve, repeat steps 2 and/or 3, and identify barriers to and enablers of effective implementation.

Step 5. Sustain

Determine how you will sustain acceptable fidelity with all clients

- Create workplace strategies to ensure treatment fidelity with all clients is sustained.
- Set up journal alerts on the named intervention approach, so that when anything is published, you can add further depth to your understanding and implementation of the approach.
- Continue to engage in continuing education activities on the evidence-based management of SSD in children.

Figure A26.1 Steps for achieving acceptable treatment fidelity when implementing interventions for children with speech sound disorders. (Adapted from Baker & Williams, 2021).

Second, preparations are necessary to learn the intervention approach (e.g., the underlying theoretical principles driving target selection, cues used in teaching moments, procedures, and service delivery) (Baker et al., 2018). Depending on the SLP's/SLT's knowledge and prior experience, this step may take some time. The time required for learning can also depend on the element concentration (number of elements), flexibility (proportion of elements that are required versus optional), and distinctiveness (proportion of rare and omitted common elements relative to sum of the elements) within the intervention approach (Baker et al., 2018). With respect to element type, it is also important to appreciate that some elements may be easy to learn and implement with acceptable fidelity whereas others may require more knowledge, skill, and/or practice (Baker et al., 2020). At this step, student, CFY or new graduate SLPs/SLTs may also need to factor in

(a) learning practical strategies such as how to engage, motivate, and encourage children during intervention sessions, (b) gathering practical resources for implementation, and (c) developing organizational skills to multitask during intervention sessions (e.g., keeping children engaged while ensuring an optimal session pace, collecting relevant data, and adhering to or adjusting the session plan considering children's responses).

The third step involves trial implementation. At this point the SLP/SLT wants to have strategies in place to measure the treatment fidelity such as a self- and peer-completed checklist of the elements comprising the intervention. The fourth step entails a focus on evaluating intervention fidelity, intervention outcomes, and the client experience. Depending on the findings, the SLP/SLT may decide to revise steps 2 and 3 until they achieve an acceptable level of fidelity. Sugden et al. (2020) provide an example of SLP/SLT and parent/caregiver fidelity of implementation for Williams (2000) multiple oppositions intervention. Hayden et al. (2015) specify guidelines for measuring treatment fidelity of PROMPT. Having achieved acceptable fidelity, the fifth and final step involves putting strategies in place to ensure that acceptable fidelity is sustained, and optimal outcomes are achieved with all clients.

Reason-based Practice and Data, and Research Dissemination

> ... the CSD discipline will need to recognize that there may not always be applicable and sufficient external scientific evidence for SLPs. In these cases, SLPs will need to be trained to use reason-based practice and data that they collect from their individual clients to make informed clinical decisions. SLPs can monitor client progress and validate treatments for individual clients until other sources are available. Also, it is important that the field consider other dissemination strategies, as peer-reviewed journal articles are typically written with other scientists in mind and not clinicians (Harold, 2019).
>
> Fulcher-Rood et al., 2020, p. 701

The authors of the fifth and final quotation, Fulcher-Rood et al. (2020) point their readers to Harold (2019), a free article in the *ASHA Leader*. It is a thoughtful piece that comes with a provocative subtitle, and a line that jumped out at me: *Clinicians desperately want research that is well-aligned with clinical reality. But what they perhaps don't realize is—scientists desperately want this, too!*

Fulcher-Rood and colleagues also encourage alternative vehicles for research dissemination that are more clinician-friendly. One avenue, already tapped, is blogging and microblogging via social media platforms, and website construction software. These are briefly discussed in Chapter 11 and include Blogspot (e.g., blogs by Dorothy Bishop, Sharynne McLeod, and Pamela Snow), Joomla (e.g., my website), Linkedin, SlideShare, and Wordpress (e.g., ResNetSLT led by Hazel Roddam, and Susan Rvachew's blog).

References

Apel, K. (1999). Checks and balances: Keeping the science in our profession. *Language, Speech, and Hearing Services in Schools, 30*(1), 98–107. https://doi.org/10.1044/0161-1461.3001.98

Apel, K. (2009). Can clinicians be scientists? *Language, Speech, and Hearing Services in Schools*, *40*(1), 3–4. https://doi.org/10.1044/0161-1461(2009/ed-01)

Baker, E. (2010). The experience of discharging children from phonological intervention. *International Journal of Speech-language Pathology*, *12*(4), 325–332. https://doi.org/10.3109/17549507.2010.488326

Baker, E., Masso, S., Huynh, K., & Sugden, E. (2022). Optimizing outcomes for children with phonological impairment: A systematic search and review of outcome and experience measures reported in intervention research. *Language, Speech, and Hearing Services in Schools*, *53*(3), 732–748. https://doi.org/10.1044/2022_LSHSS-21-00132

Baker, E., McCauley, R. J., Williams, A. L., & McLeod, S. (2020). Elements in phonological intervention: A comparison of three approaches using the phonological intervention taxonomy. In E. Babatsouli & M. J. Ball (Eds.), *On under-reported monolingual child phonology* (pp. 375–399). Multilingual Matters.

Baker, E., & Williams, A. L. (2021). Implementing interventions. In A. L. Williams, S. McLeod, & R. J. McCauley (Eds.), *Interventions for speech sound disorders in children* (2nd ed., pp. 23–31). Paul. H. Brookes Publishing.

Baker, E., Williams, A. L., McLeod, S., & McCauley, R. (2018). Elements of phonological interventions for children with speech sound disorders: The development of a taxonomy. *American Journal of Speech Language Pathology*, *27*(3), 906–935. https://doi.org/10.1044/2018_ajslp-17-0127

Breitenstein, S. M., Gross, D., Garvey, C. A., Hill, C., Fogg, L., & Resnick, B. (2010). Implementation fidelity in community-based interventions. *Research in Nursing & Health*, *33*(2), 164–173. https://doi.org/10.1002/nur.20373

Carrigg, B., Baker, E., Parry, L., & Ballard, K. (2015). Persistent speech sound disorder in a 22-year-old male: Communication, educational, socio-emotional, and vocational outcomes. *Perspectives of the ASHA Special Interest Groups*, *16*(2), 37–49. https://doi.org/10.1044/sbi16.2.37

Clark, H. M. (2003). Neuromuscular treatments for speech and swallowing: A tutorial. *American Journal of Speech-Language Pathology*, *12*(4), 400–415. https://doi.org/10.1044/1058-0360(2003/086)

Crosbie, S., Holm, A., & Dodd, B. (2005). Intervention for children with severe speech disorder: A comparison of two approaches. *International Journal of Language & Communication Disorders*, *40*(4), 467–491. https://doi.org/10.1080/13682820500126049

Davidson, M. M., Alonzo, C. N., Barton-Hulsey, A., Binger, C., Bridges, M., Caron, J., Douglas, N. F., Fuererstein, J. L., Olswang, L., Oshita, J. Y., Schliep, M. E., Quinn, E., & Morris, M. A. (2022). Prologue: Implementation science in CSD and starting where you are. *American Journal of Speech-Language Pathology*, *31*(3), 1023–1025. https://doi.org/10.1044/2022_AJSLP-22-00009

Davidson, M. M., & Morris, M. M. (2022). Epilogue: Implementation science in CSD and starting where you are. *American Journal of Speech-Language Pathology*, *31*(3), 1179–1187. https://doi.org/10.1044/2022_AJSLP-22-00010

De Thorne, L. S., Johnson, C. J., Walder, L., & Mahurin-Smith, J. (2009). When 'Simon Says' doesn't work: Alternative to imitation for facilitating early speech development. *American Journal of Speech-Language Pathology*, *18*(2), 133–145. https://doi.org/10.1044/1058-0360(2008/07-0090)

Donohue, C., Carnaby, G., & Garand, K. L. F. (2022). How to interpret and evaluate a meta-analysis in the field of speech-language pathology: A tutorial for clinicians. *American Journal of Speech-Language Pathology*, *31*(2), 664–677. https://doi.org/10.1044/2021_AJSLP-21-00267

Donohue, C., Carnaby, G., & Garand, K. L. F. (2023). A clinician's guide to critically appraising randomized controlled trials in the field of speech-language pathology. *American Journal of Speech-Language Pathology*, *32*(2), 411–425. https://doi.org/10.1044/2022_AJSLP-22-00180

Dodd, B. (2007). Evidence-based practice and speech-language pathology: Strengths, weaknesses, opportunities and threats. *Folia Phoniatrica et Logopaedica*, *59*(3), 118–129. https://doi.org/10.1159/000101770

Douglas, N. F., & Burshnic, V. L. (2019). Implementation science: Tackling the research to practice gap in communication sciences and disorders. *Perspectives of the ASHA Special Interest Groups*, *4*(1), 3–7. https://doi.org/10.1044/2018_PERS-ST-2018-0000

Douglas, N. F., Feuerstein, J. L., Oshita, J. Y., Schliep, M. E., & Danowski, M. L. (2022). Implementation science research in communication sciences and disorders: A scoping review. *American Journal of*

Speech-Language Pathology, 31(3), 1054–1083. https://doi.org/10.1044/2021_AJSLP-21-00126

Finestack, L. H., & Betz, S. K. (2021). Professional issues: A view from history. In M. W. Hudson & M. DeRuiter, *Professional Issues in Speech-Language Pathology and Audiology* (5th ed., pp. 165–183). Plural Publishing.

Finestack, L. H., & Fey, M. E. (2017). Translation and implementation research in the development of evidence-based child language intervention. In R. G. Schwartz (Ed.), *Handbook of child language disorders* (2nd ed.). Psychology Press.

Fixsen, D. L., Van Dyke, M., & Blasé, K. A. (2019). *Science and implementation.* Active Implementation Research Network.

Fulcher-Rood, K., Castilla-Earls, A., & Higginbotham, J. (2020). What does evidence-based practice mean to you? A follow-up study examining school-based speech-language pathologists' perspectives on evidence-based practice. *American Journal of Speech-Language Pathology, 29*(2), 688–704. https://doi.org/10.1044/2019_AJSLP-19-00171

Gallagher, A., Murphy, C. A., Fitzgerald, J., & Law, J. (2022). Addressing implementation considerations when developing universal interventions for speech, language and communication needs in the ordinary classroom: A protocol for a scoping review. *HRB Open Research, 4*(41), 1–21. https://doi.org/10.12688/hrbopenres.13249.1

Gansle, K. A., & Noell, G. H. (2007). The fundamental role of intervention implementation in assessing response to intervention. In S. R. Jimerson, M. K. Burns, & A. M. VanDerHeyden (Eds.), *Handbook of response to intervention: The science and practice of assessment and intervention* (pp. 244–251). Springer US. https://doi.org/10.1007/978-0-387-49053-3_18

Glasgow, R. E., Vinson, C., Chambers, D., Khoury, M. J., Kaplan, R. M., & Hunter, C. (2012). National institutes of health approaches to dissemination and implementation science: Current and future directions. *American Journal of Public Health, 102*(7), 1274–1281. https://doi.org/10.2105/AJPH.2012.300755

Greenhalgh, T. (2019). *How to read a paper: The basics of evidence-based medicine and healthcare* (6th ed.). Wiley-Blackwell.

Greenwell, T., & Walsh, B. (2021). Evidence-based practice in speech-language pathology: Where are we now? *American Journal of Speech-Language Pathology, 30*(1), 186–198. https://doi.org/10.1044/2020_AJSLP-20-00194

Harold, M. P. (2019). The research translation problem: A modest proposal: Enough with the EBP blame game. Effectively putting research into practice requires empathy from all those involved. *ASHA Leader, 24*(7), 52–61. http://dx.doi.org/10.1044/leader.FTR2.24072019.52

Hayden, D., Namasivayam, A. K., & Ward, R. (2015). The assessment of fidelity in a motor speech-treatment approach. *Speech, Language and Hearing, 18*(1), 30–38. https://doi.org/10.1179/2050572814Y.0000000046

Hersh, D. (2010). I can't sleep at night with discharging this lady: The personal impact of ending therapy on speech-language pathologists. *International Journal of Speech-Language Pathology, 12*(4), 283–291. https://doi.org/10.3109/17549501003721072

Jasso, J., & Potratz, J. R. (2020). Assessing speech sound disorders in school-age children from diverse language backgrounds: A tutorial with three case studies. *Perspectives of the ASHA Special Interest Groups, 5*(3), 714–725. https://doi.org/10.1044/2020_PERSP-19-00151

Kaderavek, J. N., & Justice, L. M. (2010). Fidelity: An essential component of evidence-based practice in speech-language pathology. *American Journal of Speech-Language Pathology, 19*(4), 369–379. https://doi.org/10.1044/1058-0360(2010/09-0097)

Krueger, B. I. (2019). Eligibility and speech sound disorders: Assessment of social impact. *Perspectives of the ASHA Special Interest Groups, 4*(1), 85–90. https://doi.org/10.1044/2018_PERS-SIG1-2018-0016

Ludemann, A., Power, E., & Hoffmann, T. C. (2017). Investigating the adequacy of intervention descriptions in recent speech-language pathology literature: Is evidence from randomized trials useable? *American Journal of Speech-Language Pathology, 26*(2), 443–455. https://doi.org/10.1044/2016_AJSLP-16-0035

McCormack, J., Baker, E., Masso, S., Crowe, K., McLeod, S., Wren, Y., & Roulstone, S. (2017). Implementation fidelity of a computer-assisted intervention for children with speech sound disorders. *International Journal of Speech-Language Pathology, 19*(3), 265–276. https://doi.org/10.1080/17549507.2017.1293160

McCormack, J., McLeod, S., Harrison, L. J., & Holliday, E. L. (2022). Drawing talking: Listening to children with speech sound disorders. *Language, Speech, and Hearing Services in Schools*, *53*(3), 713–731. https://doi.org/10.1044/2021_LSHSS-21-00140

McLeod, S., Baker, E., McCormack, J., Wren, Y., Roulstone, S., Crowe, K., Masso, S., White, P., & Howland, C. (2017). Cluster-randomized controlled trial evaluating the effectiveness of computer-assisted intervention delivered by educators for children with speech sound disorders. *Journal of Speech, Language, and Hearing Research*, *60*(7), 1891–1910. https://doi.org/10.1044/2017_JSLHR-S-16-0385

Nicoll, A., Maxwell, M., & Williams, B. (2021). Achieving 'coherence' in routine practice: A qualitative case-based study to describe speech and language therapy interventions with implementation in mind. *Implementation Science Communications*, *2*(1), 56. https://doi.org/10.1186/s43058-021-00159-0

Noell, G. H., & Gansle, K. A. (2014). Research examining the relationships between consultation procedures, treatment integrity, and outcomes. In W. P. Erchul & S. M. Sheridan (Eds.), *Handbook of research in school consultation* (2nd ed., pp. 386–408). Routledge.

Olswang, L. B., & Prelock, P. A. (2015). Bridging the gap between research and practice: Implementation science. *Journal of Speech, Language, and Hearing Research*, *58*(6), S1818–S1826. https://doi.org/10.1044/2015_JSLHR-L-14-0305

Roberts, M. Y., Sone, B. J., Zanzinger, K. E., Bloem, M. E., Kulba, K., Schaff, A., Davis, K. C., Reisfeld, N., & Goldstein, H. (2020). Trends in clinical practice research in ASHA journals: 2008-2018. *American Journal of Speech-Language Pathology*, *29*(3), 1629–1639. https://doi.org/10.1044/2020_AJSLP-19-00011

Schleif, E. P., Mason, K., & Perry, J. L. (2021). English-only treatment of compensatory speech errors in a bilingual adoptee with repaired cleft palate: A descriptive case study. *American Journal of Speech-Language Pathology*, *30*(3), 993–1007. https://doi.org/10.1044

Schlosser, R. W. (2002). On the importance of being earnest about treatment integrity. *Augmentative and Alternative Communication*, *18*(1), 36–44. https://doi.org/10.1080/aac.18.1.36.44

Secord, W., Boyce, S. E., Donohue, J. S., Fox, F. A., & Shine, S. E. (2007). *Eliciting sounds: Techniques and strategies for clinicians* (2nd ed.). Thomson Delmar Learning.

Sugden, E., Baker, E., Munro, N., Williams, A. L., & Trivette, C. M. (2018). Service delivery and intervention intensity for phonology-based speech sound disorders. *International Journal of Language & Communication Disorders*, *53*(4), 718–734. https://doi.org/10.1111/1460-6984.12399

Sugden, E., Baker, E., Williams, A. L., Munro, N., & Trivette, C. M. (2020). Evaluation of parent- and speech-language pathologist delivered multiple oppositions intervention for children with phonological impairment: A multiple-baseline design study. *American Journal of Speech-Language Pathology*, *29*(1), 111–126. https://doi.org/10.1044/2019_AJSLP-18-0248

Thome, E. K., Loveall, S. J., & Henderson, D. E. (2020). A survey of speech-language pathologists' understanding and reported use of evidence-based practice. *Perspectives of the ASHA Special Interest Groups*, *5*(4), 984–999. https://doi.org/10.1044/2020_PERSP-20-00008

Topbaş, S., & Ünal, O. (2010). An alternating treatment comparison of minimal and maximal opposition sound selection in Turkish phonological disorders. *Clinical Linguistics & Phonetics*, *24*(8), 646–668. https://doi.org/10.3109/02699206.2010.486464

Utianski, R. L., Spencer, T. D., & Wallace, S. E. (2022). Clinical impact requires clinical practice research. *Perspectives of the ASHA Special Interest Groups*, *7*(2), 651–662. https://doi.org/10.1044/2021_PERSP-21-00197

Verkerk, E. W., Tanke, M. A. C., Kool, R. B., van Dulmen, S. A., & Westert, G. P. (2018). Limit, lean or listen? A typology of low-value care that gives direction in de-implementation. *International Journal for Quality in Health Care*, *30*(9), 736–739. https://doi.org/10.1093/intqhc/mzy100

Williams, A. L. (2000). Multiple oppositions: Theoretical foundations for an alternative contrast intervention approach. *American Journal of Speech-Language Pathology*, *9*(4), 282–288. https://doi.org/10.1044/1058-0360.0904.282

Williams, A. L. (2012). Intensity in phonological intervention: Is there a prescribed amount? *International*

Journal of Speech-Language Pathology, *14*(5), 456–461. https://doi.org/10.3109/17549507.2012.6 88866

Williams, A. L., McLeod, S., & McCauley, R. (2021). *Interventions for speech sound disorders in children* (2nd ed.). Paul H. Brookes Publishing.

Williams, N. J., & Beidas, R. S. (2019). Annual research review: The state of implementation science in child psychology and psychiatry: A review and suggestions to advance the field. *Journal of Child Psychology and Psychiatry*, *60*(4), 430–450. https://doi.org/10.1111/jcpp.12960

Chapter 7
Phonological Disorders and CAS
Characteristics, Goals, and Intervention

Chapter 7 is about the dynamic assessment, differential diagnosis, and treatment of children with:

1. Moderate and severe phonological disorder.
2. Childhood apraxia of speech (CAS).
3. Suspected CAS (sCAS).
4. Cooccurring SSDs.

It comprises suggestions and discussion around intervention goals, and intervention approaches, procedures, techniques, and activities for these groups. The first topic builds on the proposition that phonological disorder and CAS have at least six inter-related characteristics in common (Velleman, 2005a) and that, in everyday practice, we find ourselves treating symptomatically, while still taking the primary diagnosis into account. In that sense, we 'treat the symptoms, not the label'.

Treat the Symptoms, Not the Label

As a motor speech disorder, CAS is a discrete diagnostic subtype of childhood SSD. There is a conservative consensus view that CAS is best characterized as a symptom complex, and not as a unitary disorder nor as a syndrome. It is also largely agreed that it may affect, to varying degrees, some combination of non-speech motor behaviours; speech motor behaviours; production of speech sounds (consonants, clusters, and vowels) and structures (word and syllable shapes); moving from sound-to-sound, and from syllable-to-syllable within words; prosody (the suprasegmentals of intonation, loudness, syllable and word stress, rate, resonance, and rhythm); language; metalinguistic/phonemic awareness; and literacy (ASHA, 2007b).

In 1997, Shriberg et al. determined that, whereas late speech onset and slow speech development were usual in CAS, neither a typical phonological developmental pathway nor a distinguishing phonological profile for children with sCAS had been found, and CAS itself had no phonological features that are uniquely its own (see, Maassen, 2002 for discussion). The 1997 finding stands, so it follows that many 'CAS characteristics' appear in other subtypes of SSD. As Velleman and Strand (1994) said, these commonalities, *'may result in a variety of motor, phonologic, linguistic or neurologic signs or*

Children's Speech Sound Disorders, Third Edition. Caroline Bowen.
© 2023 John Wiley & Sons Ltd. Published 2023 by John Wiley & Sons Ltd.

symptoms and in fact inconsistency among symptoms may be expected as typical'. If that were not sufficiently complicated, CAS and phonological disorder can occur in the same child.

Intervention for SSD, therefore, is informed by the overlap of symptoms, and the overlap of treatment methodologies, for children with CAS, children with phonological disorder, and children with articulation disorder. In keeping with this view, a common-sense (to some) symptomatic approach to treatment has emerged. Contemplating this development, Velleman wrote:

> *CAS is different from "regular" phonological disorders, but there are still patterns to be found and treated. There is a great deal of overlap in the symptoms of CAS and the symptoms of other phonological disorders, so it is often difficult to decide whether a diagnosis of CAS is appropri-*

> *ate. But, in a sense, that does not matter. Treat the symptoms, not the label.*
>
> (Velleman, 2005a, p. 3)

But, in an area that enjoys its spirited controversies, this idea does not appeal to all!

Testing for the Six, Interrelated, Common Characteristics

The left-hand column of Box 7.1 contains the 6 characteristics, or 'symptoms' in medical model parlance, of phonological disorder, and then 4 diagnostic signs, with corresponding cells on the right containing the tests that might be used to test for them. Similarly, in Box 7.2, the characteristics of CAS, and suggested tests are shown.

Box 7.1   Testing for phonological disorder: 6 Characteristics (Grunwell, 1989) and 4 Signs

Characteristics	Tests employed in examining for Phonological Disorder
1. Static speech sound system	TEST: Relational Analysis. Look for stable PCC and stable percentage of occurrence of processes over time (6–12 weeks should do).
2. Variability without gradual improvement	TEST: Inconsistency Assessment: what *kind* of inconsistency? The DEAP Inconsistency Assessment uses single words; it is important *also* to observe connected speech if possible.
3. Persisting phonological processes	TEST: Relational Analysis. Identify phonological processes/patterns that 'should have been' eliminated in terms of normative expectations.
4. Chronological Mismatch	TEST: Study inventories for later sounds and absent earlier sounds.
5. Idiosyncratic rules	TEST: Relational Analysis—look for atypical patterns.
6. Restricted use of contrast	TEST: Contrastive Assessment; Phoneme Collapses.
Four Diagnostic Signs 7. Puzzle phenomenon	TEST: Look at phonetic mastery relative to phonemic organization.
8. Unusual errors	TEST: Observations of Conversational Speech if possible. Look for unusual error-types and systematic sound preference, including the child's 'favourite sound'; 'favourite place'; 'favourite manner' of articulation.
9. Marking	TEST: Look for marking with *nasality* and marking with *vowel length*.
10. Relatively ready stimulability cf. CAS	TEST: Stimulability testing to 2 syllable positions.

Box 7.2   Testing for childhood apraxia of speech

Characteristics	Tests employed in examining for CAS
	NOTE: Use the DEMSS (Strand & McCauley, 2019a, 2019b) with very young children with low volubility and for children with severe CAS/sCAS (Strand, A31)
Receptive-expressive gap	Administer any language test procedure(s) the child can manage. Formal testing may not be possible for some children (because it is too difficult for them).
Delayed syllable / word structure development	Use a process analysis (e.g., DEAP (Dodd et al., 2002), HAPP-3 Hodson, 2004), The Quick Screener (Bowen, 1996) and/or a Conversation Sample. Look for syllable structure processes, phonotactic constraints.
Deviant syllable structures and deviant word structures	Use DEAP, HAPP-3, Quick Screener, and/or a Process Analysis of a Speech Sample. Look for deviant syllable structure errors, especially Initial Consonant Deletion, schwa insertion/addition (e.g., [ˌbəˈluː ˈkeɪˌpə] for *blue cape*) and replacing a consonant with a diphthong.
Sequencing difficulties	Use motor speech examination: DEMSS (Strand & McCauley, 2019a, 2019b); Clinically Useful Words (James, 2006 and Figure 7.1); DEAP; Nuffield Centre Dyspraxia Programme (NDP-3) assessment (P. Williams & Stephens, 2004); or make informal observations of 'long words' of >2 syllables. Families often recount the long words and tricky word combinations their child often has difficulty sequencing. Look for metathesis (pasketti), word reversals (mat door), and unusual sequencing: muesli →yoomsli / yoombleese; Open it up. → Open up it.
Word stress errors; syllable stress errors; EES	Look for excessive and/or equal stress (EES) and Weak Syllable Deletion. Make a syllable stress patterns inventory. Consider an informal long words task. Note that there is evidence that EES does not occur in French speaking children with CAS (Brosseau-Lapré & Rvachew, 2017; Rvachew & Matthews, 2017), and emerging evidence that this is also true for Hebrew (Segal et al., 2022).
Vowel constraints; vowel deviations.	Look for vowel replacements that do not match adult targets. List vowel inventory/constraints; calculate Percentage of Vowels Correct if applicable. Do vowels 'wander'? The Quick Vowel Screener (Bowen, 2010a, 2010b) is available free.
Prosodic differences	Use the SCRF (Skinder-Meredith, A28). Does prosody affect intelligibility?
PA difficulties	Use Phonological Awareness Tests. Note rhyme and syllable awareness, blending.

Pause Marker (PM); Pause Marker Index (PMI)
The PM is a behavioural marker for CAS (Shriberg et al., 2017a, 2017b, 2017c, 2017d, 2017e). A PM score is the percentage of occurrence of 4 types of inappropriate between-words pauses in a continuous speech (CS) sample. A PM score is calculated by dividing the number of such pauses by the number of between-words pause opportunities. A PM score <94% from a speaker of any age meets the criterion for CAS. The PM is criterion-referenced, not norm-referenced. The PMI, which is a severity scale for CAS that divides PM scores into classifications of mild, mild-moderate, moderate-severe, and severe, is proposed as a useful research and clinical measure. The PM is any pause between words for a period of at least 150 milliseconds in which there is no speech. An inappropriate pause is 'a between-words pause that occurs either at an inappropriate linguistic place in CS and/or has one or more inappropriate articulatory, prosodic, or vocalic features within the pause or in a sound segment preceding or following the pause' (Tilkens et al., 2017, p. 5).

(Continued)

Box 7.2   (Continued)

There are four Pause-Type-1 types, as follows:
1. **ABRUPT** A pause immediately preceded or followed by a phoneme that includes a sudden strong onset of energy or sudden offset of energy. Steep-amplitude rise/fall time is the best current visual and acoustic correlate of the percept of an abrupt phoneme.
2. **ALONE** A pause that occurs at a linguistically incorrect position in an utterance, is not one of the other seven subtypes of inappropriate pauses and does not have any identifiable auditory or acoustic feature.
3. **CHANGE** A pause immediately preceded or followed by a phoneme or word that includes a significant change in amplitude, frequency, or rate.
4. **GROPE** A pause that includes visible acoustic energy in the spectrogram consistent with a lip or tongue gesture or inappropriate voicing. The gestures may include formant traces of sounds or traces of incompletely realized stop bursts.

A CAS Assessment Prompt for the Case History Interview

Box 7.3 contains reminder notes for clinicians of areas they may wish to explore in case history interviews when they suspect that a child has CAS. This 'assessment prompt' was developed over my many years of clinical practice. If provided to parents before their interview it often served to guide discussion, acting as a reminder to parents of the questions *they* wanted to ask. It is not intended as a questionnaire, but rather as a general indication of the territory to be covered in the conduct of the initial assessment and working towards a provisional diagnosis or diagnosis.

Notes for Selected Points in Box 7.3

Point 2 Development: Feeding

CAS is a *speech* diagnosis. Early feeding difficulties and fussy, picky eating are not considered to be warning signs or red flags. Involuntary motor control for chewing and swallowing is typically unimpaired unless there is an oral apraxia (E. Strand & McCauley, 1999). So, the following issues are not implicated in CAS: dysphagia; trouble latching and sucking; fighting the breast; needing input from a lactation consultant; problems drinking from a cup and/or learn to chew and swallow solids; holding food in the mouth ('mouth stuffing'), slow feeding, and quirky or conservative food tastes; excessive gag reflex, vomiting, and reflux; and failure to thrive.

Although it does not help CAS diagnosis, there *are* reasons to ask about feeding:

- In history taking, SLPs/SLTs routinely ask about developmental milestones—including feeding—to rule dysphagia in or out and gain an overall picture of the whole child in the context of his or her family and wider communicative milieu.
- Potentially, a feeding history provides insight into the mother-child relationship, and more broadly, family relationships. For example, some parents will describe an idyllic, happy period characterized by textbook progress. At the other extreme, some may remember the first few months of the baby's life as a battleground of interminable feeds, continual fretting, crying, disturbed sleep, reflux, vomiting, and failure to thrive; worrying visits to the well-baby clinic, child and family health centre, or paediatrician; unhelpful advice from family and peers, and excruciating parental tiredness. Sometimes there are added burdens of ill health (e.g., maternal mastitis) and degrees of postpartum depression and/or postpartum anxiety in either or both parents, noting that postnatal depression affects 8–10 percent of fathers.
- Discussing a challenging start can offer a natural lead-in to exploring relationships then, and now, with gentle questioning. For example, *'That sounds like a stormy start: did it take a while for you two to form a relationship? How do you get along these days?'* or *'That must have been hard, with you and [child's name] constantly pulling in different directions. Did things improve, or is behaviour still an issue?'*

Box 7.3   A 10-point CAS Assessment Prompt

Procedures and observations will vary with the child's age and stage; there is overlap between the 10 sections, and not every section will be needed for every child.

1. Hearing	Audiology report		Hearing History
2. Development	**Perinatal History** **Milestones** **Motor development**	**Cognition** Psychometric / Paediatric report	**Social Development** Wants to communicate; solitary; aloof; 'separation issues'; clingy, why? Play: who with? Nature of play? Persistent personality? Reactive personality?
	Feeding Latching issues, fighting the breast, sucking, lactation consultant, other intervention re: feeding (and/or sleep pattern), drinking from cup, chewing, gag reflex, vomiting, reflux, failure to thrive, holding food in the mouth, breast or bottle, diet, mouth as a sensor, mouth stuffing, variety of foods.	**Health/Wellbeing** Illnesses, 'always at the doctor's', accidents, injuries, ear infections, seizures, 'separation', hospital, operations, tires easily, sleep pattern; always 'on the go'.	**Intelligibility** Ask parents: can you put a percentage on it? Who understands? Does another child 'interpret'? Does the other child make mistakes in interpreting? Does the child's intelligibility vary? Worse when tired? Worse / better in certain situations? Worse with longer utterances? Uses signs or actions to help get the message across. Aware?
	Babble Quiet baby, no or late babbling; lots of babbling, lots of vocal play; all sounded the same (undifferentiated babbling); few or no consonants in babbled utterances; 'babble' mainly squeals and grunts (i.e., not true babbling). (Overby, A27) **Imitation** Tries hard to imitate all the time; little attempt to imitate sounds or words; disinterested in imitating words; refusal to imitate words; becomes upset or passive if asked to do so. Does/does not imitate play.	**Sounds/Words** Can say words that are not used in everyday speech. How many intelligible words; how many approximations; first words (when?), low vocabulary for age (parents' judgement), comparison with other children in the family and/or age-peers; one word for many meanings ('big' for all machines / vehicles). Only says words at home. Won't attempt certain words. Can't say own name. Play is very silent.	**Gesture/Grunts** Uses gesture instead of words (nods for 'yes', shakes head for 'no'). Grizzles, squeals, or uses vowels, grunts and 'urgent noises' to gain attention or request an object or action instead. **Frustration** Frustrated when not understood (or passive, or unhappy), or 'resigned' or 'adjusted' to not being a talker?
	Losing Sounds/Words Says a sound or word and it is never heard again; keeps a sound or word for a while then 'loses' it; sounds and words come and go. **Groping/Struggle** Mouthing words? Silent posturing? Articulatory struggle?	**Comprehension** 'Understands everything' / 'very bright': essential to test receptive skills, parent report may be positive, but testing tells you about co-operation and attention, possibly revealing subtle deficits in comprehension. Such findings come as a shock to parents–don't assume they already 'know'. Is the leveloof comprehension higher than output suggests (receptive-expressive gap)?	**Theories? History?** What brought you here? Ask parents, what they think the problem might be, (or what it might be 'called'). Have you wondered about a 'label', searched the web, joined an email list or discussion group, subscribed to a blog or group in social media, received advice or 'suggestions' from family, friends, online gurus, and others? Have you thought about family history?

(Continued)

Box 7.3   (Continued)

3. Language
Ask parents; Formal tests

4. Cognition
Ask parents; Formal tests

5. PA / Literacy
Ask parents. Formal tests. Story time? Consider offering ONE piece of advice during the initial consultation.

6. Neuromuscular Examination	Gait	Sensory Function
	Posture (sitting / W-sitting?)	Involuntary movements
	Muscle Tone	(if yes, query dysarthria)
	Coordination	Physiotherapist or OT reports?
	Reflexes	

7. Motor Speech Examination
DEMSS (Strand, A31 and see, Box 7.5)

8. Speech and non-speech characteristics
There is general agreement between Davis et al. (1998) and ASHA (2007)

Non-speech characteristics (Davis et al., 1998)
1. Impaired volitional oral movements
2. Reduced expressive compared to receptive language skills (receptive-expressive gap)
3. Reduced diadochokinetic rates

Speech characteristics (Davis et al., 1998)

1. Limited consonant repertoire 2. Limited vowel repertoire 3. Frequent omissions 4. High incidence of vowel errors 5. Inconsistent articulation errors 6. Altered suprasegmentals (prosody) 7. More errors occur as output becomes longer and /or more complex 8. Difficulty in imitation (groping or refusal) 9. Use of simple, but not complex, syllable shapes	Three core features of CAS (ASHA, 2007) **SEGMENTAL** Sound production inconsistency **STRUCTURAL** Difficulty with transition between syllables **SUPRASEGMENTAL** Inconsistent realization of Lexical stress/ Prosody; nasality

9. Speech Assessment
Standardised Articulation and Phonology Test if possible
Independent and Relational Analysis (Stoel-Gammon, A7)
Inconsistency Assessment (see Rvachew A9 for discussion, and Table 5.1 and related text)
Compare Single Word PCC and PVC with Conversational Speech PCC and PVC
Intelligibility Ratings (SLP/SLT, Parent(s), Familiar Listener e.g., Preschool Teacher, Unfamiliar Listener)
1: completely intelligible in conversation
2: mostly intelligible in conversation
3: somewhat intelligible in conversation
4: mostly unintelligible in conversation
5: completely unintelligible in conversation
NOTE: Subjective intelligibility ratings are unreliable, but potentially informative clinically
Use CS sample for MLUm and Structural Analysis if formal language testing is not possible
Look for silent posturing / groping
Is the prosodic contour of utterances / sentences intact on imitation?
Contrastive stress (I **WANT** one / I want **ONE** / **I** want one)
Rule dysarthria component out or in (may not be possible with children with few words)
Rule phonological component out or in (not possible with children with few words)

10. Speech Characteristics Rating
SCRF (Skinder-Meredith, A28, and see the Speech Characteristics Rating Form in Table A28.1)

- Eventually, the SLP/SLT will want the child to practice between sessions. Insights into parent-child relationships will guide home practice goals, and how homework is introduced, structured, and implemented. If a parent portrays unmanageable, acting-out, or unhappy behaviour in situations that require cooperation, then how to 'get homework happening' must be openly discussed, and referral for professional counselling or family therapy considered if necessary (Bitter, A13).

Point 2 Development: Refusal to imitate/Upset, Passive, or Sad when asked to Imitate

As with 'losing words', and groping/struggle discussed below, parents may worry greatly if their child with sCAS or CAS doggedly refuses to imitate an adult model or becomes upset, passive, or quietly sad when asked to do so.

This presents an opportunity for the SLP/SLT to positively connote the child's behaviour, in the child's hearing, treading carefully, with something along the lines of, *'How about that!* [Child's Name] *is so smart knowing exactly the things that are hard to do. Copying mouth shapes and words can be very tricky'.* Addressing the child, *'You figured that out all by yourself, didn't you? Clever you'.'* And then, *'But you know what? You don't have to do it on your own. Do you know what I do in my job? I help children make the tricky words into easy words. Children make my job easier if they help me do that. I'll show you how you can help if you like'.* That way, you shift the burden away from parents and child to where it belongs: with you.

Putting a constructive spin on the 'negative' behaviour, affirming the child's reaction as expressions of autonomy rather than noncompliance (an awful, accusatory term to avoid) can begin to turn things around. Simplistic as sounds, at a later stage, *'Thank you for helping me help you'* and *'Thank you for working with me today'* and a little reward to take home, may work wonders.

Point 2 Development: Losing Sounds/ Losing Words

Reporting on her study of the language-learning process of 18 typically developing children between one and two years of age Nelson (1973) discussed them in terms of an interactional model, analysing each child's first 50 words for grammatical form, content, and semantic structure.

Nelson found that three children (Mark, Leslie, and Ellen) 'dropped' words from their expressive vocabularies. For example, Leslie, said first-words at 12 months, and at 16 months dropped all her nine words except 'daddy' for 2 months. At 18 months, she accumulated vocabulary again (hot, up, Mommy, snow, peek-a-boo, baby, hi, and bye-bye, and five people's names). Over the next two months her word-count expanded, passing 50 words before 20 months, with short sentences appearing soon after. At 2;6 her MLU was 2.0–2.38, and at 21 months her PPVT score was 124.

SLPs/SLTs commonly ask parents to maintain a running record of their late-talking child's vocabulary growth and early word combinations. When child who is progressing slowly drops words it is readily observable, especially if they have fewer than 50–60 words. It is good to be able to reassure parents that this is a normal phenomenon in typical acquisition (*Isn't it great to see* [Child's Name] *doing what so many other children do?*) perhaps mentioning the 3/18 children in Nelson's study. At the same time, the SLP/SLT must say that they have noted the parents' concerns and will monitor progress. Recall Box 3.6 where it says losing words is not an indicator for SSD, or CAS specifically, but that in rare instances it may indicate language regression due to epilepsy (e.g., Landau–Kleffner syndrome, in which clinical seizures do not always occur; epileptiform activity; or autism spectrum disorder). Shinnar et al. (2001) found that such regression peaks in the second year of life.

Point 2 Development: Groping/struggle

One or more of the terms 'groping', 'groping with the mouth', 'articulatory struggle', 'silent posturing', and 'mouthing words' once appeared, and in some cases still appear, on checklists of indicators of CAS.

Importantly, this apparent 'feeling around' for the correct articulatory configuration does not occur in every individual with CAS, and it is interesting to consider that it is rarely apparent in very young children with sCAS and is likely a learned phenomenon. It may even be an artefact of SLP/SLT intervention, or of someone else in the child's life helping them with their speech, especially by instructing them how to position and move their articulators.

Parents may worry unnecessarily about this searching behaviour, and this presents another opportunity for positive connotation (*I see that* [Child's Name] *is a good tryer*). Parents may be reassured to know that a child's groping/articulatory struggle are signs that: (a) they know they must apply exceptional effort to improve their intelligibility, (b) they are *trying*, and possibly that (c) they have a more persistent personality. It signals a desirable combination of self-awareness, motivation, persistence, and a willingness to engage in. and persevere with trial-and-error behaviour.

Point 2 Development: Comprehension, and Point 4: Cognition

Parents often say that their child 'understands everything' or is 'very bright' and may give excellent examples of why they do. It is nonetheless essential to *test* receptive skills. Parent report may be positive, but testing tells you about co-operation and attention too, and may reveal subtle comprehension deficits. This can come as a shock to parents, requiring sensitive handling—don't assume they 'know'.

Point 5 PA/Literacy: Consider Offering One Piece of Advice

Consider offering one piece of advice in the initial visit. At this time parents are typically not ready to absorb a lot of new information, but they will usually remember one key suggestion.

Recommending a regular 5–7 minute '*story time*', '*talking time*', '*communication time*' or '*Mum/Dad and* [Child's Name] *time*' when a parent engages quietly with the child with books, pictures or 'literacy-like' activities, sends messages about the status of both literacy and 1:1 child–adult communication opportunities. Once established, these special minutes can become the basis for a speech homework routine. Suggest concrete ways that this might be accomplished even with children who don't like books, craft, or 'educational' activities, keeping the demands on the parent reasonable and practical as they adjust to their child's diagnosis or suspected diagnosis.

Observations of CAS

Shriberg et al. (2003) suggested that clinicians look for the three diagnostic signs, and eight defining characteristics (five segmental characteristics, and three suprasegmental characteristics), when CAS is a suspected, provisional, or working diagnosis.

Diagnostic Signs

1. Speech motor sequencing difficulties.
2. Prosodic / suprasegmental differences.
3. Receptive language exceeds expressive language: 'the gap'.

8 Core Defining Characteristics of CAS

Segmental Characteristics

1. Articulatory struggle, silent posturing (in *some* children with CAS).
2. Transpositional substitution errors.
3. Marked inconsistency especially token-to-token inconsistency.
4. Sound and syllable deletions.
5. Vowel/diphthong errors.

Suprasegmental Characteristics (Prosodic Characteristics)

6. Inconsistent realization of stress.
7. Inconsistent timing of speech and pauses.
8. Inconsistent oral-nasal gestures underlying the percept of nasopharyngeal resonance.

Box 7.4 holds suggested guidelines for observations of CAS that a clinician might make during differential diagnosis. They are arranged under the overlapping headings of general characteristics, phonetic characteristics/phonetic error-types, sound sequencing difficulties, timing disturbances, disturbed temporal–spatial relationships of the articulators, contextual changes in articulatory proficiency, phonological awareness, receptive language, and expressive language.

Motor Speech Examination Worksheet

In working through the motor speech examination worksheet, displayed in Box 7.5, the tasks chosen, and the order in which they are presented depend on the severity of the child's difficulties and any predictions the clinician makes regarding their likely performance. The worksheet is intended to help confirm or reject CAS as a diagnosis, noting that any determination of oral apraxia would have been made in the structural–functional examination (Skinder-Meredith, A28).

As with the 10-point CAS assessment prompt (Box 7.3), the procedures in Box 7.5 overlap, and not all will be performed with every client. There is no set order of presentation of these tasks, other than the logical hierarchy that the clinician deems appropriate for *this* child.

Multi-syllabic Words

In her study of children's acquisition of polysyllabic words (which she called 'long words') and words containing consonant clusters, James (2006) identified the 10 words, shown in Figure 7.1, as the most 'clinically useful' or most informative diagnostically. They were *ambulance, hippopotamus, computer, spaghetti, vegetables, helicopter, animals, caravan, caterpillar*, and *butterfly*.

James's use of the expression 'clinically useful' indicates that by eliciting these words the clinician may gather information about a child's speech that is useful in clinical diagnosis. For example, there is scope for the child to demonstrate

- SODA errors (from all the words)
- Syllable structure processes

- Reduplication (from all the words).
- Cluster reduction, e.g., from *ambulance, computer, spaghetti, helicopter, butterfly*.
- Initial consonant deletion Syllable Initial Word Initial: SIWI, e.g., from *hippopotamus, computer, vegetables*.
- Initial consonant deletion SIWW, e.g., from *ambulance, spaghetti, caravan*.
- Final consonant deletion SFWF, e.g., from *ambulance, animals, caravan*.
- Final consonant deletion SFWW, e.g., from *computer, vegetables, helicopter*.
- Weak syllable deletion, e.g., from *computer, animals, caravan*.
- Substitution (systemic) processes
  - Gliding of liquids, e.g., from *ambulance, caterpillar*.
  - Gliding of fricatives, e.g., from *caravan, vegetables, butterfly*.
  - Gliding of affricates, from *vegetables*.
  - Stopping of fricatives, e.g., from *spaghetti, helicopter, caravan*.
  - Velar fronting, e.g., from *computer, spaghetti, helicopter, caravan, caterpillar*.
  - Backing, e.g., from *hippopotamus, spaghetti, caterpillar, butterfly*.
  - Assimilation errors, e.g., from *ambulance, spaghetti*.
  - Deaffrication from *vegetables*.
  - Voicing/devoicing errors, (prevocalic voicing, postvocalic devoicing).
  - Schwa insertion.
  - Schwa addition.
- Vowel replacements (from all the words).
- Sequencing difficulties (from all the words).
- Excessive and/or equal stress/atypical prosody (all the words).
- Lexical avoidance.
- Difficulty applying oral-nasal resonance.
- Variability/inconsistency of production. ·
- and more.

The clinician avoids presenting the pictures and words in a confrontation naming or imitation task, like a mini-articulation-test. Rather, they are introduced individually with the aim of hearing the child produce each word several, or even many times. For example, the child might listen to the story *There's a hippopotamus on our roof eating*

Box 7.4   Suggested Guidelines for Observations of Childhood Apraxia of Speech

Diagnostic categories for speech-language problems are typically NOT discrete. They often co-occur, overlap, and influence each other. With development (and therapy) the characteristics of the disorder will change, so the label may change, and what we do in treatment will certainly change. In differentially diagnosing CAS as a motor speech disorder (a 'movement difficulty' disorder) we need to focus on speech praxis with the language/phonology aspects being regarded as 'concomitant'. We may want to give the child's disorder the right label, but the overriding clinical goal is to understand the child's issues well enough to plan intervention.

General Observations of CAS

1. Inability to imitate sounds and segments.
2. Refusal to imitate sounds and/or segments. Note: refusal is often remarkable in otherwise biddable children who cooperate when asked to do other things.
3. Decreased proprioceptive awareness of the articulators.
4. Difficulty achieving and maintaining articulatory postures and configurations.
5. Silent posturing, groping, trial-and-error articulatory behaviour. Note: this may be an artefact of therapy or other individuals 'helping' with phonetic placement.
6. Distinctive resonance. The child may have hypernasality, or mixed nasality sometimes, or all the time.
7. Prosodic disturbances; excessive stress <u>or</u> equal stress, or excessive <u>and</u> equal stress (EES). Note: this occurs in English, but not French, Hebrew and possibly not in some other languages.

Phonetic Characteristics / Phonetic error-types in CAS

1. Multiple speech sound errors: Omissions (most common), Substitutions, Distortions, Additions, Voicing / aspiration errors, Vowel errors, Errors related to complexity of articulatory adjustment.
2. Independent phonetic inventory (what the child *can* produce) is larger than the relational phonetic inventory (what the child says).

Sound Sequencing Difficulties in CAS

1. Metathesis: Brian, 23 says 'relevant' as 'revalent'; 'evolution' as 'elovution'; 'cavalry' as 'calvary'.
2. Difficulty with a phonotactic combination, although the sounds are correct in isolation or in some combinations: Max, 7;0 can say tip, rip, tipped, ripped, but not trip which he pronounces as 'prit' (transpositional error, see 5. below).
3. Sounds are correct in some sequences are erred in other, similar sound sequences: Madison, 7;2 says 'Madison' but calls 'The Radisson' 'Da Wattison'.
4. Clusters are more difficult to produce than singletons: Max, 7;0 says 'boo' and 'Lou' but not 'blue'.
5. Transposition of sounds/syllables: Daniel, 7;0 says 'accavado' for 'avocado', 'Lunderwand' for 'Wonderland', 'wentytun' for '21', 'Ligfoe' for 'Lithgow' and 'Madny' for 'Mandy'.

Timing Disturbances in CAS

1. Word and sentence durations may be longer.
2. Slope of the 2nd formant may be shallower if the tongue is taking longer to get into position.
3. Voice onset times may be longer, perhaps explaining voicing errors.

Disturbed temporal-spatial relationships of the articulators in CAS

1. There may be imprecise, non-specific 'wandering' speech gestures.
2. Palatometry indicates children with CAS do not develop the fine-tuned, precise speech movements that typically developing children have (and possibly children with other SSDs).

Expressive language and CAS

Pronoun errors are common in children with CAS. Morphemic and syntactic errors are often due to speech simplifications (omitting /s/, /z/, /t/, /d/ word finally in tenses and plural markers). Word omissions occur. Speech may be telegrammatic; might this be a strategy to reduce linguistic load?

Receptive-Expressive gap in CAS

This gap is not necessarily across the board but may vary according to the language test task. For example, single word receptive vocabulary may be age typical, but sentence comprehension may be impaired. Receptive skills for simple sentences may be age appropriate while comprehension of complex sentences is impaired. Air et al. (1989) investigated 'older' children, finding that those who appeared to have adequate comprehension in preschool to Year 2, tended to have difficulty in language processing fundamentals (categories, organization, abstract concepts) in Years 3–4.

(Continued)

Box 7.4 (Continued)

Contextual Changes in Articulatory Proficiency in CAS
Note that points 2, 6, and 7 suggest therapy strategies. *

1. Errors increase with increasing length of the word or utterance.
2. Imitation results in better articulatory performance compared with articulatory performance in spontaneous production, *except* for highly rehearsed / habituated spontaneous production. *
3. Target sounds are easier to produce in single words than in conversational speech.
4. Errors vary according to the phonetic complexity of the utterance.
5. Errors are inconsistently produced, and high token-to-token variability is a frequent finding.
6. Articulatory accuracy increases if rate is decreased—notably if vowels are lengthened. *
7. Articulatory accuracy increases with simultaneous visual and auditory models. *

Box 7.5   Motor Speech Examination Worksheet

This worksheet was designed by Edythe Strand, and is used by permission (Bowen, 2009, pp. 212–213). The stimuli used as examples in this version are from the DEMSS (Strand, A45).

(A) Observations during connected speech Example for a young child or one with very Severe impairment

	Vowels	Consonants	Typical maximum word length	Syllable shapes C, CV, VC	MLU
Conversation					
Picture description					
Narrative					

(B) Observations of elicited utterances Example for a young child or one with very Severe impairment Examine, dynamically, the child's ability to sequence movement for phonetic sequences in various contexts: (1) Vowels (2) CV VC CVC (3) Monosyllabic, bisyllabic, polysyllabic words (4) Phrases (5) Sentences of increasing length looking at the child's: **Movement accuracy**; **Vowel production**; **Consistency**; and **Prosody**, and the level of support required. You don't have to use the DEMSS stimuli (below); use stimuli that 'suit' the child.

	Immediate repetition	Repetition after delay—no cues	Simultaneous production needed	Gestural/tactile cues needed
Isolated vowels				
CV me hi				
VC up eat				
Reduplicated syllables mama booboo				
CVC1 mom peep pop				

CVC2 mad bed hop				
Vowel errors Note the different coarticulatory contexts				
Utterances of increasing length (Note the use of *simple* words)				
Bi-syllabic 1 baby puppy				
Bi-syllabic 2 bunny happy today canoe				
Multi-syllabic banana video				
Phrases Make up stimuli to suit the child being tested Me too; Big boy				
'Sentences' Make up stimuli of increasing length to suit the child. Dad. Hi dad. Hi daddy.				

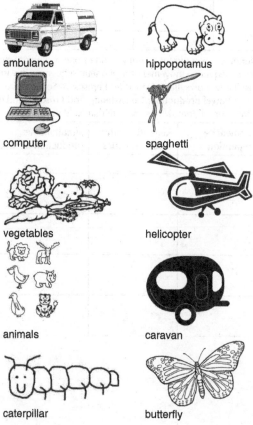

ambulance   hippopotamus

computer   spaghetti

vegetables   helicopter

animals   caravan

caterpillar   butterfly

Figure 7.1 Debbie's 10 long clinically useful words (Vardan / Adobe Stock).

cake and then play a game involving hippopotamus figurines (e.g., from a set of plastic zoo or jungle animals). The SLP/SLT, and/or a parent, would encourage as many 'repeats' of the assessment target as possible via modelling and vocal play, and the SLP/SLT would transcribe them using fine transcription, including the symbols for disordered speech if necessary. Then, not necessarily in the same session, another word, e.g., *ambulance*, would be targeted.

Characteristics Common to Phonological Disorder and CAS

The six characteristics that may be evident (note, *may* be evident, not *will* be evident) in either disorder, or that *may* be present when CAS and phonological disorder co-occur in a child, are displayed in Table 7.1, and in the first column of Table 7.2.

CAS and Phonological Disorder: Treatment Goals in Common

Column 1, Row 1 of Table 7.2 shows that the first characteristic error type in common is missing consonants, missing vowels, and missing phonotactics—in other words, consonant, vowel, and syllable shape inventory constraints. Columns 2 and 3

Table 7.1 Phonological Disorder and CAS: 6 Characteristic Error Types in Common.

1	Consonant, vowel, and phonotactic inventory constraints: that is, consonants, vowels, and syllable-word shapes are missing from their respective inventories.
2	Omissions of segments and structures: that is, omissions of consonants, vowels and syllable shapes that are already present in the child's repertoire.
3	Vowel errors including vowel replacements (substitutions) and vowel distortions.
4	Altered suprasegmentals: that is, atypical prosody.
5	Errors increase with increased errors utterance length and/or complexity.
6	The use of simple, but not complex, syllable and word shapes.

show the typical consonant, vowel, and phonotactic inventory errors in phonological disorder and CAS respectively, and in Column 4 are typical intervention goals in common.

Table 7.2, Column 2 shows that in phonological disorder, these inventory constraints manifest as:

- Systemic simplifications (also called substitution processes), such as stopping, gliding, and fronting, where one sound replaces another.
- Syllable structure processes (also called structural processes) where the structure of the syllable changes. Another way of putting this is to say that the structure of the syllable is simplified. Examples include initial consonant deletion (ICD), final consonant deletion (FCD), cluster reduction (CR), and weak syllable deletion (WSD), schwa insertion (e.g., [fɪləm] for *film*, [təˈɹu] for *true*, [ˌbəˈɹɪŋ] for *bring*), and schwa addition (e.g., [koutə] for *coat*, [bɪɡə] for *big*).

Then, in Column 3 we find that in CAS, the consonant and vowel inventory constraints may manifest as the *same* sorts of systemic and structural *simplification* errors found in phonological disorder, but in addition to these, in CAS, errors that involve increased phonetic *complexity* are found. For example, Costa, 5;8, with CAS and high levels of inconsistent word production, referred to *Henry the green engine* which has 10 consonants, as [ˈdʒendˌɹi vɜ ˈdʒɹˠwind ˈenˌdʒɹənd] which has 15. Other examples of his 'complexification' are listed below.

Word	Costa 5;8	Word	Costa 5;8
jump	ˈdʒɪʌːˌmpə	Mrs. Oates	ˈmɪtʃˌʌz ˌoutˈʃəz
twin	ˈtʃəɹɪndᵇ	real	ˈbəɹiʊʷdə
fastest	tʃəˈɹatˌsɪst	fishing	ˈtʃɪˌtʃɪŋ
blackout	ˈvəɹakˌʒout	creepy-crawly	ˈkəlɪbˌɹiˈɡlɔˌɹid
kilometre	klɪləˌməməˈlitlə	twice	tʃəˈɹaɪtəs
Costa	ˈklɒtˌstaˑ	Georgiades	ˈdɹiːɔˌdɹiːˌ dɹaːˌdʒidz

Costa's complexity errors included schwa addition and insertion (both occurred in [bəɹiʊʷdə] for *real*), affricates replacing stops, e.g., *top* pronounced as [dʒɒbə] or [dzɒptə];

Table 7.2 Phonological Disorder (PD) and CAS Typical Errors and Typical Goals in Common.

1. PD and CAS	2. PD	3. CAS	4. PD and CAS
6 Characteristic error types in common	**Typical errors in phonological disorder (PD)**	**Typical errors in Childhood Apraxia of Speech (CAS)**	**Typical intervention goals in common**
(1) Missing Consonants; Missing Vowels; Missing Phonotactics (syllable shapes).	Simplifications: (a) systemic or substitution processes e.g., stopping, gliding; (b) syllable structure processes e.g., FCD, CR, WSD.	Simplifications AND increased segmental complexity: e.g., affricates replacing stops; clusters replacing singletons; diphthongs replacing vowels.	1. Consonant inventory expansion. 2. Vowel inventory expansion. 3. Phonotactic inventory expansion.
(2) Omissions of consonants, vowels and syllable shapes that are *already* in the inventory.	Simplifications in the form of syllable structure processes and phonotactic errors: e.g., ICD, FCD, CR, WSD	Simplification AND increased structural complexity e.g., epenthesis (schwa insertion) /səked/ for 'scared'.	4. Syllable shape inventory expansion. 5. Word shape inventory expansion. 6. Increased accuracy of production of target structures.
(3) Vowel errors.	Vowel errors are less common in children who do not have CAS	Vowel errors are more common, and more persistent in CAS	7. More complete vowel repertoire. 8. More accurate vowel production.
(4) Altered suprasegmentals.	Weak syllable deletion	Excessive and equal stress	9. Production of strong and weak syllables. 10. Differentiation of strong and weak syllables.
(5) More errors with longer and or / more complex utterances, including 'SODA' errors.	SODA, process errors, and segmental complexity errors increase as contexts become more difficult, reducing intelligibility.	SODA, process errors, and segmental complexity errors increase as contexts become more difficult. This is *more* obvious in children with CAS.	11. Generalization of new consonants, vowels, syllable structures, and word structures, to more challenging contexts.
(6) Use of simple, but not complex, syllable shapes and word shapes.	Syllable structure processes: ICD, FCD, CR, WSD, and Reduplication	Syllable structure processes are more prevalent and persistent, even when phonetic repertoire is apparently adequate.	12. More complete phonotactic repertoire. 13. More varied use of phonotactic range within syllables and words. 14. Improved accuracy.

ICD = Initial Consonant Deletion; FCD = Final Consonant Deletion; CR = Cluster Reduction; WSD = Weak Syllable Deletion; SODA = Errors involving Substitution Omission Distortion Addition.

clusters replacing singletons, for example, *rabbit* pronounced as [bɹæbɪt] or [dɹæbɪt]; and diphthongs replacing vowels, e.g., *bed* pronounced as [baɪd] or [biːəd].

Sam, 4;9 was also diagnosed with CAS. He exhibited complexification but, his errors were usually consistent; both *red* and *bed* were produced homonymously as ['bɹend] and *rabbit* was ['bɹæˈbɪnt].

Phonetic transcription for Australian English		
Word	Adult target	Sam 4;9
red	ˈɹed	ˈbɹend
bed	ˈbed	ˈbɹend
rabbit	ˈɹæbɪt	ˈbɹæˈbɪnt
school	ˈsklɐʉl	ˈsklɐʉləd
Myers	ˈmɑeəz	ˈmɹˈɑedɹəz
Coles	ˈkoʊlz	ˈgloʊdz
Ikea	ˌɑeˈkɪə	ˌɑeˈklɪə
Freedom Furniture	ˌfɹiːˈdəm ˈfɜːnɪtʃə	ˌfɹiːˈdɹəmd ˈfɹɜːntʃəˌfdɹə

Sam talked about his mother as 'always shopping' and himself as 'shopping a lot'. He mentioned retailers often, hence *Myers* a department store, *Coles* a supermarket, and *Ikea* and *Freedom Furniture* which are homeware and furniture chains.

Still viewing the first row of Table 7.2, we see in Column 4 that the typical therapy goals in common are consonant, vowel, and phonotactic inventory expansion to give the child 'more to work with'. The same format is used in the following five rows of Table 7.2. If the clinician determines that a characteristic is present, their next task is to decide how best to pursue the corresponding goals, given the child's overall presenting picture. This question of 'how' is addressed later in this chapter, and the reader who cannot stand the suspense is referred to Tables 7.3 and 7.4.

CAS Diagnosis by Someone Other than an SLP/SLT

A difficulty associated with the overlap of characteristics between phonological disorder and CAS is that, when families with no background in SLP/SLT seek information without appropriate professional guidance, suspecting or convinced that their child has CAS, they will often perceive enough 'features' of CAS to be sure that they have identified their child's speech problem. They may reach this conclusion without knowing that those same symptoms are *far* more likely to signal phonological disorder, given the comparatively low incidence of CAS.

Compounding this problem, when lay people turn to the internet for elucidation, they find a disproportionately high number of electronic media (e.g., Blogs, Facebook groups, and YouTube videos) dealing with CAS, the less frequent SSD, and these may contain inaccurate information. Some of the misleading sites present as fact: wishful thinking, unsubstantiated opinion, and supposition. Often the content is associated with time, and money-wasting products (e.g., dietary supplements, 'special diets' such as the Speech Diet, and non-evidence-based intervention approaches such as the Verbal Motor Learning or VML treatment for apraxia, and Ayurvedic drugs), services (e.g., non-evidence-based online treatment), tools and toys, for example chewy tubes, straw and horn hierarchies, the Myomunchee appliances, and other products related to non-speech oral motor therapy (Lof, A24) and other mouth exercises. By contrast, few sites deal explicitly and accurately with phonological disorder, the more common SSD.

It may not be obvious to lay people that SSD affects about 7 children in every 100, and that within that population the prevalence of Childhood Apraxia of Speech is 2.4%, Childhood Dysarthria 3.4%, Speech Delay comprising phonological disorder and/or articulation disorder 82.2%, and Speech Delay and Concurrent Motor Speech Disorder 17.8% (see Table 2.3 and related discussion).

A reliable internet source of CAS information for consumers and clinicians is the Childhood Apraxia Association of North America (CASANA) website, Apraxia-KIDS (https://www.apraxia-kids.org). Apraxia-KIDS was founded in 1994 as a non-profit by the parent of a child with CAS, Sharon Gretz. An articulate advocate, she gathered in like-minded parents, professionals, and other dedicated supporters to work with her. Gretz became Executive Director of CASANA from its foundation at the end of 1999 to the end of 2017 when she left the organization to take up the Directorship of the Osher Lifelong Learning Institute at the University of Pittsburgh.

Aspects of Gertz's legacy include increased accuracy of information about speech development and disorders circulating on the Web, 'more equal' relationships between consumers and professionals, and sharper appreciation of the effects of communication disorders on affected individuals and their families. An added benefit may have been to fine tune SLPs'/SLTs' skills both as counsellors and knowing when and how to refer to a professional counsellor (Bitter,

A13; Stoeckel, A14). In 2022, under the leadership of Angela Grimm (Apraxia-KIDS Executive Director), Laura Moorer (Vice President of Programs), and Amy Salera (parent of a child with CAS and Community Engagement Manager) Apraxia-KIDS launched a supportive, informational Parent Portal (https://parent.apraxia-kids.org).

Longer Term Consequences of SSD, Particularly CAS

Among the issues and concerns that arise in parent and family interviews, information-sharing, and counselling, and in counselling older children and young people with persisting SSD, are the potential long-term effects of these conditions. Gierut (1998) indicated that some individuals with SSD can expect lifetime challenges with retrieval, manipulation, and comprehension of linguistic information; expressive language capabilities; and education and work choices.

In timely and more recent research, Miller et al. (2019), Cassar et al. (2023) and Turner et al. (2019) provide important insights into the lifelong speech, literacy, and psychosocial consequences for adults with CAS, a topic elaborated by McCabe (A34). Also welcome is a study exploring the issues of concern for families of children aged 3 to sixteen with primary diagnoses of CAS (Rusiewicz et al., 2018), and an investigation of and parents' adjustment to their child's apraxia diagnosis and its impacts (Miron, 2012).

Dr. Colleen Miron, an Educational Psychologist, interviewed, in-depth, eleven parents who were white, highly educated, middle- to upper-middle-class, Apraxia-KIDS supporters, and active advocates for CAS, who had volunteered as participants. They included 3 husband/wife couples who were interviewed together, 4 mothers in nuclear families, and a divorced single mother, interviewed individually. Miron afforded them the opportunity to frame their own emotional and practical experiences of CAS, their decision-making processes, and their self-concepts and identities as parents of children with CAS (Miron, 2012, 2013). She found that, at least for this privileged group, having a child with CAS set in motion several stages of adaptation, culminating in healthy adjustment and positive outcomes.

Discussing her conclusions, Miron (2012) wrote: *critical positive encounters with professionals are vital to facilitating positive parent adaptation. These encounters are significant enough that one positive encounter appears to be powerful enough to negate dozens of negative experiences and spark a lasting attitude of optimism and advocacy for parents.* Her recommendations directed to clinicians and researchers, warrant our consideration, that professionals recognize that:

1. For the most part, parents view their interactions with the medical and educational communities as disheartening, unhelpful, and at times, adversarial.
2. Critical positive encounters with key professionals were the most significant trigger for a positive adaptation experience for parents, and that further research focus on the specific aspects of those encounters, encompassing questions such as:
   - What characteristics must be present for it to be a 'critical encounter'?
   - How do short-term interactions and long-term relationships differ in their effect on parents' adaptation process?
   - How do professionals perceive these encounters?
   - What skills or techniques can professionals use or improve on to increase the likelihood that they can facilitate a critical encounter with parents?

Case History Interviewing

The short-term and lifelong implications of SSD in general, and phonological disorder and CAS specifically, impact the assessment, diagnosis, intervention, and discharge process, from the opening moments of the initial consultation or case history interview.

There is more to gathering a history than completing the sections on a form. Case history interviewing is a *procedure* in which the interviewer—in this case an SLP/SLT—finds out about another. The 'other' is a client with, or thought to have a communication disorder, or their family member or caregiver, typically a parent. Interviewing is also a *skill*. It can be taught, and has scope over time, for refinement and improvement through additional training and relevant interviewing experience with interviewees with diverse stories, and in various service delivery models: e.g., in-the-flesh, or via telehealth. While the two bear similarities, and are often taught together at university, interviewing differs from counselling (Bitter, A13; Holland & Nelson, 2020, pp. 14–15).

As a skill, interviewing requires sensitive, perceptive questioning for information gathering; active listening; informed observations based on the SLP/SLT knowledgebase and a degree of common sense; well-paced exchanges allowing time for interviewees to collect their thoughts and address questions; a supportive, empathetic, non-judgemental, stance; and an openness to answering *their* questions, incorporating *their* feedback, and respecting and overtly acknowledging *their* needs and preferences.

The goal of the case history interview is to provide the clinician with valid, pertinent, and helpful information that enlightens the clinical process, including the application of appropriate assessment, intervention, and case management approaches, procedures, and activities.

Intervention Principles

Box 7.6   Intervention Principles for Phonological Disorder

Phonological Principles

1. Intervention is based on the systematic nature of phonology.
2. Intervention is characterized by conceptual activities rather than motor activities.
3. Intervention has generalization as its end-goal, promoting intelligibility. In explicitly targeted therapy it should be unnecessary to work on all possible targets.

10 Points to Consider in Intervention

1. If using a 3-position SODA test transcribe entire words to see error patterns more readily.
2. Work at word (meaning) level.
3. Work towards functional generalization.
4. Treat a pattern, or patterns, of errors.
5. Teach appropriate contrasts.

3-5 Minimal Pairs!
Elbert et al. (1991) found that they could teach as few as 3 to 5 minimal pairs. Their participants showed spontaneous generalization to other words containing the target sounds.

6. Direct the child's attention to the way that different sounds make different meanings. Make this apparent to parents too, e.g., give them examples of their own child's homonymy.
7. Use naturalistic contexts that have *meaning* (hold interest) for the child, because this helps demonstrate to the child that the function of phonology is to make meaning (to communicate).
8. Stack the 'therapy environment' with several exemplars of each individual target word so the child can self-select activities, e.g., for work on eliminating Velar Fronting, for the target words: car, key, core, cow, have available several different cars, car keys, etc. activities such as picture cards, a game with toys, a board game, a story, alliterative input, listening lists, drill and drill play.
9. Select targets with an eye to their potential impact on the child's system.
10. Carefully select exemplars of an error pattern / phonological rule. With clever exemplar-choices, the rule is learned, and carries over (generalizes) to the other targets.

Box 7.7   Intervention Principles for Childhood Apraxia of Speech

'CAS Therapy' Principles

1. Intervention is based on the principles of motor learning.
2. Intervention is characterized by motor activities rather than conceptual activities.
3. Intervention has habituation <u>and then</u> automaticity as its end-goal, promoting intelligibility.

15 Points to Consider in Intervention

1. Use paired auditory and visual stimuli in intensive practice trials.
2. Train sound combinations (CV VC CVC etc.) rather than isolated phones.
3. Keep the focus in therapy (and at home) on movement performance drill.
4. Use repetitive production trials / systematic drill as intensively as possible.
5. Carefully construct hierarchies of stimuli, using small steps.
6. Use reduced production rate with proprioceptive monitoring (child's self-monitoring).
7. Use *simple* carrier phrases and *simple* cloze tasks.
8. Pair movement sequences with suprasegmental facilitators: including stress, intonation, and rhythm. Be thinking 'prosodic contour' of the utterance all the time!
9. Use singing, whispering and loudness judiciously.
10. Establish a core vocabulary or a small number functional 'power words' (that make things happen) early in therapy, especially for non-verbal or minimally verbal children.

11. Use sign / AAC to facilitate communication, intelligibility, and language development, and to reduce frustration. Reassure families that AAC will not get in the way of learning to speak.
12. Be flexible. Treatment changes over time. Signal changes and explain them to parents, lest they be misinterpreted. Note that unexplained changes can leave parents with a worrying false impression that the child's speech challenges are more severe than first though; that the SLP/SLT was 'on the wrong track'; or that the SLP/SLT is grasping at straws with a 'difficult case'.
13. Present regular, consistent, effective homework as a 'given', within reason.
14. Expect 'good days and bad days' in terms of the child's performance.
15. The principles of motor learning apply to CAS dynamic assessment and therapy.

Intervention Techniques, Procedures and Activities

To recap, Table 7.1 displays the six characteristic error types found in phonological disorder *and* CAS. In Table 7.2 the same errors are listed, with a comparison in columns two and three of how they manifest in phonological disorder and the different ways they manifest in CAS. In column 4 of Table 7.2 are 14 treatment goals common to these two SSDs.

Table 7.3, below, shows the six characteristic error types and goals once again, but this time with 20 corresponding approaches, strategies, and techniques suggested in the third column for 'how to' address the goals. Then, in Table 7.4 the 20

approaches, strategies, and techniques are listed in the left-hand column with the types of approaches, techniques, procedures, strategies, and activities to use to achieve the typical goals are listed in the right-hand column.

In the section that follows Table 7.4, the intervention approaches, techniques, procedures, strategies, and activities are either described briefly or the reader is directed to relevant sections in other chapters. Note that stimulability training, pre-practice, phonemic placement techniques, shaping, phonotactic therapy, progressive approximations, and techniques to encourage self-monitoring are all mentioned in relation to more than one goal, and each is discussed under one heading.

Approaches, Techniques, Procedures, Srategies, Activities

1. Pre-practice

Pre-practice is an early step in motor learning that occurs prior to the practice phase. Pre-practice, combining stimulability training, phonetic placement techniques and shaping, has an important role in consonant and vowel inventory expansion (increasing the phonetic inventory). This goes beyond learning new phones in isolation into pre-practice for new syllable shapes, words including multisyllabic words, and longer utterances. The client is taught how to reliably produce the target, or an acceptable (in terms a clinical judgement of what they

Table 7.3 Phonological Disorder and Childhood Apraxia of Speech.

Typical Errors and Goals in Common and Suggested Ways to Achieve those Goals

6 Typical Errors	14 Typical Goals	20 Approaches, Strategies and Techniques
(1) Consonant inventory constraints; vowel inventory constraints; and phonotactic inventory constraints.	1. Consonant inventory expansion 2. Vowel inventory expansion 3. Phonotactic inventory expansion	1) Stimulability training 2) Pre-practice 3) Phonemic placement techniques 4) Shaping
(2) Omissions of consonants, vowels and syllable shapes that are *already* in the inventory.	4. Syllable shape inventory expansion 5. Word shape inventory expansion 6. Increased accuracy of production of target structures	5) CV syllable and word drills 6) Phonotactic therapy 7) Metalinguistic approaches 8) Reading

Typical Errors and Goals in Common and Suggested Ways to Achieve those Goals

6 Typical Errors	14 Typical Goals	20 Approaches, Strategies and Techniques
(3) Vowel errors.	7. More complete vowel repertoire 8. More accurate vowel production	o Stimulability training o Pre-practice o Phonemic placement techniques o Shaping 9) Auditory Input Therapy / Naturalistic Recast Intervention 10) Minimal contrasts therapy
(4) Altered suprasegmentals.	9. Production of strong and weak syllables. 10. Differentiation of strong and weak syllables	o Phonotactic therapy 11) Melodic Intonation therapy 12) Singing
(5) More errors with longer and or / more complex utterances, including the so-called 'SODA' errors of substitution, distortion, and addition.	11. Generalization of new consonants, vowels, syllable structures, and word structures, to more challenging contexts	13) Prolongation of vowels 14) Slowed rate of production 15) Progressive approximations 16) Single word (SW) production drill 17) Techniques to encourage self-monitoring
(6) Use of simple, but not complex, syllable shapes and word shapes.	12. More complete phonotactic repertoire. 13. More varied use of phonotactic range within syllables and words 14. Improved accuracy	o Phonotactic therapy o Progressive approximations 18) SW and Connected Speech production drill 19) Backward build-ups 20) Backward chaining o Techniques to encourage self-monitoring

Table 7.4 Phonological Disorder and Childhood Apraxia of Speech.

Intervention and Approaches, Techniques, Procedures, and Strategies, with Examples

20 Approaches, Strategies and Techniques	Examples of Approaches, Techniques, Procedures, Strategies, and Activities to use to Achieve the Typical Goals
1) Stimulability training 2) Pre-practice 3) Phonemic placement techniques 4) Shaping 5) CV syllable and word drills	Stimulability Training, Miccio's Stimulability Therapy (Miccio A17) (evidence-based for phonological disorder), Pre-Practice, Phonemic Placement Techniques, Shaping and CV Syllable and Word Drills all overlap, usually incorporating metalinguistic 'cues' (Table 4.1 and related text) elements of Traditional Articulation Therapy / 'phonetic approaches' (Van Riper & Irwin, 1958). https://speech-language-therapy.com/pdf/ppsxtraditionalartictx.ppsx You can use: • Miccio's Stimulability Therapy program • Phonetic Approaches / 'Traditional' articulation therapy • Baba Board (Velleman, 2003), Word Flips (Granger, 2005) • Nuffield Sequences, starting at syllable level, not b-b-b-, b-p-k-b-p-k... (P. Williams & Stephens, 2004) • Colleagues' suggestions in social media e.g., https://www.facebook.com/groups/E3BPforSSD • Shaping (Bleile, 2017, 2019; Secord et al.,2007)

Intervention and Approaches, Techniques, Procedures, and Strategies, with Examples

20 Approaches, Strategies and Techniques	Examples of Approaches, Techniques, Procedures, Strategies, and Activities to use to Achieve the Typical Goals
6) Phonotactic therapy (for syllable structure)	Immature phonotactic patterns require us to focus on the syllable level. Therapy that addresses syllable shapes will generalize well beyond the specific sound or sounds targeted in a syllable position (Velleman, 2002).

7) Metalinguistic approaches	Metalinguistic Cues: imagery, gesture, and touch cues
	• Metaphon: puzzling, reflection, guided discussion
	• PACT Multiple Exemplar Training (Bowen and Cupples,1999)
	• Phonemic Awareness Intervention (Hesketh, 2010)
	• Imagery Therapy (Klein, 1996)
	• Slideshows at www.speech-language-therapy.com
	  – Modelling and Recasting/Frequent Recasting
	  – Fixed-up-One Routine Slideshow
	  – Many Repeats (Drill for Beginning Beginners)

8) Reading	'Syllabification' and 'Clusters' (games from Smart Kids); Reading games Phonological Awareness activities (McNeill, A22; Neilson, A49)
9) Auditory Input therapy Thematic play Auditory Bombardment	In auditory input therapy multiple exemplars of targets are provided in INPUT during play activities. It aims for many minimal pair exemplars of the TARGET. When contrasts are used the feature difference usually minimal. e.g.: • Stories: e.g., Jeff's scarf (Figure 7.6) • Alliterative children's games, stories, and rhymes e.g., a Surf Smurf jumps off a roof. • Auditory Bombardment (Focused Auditory Input) / Listening Lists (Hodson, 2011) • Alliterative input (Bowen & Rippon, 2013
10) Minimal Pair therapies	See Chapter 4: 1. Conventional Minimal Pairs (Weiner, 1981) 2. Maximal Oppositions (Gierut, 1989) 3. Multiple Oppositions (A. L. Williams & Sugden, 2021) 4. Empty Set (Gierut, 1989)
11) Melodic Intonation therapy (MIT) 'Chanting Therapy' Combine MIT with other Approaches and Strategies	Developed by Helfrich-Miller (1983), Helfrich-Miller (1984, 1994) for children with CAS, MIT is based on the three elements of prosody: melody, rhythm, and stress. Although it has been validated as a short-term intervention demonstrating qualitative improvement in the speech of adults with Broca's Aphasia (Benson et al., 1994) its efficacy with children with CAS is inconclusive. It was never intended as a stand-alone therapy (Helfrich-Miller, 1994). When used in conjunction with kindred approaches and strategies of (e.g., Integral Stimulation, singing, vowel prolongation) it appears to have clinical utility. In MIT an intoned utterance, is lengthened and the rhythm and stress are exaggerated, while the pitch is held constant for several whole notes. In such intoned or chanted 'stylised' utterances pitch typically varies by only one whole note. Its focus is not on the segmental level, but rather on prosody, and its role is in helping children to produce and differentiate strong and weak syllables and vary the length of notes (vocalizations) at will. The clinician uses rhythmical stories as well as songs, nursery rhymes, etc.

Intervention and Approaches, Techniques, Procedures, and Strategies, with Examples

20 Approaches, Strategies and Techniques	Examples of Approaches, Techniques, Procedures, Strategies, and Activities to use to Achieve the Typical Goals
12) Singing	Slow Sing-along Songs Karaoke, in YouTube Lullabies: e.g., Bye-bye baby, bye-bye-bye to the tune of Substitute the words of 'There is a tavern in the town' with word-sequences such as: • Bye-bye bye baby, bye bye-bye • Mum Mum Mumma, Mumma Mum • Dad Dad Dadda Dadda Dad • Pop Pop Poppa Poppa Pop • Nan Nan Nanna Nanna Nan
13) Prolongation of vowels	Model 'see' as 'seeeeee', not 'sssssee', even though this seems counter-intuitive. Gradually reduce vowel length.
14) Slowed rate of production	Encourage metalinguistic awareness of 'normal rate' and 'slow rate' rather than 'slow' vs. 'fast'. There is no advantage in encouraging 'talking fast'. Model a slower rate with *slightly* prolonged vowels, then gradually reduce the prolongation in response to the child's success. This can be difficult to do, and parents and the SLP/SLT may need to practise before modelling in this way.

15) Progressive approximations	Kaufman Speech Praxis Workout Book https://www.northernspeech.com/apraxia-childhood/kaufman-k-slp-workout-book-3rd-edition
	Slideshows at www.speech-language-therapy.com
	• How Jessica Learned to Say Yellow
	  https://www.speech-language-therapy.com/pdf/yellow.pptx
	• How Max Learned to Say Leura Public
	  https://www.speech-language-therapy.com/pdf/max.ppsx

16) Single-word production drill	Word Flips (Granger, 2005) Nuffield words (P. Williams & Stephens, 2004) Intervention Resources at: www.speech-language-therapy.com Smart Chute and picture cards—drill, drill play Speech Sounds on Cue (Apple App Store) Black Sheep Press materials www.blacksheeppress.co.uk
17) Techniques to encourage self-monitoring	Fixed-up-One Routine worksheets at www.speech-language-therapy.com 'You can't say roo if you mean roof, you can't say nigh if you mean knife, …' Frequent Recasting (12–18 recasts in a minute for a few minutes of the day)
18) SW and CS production drill	Stimulus and probe items used by Kostner and Jakielski (2004) for a girl 8;9 with CAS. I go play outside with Emma. I want to sit by her. Leave me alone, please. I don't think so! I want to read to you. I go to that house. I write on the board. I want to ride my bike. I sing at church. I want to eat. Who will pick me up?

Intervention and Approaches, Techniques, Procedures, and Strategies, with Examples

20 Approaches, Strategies and Techniques	Examples of Approaches, Techniques, Procedures, Strategies, and Activities to use to Achieve the Typical Goals
19) Backward build-ups	Backward build-ups have been used in foreign language teaching for a long time. Velleman (2003) advocates using them for multi-syllabic words, especially with children with CAS. Start with as much of the end of the word a child can say. This might even be the entire word except the first syllable.
20) Backward chaining	Backward chaining is a technique that has been around for a long time too, and it can be used to facilitate the production of two-syllable words in children who only produce monosyllables.

can produce) approximation, *before* entering the practice phase. The child is given frequent models and feedback about their movement performance (i.e., 'knowledge of performance' or KP feedback) during pre-practice. Once in the practice phase, KP feedback is given only when necessary (i.e., if production accuracy drops off), and feedback is around 'knowledge of results' (KR feedback) and the child adjusts production independently with minimal, or no, clinician modelling (Shriberg & Kwiatkowski, 1990; Maas et al., 2012).

2. Stimulability training

The late Adele Miccio (A17) describes a rationale and a program for stimulability training. Miccio's treatment (Miccio, 2005; Miccio & Elbert 1996) was evaluated as a stand-alone treatment with children with phonological disorder, but not CAS. It has immediate relevance, however, to all children with depleted phonetic and phonemic inventories. Furthermore, Iuzzini and Forrest (2010) reported successful treatment outcomes for four children diagnosed with CAS who received intervention that combined stimulability training, Core Vocabulary Therapy (see Chapter 5) and complex phonological targets (Krueger, A35).

3. Phonetic placement techniques

There are several helpful published sources of techniques for phonetic placement, particularly Bleile (2017, 2019), Flipsen Jr. (2022), and Secord et al. (2007). Phonetic placement is precisely what it sounds like—the physical positioning of the client's articulators into the correct place of articulation and associating it with the correct manner

of articulation (and of course, voicing). Phonetic placement techniques may incorporate a variety of models provided by the clinician or other helper for immediate, or delayed, or simultaneous imitation. Imagery names, simple verbal cues and reminders and iconic gesture cues, as displayed in Table 4.1, are also employed.

4. Shaping

Shaping involves altering a sound in the child's repertoire to facilitate acquisition of a new sound. For example, a prolonged, 'fricated' [t] might be shaped into /s/; [t] closely followed by [ʃ] might be shaped into /tʃ/; saying *to-you-to-you-to-you* briskly many times might also be used to elicit /tʃ/ (via [tj]); or the voiceless velar fricative /x/ (the final consonant in *Bach* /bɑx/) can be prolonged and then 'stopped' to elicit /k/.

The question of evidence for phonemic placement and shaping cues

The question of whether phonemic placement and shaping cues are 'evidence based' and requests for peer reviewed, published evidence for them arise in CPD events, social media, and correspondence. The Butterfly Procedure provides an example. It is described in detail at www.speech-language-therapy.com, (see https://www.speech-language-therapy.com/pdf/metalinguisticcues.pdf) as a stimulability technique that involves phonemic placement, shaping and imagery to remediate lateral /s/ and /z/ and fricatives and affricates produced with tongue-palate contact. Before the therapist can proceed with it, children must be able to produce

/t/ and/or /d/ and /i/. Then the SLP/SLT can help him or her assume the 'butterfly position' (the alveolare place of articulation for /s/ and /z/) and understand the associated imagery in which the tongue is imagined as a butterfly with a central groove and its wings 'braced' against the teeth.

The technique is tried and clinically tested, dating back to at least the 1940s. It has been on my website since 1998 because in my clinical experience it has usually 'worked'. It is associated with modest Level IV Evidence, *viz.* 'Expert committee report, consensus conference and clinical experience of respected authorities' (American Speech-Language-Hearing Association, 2004, adapted from the Scottish Intercollegiate Guidelines Network), and displayed in Table 7.5.

The Butterfly Procedure stirs questions from SLPs/SLTs and students, such as this in 2022: '*I am currently a student with my very first client who has a lateral lisp. I came across the "butterfly procedure" on your website, which I think may be helpful for my client to be successful. I was trying to find empirical evidence for this technique and was not successful in my search. I am curious to know if you are aware of such evidence?*'

This is a reasonable, frequently asked question, and the answer is that there is no empirical evidence in support of the Butterfly Procedure *per se*. Rather, we know from collective clinical experience of clients' progress that phonemic placement

Table 7.5 Levels of Evidence Scottish Intercollegiate Guidelines Network www.sign.ac.uk (ASHA, 2004).

Level	Description
Ia	Well-designed meta-analysis of >1 randomized controlled trial
Ib	Well-designed randomized controlled study
IIa	Well-designed controlled study without randomization
II	Well-designed quasi-experimental study
III	Well-designed non-experimental studies, i.e., correlational and case studies
IV	Expert committee report, consensus conference, clinical experience of respected authorities

techniques, shaping techniques and facilitative contexts *such as* the Butterfly Procedure, with imagery that is meaningful for the child with SSD, *may* help their stimulability. What works with one child-family-clinician combination may not be effective with the next and as clinicians we may need try various alternatives, applying clinical reasoning, before settling on an optimal strategy for a client, or one that is most comfortable for us to use.

5. CV syllable and word drills

CV-syllable drill and CV-word drill involve repetitive practice of spoken, chanted, or sung syllables, such as 'many repeats' of *bye-bye-bye*, or *bay-bee-bay-bee-bay-bee*, or rehearsal of a list of CV syllables with a common phonetic or structural characteristic, such as *fee-fie-foe-fum* or *ha-ha-hee-hee-ho-ho-hoo-hoo-hi-hi* or *up-up-up-up* or *off-off-off-off-off* or *go-go-go-go-go*. Returning to the idea of a clinician being 'comfortable' with a technique, for some SLPs/SLTs singing in therapy sessions is an embarrassing undertaking that we don't have to experience if we do not wish to.

The term 'drill play' implies that syllable and word drills are performed in the context of play activities. These can be presented via conventional toys and games, electronically on CD-ROM, as Apps (e.g., *Say Bananas* by Dr. Kirrie Ballard and Dr. Beena Ahmed: https://www.youtube.com/watch?v=4Unh1uKJWwA), or in slides (e.g., using Apple Keynote or Microsoft PowerPoint). Drill and drill play can be accomplished with card games such as *Go Fish* and *Snap*, board games like *Snakes and Ladders*, and toys such as posting boxes, *Pop Up Pirate*, *Coco Crazy* and *Monkeying Around*, flip-over easel books such as *Word Flips* (Granger, 2005): https://www.superduperinc.com/word-flips.html, card chutes (e.g., *Smart Chute*: www.smartkids.com.au), and dedicated speech therapy programs, notably the P. Williams and Stephens (2004) Nuffield worksheets, and games invented by child, parent and clinician like variations of *I Spy*, *Simon Says*, and *hide-and-seek* and pen and paper games.

6. Phonotactic therapy

Velleman (2002) described a non-linear intervention framework, dubbing it 'Phonotactic Therapy'. She noted that immature phonotactic (syllable shape) patterns require intervention focusing syllables, noting that this may evoke generalization well beyond the targeted sound, or sounds, or syllable position. Undue persistence of the syllable structure processes/patterns in Table 4.3 occurs in children with phonological disorder, CAS, or both. They may include initial consonant deletion, final consonant deletion, replacement of a VC (e.g., /iːz/ in *keys*) with a diphthong (to make [kiə]), reduplication, weak syllable deletion, reduction of multisyllabic words, and cluster reduction. Also, children with such difficulties may also only ever produce monosyllables, and they may produce erroneous word stress patterns. Strategies and resources to use to address these difficulties, mostly inspired by Velleman (2002), Velleman (2003), are suggested below.

6a. Initial consonant deletion

In children with initial consonant deletion (ICD), reinforce any initial consonants in CV syllables irrespective of accuracy, starting with consonants already in the child's inventory. VC combinations, in strings, can be used to facilitate CV syllable shapes. For example, *oak-oak-oak-oak-oak* might be repeated and shaped into *coke-coke-coke-coke* and finally *Coke*, or *um-um-um-um* might be used to gradually elicit *mum-mum-mum-mum*, and ultimately *Mum*.

6b. Final consonant deletion

Final consonant deletion (FCD) past about the age of 2;10 is cause for concern in most languages (see Box 3.7), including English. Most consonants in English are mastered first SIWI, but velars and fricatives are mastered first SFWF. English has many final consonants, many CVC words, and many CVC syllables. The most prevalent final consonants are velars, fricatives, and voiceless stops. To facilitate development of final consonants, the clinician can reward *any* final consonant, irrespective of accuracy at first, focusing on sounds already in the child's inventory, favouring the prominent final consonants in the language—fricatives, velars, and voiceless stops.

It is helpful also to know that, in typical development, children produce their first instances of final consonants (codas) after short (lax) vowels, so their success may be optimized by target-word choices such as *buck, dove* (the

bird) and *foot*, where the vowel is short, rather than *beak, bike, bake, Dave, feet* and *fête*, where the consonants are the same but the word contains a long vowel (as in *feet*), or a diphthong (as in *fête*). Picture and word work sheets (#1–3 below), and a word list (#4 below) with word-final fricatives in CVCs with short vowels are available to download.

1. **Final fricatives with short vowels (pictures and words)**
   www.speech-language-therapy.com/pdf/ shortvowels_fricatives.pdf
   miss kiss Liz fizz whiff biff live give wish dish mess guess says eff rev chef mesh gas mass jazz Rav cash bus cuff buzz dove rush wash cough mash posh of moss boss Oz glove

2. **Final velars with short vowels (pictures and words)**
   www.speechlanguage-therapy.com/pdf/short vowels_velars.pdf
   pick wick fig twig wing lick sing peck neck peg beg pack back-pack wag bag bang fang tuck luck bug mug bung rung lock knock fog log song pig book buck wok gong king long

3. **Final voiceless stops with short vowels (pictures and words)**
   www.speech-language-therapy.com/pdf/ shortvowels_voicelessstops.pdf
   zip dip mitt hit wick sick yep Shep net pet neck deck nap lap bat pat yak pack cup pup nut hut luck buck hot dot wok sock

4. **'Favoured' final consonants and short vowels (words with no pictures)**
   Note that in Table 7.6, under /ʌ/ and /ʊ/ the words listed are the same to reflect different varieties of English (*bus, fuss, buzz* etc. pronounced with the vowel /ʌ/ and the same words pronounced with the vowel /ʊ/).

Non-linear Represenation of the Contents of a Syllable

There are two ways of representing the contents of a syllable non-linearly: with an onset and rime (rhyme) syllable tree (Figure 7.2), or a mora syllable tree (Figure 7.3).

Table 7.6 Favoured final consonants with short vowels www.speech-language-therapy.com/pdf/shortvowels.pdf.

	I	e	æ	ʌ	ɒ	ʊ
Fricatives SFWF Mastered first word finally	miss	mess	mass	bus	moss	bus
	kiss	guess	gas	fuss	boss	fuss
	Liz	says	jazz	buzz	Oz	buzz
	fizz	Des	has	fuzz	was	fuzz
	whiff	eff	gaffe	cuff	cough	cuff
	biff	chef	graph	tough	off	tough
	live	rev	have	dove	of	dove
	give	Bev	Rav	glove	Dov	glove
	wish	mesh	cash	rush	posh	rush
	dish	flesh	mash	hush	wash	hush
Velars SFWF Mastered first word finally	pick	peck	pack	tuck	lock	tuck
	wick	neck	back	luck	knock	luck
	fig	check	wag	bug	fog	bug
	twig	peg	bag	mug	log	mug
	wing	beg	bang	bung	song	bung
	sing	leg	fang	rung	long	rung
Voiceless Stops SFWF	zip	yep	nap	cup	top	cup
	dip	Shep	lap	pup	pop	pup
	mitt	net	bat	nut	hot	nut
	hit	pet	pat	hut	dot	hut
	wick	neck	yak	luck	wok	luck
	sick	deck	pack	buck	sock	buck

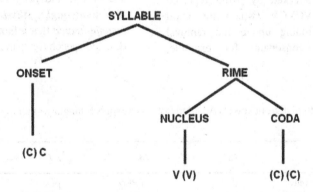

Figure 7.2 Onset and rime syllable tree.

In an onset and rime syllable tree, the onset is an initial consonant if any. Note that in this tree, (C) and (V) in parentheses mean there is no consonant or no vowel, respectively. The onset is followed by the rime, which is the rest of the syllable. The rime is further divided. The first division is the nucleus, comprising a vowel or vowels. Here, 'vowels' means a diphthong or triphthong. The second division is the coda comprising the final consonant or consonants, if any.

In a mora syllable tree, the portion of the syllable that follows the onset consists of one or more moras. Each mora is a unit of syllable time, or 'weight', and each one is a consonant (C) or vowel (V). Typically,

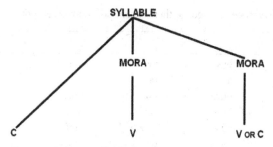

Figure 7.3 Mora syllable tree.

the first mora of the syllable is a vowel. A diphthong is recorded as two vowels (VV) and a triphthong, three (VVV).

6c. Replacement of a word-final VC with a diphthong

If we think about mora syllable trees rather than onset and rhyme, it helps us to see why some children with SSD replace a final VC with a diphthong. The do so because of a weight unit constraint, causing them to produce CVC words such as *bush* as [buə], *keep* as [kɪə] or [kiə]), and *walk* as [wɔə], evidently 'knowing' that something is needed after first vowel but making a mistake about its consonantal nature.

This can be attacked by using repeated sequences of CVCVCV (which the child *can* produce) building up to the removal of the second consonant, for example,

[pʌpʌ-pʌpʌ-pʌpʌpʌpʌ-pʌpʌ-pʌp]. Ideal early targets are 'harmony words' or 'palindrome words' with short vowels and the same initial and final consonants, such as *Bob, bub, cook, dad, kick, mum, nan, none, pip, pop, pup*, and *sis* which are available here: www.speech-lan guagetherapy.com/pdf/palindromes.pdf

6d. Reduplication

Reduplication is the tendency for typical early language learners and older children with SSD to repeat the first syllable of a two-syllable word or utterance so that *daddy* becomes ['dʌ'dʌ], *water* is pronounced ['wɔ'wɔ] and *me too* becomes ['mi'mi]. In remediating this in children with SSD, it is useful to know that a natural phonological tendency is for toddlers to produce the high front vowel /i/ as the second vowel of CVCV babble, or CVCV words (e.g., diminutization such as *blankie, doggie*, and *cuppy*). In intervention, we can take advantage of this tendency by choosing two syllable words with alveolar consonants, and /i/in the second syllable, like the words in Table 7.7, because high front vowels and alveolars tend to co-occur in English, making these contexts facilitative. Early targets could include *buddy, busy, body* and *messy*, and baby expressions and words like *nighty-night, silly-billy, funny-bunny* and *meanie-beanie* that a family might use in child directed speech (or 'parentese').

Table 7.7 Alveolars with high front vowels Adapted from www.speech-language-therapy.com/pdf/high_front_vowels.pdf.

/t/	/t/	/d/	/d/	/s/	/s/
pretty	itty-bitty	daddy	Noddy	pussy	horsie
party	tutti frutti	tidy	lady	messy	wussy
auntie	empty	body	baddy	bossy	teensy weensy
dirty	footy	buddy	teddy	fussy	kissy kissy
/z/	/z/	/n/	/n/	/l/	/l/
busy	buzzy	meanie beanie	pony	silly	silly billy
easy	lazy	tiny	funny	billy	telly
cosy	mozzie	shiny	bunny	dolly	lolly
noisy	daisy	Winnie	money	jelly	chilly

6e. Children who only produce of monosyllables

To increase the number of syllables a child can produce in a word or longer utterance, *known* vocabulary can be employed in a reduplication strategy. For example, suppose the child can already say *bye*. This might be repeated (modelled and imitated) many times in the context of a fun, silly song, perhaps to the tune of 'There is a tavern in the town' or the 'Colonel Bogey March', both 'searchable' and available free as MP3s and YouTube videos on the internet. For parents and clinicians who do not fancy singing, it could be chanted or spoken. When the child can say sequences *bye-bye-bye-bye-bye-bye* ('evenly' and deliberately at first) the clinician changes the timing (*bye-bye | bye-bye | bye-bye*), gradually building up to the child being able to say *bye-bye* once.

Not every family (or clinician) will be able to endure words like *poo, pee, foo-foo, kaka* and *wee* said many times, but where they are tolerable, they are useful as early targets for increasing the number of syllables a child can say, not least because the children themselves are often fascinated by 'rude' words, and their siblings in the younger age group may be delighted to reinforce them! Advantageous early targets are *boo-boo, hoho-ho, dah-dah, no-no, Noo-noo* (naughty Noo-Noo is the vacuum cleaner in Teletubbies) and similar reduplicated combinations. Once a child is producing a range of these easily, a consonant or a vowel in one syllable can be changed to produce a new (real) word or onomatopoeic effect. For example, *weewee* might change to *peewee* or *pee-pee* might be changed to *peepaw* for a fire-engine sound effect, and then *pawpaw*.

SLPs/SLTs have a history of adapting card, board, and other games such as lotto, go-fish, snap, snakes and ladders, dominoes, I spy, tiddlywinks, and matching, sorting, posting, and stacking games, to target speech goals. The card game Spotty Snap (https://www.speech-language-therapy.com/pdf/spottysnap.pdf) for example, is an adaptation of Snap in which you say 'Spotty!' instead of 'snap' when two spotty things pictured on cards match. Once the child can say 'spotty' (perhaps with cluster reduction) the clinician can introduce a different activity with new vocabulary in the form of more 2-syllable adjectives with an alveolar followed by /i/ (*dirty, naughty, pretty, funny, silly, fussy, messy, easy*). In addition, spondees (words with two strong syllables) can be targeted to encourage the addition of a second syllable. *Coco, choo-choo, tutu, pawpaw, bye-bye, dodo, Noo-noo, cha-cha, yoyo, La-La, weewee, bonbon, Bambam* and others are pictured here: https://www.speech-language-therapy.com/pdf/metre/spondees.pdf

6f. Weak syllable deletion and reduction of multi-syllabic words

Some children only delete weak syllables if the word or word combination is iambic; that is, if the stress pattern is weak–strong (WS) as in '*around*' or weak-strong-weak-strong (WSWS) as in '*a roundabout*'. So, for example, they can say the trochaic words *monkey, hoping, single* and *fussy* (SW) but not iambic *giraffe, delay, amount,* and *command* (WS). This tendency is exacerbated if a weak syllable precedes the iambic word or phrase, as it the following examples with WSWWS stress: 'I saw a guitar'; 'we found a balloon'. The weak-strong-weak-weak-strong stress pattern (metre) feeds the tendency for the child to pronounce *guitar* as [ta] and *balloon* as [bun].

For carrier phrases in drill or drill play, and for preference, in functional, meaningful contexts for the child, these WS words are easier for the child to say if the therapist makes the whole utterance iambic, with the insertion of a stressed word. The resultant weak-STRONG-weak-STRONG-weak-STRONG metre, uttered in a sing-song manner, 'carries' the utterance, rhythmically facilitating the child's production of it: 'I *saw* a *big* guitar'; 'I *saw* a *nice* guitar'; 'I *saw* a *red* guitar'; 'I *saw* a *great* guitar'; 'I *saw* a *cool* guitar'; and 'We *got* a *long* balloon'; 'We *got* a *round* balloon'; 'We *got* a *square* balloon'; 'We *got* a *weird* balloon'; Functional utterances might include: 'I *want* to *read* a book'; 'We *went* down *to* the lake'; 'He *put* it *back* in there'; Dad *thought* it *was* so good'; 'I *like* it *very* much'; I *thought* I *heard* a dog', 'Your *keys* are *in* the car'; 'Are *you* as *tall* as her?' and 'We *flew* across to Perth'.

6g. Increasing the number syllables a child can produce

Pursuing the goal of increasing the number of syllables a child can produce in a word or longer utterance, we can capitalize on the natural tendency in development for trochees (SW) to be easier for children to say. To this end, we can target trochaic words and sequences first, gradually adding a few of the harder (WS) sequences (*giraffe*) and WSW (*volcano*) sequences when the child is ready. Fun trochaic sequences that lend themselves to word play and promote repetition might include *silly billy* (SWSW), *polly wolly, dilly dally* and *teeter totter;* and *water pistol, Peter Parker, Wonder Woman, Reader Rabbit, Buster Keaton, Mister Fixit, Henny Penny, Foxy Loxy* and *Lego Island.* An example of pictures and words for trochaic sequences is displayed in Figure 7.4 and four worksheets are available on my website, as follows.

Trochees 1 www.speech-language-therapy.com/ pdf/metre/trochees1.pdf

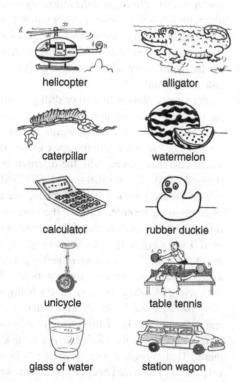

Figure 7.4 Trochaic sequences. Pictures by Helen Rippon, Speech and Language Therapist.

Helicopter, locomotive, caterpillar, watermelon, kookaburra, motorcycle, grand piano, alligator, mashed potato, Easter Bunny, creepy crawly, cheeky monkey, clever puppy, birthday present, picking apples, big banana, camel rider, ballerina, taxi driver, soccer player, underwater, hula dancer, television, Humpty Dumpty, finger painting, escalator

Trochees 2 www.speech-language-therapy.com/ pdf/metre/trochees2.pdf

Letterboxes, tiger lily, very windy, scary monster, service station, stripy tiger, hungry kitty, cosy jacket, clever lady, aviator, tractor driver, unicycle, shopping basket, stacking boxes, supermarket, calculator, shopping trolley, nice tomatoes, laundry basket, rubber duckie, pillowcases, dictionary, competition, excavator, chocolate crackles, agapanthus, Persian carpet, Cookie Monster, grand piano, tiny pencil

Trochees 3 www.speech-language-therapy.com/ pdf/metre/trochees3.pdf

Pencil sharpener, birthday candles, tape recorder, suit of armour, asthma puffer, graduation, Viking helmet, Hello Kitty, pressure cooker, motor scooter, airline pilot, ballroom dancing, table tennis, ten pin bowling, table tennis, exercising, scuba diving, entertainer, ballerina, hula dancer, opera singer, film director, portrait painter, carpet layer, fortune teller, respirator, coffee maker, vacuum cleaner, concertina

Trochees 4 www.speech-language-therapy.com/ pdf/metre/trochees4.pdf

Ukulele, movie camera, tennis player, toilet paper, salad sandwich, bunch of roses, fortune cookie, apple blossom, window cleaner, paper hanger, teeter totter, vaccination, milk and cookies, bunch of daisies, station wagon, music teacher, salad dressing, taxi driver, glass of water, education, swimming lesson, synthesizer, stormy weather, consultation, swimming teacher, exclamation, animation, plastic bottle, four-leaf clover, end of freeway

It is relatively easy to think of trochaic and non-trochaic sequences related to children's interests. For example, a child who likes the media franchise character Ben 10 might enjoy trochees such as *Alan Albright, Armodrillo, Charm of Bezel, Code of Conduct, Colonel Rozum,*

Cooper Daniels, Doctor Viktor, Kevin Levin, Mr. Smoothy, Spidermonkey, Water Hazard and *Yamamoto* targeted first, before moving on to non-trochaic sequences, e.g., *Omnitrix, Alien Swarm, Amp-Fibian, Rust Bucket III* and *XLR8*.

6h. Cluster reduction

Remarkably, English-learning 2-year-olds typically produce some combination of clusters SIWI, SFWF, or both, and by the age of 3;5, full clusters are produced at least 75% of the time! The general trend in acquiring clusters is from complete deletion (which, like ICD, is rare in English), such as [ɪm] for *swim*, to deletion of one element, for example, [wim] for *swim*, to substitution of one element, for example, [fwim] for *swim*, to correct production, that is, [swɪm] for *swim*. When an element of a two-element cluster is deleted, it is typically, but not always, the most marked one, that is, the one that is most *uncommon* in the languages of the world. For example, /s/ is deleted from *snail* and *squash*, and liquids are deleted from *blue* and *drop*. Similarly, /s/ is deleted from the adjuncts /sp/, /st/, and /sk/. Note that for some linguists, /sm/ and /sn/ sit somewhere between 'true clusters' (complex onsets) and adjuncts.

There is an argument in favour of prioritizing more marked clusters to evoke generalization to less marked ones. It invites us to put three element clusters (e.g., /spl, stɹ/) or two element clusters with small sonority difference scores, such as /fl, sl, ʃɹ/, first (for picture and word resources for this see, Bowen & Rippon, 2013). Worksheets with captioned pictures of 2-element clusters with low sonority differences of 2, 3 or 4: /sm/, /sn/, 'ʃɹ' /fl/ /fɹ/ 'θɹ' /sl/ /bl/ /bɹ/ /dɹ/ /gɹ/ and /sw/; cluster minimal pairs; and pictures for 3-element clusters are available free at www.speech-language-therapy.com

Morrisette et al. (2006) postulate that initial /s/+ stop 'clusters' are adjuncts and not 'true clusters', showing that they are not subject to the implicational relationships amongst clusters with respect to sonority (and generalization). Although Gierut (2007) advised against targeting adjuncts because they did not promote system-wide change, it may be tempting, and justifiable, to bend the rules. Because /sp/ and /

st/are 'visible' or easily modelled for children, a clinician may make a reasoned decision to target them early on in therapy for a child with no or few clusters, not with a view to system-wide generalization, but to give the child 'the idea' of a 'two-step sound' (see Table 4.1).

7. Metalinguistic approaches, procedures, and activities

In child speech intervention, working at metalinguistic levels involves the child talking about and reflecting upon:

a. **The properties of phonemes**. These include the place, voice, and manner (PVM) features displayed in Figure 2.1. The properties are given age-appropriate names. For example, /t/, /d/, /n/ and /l/ are called 'tongue up' sounds to denote coronal (palatal and palate-alveolar) **place**; /s/, /z/, /ʃ/ and /ʒ/ are called hissy sounds indicating fricative **manner**; and for **voice**, /s/ and /ʃ/ are called quiet hissy sounds to imply voicelessness, /z/ and /ʒ/ might be buzzy hissy sounds to suggest voicing.

b. **The structures of syllables**. For example, a toy steam locomotive (steam engine) and a tender (coal-car) might be used to contrast near minimal pairs for final consonant inclusion/deletion, in a child exhibiting Final Consonant Deletion (FCD). Using a choice of three to five pairs such as *go-goat, bow-boat, dough-dome, hoe-hose, row-road, no-nose,* and *toe-toad*, the SLP/SLT demonstrates, by detaching and attaching the two components, that *go* does not have a tender (final consonant) and *goat* does. Production practice in the form of drill and drill play might follow once the child can sort the pairs according to their tender-vs-no-tender status. The tender-no-tender metaphor could be reversed for a child with Initial Consonant Deletion (ICD) and the engine representing the rest of the word, using near minimal pairs such as those depicted in Figure 7.5. They are: *eight-fête, aisle-file, ox-fox, arm-farm,* and *eel-feel*. In this case, the child would judge the engine-no-engine status of the word under consideration (*eight* does not have an engine, *fête* does). Note that

No initial consonant vs. /f/ SIWI

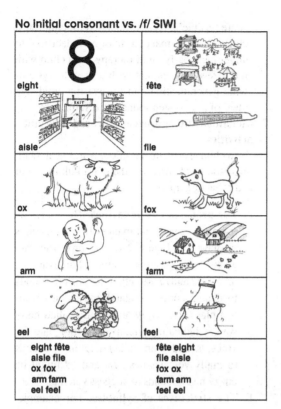

eight	fête
aisle	file
ox	fox
arm	farm
eel	feel

eight fête	fête eight
aisle file	file aisle
ox fox	fox ox
arm farm	farm arm
eel feel	feel eel

Figure 7.5 No initial consonant versus /f/ SIWI. Drawing by Helen Rippon, Speech and Language Therapist www.blacksheeppress.co.uk

the written word, in lower case unless it is a proper noun, accompanies all the pictures.

c. **Communicative effectiveness, incorporating homophony confrontation, judgement of correctness, and making revisions and repairs**. For example, clinician and child could engage in a homophony confrontation task. They might take turns to request pictures (e.g., from a choice of *fun sun, feet seat, foal sole, fox socks, foot soot*) with the SLP/SLT handing the child the picture that corresponded to what they *said*, and not necessarily the one the child *meant*. For example, if the child said [siːt] for *feet*, the clinician would hand over *seat*, and then ask the child, '*Did you really want seat with a s..., or feet with a bunny rabbit sound, f...?*', followed by guided discussion, modelling, phonemic placement input, and for the child, another attempt at saying *feet*.

If the child is able (this usually means 'old enough'), reading and/or phonological awareness (McNeill, A22; Neilson, A49) are incorporated into metalinguistic approaches. All the interventions described in Chapters 1, 4, 5, 8, 9, and 11 incorporate metalinguistic elements. The interventions, in order of appearance in this text, include The Cycles Phonological Patterns Approach, Auditory Discrimination Training as a component of Traditional Articulation Intervention, Stimulability Intervention, Conventional Minimal Pairs Intervention, Perception-Production Minimal Pairs Intervention, Maximal Oppositions and Empty Set Intervention, Multiple Oppositions Intervention, Vowel Intervention, Intervention based on Grunwell's Guidelines, Auditory Input Therapy, Naturalistic Recast Intervention, *Metaphon*, Whole Language based Intervention, Core Vocabulary Intervention, Intervention based on the Psycholinguistic Framework, Parents and Children Together, the Speech Systems Approach for Developmental Dysarthria, Integral Stimulation, Dynamic Temporal and Tactile Cueing, the Rapid Syllable Transition Treatment, The Nuffield Dyspraxia Programme, Phonotactic Intervention, and Visual Biofeedback Interventions: electropalatography (EPG) and ultrasound.

8. Reading

Reading and spelling are sophisticated metalinguistic task which can facilitate work on syllable shape inventory expansion, word shape inventory expansion, and increased accuracy of production of target structures, whether the child is being read to, or is doing the reading. Story reading, and spelling and reading games, can help young readers with speech impairment to increase their awareness of the structures of syllables, and the sequences in which sounds occur, while alphabet letters (graphemes) and printed words provide needed cues and prompts. Games that involve letter manipulation, word assembly and word building with concrete media such as letter-tiles, and similar activities are straightforward to incorporate into therapy sessions (Carson et al., 2013; McNeill, A22; Neilson, A49).

9. Auditory input therapy; AIT, and Naturalistic Recast Intervention

Two intervention approaches, **Auditory Input Therapy: AIT** (Flynn & Lancaster,

1996; Lancaster, 2015; Lancaster et al., 2010; Lancaster & Pope, 1989), and **Naturalistic Recast Intervention** (Camarata, 2021, and see Chapter 5) formerly called **Naturalistic Intervention for Speech Intelligibility and Speech Accuracy** (Camarata, 2010) are broadly similar. In both interventions, multiple exemplars of targets and contrasts are provided, naturalistically, in input, while the child *listens*, or preferably *watches* and listens, during activities that are enjoyable for them, such as imaginative play. There is little or no requirement for the child to imitate adult models or name objects associated with the activity.

Originally described by Flynn and Lancaster (1996) in a workbook that included many ideas for suitable activities, AIT is an important ingredient of PACT (Bowen & Cupples, 1999), and is based on the principle that repeated exposure to a word target enhances saliency, thereby increasing its learnability.

Figure 7.6 provides an example of a story a child might be told with /f/ SFWF as the target. Once the story has been read, it is easy to pursue the goal of 'immersing' the child in /f/ SFWF by developing games related to the story. For example, the child might cut up fabric to make *scarf* after *scarf* for his or her soft toys or play a game involving zoo animals crowding onto a *roof* one by one to be *safe* from a marauding *wolf*.

Other activities for final-f related or unrelated to the story might see the child *stuff* a stocking or long sock to make a caterpillar, carefully cutting lengths of plastic string exactly in half, or feeding a giraffe leaf by leaf, or work with the words depicted in Figure 5.8 A favourite final-f game is to have one *Surf Smurf* after another *surf off* a *roof* (or a *cliff*, or a *wharf*) and into a *trough* of water. It can messy but it's fun! Phonemic contrasts can be introduced in input by saying things like, 'I like this *Smurp*—oops I like this *Smurf*' and reflecting about it aloud, 'You can't say *Smurp* when you mean *Smurf*'.

A game some very young children enjoy is to 'refuse' to place a picture or object in a certain spot unless the adult says its name properly ('Give me the *Smurf*' vs. 'Give me the *Smurp*'), or to put words said correctly by the adult into a container marked 'right' (e.g., ✓ or ☺), and

those said incorrectly in a container marked 'wrong' (e.g., ✗, or ☹).

10. **Minimal contrast therapy**

The attributes of four minimal pair approaches, or minimal contrast therapies (Conventional Minimal Pairs, Maximal Oppositions, Multiple Oppositions and Empty Set), are contrasted in Table 7.8 and described in Chapter 4, and in Storkel (2022).

Music and musical elements in SSD intervention

The next two procedures, 11) Melodic intonation therapy (MIT), and 12) Singing, incorporate music and musical elements, while 13) Prolongation of vowels is sometimes combined with MIT, particularly in the implementation of DTTC (Strand A31). The chanted, sung, and intoned components of MIT can be, and often are, integrated with 14) Slowed rate of production, 15) Progressive approximations, and 16) Single word production drill.

It should be noted, however, that Van Tellingen et al. (2022) reviewed eight studies of music-based interventions for SSD, concluding that evidence of effectiveness of the use of music in SSD treatment is limited. The researchers behind seven of the studies reported positive outcomes, but their findings were based on such weak methodologies that they could not be counted as evidence. Many SLPs/SLTs are drawn to music-based interventions and the opportunity to collaborate with Music Therapists, so the suggestions for future research in this tantalizing area that Van Telligen et al. provide are welcome.

11. **Melodic intonation therapy (MIT)**

Melodic intonation therapy (MIT) might be termed a 'prosodic approach' as it is based on three elements of prosody: the melodic line, tempo and rhythm, and points of stress, and employs intoned utterance and 'visible clues' (i.e., Signed English). Helfrich-Miller, who adapted the approach for Developmental Apraxia of Speech (DAS) in seven- and eight-year-old children with moderate or marked DAS, cautions: '*In an intoned utterance, the tempo is lengthened, the rhythm and stress are exaggerated, and the constantly varying pitch of speech is reduced and stylized into a pattern*

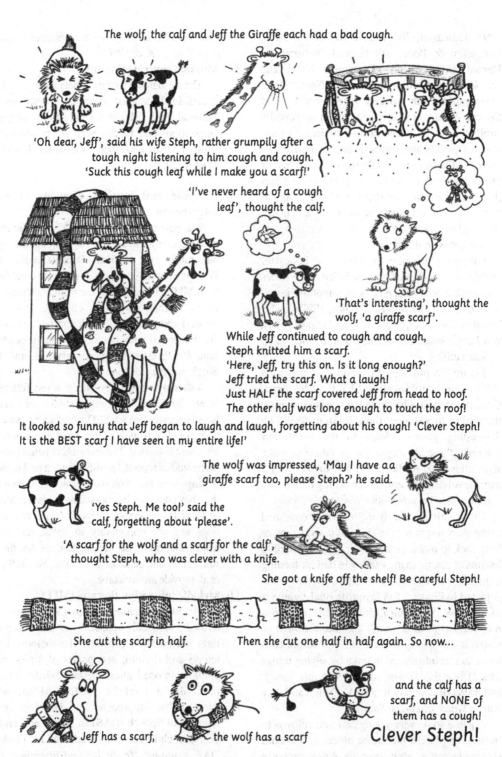

The wolf, the calf and Jeff the Giraffe each had a bad cough.

'Oh dear, Jeff', said his wife Steph, rather grumpily after a tough night listening to him cough and cough. 'Suck this cough leaf while I make you a scarf!'

'I've never heard of a cough leaf', thought the calf.

'That's interesting', thought the wolf, 'a giraffe scarf'.

While Jeff continued to cough and cough, Steph knitted him a scarf. 'Here, Jeff, try this on. Is it long enough?' Jeff tried the scarf. What a laugh! Just HALF the scarf covered Jeff from head to hoof. The other half was long enough to touch the roof!

It looked so funny that Jeff began to laugh and laugh, forgetting about his cough! 'Clever Steph! It is the BEST scarf I have seen in my entire life!'

The wolf was impressed, 'May I have a a giraffe scarf too, please Steph?' he said.

'Yes Steph. Me too!' said the calf, forgetting about 'please'.

'A scarf for the wolf and a scarf for the calf', thought Steph, who was clever with a knife.

She got a knife off the shelf! Be careful Steph!

She cut the scarf in half.

Then she cut one half in half again. So now...

Jeff has a scarf,   the wolf has a scarf   and the calf has a scarf, and NONE of them has a cough!

Clever Steph!

Figure 7.6 Jeff's scarf. Drawing by Helen Rippon, Speech and Language Therapist www.blacksheeppress.co.uk

Table 7.8 Comparison of Four Minimal Pair Approaches: described in Chapter 4.

Principle	Homonymy	Saliency	Homonymy	Saliency
	Conventional Minimal Pairs	**Maximal oppositions**	**Multiple oppositions**	**Empty set / Unknown set**
References	Weiner (1981).	Gierut (1989).	Williams (2003).	Gierut (1989).
Contrasts	**Error-Target** The child's customary error is paired with the target.	**Correct-Target** The child's target sound (one that they cannot say) is paired with a sound the child 'knows' (one they can say). The two sounds are maximally distinct.	**Error-Targets** Up to 4 of the child's targets (sounds they cannot say) are contrasted with their 'collapse'. Target choices are based on phoneme collapses where the child replaces several different sounds with one sound.	**Error-Error** Two errors (two sounds the child does not know) are paired as treatment targets. The child knows neither of the two sounds. The two are maximally distinct.
Feature difference	Minimal or maximal, but usually minimal.	Maximal.	Minimal to maximal across a treatment set	Maximal.
Rationale	Eliminate homonymy by inducing a phonemic contrast.	Increased phonemic saliency facilitates learnability.	Eliminate homonymy by inducing multiple phonemic contrasts.	Increased phonemic saliency facilitates learnability.
Severity	Mild and low moderate.	High moderate and severe.	Severe.	Severe.
Approach	Linguistic.	Linguistic.	Linguistic.	Linguistic.

involving the constant pitch of several whole notes. It is important to avoid using patterns that are [like] *popular songs, because clients often revert to the words contained within the songs instead of the intoned utterance*' (Helfrich-Miller, 1984, p. 120).

Reporting 'encouraging results' with children aged four and five, she noted that MIT required three or four treatments per week over 10–12 weeks, targeting 10–20 phrases per session. It has stringent requirements for advancing through its three levels. A child moves up a level, with more complex targets and less therapist support, when they achieve 90% accuracy in 10 consecutive sessions. Examples of phrases targeted include Level 1 (with slow tempo and exaggerated rhythm and stress): *more money; buy pop; need pen*; Level 2: *You make me mad; Give it me; I don't like*

you; Level 3 (with more natural prosody): *I want more water; I want you to leave; I need some more money.*

Although validated as a short-term intervention evoking qualitative speech improvements in adults with Broca's aphasia (Benson et al., 1994), its efficacy with children with CAS remains inconclusive (Van Tellingen et al., 2022).

MIT was never intended as a stand-alone therapy (Helfrich-Miller, 1994). When used with the kindred techniques embedded in Integral Stimulation (see Chapter 8), such as prolongation of vowels, singing, and tactile cues, it appears to hold promise of clinical utility. Interestingly, Martikainen and Korpilahti (2011) provide evidence, in a single case study of a girl with CAS aged 4;7, of effective treatment composed of 6 weeks of MIT, 6 weeks break from intervention, and 6 weeks of a touch-cue method (Bashir et al., 1984).

12. Singing

Singing lends itself to decreased rate of production (via vowel prolongation), so it may make proprioceptive monitoring easier for some children and allow children who have difficulty 'keeping up' with the words of songs to cope better. 'Slowed down' versions of children's songs and nursery rhymes, such as those on a CD-ROM called *Time to Sing* (https://www.pkcomp.com/apraxiakids/SKUDetailsAPR2FAPR9125.asp) offer an invaluable, entertaining resource for younger children, especially those who are minimally verbal. As well as potentially facilitating self-monitoring, the clinician can run a 'visual check' to see that the child has optimal symmetry and the best possible articulatory configurations while producing the 'sung' words.

For older children, slow karaoke is an appealing vehicle for practice. Suitable songs are available in YouTube and via web searches for 'slow karaoke'. Singing can be incorporated into several of the strategies already described, particularly the reduplication strategy (6d above) for increasing the number of syllables a child can produce, and auditory input therapy. Combining singing with the reduplication strategy, a word sequence such as bye-bye can be repeated many times to slow tunes or lullabies (e.g., Bye-bye baby, bye-bye-bye to *Doeler* a traditional tune for the Christian hymn *Loving shepherd of thy sheep*) (www.youtube.com/watch?v=uGeKNfDTxak), or to the tune of *There is a tavern in the town* (www.youtube.com/watch?v=VstQHnmtJoI). While some families and SLTs/SLPs may not like the words of this rollicking 'drinking song', the tune of *There is a tavern in the town*, at moderate tempo, is conducive to *Bye-bye bye baby, bye bye-bye, Mum Mum Mumma, Mumma Mum, Dad Dad Dadda Dadda Dad, Nan Nan Nanna Nanna Nan*, and similar sequences, with a few tiddly poms added for laughs.

13. Prolongation of vowels

Clinicians can encourage new consonants and vowels, and new syllable structures and word structures to generalize to more challenging contexts by slowing children's utterance rate. For example, model, and have the child say *sat* as [sæ :::t] as in DTTC (see Strand, A31 in Chapter 8), prolonging the vowel, rather than [s:::æt], prolonging the onset consonant. Vowel prolongation is a helpful strategy to apply when a word that is difficult for the child to produce is introduced, such as a significant name. This might be the surname of a new teacher that the child badly wants to say properly. Singing can be incorporated into this technique, and into 14, 15, and 16 below.

14. Slowed rate of production

Within *Temporal and Tactile Cueing (DTTC)* (Strand, A31), and in intervention generally, when the aim of an activity is generalization of newly acquired segments and structures to more difficult contexts for the child (L. D. Shriberg & Kwiatkowski, 1990), it can be helpful to instate a 'slow talking time' as part of daily practice. The clinician can model 'slow talking'—explaining its purpose to parents and other helpers—and providing models and instruction as well as opportunities for rehearsal *with* the child. It is important not to contrast 'slow talking' with 'fast talking'. It is rarely desirable to have a child with moderate or severe SSD to speak *rapidly*, and it is preferable to suggest to parents that they contrast slow rate with 'normal rate' or even 'ordinary rate' (or 'normal talking' and 'ordinary talking'). This may prevent the child from getting the idea that talking quickly is clever. In practice, it is a risky undertaking for many children with moderate and severe SSD because their intelligibility may deteriorate as they gather speed (Klopfenstein, 2009).

15. Progressive approximations

The technique of progressive approximations (Van Riper, 1963), sometimes called successive approximations (Kaufman, 2005; McCurry & Irwin, 1953), is used with shaping, cuing, and other feedback to 'convert' an utterance that the child can already produce into a 'better version' of the utterance (Shriberg, 1975). Usually the improved utterance is not 'perfect' but rather a reasonable approximation to the intended target, intelligible to a familiar or motivated listener. It was used with my client Simon, 19;0 who had Down syndrome. He was learning to travel independently by train and needed to ask for a ticket to Lindfield where his sheltered workplace was. *Lindfield* was beyond his capabilities, but he knew *Lynn* who helped at his school for many years, and associated *peel* with her name because one of her jobs was to assist students to peel and cut up fruit for morning tea. He was trained to say *Lynn-peel* for *Lindfield*, and in the context of the railway station, this was fully intelligible to the ticket seller.

In another example, Max, 6;0, was a late school starter who had CAS, and developmental language disorder associated with cognitive impairment. He wanted to say the name of his school, *Leura Public* /ˈluˌɹə ˈpʌbˌlɪk/, but was calling it [ˈpʌbˌwiˈluˌwə]. Producing /ɹ/ was beyond him, so we compromised and aimed for /ˈluˌwə ˈpʌbˌlɪk/ (the customary pronunciation of many of his age peers). He learned to sequence it correctly, with picture cues in a slide show representing *loo* (lavatory) *wah* (a crying baby) *pub* (a hotel) and *lick* (a person licking an ice-cream) for the syllable sequence *loo-wah-pub-lick* (see http://www.speech-language-ther apy.com/pdf/max.ppsx). Note that his parents were asked for, and after some thought gave, permission to use the words *loo* and *pub*.

16. **Single word production drill**

It is manifest in working with children with moderate and severe SSD, particularly children with CAS that 'practice makes perfect' or at least 'practice makes good enough', and as Thomas et al. (2022) said in the title of a conference paper, '*less frequent is less good*'. Production practice of single words containing target sounds and/or syllable shapes, or practice of 'difficult' or polysyllabic words, facilitates generalization of newly learned speech skills. The child might practice a few pictured words with a common phonetic feature, such as the final-f words (*knife*, *scarf*, *off*, *roof*, etc.) displayed in Figure 7.7.

17. **Techniques to encourage self-monitoring of speech production**

Tasks and techniques to encourage children to self-monitor are embedded in several treatment approaches (Bernthal et al., 2022; Ruscello, A38,

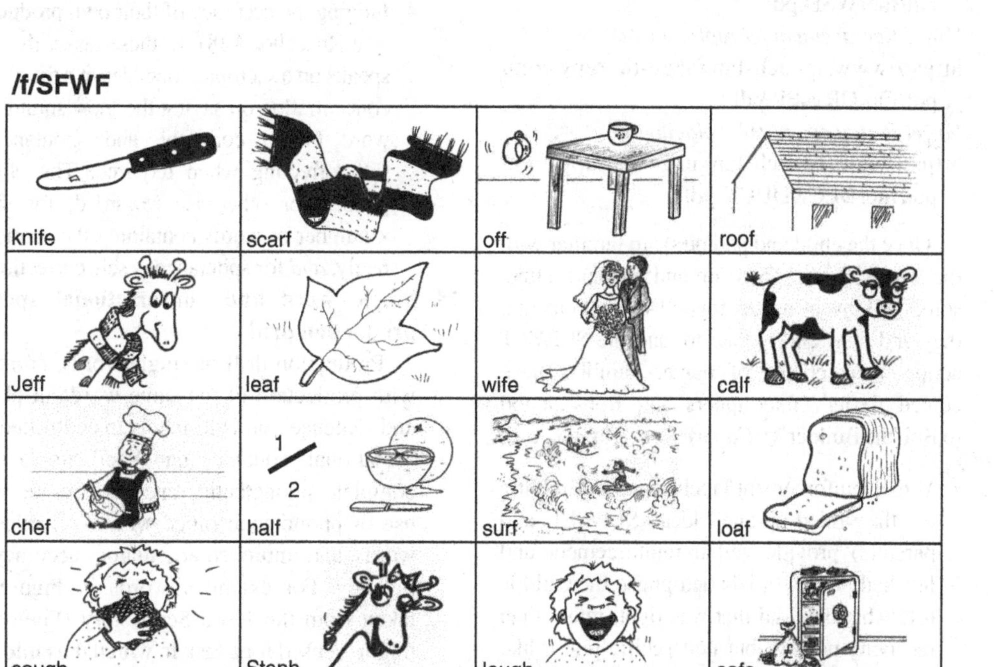

/f/SFWF

knife	scarf	off	roof
Jeff	leaf	wife	calf
chef	half	surf	loaf
cough	Steph	laugh	safe

Figure 7.7   /f/ SFWF—knife, scarf, off, roof, Jeff, etc. Drawing by Helen Rippon, Speech and Language Therapist www.blacksheeppress.co.uk

Shriberg & Kwiatkowski, 1987, Shriberg & Kwiatkowski, 1990). They include the client:

- Judging or discriminating their own correct and incorrect productions of targets during production practice (Baker & McCabe, 2010).
- Judging or discriminating the correct and incorrect productions of targets by another speaker such as the SLP/SLT or a caregiver.
- Working through relevant Fixed-up-one Routine worksheets like the one in Figure 5.7. Several worksheets are available at www.speech-language-therapy.com, e.g.:

Interdental /s/ and /z/
https://www.speech-language-therapy.com/ pdf/fuorINTERDENTALsz.pdf
Velar Fronting
https://www.speech-language-therapy.com/ pdf/fuorVELARFRONTING.pdf
Cluster Reduction (of /sn/)
https://www.speech-language-therapy.com/ pdf/fuorSN.pdf
Weak Syllable Deletion
https://www.speech-language-therapy.com/ pdf/fuorWSD.pdf
Vowel Replacement /ɔ/ replacing /ɜ/
https://www.speech-language-therapy.com/ pdf/fuorORvsER.pdf
Vowel Replacement /ʌ/ replacing /ɛ/
https://www.speech-language-therapy.com/ pdf/fuorDECKDUCK.pdf

Once the child and parent(s) are familiar with the 'fixed-up-one' (revision and repair) routine, some will invent names for self-corrections that they and their child relate to, and the SLP/SLT adopts their choice of name. Families have coined 'fix-its', 'fixer uppers' and 'Bobs', a nod to Bob the Builder's, *'Can we fix it? Yes, we can'*.

- Verbal reinforcement/labelled praise. Building on the 'fixed-up-one' idea, SLP/SLT and parent(s) provide verbal reinforcement and labelled praise. In labelled praise the child is told what they did that was right, rather than receiving positive but nonspecific praise like *'good job'*, *'well done'*, *'great'*, etc., e.g.,

- *'Well done! You fixed that one up all by yourself. First you said dote, and then you reminded yourself and said goat. That was so cool'.*
- *'Oh wow! You said date, and quickly reminded yourself about gate. I like the way you remembered to fix-it-up without anyone telling you to.'*
- *'Terrific! You said dressing down, and quick as a flash reminded yourself and said dressing gown. Great fixed-up-one. It is dressing gown, isn't it?'*
- *'We talked for five minutes, and I heard you do LOTS of fixed-up ones. You changed billy dote to billy goat, shut the date to shut the gate, and dressing down to dressing gown. It's fantastic that you fixed them up all by yourself'.*

It is impressed on the child's family that, once work on a new sound or structure reaches this stage, it is as important to praise revisions and repairs as it is to praise correct word production, and to try to create a 50:50 balance between the two.

- Judging the accuracy of their own productions (see Ruscello, A38). In these tasks, the client speaks on a set topic, 'one idea at a time' while concentrating on saying the 'new sound' (in a word target) correctly, and spontaneously self-correcting when required. The child is praised, or otherwise rewarded, for saying x-number of words containing the sound correctly, *and* for spontaneous self-corrections.

18. Single word and conversational speech production drill

Production drill of single words, combined with production of the same words in phrases and sentences, and ultimately in controlled conversational contexts can facilitate a more complete phonotactic repertoire, more varied use of phonotactic range within syllables and words, and improved articulatory accuracy and prosody. For example, words in Figure 7.7, taken from the Jeff's Scarf story (Figure 7.6) might be used for a task in which the child must say the words in short phrases. Similarly, the child might be asked to formulate short sentences with the words in Figure 7.5 to highlight meaning differences. This could be something quite simple, e.g., having the child say, 'You can't say *eight* if you mean *fête;* You can't say *aisle* if you mean *file*; You can't say *ox* if you mean *fox*' etc., or having them instruct an adult to 'Point to *la*; Point to *laugh*'; etc.

19. **Backward build-ups**

Backward build-ups have long been used in foreign language teaching. Velleman (2003) advocates their use teaching multi-syllabic words, especially with children with CAS. They are also handy for the shorter but 'tricky words', like *yellow*, which may exist as erred fossilized forms. The clinician starts with as much of the *end* of the word a child can say. This might even be all the word except the first syllable. For example, to teach *dictionary*, the clinician starts by having the child rehearse and strengthen production of *arry*, then *shun-arry*, and finally *dick-shun-arry*, after which the word stress and timing are adjusted until the child is saying *dictionary*, naturally with appropriate prosody. *California* might go: *yuh*, then *forn-yuh*, then *lee-forn-yuh*, then *callie-forn-yuh*, and ultimately *California*.

20. **Backward chaining**
    2-syllable words

Backward chaining is a technique that can be used to facilitate the production of two-syllable words in children who only produce monosyllables. The child produces the second syllable frequently (e.g., the *king* in *making* or the *key* in *donkey*) until they can say it easily. The words can be presented on worksheets, cards, or slides, for example:

'King words'
https://www.speech-language-therapy.com/
     pdf/chaining-king.pdf
'Key words'
https://www.speech-language-therapy.com/
     pdf/chaining-key.pdf
'Low words' How Jessica learned to say 'yellow'
https://www.speech-language-therapy.com/
     pdf/yellow.pptx

Then, the highly rehearsed, habituated second syllable is alternated with several potential first syllables. For example, the child might practice *king may king way king tay king*, etc. At first, the child is saying *king-may, king-way, king-tay*, etc., but then the stress is gradually shifted so that they are saying, *making, waking, taking, looking, poking*, etc. It may be necessary to provide simultaneous models at first, and then 'fade' the model, Integral Stimulation style, using DTTC (Strand, A31) if required.

Velar stops SIWI and SIWW

It is quite common to find children with SSD who can produce stops (plosives) word finally (SFWF) and syllable finally within words (SFWW) but not word initially (SIWI) and at the beginnings of syllables within words (SIWW). This is particularly the case for /k/ and /g/, where a child can say the velars in *bag, back, zigzag* and *tic-tac*, but not, for example, in *key* and *go*. A variation of backward chaining can be used to address this difficulty by using final velars that the child *can* already produce, to facilitate initial velars. For example, using the 'King words' and 'Key words' worksheets, linked above, to elicit *king* and *key*, the child rehearses *mong*-key, *dong*-key, *bling*-key and so on, emphasizing the first syllable. The stress on the first syllable is gradually reduced and shifted to the second syllable, making it more prominent: mong-*key*, dong-*key*, bling-*key*, etc., and then the lexical stress shifts to the first syllable and a little 'gap' is inserted between the syllables: *monkey, donkey, Blinky*. Note that the /ŋ/ SFWW in these words is facilitative.

Moving at the child's pace, the clinician works towards just mouthing or cueing the first syllable of *monkey, Blinky, donkey*, etc. (silently), so that the child is saying *key* on his or her own with a strong onset, but not a distorted /k/. Once *key* is well established, the child can be encouraged to practice strings of *key-keep, key-keys, key-keen, key-keel, key-quiche*, etc., (see https://www.speech-language-therapy.com/pdf/key_Keith.pdf) before introducing initial /k/ in combination with vowels other than /i/.

More to Come

The available repertoire of approaches and techniques to apply in the symptomatic treatment of SSD does not stop here. There is more to come in Chapter 8, where the focus is on intervention specifically for CAS; and in Chapter 9, which covers a range of 'tips' for target selection and intervention for phonological disorder.

References

Air, D. H., Wood, A. S., & Neils, J. R. (1989). Considerations for organic disorders. In N. A. Creaghead, P. W. Newman, & W. A. Secord (Eds.), *Assessment and remediation of articulatory and phonological disorders* (2nd ed., pp. 265–301). Merrill Publishing Company.

American Speech-Language-Hearing Association. (2004). *Evidence-based practice in communication disorders: An introduction* [Technical Report]. Available from www.asha.org/policy [https://www.asha.org/policy/tr2004-00001]

American Speech-Language-Hearing Association. (2007). *Childhood apraxia of speech* [Position Statement]. Available from www.asha.org/policy

Baker, E., & McCabe, P. (2010). The potential contribution of communication breakdown and repair in phonological intervention. *Canadian Journal of Speech-Language Pathology, 34*(3), 193–204. https://cjslpa.ca/detail.php?ID=1029&lang=en

Bashir, A. S., Graham-Jones, F., & Bostwick, R. Y. (1984). A touch-cue method of therapy for developmental verbal apraxia. *Seminars in Speech and Language, 5*(2), 127–137. https://doi.org/10.1055/s-0028-1082519

Benson, D. F., Dobkin, B. H., & Gonzalez, L. J. (1994). Assessment: Melodic intonation therapy. Report of the therapeutics and technology assessment subcommittee of the American Academy of Neurology. *Neurology, 44,* 566–568. https://doi.org/10.1212/wnl.44.3_part_1.566

Bernthal, J. E., Bankson, N. W., & Flipsen, P., Jr. (2022). *Speech sound disorders: Articulation and phonological disorders in children* (9th ed.). Paul H. Brookes Publishing.

Bleile, K. M. (2017). *The late eight* (3rd ed.). Plural Publishing.

Bleile, K. M. (2019). *Speech sound disorders: For class and clinic* (4th ed.). Plural Publishing.

Bowen, C. (1996). The quick screener. Available from www.speech-language-therapy.com

Bowen, C. (2009). *Children's speech sound disorders.* Oxford: Wiley-Blackwell.

Bowen, C. (2010a). The quick vowel screener. Available from www.speech-language-therapy.com

Bowen, C. (2010b). The vowel quick screener pictures. https://speech-language-therapy.com/pdf/vowelscreenercolnosymbols.pdf

Bowen, C., & Cupples, L. (1999). Parents and children together (PACT): A collaborative approach to phonological therapy. *International Journal of Language and Communication Disorders, 34*(1), 35–55. https://doi.org/10.1080/136828299247603

Bowen, C., & Rippon, H. (2013). *Consonant clusters: Alliterative stories and activities for phonological intervention.* Black Sheep Press.

Brosseau-Lapré, F., & Rvachew, S. (2017). Underlying manifestations of developmental phonological disorders in French-speaking pre-schoolers. *Journal of Child Language, 44*(6), 1337–1361. https://doi.org/10.1017/S0305000916000556

Camarata, S. M. (2010). Naturalistic intervention for speech intelligibility and speech accuracy. In A. L. Williams, S. McLeod, & R. J. McCauley (Eds.), *Interventions for speech sound disorders in children* (pp. 381–405). Brookes Publishing Co.

Camarata, S. M. (2021). Naturalistic recast intervention. In A. L. Williams, S. McLeod, & R. J. McCauley (Eds.), *Interventions for speech sound disorders in children* (pp. 227–361). Brookes Publishing Co.

Carson, K., Gillon, G., & Boustead, T. (2013). Classroom phonological awareness instruction and literacy outcomes in the first year of school. *Language Speech, and Hearing Services in Schools, 44*(2), 147–160. https://doi.org/10.1044/0161-1461(2012/11-0061)

Cassar, C., McCabe, P., & Cumming, S. (2023). "I still have issues with pronunciation of words": A mixed methods investigation of the psychosocial and speech effects of Childhood Apraxia of Speech in adults. *International Journal of Speech-Language Pathology, 25*(2), 193–205. https://doi.org/10.1080/17549507.2021.2018496

Davis, B., Jakielski, K., & Marquardt, T. (1998). Developmental apraxia of speech: Determiners of differential diagnosis. *Clinical Linguistics & Phonetics, 12*(1), 25–45. https://doi.org/10.3109/02699209808985211

Dodd, B., Crosbie, S., Zhu, H., Holm, A., & Ozanne, A. (2002). *Diagnostic evaluation of articulation and phonology (DEAP)*. Psychological Corporation.

Elbert, M., Powell, T. W., & Swartzlander, P. (1991). Toward a technology of generalization: How many exemplars are sufficient? *Journal of Speech and Hearing Research*, *34*(1), 81–87. https://doi.org/10.1044/jshr.3401.81

Flipsen, P., Jr. (2022). *Remediation of /r/ for SLPs*. Plural Publishing, Inc.

Flynn, L., & Lancaster, G. (1996). *Children's phonology sourcebook*. Winslow Press.

Gierut, J. (1989). Maximal opposition approach to phonological treatment. *Journal of Speech and Hearing Disorders*, *54*(1), 9–19. https://doi.org/10.1044/jshd.5401.09

Gierut, J. A. (1998). Treatment efficacy: Functional phonological disorders in children. *Journal of Speech, Language, and Hearing Research: JSLHR*, *41*(1), S85–S100. https://doi.org/10.1044/jslhr.4101.s85

Gierut, J. (2007). Phonological complexity and language learnability. *American Journal of Speech-Language Pathology*, *16*(1), 6–17. https://doi.org/10.1044/1058-0360(2007/003)

Granger, R. (2005). *Word flips*. Super Duper Publications.

Grunwell, P. (1989). Developmental phonological disorders and normal speech development: A review and illustration. *Child Language Teaching and Therapy*, *5*(3), 304–319. https://doi.org/10.1177%2F026565908900500305

Helfrich-Miller, K. R. (1983). The use of melodic intonation therapy with developmentally apractic children: A clinical perspective. *Journal of the Pennsylvania Speech-Language-Hearing Association*, 1–15.

Helfrich-Miller, K. R. (1984). Melodic intonation therapy with developmentally apraxic children. *Seminars in Speech and Language*, *5*(2), 119–125. https://doi.org/10.1055/s-0028-1082518

Helfrich-Miller, K. R. (1994), Clinical perspective: Melodic intonation therapy for developmental apraxia. *Clinics in Communication Disorders*, *4*(3), 175–182. PMID: 7994292.

Hesketh, A. (2010). Metaphonological intervention. In A. L. Williams, S. McLeod, & R. J. McCauley (Eds.), *Interventions for speech sound disorders in children* (pp. 247–274). Brookes Publishing.

Hodson, B. (2004). *HAPP-3: Hodson assessment of phonological patterns* (3rd ed.). Pro-Ed.

Hodson, B. (2011, April 05). Enhancing phonological patterns of young children with highly unintelligible speech. *The ASHA Leader*, *16*(4), 16–19. https://doi.org/10.1044/leader.FTR2.16042011.16

Holland, A. L., & Nelson, R. L. (2020). *Counseling in communication disorders: A wellness perspective* (3rd ed.). Plural.

Iuzzini, J., & Forrest, K. (2010). Evaluation of a combined treatment approach for childhood apraxia of speech. *Clinical Linguistics & Phonetics*, *24*(4–5), 335–345. https://doi.org/10.3109/02699200903581083

James, D. G. H. (2006). Hippopotamus is so hard to say: Children's acquisition of polysyllabic words. *Unpublished PhD thesis, University of Sydney*. http://hdl.handle.net/2123/1638

Kaufman, N. (2005). *Kaufman speech praxis workout book*. Northern Speech Services.

Klein, E. S. (1996). Phonological/traditional approaches to articulation therapy: A retrospective group comparison. *Language, Speech and Hearing Services in Schools*, *27*(4), 314–323. https://doi.org/10.1044/0161-1461.2704.314

Klopfenstein, M. (2009). Interaction between prosody and intelligibility. *International Journal of Speech-Language Pathology*, *11*(4), 326–331. https://doi.org/10.1080/17549500903003094

Kostner, T. L., & Jakielski, K. J. (2004). Efficacy of integral stimulation intervention for CAS: A case study. Results of integral stimulation intervention in three children. *Paper presented at the American Speech-Language-Hearing Association Convention*, ASHA, *Philadelphia*, PA.

Lancaster, G. (2015). Auditory input therapy. In C. Bowen, *Children's speech sound disorders* (2nd ed., pp. 184–188). Wiley-Blackwell.

Lancaster, G., Levin, A., Pring, T., & Martin, S. (2010). Treating children with phonological problems: Does an eclectic approach to therapy work? *International Journal of Language and Communication Disorders*, *45*(2), 174–181. https://doi.org/10.3109/13682820902818888

Lancaster, G., & Pope, L. (1989). *Working with children's phonology*. Winslow Press.

Maas, E., Butalla, C. E., & Farinella, K. A. (2012). Feedback frequency in treatment for childhood apraxia of speech. *Journal of Speech, Language, and Hearing Research*, *55*(2), 561–578. https://doi.org/10.1044/1058-0360(2012/11-0119)

Maassen, B. (2002). Issues contrasting adult acquired versus developmental apraxia of speech. *Seminars in Speech and Language*, *23*(4), 257–266. http://dx.doi.org/10.1055/s-2002-35804

Martikainen, A., & Korpilahti, P. (2011). Intervention for childhood apraxia of speech: A single-case study. *Child Language Teaching and Therapy*, *27*(2), 9–20. https://doi.org/10.1177%2F0265659010369985

McCurry, W. H., & Irwin O. C. (1953). A study of word approximations in the spontaneous speech of infants. *The Journal of Speech and Hearing Disorders*, *18*(2), 133–139. https://doi.org/10.1044/jshd.1802.133

Miccio, A. W. (2005). A treatment program for enhancing stimulability. In: Kamhi, A. G., & Pollock, K. E. (Eds.), *Phonological disorders in children: Clinical decision making in assessment and intervention* (pp. 163–173). Paul H. Brookes Publishing Co.

Miccio, A. W., & Elbert, M. (1996). Enhancing stimulability: a treatment program. *Journal of Communication Disorders*, *29*(4), 335–351. https://doi.org/10.1016/0021-9924(96)00016-0

Miller, G. J., Lewis, B., Benchek, P., Freebairn, L., Tag, J., Budge, K., Iyengar, S. K., Voss-Hoynes, H., Taylor, H. G., & Stein, C. (2019). Reading Outcomes for individuals with histories of suspected childhood apraxia of speech. *American Journal of Speech-Language Pathology*, *28*(4), 1432–1447. https://doi.org/10.1044/2019_AJSLP-18-0132

Miron, C. (2012). The parent experience: When a child is diagnosed with childhood apraxia of speech. *Communication Disorders Quarterly*, *33*(2), 96–110. https://doi.org/10.1177%2F1525740110384131

Miron, C. (2013). *The critical encounter: Facilitating positive parent adaptation to CAS.* Apraxia Kids. CASANA. https://www.apraxia-kids.org/apraxia_kids_library/giving-the-news-how-to-talk-to-parents-about-the-apraxia-diagnosis

Morrisette, M. L., Farris, A. W., & Gierut, J. A. (2006). Applications of learnability theory to clinical phonology. *International Journal of Speech-Language Pathology*, *8*(3), 207–219. https://doi.org/10.1080/14417040600823284

Nelson, K. (1973). Structure and strategy in learning to talk. *Monographs of the Society for Research in Child Development*, *38*(1/2), 1–135. Stable URL https://www.jstor.org/stable/1165788

Rusiewicz, H. L., Maize, K., & Ptakowski, T. (2018). Parental experiences and perceptions related to childhood apraxia of speech: Focus on functional implications. *International Journal of Speech-Language Pathology*, *20*(5), 569–580. https://doi.org/10.1080/17549507.2017.1359333

Rvachew, S., & Matthews, T. (2017). Using the syllable repetition task to reveal underlying speech processes in childhood apraxia of speech: A tutorial. *Canadian Journal of Speech-Language Pathology and Audiology*, *41*(1), 106–126. http://www.cjslpa.ca/detail.php?ID=1207&lang=en

Secord, W., Boyce, S., Donohue, J., Fox, R., & Shine, R. (2007). *Eliciting sounds: Techniques and strategies for clinicians* (2nd ed.). Delmar Cengage Learning.

Segal, O., Tubi, R., & Ben-David, A. (2022). Lexical stress in Hebrew-speaking children with and without Childhood apraxia of speech. *Paper presented at the American Speech, Language, Hearing Association Convention*, ASHA, New Orleans, Louisiana.

Shinnar, S., Rapin, I., Arnold, S., Tuchman, R. F., Shulman, L., Ballaban-Gil, K., Maw, M., Deuel, R. K., & Volkmar, F. R. (2001). Language regression in childhood. *Pediatric Neurology*, *24*(3), 183–189. https://doi.org/10.1016/s0887-8994(00)

Shriberg, L., & Kwiatkowski, J. (1987). A retrospective study of spontaneous generalization in speech-delayed children. *Language, Speech and Hearing Services in Schools*, *18*(2), 144–157. https://doi.org/10.1044/0161-1461.1802.144

Shriberg, L. D. (1975). A response evocation program for /ɚ/. *Journal of Speech and Hearing Disorders*, *40*(1), 92–105. https://doi.org/10.1044/jshd.4001.92

Shriberg, L. D., Aram, D. M., & Kwiatkowski, J. (1997). Developmental apraxia of speech: III. A subtype marked by inappropriate stress. *Journal of Speech, Language, and Hearing Research*, *40*(2), 313–337. https://doi.org/10.1044/jslhr.4002.313

Shriberg, L. D., Campbell, T. F., Karlsson, H. B., McSweeney, J. L., & Nadler, C. J. (2003). A diagnostic marker for childhood apraxia of speech: The lexical stress ratio. *Clinical Linguistics & Phonetics*, *17*(7), 549–574. https://doi.org/10.1080/0269920031000013812

Shriberg, L. D., & Kwiatkowski, J. (1990). Self-monitoring and generalization in preschool speech-delayed children. *Language Speech and Hearing Services in Schools*, *21*(3), 157–170. https://doi.org/10.1044/0161-1461.2103.157

Shriberg, L. D., Strand, E. A., Fourakis, M., Jakielski, K. J., Hall, S. D., Karlsson, H. B., Mabie, H. L., McSweeny, J. L., Tilkens, C. M., & Wilson, D. L. (2017a). A diagnostic marker to discriminate childhood apraxia of speech from speech delay: Introduction. *Journal of Speech, Language, and*

Hearing Research, *60*(4), S1094–1095. https://dx.doi.org/10.1044%2F2016_JSLHR-S-16-0148

Shriberg, L. D., Strand, E. A., Fourakis, M., Jakielski, K. J., Hall, S. D., Karlsson, H. B., Mabie, H. L., McSweeny, J. L., Tilkens, C. M., & Wilson, D. L. (2017b). A diagnostic marker to discriminate childhood apraxia of speech from speech delay: I. Development and description of the Pause Marker. *Journal of Speech, Language, and Hearing Research*, *60*(4), S1096–S1117. https://doi.org/10.1044/2016_jslhr-s-15-0296

Shriberg, L. D., Strand, E. A., Fourakis, M., Jakielski, K. J., Hall, S. D., Karlsson, H. B., Mabie, H. L., McSweeny, J. L., Tilkens, C. M., & Wilson, D. L. (2017c). A diagnostic marker to discriminate childhood apraxia of speech from speech delay: II. Validity studies of the Pause Marker. *Journal of Speech, Language, and Hearing Research*, *60*(4), S1118–1134. https://doi.org/10.1044/2016_jslhr-s-15-0297

Shriberg, L. D., Strand, E. A., Fourakis, M., Jakielski, K. J., Hall, S. D., Karlsson, H. B., Mabie, H. L., McSweeny, J. L., Tilkens, C. M., & Wilson, D. L. (2017d). A diagnostic marker to discriminate childhood apraxia of speech from speech delay: III. Theoretical coherence of the Pause Marker with speech processing deficits in Childhood Apraxia of Speech. *Journal of Speech, Language, and Hearing Research*, *60*(4), S1135–1152. https://doi.org/10.1044/2016_jslhr-s-15-0298

Shriberg, L. D., Strand, E. A., Fourakis, M., Jakielski, K. J., Hall, S. D., Karlsson, H. B., Mabie, H. L., McSweeny, J. L., Tilkens, C. M., & Wilson, D. L. (2017e). A diagnostic marker to discriminate childhood apraxia of speech from speech delay: IV. The Pause Marker Index. *Journal of Speech, Language, and Hearing Research*, *60*(4), S1153–1169. https://doi.org/10.1044/2016_jslhr-s-16-0149

Storkel, H. L. (2022). Minimal, maximal, or multiple: Which contrastive intervention approach to use with children with speech sound disorders? *Language, Speech, and Hearing Services in Schools*, *53*(3), 632–645. https://doi.org/10.1044/2021_LSHSS-21-00105

Strand, E., & McCauley, R. J. (1999). Assessment procedures for treatment planning in children with phonologic and motor speech disorders. In A. Caruso & E. Strand (Eds.), *Clinical management of motor speech disorders in children* (pp. 73–107). Thieme-Stratton.

Strand, E. A., & McCauley, R. J. (2019a). *Dynamic evaluation of motor speech skill*. Paul Brookes Publishing Co. https://bit.ly/DEMSS

Strand, E. A., & McCauley, R. J. (2019b). *Dynamic evaluation of motor speech skill (DEMSS) manual*. Paul Brookes.

Thomas, D. C., Murray, E., Przulj, M., & McCabe, P. (2022, July). Less frequent is less good: A single case experimental design study of once weekly ReST therapy. *Paper presented at the Apraxia-Kids Research Symposium*, CASANA, Las Vegas.

Tilkens, C. M., Karlsson, H. B., Fourakis, M., Hall, S. D., Mabie, H. L., McSweeny, J. L., … Shriberg, L. D. (2017). A diagnostic marker to discriminate childhood apraxia of speech (CAS) from Speech Delay (SD). *(Technical Report 22)*. Waisman Center. https://www.waisman.wisc.edu/phonology

Turner, S. J., Vogel, A. P., Parry-Fielder, B., Campbell, R., Scheffer, I. E., & Morgan, A. T. (2019). Looking to the future: Speech, language, and academic outcomes in an adolescent with childhood apraxia of speech. *Folia Phoniatrica et Logopaedica*, *71*(5–6), 203–215. https://doi.org/10.1159/000500554

Van Riper, C., & Irwin, J. V. (1958). *Voice and articulation*. Prentice Hall.

Van Riper, C. (1963). *Speech correction: Principles and methods*. Prentice Hall.

van Tellingen, M., Hurkmans, J., Terband, H., Jonkers, R., & Maassen, B. (2022). Music and musical elements in the treatment of childhood speech sound disorders: A systematic review of the literature. *International Journal of Speech-Language Pathology*, 1–17. Advance online publication. https://doi.org/10.1080/17549507.2022.2097310

Velleman, S. (2002). Phonotactic therapy. *Seminars in Speech and Language*, *23*(1), 43–57. https://doi.org/10.1055/s-2002-23510

Velleman, S. L. (2003). *Resource guide for childhood apraxia of speech*. Delmar Thomson Learning.

Velleman, S. L. (2005a, November 19). Apraxia and phonology. In L. Flahive, S. L. Velleman, & B. W. Hodson, *Mini-seminar handout*. ASHA National Convention.

Velleman, S. L., & Strand, K. (1994). Developmental verbal dyspraxia. In J. E. Bernthal & N. W. Bankson (Eds.), *Child phonology: Characteristics, assessment, and intervention with special populations* (pp. 110–139). Thieme Medical Publishing, Inc.

Weiner, F. (1981). Treatment of phonological disability using the method of meaningful contrast: Two case studies. *Journal of Speech and Hearing Disorders*, *46*(1), 97–103. https://doi.org/10.1044/jshd.4601.97

Williams, A. L. (2003). *Speech disorders: Resource guide for preschool children*. Thomson Delmar Learning.

Williams, A. L., & Sugden, E. (2021). Multiple oppositions intervention. In A. L. Williams, S. McLeod, & R. J. McCauley (Eds.), *Interventions for speech sound disorders in children* (2nd ed.), 1689-361. Brookes Publishing Co.

Williams, P., & Stephens, H. (Eds.). (2004). *The nuffield centre dyspraxia programme* (3rd ed.). Nuffield Centre Dyspraxia Programme Ltd.

Chapter 8
Motor Speech Disorders

This chapter is about children, young people, and adults with the Motor Speech Disorders (MSD) Childhood Apraxia of Speech (CAS) and Developmental Dysarthria, also known as Childhood Dysarthria. It begins with a summary of the principles of motor learning (PML) defined as 'a set of processes associated with practice or experience leading to relatively permanent changes in the capability for movement' (Schmidt & Lee, 2011; Schmidt et al., 2019, p. 410; and see; Maas et al., 2008). These principles are central to the dynamic assessment (DA) and evidence-based treatment of CAS. Then follow eight contributions, A27 to A34.

Assessing MSD

In A27 is Dr. Megan Overby's account of her work on a clinically applicable early warning system for speech delay. She studies early vocalisations and speech sound development of infants who are later assessed and diagnosed with SSD. Then, in A28, Dr. Amy Skinder-Meredith surveys diagnostic evaluations that go beyond segmental errors to consider the suprasegmental and physiological aspects of speech. Next, in A29, Dr. Kristen Allison explains intelligibility measurement, via word identification approaches, and scaled rating approaches (Allison, 2020) in children with MSD.

Intervention for MSD

Moving on to intervention, Dr. Lindsay Pennington (A30) unpacks the principles and practice of the Speech Systems Approach. This evidence based short-term motor learning intervention is demonstrably effective in improving intelligibility in 6- to 18-year-olds with developmental dysarthria. It is delivered 1-to-1, three times per week for 6 weeks, targeting speech intensity and rate. This is followed by Dr. Edythe Strand (A31) who updates readers on her influential work in assessing children with MSD, covering the *Dynamic Evaluation of Motor Speech Skill: DEMSS*, and intervening with the *Dynamic Temporal and Tactile Cueing: DTTC* approach. In another progress report on a constantly developing treatment approach for CAS, Dr. Patricia McCabe (A32) describes continual advances with the *Rapid Syllable Transition Treatment: ReST*. There is a river of ReST research, with so many tributaries, issuing from ReST-HQ in Sydney, Australia that it is almost impossible to stay abreast of its progress. Readers are advised to visit https://rest.sydney.edu. au periodically for a research and resources update. Dr. Pam Williams (A33) follows, reviewing the current iteration of the *Nuffield Centre Dyspraxia Programme: NDP3*, which is also carefully refined, revised, and expanded in response to collaborative research evidence.

CAS in Children and across the Lifespan

To date, DTTC, NDP3, ReST, and Integrated Phonological Intervention: IPA are the only four interventions for CAS that are supported by robust research evidence. Each has been developed for children in different age-ranges, and different severities of involvement, ability levels, and treatment needs. All these factors can change over time, and children – and ultimately, adolescents and adults – may make one or more transitions from one form of intervention to another.

DTTC is suited to younger children with moderate to severe CAS who are just embarking on treatment. NDP3 is designed for 4- to 12-year-olds with mild to severe MSD, including CAS, often called Developmental Verbal Dyspraxia (DVD) in the UK, where the NDP3 originated. ReST was developed for 4- to 13-year-olds with a primary diagnosis of 'less severe' CAS with no concomitant speech and language issues. IPA (Gillon & McNeill, 2007 see https://tinyurl.com/ IPAintegratedApraxia; Gillon & Moriarty, 2007; Moriarty & Gillon, 2006) is designed for 4- to 7-year-olds with 'less severe' CAS to improve their speech production, phonological awareness, and letter-sound knowledge.

The contributions in this chapter conclude with Dr. Patricia McCabe in A34 where she delivers details of nascent research into the lifelong speech and psychological consequences of CAS, with suggestions for both (a) informing families and individuals diagnosed with CAS as children, and (b) ongoing transdisciplinary management.

Principles of Motor Learning

The precursors to motor learning, including speech motor learning are

1. Motivation.
2. Focused attention.
3. Pre-practice before entering the practice phase.

If a child cannot accomplish the three precursors, the clinician and parents may need to consider a behaviour management plan, implemented by a suitably qualified professional (Bitter, A13; Stoeckel, A14). Such a management plan may be helpful for children who

- cannot focus or co-operate easily in sessions,
- are unduly reluctant candidates for therapy with limited motivation,
- find it difficult or impossible to attend and stay on task,
- have behaviours of concern,
- are otherwise unable to engage in intervention, particularly in pre-practice.

It is essential for parents (and us) to know that simply attending intervention sessions will have little or no impact on the speech of children with CAS unless they participate adequately in activities associated with motor learning. It is also important that we recognise the limits of our professional expertise and not attempt to address issues, such as behaviour of concern (Chan et al., 2012) that are best managed by a paediatrician, counsellor, clinical psychologist, or other professional, or indeed, by the child's family.

The conditions of practice for motor learning, including speech motor learning are

1. Motivation.
2. Goal and target setting (what will be practiced, and how many times).
3. Instructions (how directions will be delivered).
4. Modelling (e.g., simultaneous production/ immediate imitation/delayed imitation as in DTTC; with a written/print component as in ReST).
5. The setting and with whom (i.e., where the practice occurs and who will be present).
6. Feedback (e.g., KP and KR feedback, explained below).

Other factors may arise specific to a client. For example, the reinforcement (praise) used should not take up too much time, make too much noise, 'interrupt' the session, or distract the child. It is usually necessary to guide parents in how to deliver reinforcement, providing explicit modelling, practice, and feedback in sessions.

Learning the skills of modelling and reinforcement is facilitated if the parent works *with* the child while the clinician takes a coaching role 'on the sidelines', *showing* the parent, rather than *telling* them what to do, fine-tuning the parents' performance, and explaining why delivering modelling and reinforcement in certain ways may be most effective (e.g., https://www.speech-language-therapy.com/pdf/ppsxmodelling.ppsx).

It is also necessary to choose and develop appealing but uncomplicated activities for the child (and to an extent for the parents) that will facilitate and invite repeated opportunities for production practice. In doing this, use simple carrier phrases to keep the linguistic load manageable for the child. Sometimes, by trying to generate 'interesting' or 'educational' stimuli and activities, carrier phrases, word targets, phrases and sentence targets, the child's tasks can become needlessly complex linguistically and/or conceptually, so distracting the child from the speech task they must learn, and then practice repeatedly.

Repetitive Practice (Motor Drill)

The type of practice SLPs/SLTs aim for is repetitive practice, sometimes called motor drill. There *must* be sufficient trials (or 'repeats' of the target behaviour) within a practice session for any motor learning to take place and for it to become habituated. Habituation is a step towards more automatic speech output processing.

Practice Schedules

There are four types of practice schedule, each with advantages and disadvantages. SLPs/SLTs soon realise that in the 'real world' we may not *have* the luxury of choice regarding practice distribution. Nonetheless we *must* decide which targets to select

and how many will be addressed concurrently or sequentially and communicate this clearly to those concerned: the parents and any other helpers implementing practice away from the treatment room (if practice between sessions is desirable for *this* child) and communicated clearly to the child. The options are massed practice versus distributed practice and random practice versus blocked practice.

Massed Practice Versus Distributed Practice

Massed practice involves fewer practice sessions, but the sessions themselves are longer. This promotes quick development of skills, but poor generalisation. Distributed practice, on the other hand, has the same duration, in aggregate, distributed across more sessions. Distributed practice takes longer, and can become tedious, but has the advantage of promoting better motor learning and may be more motivating over time.

Blocked Practice Versus Random Practice

In blocked practice, all practice trials ('repeats' of the behaviours) of a stimulus (target) are done in one time block before moving to the next target. This arrangement tends to lead to better performance. By contrast, in random practice, the order of presentation of all stimuli is randomized through the session, and this fosters better retention, better motor learning, and, in many instances, higher levels of motivation.

KP and KR Feedback to the Child

It is essential during motor drill to give a child frequent information about his or her movement performance, building their 'knowledge' of what the speech motor apparatus is capable of, what it is doing 'right now', and what it did a moment before ('just then').

There are reports in the cognitive motor literature that adults derive most benefit from finely specified feedback. Conversely, if feedback to children is too specific, their performance can decline. Skilled observations by the SLP/SLT allow the frequency of feedback to be tailored to suit, remembering that it can distract some children and, for some, saving any reward until the end of a session is the most efficient way to proceed.

KP Feedback during the Pre-practice Phase

During pre-practice the clinician models the utterance and provides detailed feedback on 'movement performance' to shape correct responses, and to prepare the child for the practice phase. This style of feedback is called **knowledge of performance** (KP) feedback. In the practice phase that follows pre-practice, the child should be able to adjust productions independently in the absence of both models and KP feedback.

KR Feedback during the Practice Phase

In the practice phase, the clinician minimizes the instances of modelling, really aiming to provide no models. Instead, **knowledge of results** (KR) feedback that diminishes over the course of treatment is provided. This KR feedback is delivered in response to about 80% of the child's responses at first, either in a session or over several sessions, diminishing to 10% as the client's capacity for self-monitoring, instating revisions and repairs, and engaging in self-reinforcement builds. If the child is not doing well in a practice session with KR feedback only, then some KP feedback may be introduced to get him or her back on track.

Rate of Production Trials

There is usually a trade-off between production rate and production accuracy. A slower production rate will, up to a point, increase accuracy. *Varying the expected production rate* can be an effective

technique to incorporate into motor drill, using speech, chanting (Melodic Intonation Therapy) and singing, because it encourages habituation of articulatory movement accuracy while working towards automaticity, a natural rate and natural prosody.

Prelinguistic Indicators of SSD

Since there are no biomarkers for SSD, assigning a child's speech to a diagnostic category is typically achieved by observing characteristics that are known to (or thought to) be coupled with a particular label. The early indicators of SSD, including CAS, that may be observed in infants and very young children, is a longstanding research interest of Dr. Megan Overby's.

Dr. Megan Overby, formerly an Associate Professor at Duquesne University who specializes in childhood apraxia of speech (CAS), speech sound disorders, and literacy. Her publications have addressed potential early red flags of CAS, its social consequences, and associations between CAS and literacy development. She is a member of the Apraxia-Kids Professional Advisory Council.

Q27.   Megan Overby: Listening to Infants at Risk: Vocal Play, Babbling and Sounds

The ability to identify probable features of atypical vocal play, babbling and emerging prelinguistic speech sounds can allow SLPs/SLTs to 'get in early', advising parents and caregivers and implementing timely counselling, assessment, and intervention. The advantage of doing so can, potentially, minimize the impact of eventual difficulties with speech, language, and literacy. In the context of communication development and disorders, what does the term 'at-risk' mean, and what does the available literature – including your own work and findings – tell us to look for in the very young age group?

A27. Megan Overby: Early Vocalisations and Speech Sound Development in Infants and Toddlers Later Diagnosed with Speech Sound Delay

Vocal exploration and canonical babbling (CB) are important precursors to eventual speech sound acquisition (McCune & Vihman, 2001; Newman et al., 2016; Stoel-Gammon & Cooper, 1984). Vocal exploration is infants' experimentation with sounds, pitch, intonation, and loudness as well as varied alterations of squeals, growls, and other manipulations of the vocal tract. Canonical babbling is the production of well-formed rhythmic syllables comprising at least one consonant and one vowel, with a rapid and audibly undetectable transition between the two sounds. The onset of CB is usually around 6 months of age (Cobo-Lewis et al., 1996; Eilers et al., 1993) but may be as late as 10 months old (Oller et al., 1998).

During CB and vocal play, prelinguistic infants learn about the relationships among auditory, proprioceptive, and verbal feedback, thereby creating systemic mappings between articulatory movements and their auditory consequences (Guenther et al., 1998; Maassen, 2002). As a result of these systemic mappings, the infant can build the phoneme-specific mappings that lay the foundation for the phonemic categories of the infant's ambient language. This mapping process may partially explain the strong phonetic similarities between an infant's late babbling and early meaningful speech. If vocal exploration is reduced, as might occur in the case of a communication disorder, evidence of these disrupted mappings should appear in an affected infant's prelinguistic vocalisations as changes in the quantity and quality of babbling (Highman et al., 2012; Maassen, 2002). Evidence of CB delays is likely a robust indicator of later developmental disorders (Lang et al., 2019; Oller et al., 1999).Early Speech Sound Development

Findings of atypical prelinguistic speech sound development have been reported in some infants with hearing impairment as well as some infants later diagnosed with either childhood apraxia of speech (CAS) or a non-motor speech sound disorder (SSD) (e.g., a phonetically based articulation or phonemically based phonological disorder). Recognizing potential characteristics of atypical early speech sound development in infants can assist speech-language pathologists/speech-language therapists (SLPs/SLTs) in identifying at-risk infants, leading to potentially early treatment and minimizing long-term communication challenges.

Hearing Impairment

Although the degree of hearing loss experienced by an infant affects the type and nature of vocalisations the infant will produce (von Hapsburg & Davis, 2006), delays in the onset of canonical babbling are nevertheless a well-documented risk to the infant's later communication competency (Iyer & Oller, 2008; Oller et al., 1998; Persson et al., 2020). In the case of profound hearing loss, unaided infants either do not engage in babble-like vocalisations (Oller & Eilers, 1988) or demonstrate CB onset much later than their typical hearing peers (Iyer & Oller, 2008). Differences in the characteristic rhythmic cadence of typical babbling may appear, such that infants with hearing loss may prolong one of the sounds in the babble or produce poorly timed vocalisations (Oller & Eilers, 1988). However, some unaided infants with moderate-severe hearing loss have been observed to babble on time (Davis et al., 2005; Moeller et al., 2007).

Some studies have reported that infants with hearing loss vocalise as frequently (that is, have similar volubility) as their hearing peers (Iyer & Oller, 2008; Nathani et al., 2007) but differences in vocalisation sampling and methodology constrain our understanding of the effect of hearing loss on volubility (Roberts & Hampton, 2018). Furthermore, many infants with hearing loss are identified in newborn screening programs and consequently, parents of infants with hearing loss may interact differently with their infant with a hearing impairment than they do with those with typical hearing, thereby stimulating infant volubility so that volubility is minimally affected by hearing loss.

Infants with hearing loss may also demonstrate differences from typically developing infants in early consonant development (Iyer & Oller, 2008; Moeller et al., 2007), using more labials (e.g., /p b m w f v/) than their typically hearing infant peers, perhaps due to the visual accessibility of these sounds, and more nasals (e.g., /m n ŋ/) (Davis et al., 2005). Infants with hearing loss are slower to expand their phonetic repertoire than typically hearing infants, with fricatives notably reduced until at least 24 months of age (Moeller et al., 2007).

Speech Sound Disorder

There is little information on the early speech sound development of infants later identified with a non-motor SSD, such as an articulation or phonological disorder. Suggested indicators of non-motor SSD at 24 months of age have included: a final consonant inventory larger than that for initial consonants; a phonetic inventory lacking in stops, nasals, and glides; velars but no labials or alveolars; extensive syllable-initial consonant deletions; glottal replacement (e.g., [ʔ] replacing /t/); and fewer than four different consonants (Stoel-Gammon, 1991). Williams and Elbert (2003) examined five late-talkers (two aged 22 months and three aged 30- to 31-months) over 10–12 months and reported that a limited phonetic inventory and chronological mismatch at 33 months could help identify children with non-motor SSD.

Retrospective home-video study (from birth–24 months old) of vocalisations from infants (n = 4) identified with a non-motor SSD as an older child revealed no differences from typically developing infants (n = 6) in either volubility or the canonical babbling ratio (CBR; calculated by dividing the total number of canonical babbles by the total number of babbles; Overby, Belardi et al., 2019). However, even though attainment of 0.15 CBR is an important indicator of CB onset, only 50% (2/4) of infants later identified with a non-motor SSD achieved a CBR of .15 between 7–12 months of age, compared to 67% (4/6) of the typically developing group.

In a different retrospective home-video investigation, Overby, Caspari et al. (2019) compared the longitudinal consonant development (birth–24 months old) of five infants later identified with a non-motor SSD to five typically developing infants. The infants later identified with a non-motor SSD often were often slower to acquire consonants than their typical peers and tended to trail behind their peers in phonological acquisition, although between-group statistical differences were not observed, perhaps due to wide variability of the experimental group. Overby and colleagues suggested that slower overall phoneme acquisition in the experimental group implied that emerging articulatory and/or phonological impairment in infants may be expressed via a broad subtle dampening effect on overall infant speech sound development, although any such effect appeared to be short-lived within the time frame of the study.

Similar findings were reported in a retrospective between-group case-controlled study using home-videos (birth–24 months) comparing three infants who later demonstrated lateralized alveolar fricatives to three typically developing infants (Overby et al., 2020). Although there was no between-group difference in volubility or the age at which erred [s] and [z] emerged, there was a statistically significant between-group difference and small-moderate effect size in the frequency of fully formed consonants. In addition, none of the infants in the experimental group attained CB onset between 7–12 months of age, whereas all the typically developing infants did. Delays in CB onset reduced the frequency with which infants in the experimental group produced syllable sequences, so that the infants favoured the production of singleton consonants or consonant-vowel productions over other phonotactic structures.

Childhood Apraxia of Speech (CAS)

Many (41%–42%) parents of infants later identified with CAS report that that their child struggled to speak or had minimal speech as an infant or toddler (Teverovsky et al., 2009). A retrospective home-video study (birth–24 months old) between infants later identified with CAS (n = 4) and typically developing infants (n = 2) revealed significant between-group differences in volubility of fully formed consonants, but not in overall volubility (Overby & Caspari, 2015). Similar results were reported in a study with a slightly larger sample size group; there was no significant between-group difference in overall volubility between seven infants later identified with CAS and five typically developing control group infants (Overby, Caspari et al., 2019). Yet between-group differences for volubility for fully formed consonants approached significance (p = .64) and Glass's effect size was large (Δ = .95).

Parents of infants later identified with CAS have also reported that their child babbled less than expected (Aziz et al., 2010; Highman et al., 2008) with few variegated syllable structures (Highman et al., 2008). In a study of infant canonical babbling, only 1 of 10 infants later diagnosed with CAS achieved a CBR ≥.15 between 7–12 months old compared to 4/6 for the typically developing infants (Overby, Belardi et al., 2019).

In a longitudinal study of the pre-linguistic skills of siblings of children with CAS, lack of consonant-vowel babble and a limited phonetic repertoire was reported to suggest pre-linguistic CAS (Highman et al., 2013). One infant sibling later diagnosed with CAS produced no consonants at 9 months of age, only three consonants at 12 months of age (/d/, /b/, and /m/), and used limited vowels. Two other studies, both analysing vocalisations from retrospective home-videos between birth–24 months of age of infants later identified with CAS, found that a limited phonetic inventory may be a possible red flag for CAS, specifically the acquisition of three or fewer consonants between 8–16 months, five or fewer consonants between 17–24 months of age, or acquiring the first consonant after age 12 months (Overby & Caspari, 2015; Overby, Caspari et al., 2019).

Despite these converging data, few studies have explored treatment options for infants demonstrating at-risk characteristics for CAS. A quasi-experimental 10-week investigation of 32 toddlers with possible CAS (Mean age = 29.7; SD = 3.44) provided parent education and parent-child activities focused on imitation of word shapes and sounds and reported post-test gains in participants' sound repertoires and imitative skills (Kiesewalter et al., 2017). Findings from a Babble Boot Camp between 2–24 months of age for four infants at high-risk for speech-language delay due to classic galactosemia revealed that when parents stimulated their infant five minutes a day in activities such as reinforcing babbling, engaging in joint book reading, and expanding utterances, infant babbling and meaningful speech was increased over the single control infant (Peter et al., 2020). Children with galactosemia are at particular risk for CAS, with prevalence estimates at 24%, which is 180 times more than estimates for idiopathic CAS (Shriberg et al., 2011).

Clinical Implications for SLPs/SLTs

When considering the communication status of infants and/or toddlers, SLPs/SLTs should evaluate whether there is evidence of reduced babbling and/or limited phonetic repertoire, as these may be possible indicators of later impaired speech sound development. If reduced babbling and/or a limited phonetic repertoire are identified, either through parent questionnaire or direct observation, clinicians may wish to initiate treatment via parent stimulation of canonical babbling and sound production, though clinicians should bear in mind that evidence of the success of such programs is limited.

Early identification and treatment of a communication disorder may take advantage of the brain's neural plasticity and have a significant impact on a child's early learning and development (Bruder, 2010; Zwaigenbaum et al., 2013), but additional studies are needed to guide clinicians with a stronger evidence base for their decisions. Moreover, additional study of the developmental trajectories of pre-linguistic infants later identified with different types of speech sound disorders could lead to standardized profiles of the early emergence of these disorders, as has been done in autism (Roche et al., 2018; Zwaigenbaum et al., 2013).

Children with Suspected Childhood Apraxia of Speech (sCAS)

Like Overby (A27) and Strand (A31) the ongoing quest for reliable means of early identification of CAS has been our next author's clinical and research interest for a long time. **Dr. Amy**

Skinder-Meredith (A28) is a Clinical Professor at Washington State University-Spokane. She is the founder and director of Camp Candoo, an intensive two-week summer program for children with CAS. She has worked with and researched children with CAS for over 20 years.

Her early work focused on characteristics of CAS, such as the trade-off between suprasegmental and segmental accuracy, voice onset time, vowel errors, formant transitions, prosody, and pauses between syllables and words. Her current focus is on incorporating phonological and phonemic awareness with motor speech approaches in treatment. She is on the Professional Advisory Council for Apraxia-Kids and has presented nationally and internationally on assessment and management of CAS. She is passionate about service learning locally and globally, and has led several Mission Trips to Zacapa, Guatemala with *Hearts in Motion*, to provide SLP services with her students.

Q28. Amy Skinder-Meredith: Observing and Rating the Speech Characteristics of sCAS

Readers of previous editions of this book have been enthusiastic about your speech characteristics rating form: SCRF (Skinder, 2000) finding it efficient and practical during differential diagnosis of children with suspected Childhood Apraxia of Speech (sCAS). In implementing it, the clinician records, on a series of 5-point scales displayed in Table A28.1, gaining and recording quick but detailed observations of speech prosody, fluency and rate, voice quality, loudness, pitch, and resonance. Can you lead the reader through this process, discussing these and other suprasegmental aspects of speech output, and the segmental aspects that you would include in your descriptive analysis? The nature of assessment for sCAS varies with the age, cognitive capacity, attention span, and compliance of the child. In general, with a child who can cooperate well with testing, in an initial diagnostic workup at say, 3;0, 5;0, and 9;0 years of age, what procedures do you regard as essential components of a test battery? With children whose ability to cope with formal testing is compromised, what advice would you offer clinicians in terms of the observations they can make in the assessment process?

A28. Amy Skinder-Meredith: Assessment of SSD Beyond the Segmental Errors

Assessments for SSDs primarily focus on articulation and phonology, the segmental aspects of speech. Given that most SSDs are functional in nature (Shriberg et al., 2019), this is understandable. However, if a child has an SSD that includes an organic component, we need to also look at the suprasegmental and physiological aspects of speech. This requires tools that allow us to focus on prosody, lexical stress patterns, co-articulation, voice, loudness, pitch, and resonance. The speech characteristics rating form (SCRF, displayed in Table A28.1) is an adaptation of the SCRF that appeared in Skinder-Meredith (2015) and can be used to judge these characteristics in connected speech.

Connected speech samples can be elicited by having the child tell a story that goes with a wordless picture book or describing a picture. Patel and Connaghan (2014) created a park play scene for a picture description task to elicit words in sentences that contain a variety of syllable lengths, syllable shapes, and sounds. If a child cannot provide a connected speech sample, repetition of multi-syllabic words and short phrases may also yield enough stimuli to use with the SCRF. It will be important to video record the speech sample so that you can re-listen to pay closer attention to each of the areas listed. SLPs/SLTs are trained well in listening to the segmental errors, but often need more time to attend to suprasegmental differences (Hawthorne & Fischer, 2020).

Table A28.1 Speech Characteristics Rating Form (SCRF).

Speech Characteristics Rating
Circle the number that you judge, best correlates with the corresponding speech characteristic:
1-never present 2-rarely present 3-sometimes present 4-frequently present 5-always present

Speech characteristics		Rating scale				
PROSODY		never	rarely	sometimes	frequently	always
1	**Incorrect stress pattern (equal stress, wrong lexical stress)**	1	2	3	4	5
2	**Segmented/syllable segregation – poor co-articulation between sounds and syllables**	1	2	3	4	5
3	**Hyperprosodic (sing-song)**	1	2	3	4	5
4	**Appropriate prosody, stress, and co-articulation**	1	2	3	4	5
Comment						
VOICE QUALITY / RESONANCE						
1	**Hoarse voice quality**	1	2	3	4	5
2	**Breathy voice quality**	1	2	3	4	5
3	**Glottal fry**	1	2	3	4	5
4	**Appropriate voice quality**	1	2	3	4	5
5	**Hypernasal**	1	2	3	4	5
6	**Hyponasal / Denasal**	1	2	3	4	5
7	**Appropriate resonance**	1	2	3	4	5
Comment						
PITCH / LOUDNESS						
1	**Mono-pitch**	1	2	3	4	5
2	**Appropriate pitch**	1	2	3	4	5
3	**Loud voice**	1	2	3	4	5
4	**Soft voice**	1	2	3	4	5
5	**Appropriate loudness**	1	2	3	4	5
Comment						
RATE / FLUENCY						
1	**Slow rate**	1	2	3	4	5
2	**Fast rate**	1	2	3	4	5
3	**Appropriate rate**	1	2	3	4	5
4	**Dysfluent**	1	2	3	4	5
5	**Appropriate fluency**	1	2	3	4	5
		never	rarely	sometimes	frequently	always
Comment						

Prosody

Children with functional SSDs typically have normal prosody. English-speaking children with CAS are noted to use equal-excessive stress patterns, where typically unstressed syllables receive stress (e.g., ['bʌ.'næ.'nʌ] for /bə.'næ.nə/) or may omit the weak syllable to preserve a strong-weak stress pattern (e.g., ['næ.nə] for /bə.'næ.nə/) (Kopera & Grigos, 2020; Velleman & Shriberg, 1999). Their prosody is also impacted by poor co-articulation, which can result in their speech sounding more segmented with inappropriate silent intervals between words (Shriberg et al., 2017). This silent interval is called a pause marker and is theorized to be due to the difficulty with both auditory-perceptual and memory elements of representational processes and transcoding (i.e., planning and programming) the movements for speech (Shriberg et al., 2017).

Voice Quality, Glottal Fry and Resonance

The intelligibility of children with CAS may reduce when they use less than optimal voice quality. Lee et al. (2004) found SLPs rarely screen for voice disorders in children, yet over a third of school-aged children have presented with hoarseness. Hoarseness is often due to misuse of the voice, as in shouting and making vocal noises during play. Both behaviours would be likely to occur for a child with CAS having difficulty being understood due to shouting out of frustration or making play sounds (e.g., revving an engine), which is easier than articulating words (Rusiewicz et al., 2018).

Glottal fry ('creaky voice' or 'pulse register'), a common physiological occurrence at the ends of sentences, manifests when a speaker is running out of air and attempting to vocalise at too low a fundamental frequency. Constant glottal fry greatly reduces intelligibility. *Some* children may be *more* at risk of producing glottal fry due to poor timing between respiration and phonation.

When listening for resonance, it helps to note words where timing of the velopharyngeal mechanism must move quickly from closed to open to closed, as in the words 'can't' or 'seventy'. Sealey and Giddens (2010) noted children with CAS had a longer time delay after the end of nasal airflow to the point of peak oral pressure, indicating that it took them more time to achieve velopharyngeal closure, resulting in more nasal resonance. It is assumed that children with CAS have difficulty planning movements of the velum, as they do with other articulators (Sealey & Giddens, 2010). Consistent with this assumption, researchers have found 50% or more of the children with CAS in their studies to have disordered resonance (Hall et al., 1990; Iuzzini-Seigel et al., 2017; Skinder-Meredith et al., 2004).

Pitch and Loudness

Many parents observe that their children with CAS have difficulty modulating loudness, and I have noted that they have similar problems with pitch. Speculatively, this might be due to poor speech monitoring or difficulty in coordinating respiration and phonation sufficiently to allow appropriate pitch and loudness variation. This can impact their ability to use the appropriate intonation pattern for a statement versus a question.

Rate and Fluency

Rate

When observing rate, note the speed-accuracy trade-off. Children speaking at fast or normal rates may omit syllables and segments. Children using slow speech-rates may be doing so deliberately to maintain segmental or structural accuracy. Skinder (2000) found that children with better segmental accuracy tended towards slower speech while children with poor segmental accuracy spoke at either a normal or fast rate. In a study comparing children with CAS to children with speech delay, Iuzzini-Seigel et al. (2017) found 50% of children with CAS exhibited a decreased rate of speech versus 20% of children with speech delay without CAS.

Fluency

Fluency is of considerable interest. Many parents report dysfluent periods as the phonetic repertoire and the length of utterance increase, and it is interesting to speculate about causes. Caruso and Strand (1999) consider stuttering to be related to motor planning and thus dysfluency and apraxia of speech could be viewed as being related. However, the dysfluencies of children with CAS may differ from those of children who stutter. Hall (2007) noted that children with CAS may sound dysfluent due to their decreased rate of speech and prolonged pauses between sounds, syllables, and words (ASHA, 2007). Hall (2007) discusses the integration of speech and language production processes possibly being a factor. Since the receptive language is often better developed than the speech production in children with CAS, the complexity of what the child is trying to say may stress the output system, leading to disruptions of fluency and prosody (Hall, 2007). I frequently observed children with CAS having a transient period of dysfluencies. Once syntax and motor speech were addressed, the dysfluencies subsided.

Assessment Varies with a Child's Presenting Characteristics

The assessments we use to determine if a child has CAS will vary depending on the age of the child, as well as the severity of their SSD and any comorbidities the child may have. Hence, the guidelines for assessment for each age group are more dependent on the child's abilities than their chronological age.

SLPs/SLTs often ask at what age can we diagnose CAS. The information in the ASHA Childhood Apraxia of Speech Practice Portal (n.d.) suggests that making a definitive diagnosis of CAS prior to age three is difficult for a variety of reasons, such as the challenge of obtaining a sufficient speech sample and potential unwillingness of the child to attempt speech targets. Hence, ASHA recommends stating 'CAS cannot be ruled out', 'signs are consistent with problems in planning the movements required for speech', or 'suspected to have CAS' prior to age three if characteristics of difficulty with motor planning and programming for speech are observed.

The Table A28.2 indicates the components of assessment that are useful at each stage of development. Children with CAS often have challenges in addition to motor programming and planning for speech (Murray et al., 2021; Rvachew et al., 2005). Thus, differential diagnosis is not as much of an 'either/or' process, as it is a method of determining the relative contribution of each communicative strength and challenge the child has.

When a child is unable to comply with a long battery of tests, the following tips may help for getting the information you need, over a shorter timeframe, to aid in differential diagnosis. For a structural functional exam, watch them eat, drink, laugh, and give their parent a kiss to observe the lips, jaw, and tongue. To determine function of the palate, elicit oral and nasal consonants in syllables (e.g., 'pop' when popping bubbles and 'mama' to get the mother's attention). Note if there is any nasal emission or nasalizing of oral sounds and if these errors are consistent or inconsistent to discern if the disordered resonance is due to structure, dysarthria, or CAS. For motor speech, engage the child in an activity that allows elicitation of three repetitions, each, of polysyllabic words. See Figure 7.1 for Debbie James's helpful list of words (James, 2006). This is an efficient way to hear key characteristics of CAS, such as syllable segregation, lexical stress errors, decreased PCC (Murray et al., 2015a), inconsistency of speech sound errors (Iuzzini-Seigel & Murray, 2017; Terband et al., 2019), and vowel errors (Lewis et al., 2004).

Table A28.2 Useful assessment components at various ages/developmental stages.

Age/Stage	Assessment Component	Purpose of Assessment
All ages	Audiological examination	Ensure that hearing acuity is optimal for speech development and that middle ear health is monitored.
Infant/ Toddler	Developmental history of early vocalization, speech and eating from birth to age 2	Characteristics often observed in children under age three with CAS include: quiet baby with little babbling, limited sound repertoire, fewer resonant consonants, limited intonation patterns, delayed first words, reduced syllable shapes and possible groping or uncoordinated feeding (Overby & Caspari, 2015; Overby, Belardi et al., 2019; and see Overby A27).
Infant/ Toddler	Observations and history of pre-linguistic behaviours	Given the high incidence of autism and the overlapping characteristics of reduced communication during the early stages of communication development, the SLP/SLT should screen for Autism. The Autism Parent Screen for Infants (APSI) is one of several Autism screeners and can be used for children 6–24 months (Sacrey et al., 2021). Behaviours characteristic of Autism include impairments in eye contact, visual tracking, responding to name, imitation, language, social development, joint attention, gestures, play, visual examination of objects, and emotional regulation (Sacrey et al., 2018).
All ages	Receptive and Expressive Language	Children with CAS have stronger receptive than expressive language skills. Knowledge of the child's language skills will help determine strengths and challenges for the child and will guide treatment. Children with CAS typically need to work on expressive language skills in addition to motor speech.
All ages	Observations of the neuromuscular condition	General observations of symmetry, strength, muscle tone, gait, and presence of involuntary movements (e.g., spasms, myoclonus, intention tremors, chorea, dystonia) will allow the SLP/SLT to note if there are neurological signs associated with a neurological pathology, such as cerebral palsy. These overt characteristics are more apt to be associated with dysarthria (Pennington, A30) than apraxia. Developmental discoordination disorder (DCD), however, has been found in approximately half of children with sCAS (Duchow et al., 2019)
Ages 3 and up	Examination of Physiological Parameters	To test for dysarthria (Pennington, A30), assess the child's phonatory and respiratory function for speech with a maximum voluntary phonation duration test. By age 3, a child can sustain phonation for an average of 5.5 seconds. As they get older, the length increases. By 7, they can sustain phonation for at least 10 seconds (Robbins & Klee, 1987). Observe voice quality during phonation. Weak, breathy, or strained voice quality, in addition to reduced duration may indicate dysarthria.
Ages 3 and up	Structural-Functional Examination (SFE)	To rule out overt structural deficits (e.g., cleft) or functional impairments (e.g., dysarthria), observe the articulatory structures at rest and during movement to judge the adequacy of the lips, tongue, jaw, and velum for speech production (Murray et al., 2015b). If there is asymmetry, reduced range of motion, speed, strength, and/or coordination, the child may have dysarthria (Pennington, A30).
Ages 3 and up	DDK	When analysing repeated productions of 'pataka', listen for reduced PCC, inconsistent sound-sequencing, lowered rate, voicing errors, and syllable segregation. Murray et al., 2015b found such errors may persist to at least age 12.
Ages 3 and up	Test for non-verbal oral apraxia (NVOA)	Have the child imitate non-verbal oral movements of increasing length to see if there is any groping or difficulty sequencing movement. For example: Pucker | Pucker-smile | Pucker-smile-blow Children with CAS may/may not have co-occurring NVOA (Iuzzini-Seigel, 2019).

Table A28.2 (Continued)

Age/Stage	Assessment Component	Purpose of Assessment
Ages 3 and up	Motor speech evaluation (MSE)	*The Dynamic Evaluation of Motor Speech Skill (DEMSS) (Strand & McCauley, 2019a, 2019b) is appropriate for children ages 3 and above with severe SSDs and reduced phonetic inventories (Strand, A31). An informal motor speech evaluation can be made for older children with a more complete phonetic inventory by systematically increasing phonetic complexity, syllable shape, syllable length and phrase length. The goal is to see where the child breaks down and if they improve with cuing, such as saying the target word simultaneously while watching the clinician and responding to tactile cues. This element of the exam is crucial for choosing appropriate targets for treatment.
Ages 3 and up	Articulation and Phonology	Assessment of articulation and phonology allows the clinician to see if sound errors are limited to just a few sounds, as is the case with an articulation disorder or if there is a consistent pattern of errors (e.g., fronting, cluster reduction, initial consonant deletion), *possibly* indicating phonological disorder. CAS phonological disorder can co-occur (Figure i.1).
Ages 4 and up	Single-Word Test of Polysyllables	Once a child can attempt multisyllabic words, this is a helpful task for differential diagnosis. Children with CAS frequently present with lexical stress errors and syllable segregation (notable gaps between syllables) even after articulatory accuracy has improved (Murray 2015b, Murray et al., 2021). These features may persist into early adolescence (Benway & Preston, 2020). Additional characteristics observed may include syllable deletion and articulation errors; however, children with functional SSDs and poor receptive vocabulary may also present with these errors (Masso et al., 2018).
Ages 4 and up	Speech Sound Inconsistency task	Elicit productions of the same word or phrase across multiple opportunities to determine inconsistency of speech sounds. There are several measures for identifying inconsistency. To differentiate CAS from other SSDs, phonemic and phonetic inconsistency measures tend to be more sensitive than token-to-token inconsistency when using words (Iuzzini-Seigel & Murray, 2017). However, using 5 repetitions of 'buy Bobby a puppy', token-to-token inconsistency was found to be more sensitive (Iuzzini-Seigel et al., 2017).
Ages 4 and up	Phonological awareness	Informal assessments of phonological awareness can start at age 3, but most formal assessments are standardized for children 4 and up. Children with CAS and language impairment also have difficulty with phonological and phonemic awareness tasks (Gillon & Moriarty, 2007; Lewis et al., 2004; Miller et al., 2019).
School-age	Reading and Writing	Children with CAS often have reading and spelling difficulties. They may have syntax and morphology errors too (Gillon & Moriarty, 2007). Children with CAS are at higher risk for reading and spelling deficits, even after motor speech skills improve (Lewis et al., 2004; Miller et al., 2019).

Objective Measurement of Intelligibility in MSD in Children

How intelligible is the child? *Despite the frequency and importance of this question in clinical practice, there is little agreement as to how it should be answered. The process of* assessing intelligibility is fraught with procedural and interpretative complications. These complications are becoming increasingly evident as intelligibility assessment is more pointedly addressed in contemporary clinical evaluations, particularly for children with hearing impairment, phonological disorders, or severe impairments of expressive language.

These are by no means the only populations of relevance, but it is with these populations that the issue of speech intelligibility has been most systematically considered.

Kent et al., 1994

Fast forward almost three decades beyond 1994 to meet our next author who has embraced the challenge of evaluating intelligibility of children with MSD, especially those with childhood dysarthria. She is **Dr. Kristen Allison**, an assistant professor in the Department of Communication

Sciences & Disorders and director of the Speech Motor Impairment and Learning (SMILe) Laboratory at Northeastern University. Her research centres on improving assessment and treatment of motor speech disorders in children, with a particular focus on paediatric dysarthria. Dr. Allison received her PhD from the University of Wisconsin-Madison and completed a postdoctoral fellowship at the Massachusetts General Hospital Institute of Health Professions (MGH IHP). Her research has been funded by the National Institutes of Health and the Cerebral Palsy Research Network.

Q29.   Kristen Allison: Comprehensibility and Intelligibility in MSD

The implementation of approaches, procedures, and techniques, designed to measure speech intelligibility in children with Motor Speech Disorders (MSD) can pose practical difficulties for SLP/SLT clinicians. This is particularly the case for practitioners who have seldom, or never, tried to do so, or who rarely engage with this client group. Clarifying the distinctions between comprehensibility and intelligibility, and the factors that can impact intelligibility – for better or worse – can you provide readers with an evidence-based explanation of the pros and cons of existing assessment methodologies? Are some methodologies that work well in laboratory settings unsuitable for use in 'ordinary' clinical settings? How do intelligibility measures relate to other speech function metrics? Finally, to round off your Intelligibility in MSD 101: are there evidence-based, clinically practicable treatments that SLPs/SLTs might use, with reasonable levels of confidence, in to increase the speech intelligibility of children with MSD on their caseloads?

A29.   Kristen Allison: Measuring Speech Intelligibility in Children with Motor Speech Disorders

Intelligibility is an important construct and outcome to measure for children with motor speech disorders (MSD). Unlike other speech sound disorders, MSD often result in difficulties with speech production that persist into adulthood, and precise production of all speech sounds may not be achievable. For children with dysarthria, impairments in respiratory, phonatory, and resonatory speech subsystems commonly occur in conjunction with articulation difficulties and these impairments contribute to distortion of the speech signal. Therefore, maximizing intelligibility is often a primary goal of treatment. Objective and reliable measurement of intelligibility is important for assessing severity (see Flipsen Jr., A8), evaluating functional limitations, and documenting progress for children with MSD.

There are several definitions of intelligibility, and in the motor speech literature it is defined as 'the degree to which the acoustic signal produced by a speaker is accurately perceived by a listener' (Yorkston et al., 1996). In contrast, comprehensibility refers to 'the extent to which a listener understands utterances produced by a speaker *in a communication context*' (Barefoot et al., 1993; emphasis added). Many contextual factors can influence how accurately listeners decipher a speaker's words. For example, gestures, facial expressions, environmental cues, and augmentative / alternative communication (AAC) devices provide listeners with additional information, typically boosting how much of a speaker's message is understood (Garcia & Cannito, 1996; Hammen et al., 1991). Intelligibility and comprehensibility provide meaningful, but slightly different, indices of communication function; comprehensibility may better reflect how well a speaker is understood in real-life settings, whereas intelligibility more directly reflects the adequacy of the speech signal. Percentage of Consonants Correct (PCC) is another commonly used metric of speech severity (Flipsen Jr., A8; Shriberg et al., 1997). PCC is a direct measure of a child's segmental accuracy but does not take listeners' comprehension into account. Although segmental errors contribute to reduced intelligibility, there is not a direct correspondence between PCC and intelligibility (Hodge et al., 2013; Shriberg et al., 1986).

There are two main approaches to intelligibility measurement: word-identification approaches and scaled rating approaches. In the following sections the measurement procedures for these approaches are reviewed, along with benefits and challenges of each. These methods are discussed in more detail in Allison, 2020.

Word-Identification Approaches

Word identification methods involve having the child produce a known set of target utterances, comprising words and/or sentences, and then having unfamiliar listeners listen to an audio recording of the child's productions and judge what they think the child said. Listeners' transcriptions are compared to the target utterance and used to calculate a percentage of words correctly identified (or %-intelligibility). General procedures for measuring intelligibility using this approach are detailed in Figure A29.8.1.

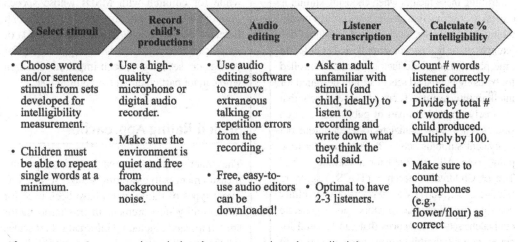

Figure A29.8.1 Summary of word-identification procedures for intelligibility measurement.

The primary benefit of measuring a child's speech intelligibility using a word-identification method is that it provides an objective index of the adequacy of the child's speech for communication exchanges, on a scale that is sensitive to change. Because this method yields a %-intelligibility score between 0–100%, incremental changes in a child's speech production abilities over time are likely to change their %-intelligibility, unless their speech impairment is mild, and their intelligibility was high at the outset. Researchers have suggested that changes in intelligibility of approximately 10–15% are clinically meaningful (Hodge & Gotzke, 2014; Pennington et al., 2010; Pennington, Roelant et al., 2013; Stipancic et al., 2018). The sensitivity of this measure makes it valuable for documenting functional progress due to therapy, or in the case of degenerative diseases, to document changes due to disease progression. Word-identification measures of intelligibility can also help with identifying MSDs in young children (Hustad et al., 2015; Hustad, Sakash, Broman, et al., 2019). For children with cerebral palsy, %-intelligibility at young ages can provide useful prognostic information about speech development (Hustad, Sakash, Natzke, et al., 2019).

Word-identification measures of intelligibility can be affected by listener factors and linguistic factors in addition to the child's speech production abilities. Listener factors include the listener's familiarity with the child (Flipsen, 1995; Kwiatkowski & Shriberg, 1992); and linguistic factors involve characteristics of the stimuli used, notably sentence length and word predictability (Allison & Hustad, 2014; Garcia & Cannito, 1996; Kalikow et al., 1977; Allison et al., 2019; Yorkston & Beukelman, 1981). Therefore, controlling these factors when choosing stimuli is crucial to ensuring that changes in a child's intelligibility over time are 'real' and not a result of differences in the listeners or stimuli used at different time points. Linguistic factors can be controlled for by using published sets of stimuli designed for intelligibility testing. There are several sets that are freely available as part of published research studies. They allow clinicians to select unique but equivalent stimulus sets at different testing time points (see, Allison, 2020 for a summary). The Test of Children's Speech + (TOCS+) software (Hodge et al., 2007) was developed to carefully control for linguistic factors and generate equivalent sets of sentences that can be used for comparing intelligibility over time, as well as to provide an interface for recording, judging, and automatic scoring of intelligibility.

To control for listener factors that can affect intelligibility measurement, it is ideal if people who are unfamiliar with the child speaker serve as listeners. In research settings, intelligibility is generally based on average accuracy of 2–3 unfamiliar listeners. In clinical settings, finding unfamiliar listeners to judge children's speech samples can be a barrier; however, there are many possible creative solutions to this problem (Allison, 2020). If different stimuli are used at each time point, as described above, the same listener can transcribe the speech samples at each time point, assuming their familiarity with the child does not change over that period (e.g., a staff member who does not work with the child, a grandparent). The child's intelligibility score should be interpreted in the context of the listeners used (e.g., familiar vs. unfamiliar listeners).

Although word-identification approaches yield objective, clinically meaningful data, editing audio recordings, acquiring listener transcriptions, and checking listener responses can be time-consuming and is not always feasible in clinical settings. Because of these barriers, word-identification approaches to intelligibility measurement are most often used in research settings. However, SLPs/SLTs who are familiar with these procedures and are willing and able to invest the time can also use this approach in clinical settings. This may be particularly worthwhile for children with MSDs whose speech intelligibility is a primary goal of treatment. Because it requires children to repeat words or sentences, this approach is not appropriate for young or severely speech-impaired children who cannot participate in a repetition task.

Scaled Rating Approaches

The other primary approach to intelligibility measurement is to use rating scales. Several different types of rating scales have been used for intelligibility measurement in paediatric motor speech research, including informal Likert scales (Hustad et al., 2012) and more formally developed, validated scales (McLeod et al., 2012, McLeod & Crowe, A42; Pennington, Virella et al., 2013). Rating scales have several advantages compared to word-identification methods for intelligibility measurement. First, they are easy and quick to administer, making them highly practicable to implement in clinical settings. They also do not require the child to participate in a structured repetition task, so they are more suitable for measuring the intelligibility of young children or those with more global impairments. In addition, rating scales are often completed by a child's caregiver, which allows for incorporation of the caregiver's perspective as part of the evaluation.

Despite these advantages, there are also several limitations to using scaled ratings to measure intelligibility. First, most rating scales index intelligibility using a small range of defined levels (e.g., 5- to 7-point scales with equal intervals), which makes them less sensitive to changes in intelligibility over time compared to more granular %-intelligibility measurements. As a result, rating scales can be less useful for documenting progress in therapy than word-identification methods. Rating scales also rely on subjective judgments of a child's intelligibility, and thus, can have limited reliability (Flipsen, Jr., 2006; A8). Use of validated rating scales, which generally have documented information about their reliability, can help alleviate this disadvantage. Unfortunately, only a few validated rating scales for intelligibility exist.

Two validated rating scales for measuring intelligibility in children are the Intelligibility in Context Scale: ICS (McLeod et al., 2012; McLeod, 2020; McLeod & Crowe, A42) and the Viking Speech Scale: VSS (Pennington, Virella et al., 2013). The ICS was developed as a screening measure for speech sound disorders in preschool-aged children. It asks parents to rate how well their child's speech is understood by different communication partners on a series of 5-point scales and provides an average score that can be compared to normative data. The scale has been validated in multiple languages and is available free under a Creative Commons license: https://www.csu.edu.au/research/multilingual-speech/ics.

The Viking Speech Scale: VSS (Pennington, Virella et al., 2013) is another validated rating scale that was developed specifically for rating severity of speech motor impairment in children with cerebral palsy. The VSS asks parents or clinicians to assign a child's speech to one of four levels between I (no speech motor impairment) and IV (no understandable speech). With only four levels, this scale classifies severity broadly; however, VSS levels positively correlate with transcription-based measures of intelligibility (Pennington & Hustad, 2019).

Although these rating scales are clinically useful for indexing the severity of a child's intelligibility impairment, their limited range makes them less sensitive to small changes in intelligibility over time, and thus less useful for tracking progress in therapy.

Summary and Intervention

Different clinical situations warrant different approaches to intelligibility measurement. If increasing intelligibility is a primary goal of intervention, word-identification methods provide the best method for detecting change in intelligibility over time and may be worth the additional time and clinical effort required for measurement. For children who cannot yet repeat words or sentences, or for whom intelligibility is not a main treatment focus, scaled ratings of intelligibility may be preferable for indexing severity of intelligibility impairment. Regardless of the type of MSD, maximizing intelligibility is meaningful and functional goal. Several intervention approaches for children with MSD have been developed that have increasing evidence bases, including Dynamic Temporal and Tactile Cueing: DTTC (Strand, 2020; Strand, A31) and Rapid Syllable Transitions Treatment: ReST (McCabe et al., 2020; McCabe, A32) for children with CAS and other paediatric MSDs; intervention based on the speech subsystems approach (Pennington, Roelant et al., 2013; Pennington, A30), the Lee Silverman Voice Treatment: LSVT LOUD® (Boliek & Fox, 2017); and Speech Intelligibility Treatment: SIT (Levy et al., 2020) for children with dysarthria. The specific therapy approach used should be based on the child's motor speech diagnosis and speech presentation; however, leveraging principles of motor learning (Maas et al., 2008) has been shown to be important for maximizing speech outcomes and intelligibility in children with MSDs. Intensive intervention is a primary component of motor-based speech treatments, which can be challenging for clinicians to get funded or approved. Objective documentation of progress on functional measures like intelligibility can help support the need for intensive speech services for children with MSDs.

Targeting Intelligibility in Childhood Dysarthria

Children with dysarthria often have shallow, irregular breathing and speak on small, residual pockets of air. They have low pitched, harsh voices, nasalized speech, and very poor articulation. Together, these difficulties make the children's speech difficult to understand.

Pennington et al., 2009, p. 1

Poor intelligibility and compromised speech naturalness are probably the most immediately observed speech characteristic of an individual with developmental dysarthria. They adversely impact the child's or adult's general presentation, functional communication, communicative competence-and-participation (Levy et al., 2020), and participation in society (Hustad, 2012; McLeod, A2). The treatment goal of improving intelligibility is relevant for all manner of SSDs, except for mild articulation disorders. In mild articulation disorders, comprehensibility and intelligibility are usually adequate, even though *social* acceptability may vary (Munson & Tripp, A40) and the blurry line between SSD and speech difference that is related to dialect or multilingual acquisition, for example, can become tangled (Clark et al., 2021; Easton & Verdon, 2021; Oetting et al., 2016).

There is no such confusion between the sometimes problematic 'difference' -vs- 'disorder', 'typical' -vs- 'atypical' or 'typical' -vs- 'acceptable' divides (McLeod & Baker, 2017, pp. 178–180) when it comes to determining where a dysarthria sits.

Rigorous, fully powered randomised controlled trials are needed to investigate if the positive changes in children's speech observed in phase I and phase II studies are generalisable to the population of children with early acquired dysarthria served by speech and language therapy services. Research should examine change in children's speech production and intelligibility. It must also investigate children's participation in social and educational activities, and their quality of life, as well as the cost and acceptability of interventions.

Pennington et al., 2016, p. 1

Dysarthric speech is unequivocally disordered speech and for parents, teachers, and SLPs/SLTs the imperative to 'do something' to improve an affected individual's articulation and intelligibility is patent. Determining how best to intervene (how to 'do something' that is both effectual and tolerable for the client) is a central component of Lindsay Pennington's research agenda. She investigates the oromotor and communication disorders that occur in childhood neurodisability, how they impinge on young people's health and well-being, and the effectiveness and acceptability of SLP/SLT interventions.

Dr. Lindsay Pennington is a Reader in Communication Disorders at Newcastle University UK and Honorary Consultant Speech and Language Therapist in the UK National Health Service (NHS). Her research focusses on oromotor disorders in childhood and the development of effective communication by children with cerebral palsy. She has led trials of parent training programs for early communication development, intensive therapy to improve speech intelligibility, and the comparative effects of drooling medications for children with neurodisability. She has also led several reviews of interventions for the Cochrane Collaboration on speech-language pathology interventions and has recently completed an evaluation of the effectiveness and feasibility of parent-delivered interventions for children with eating, drinking and swallowing difficulties for the UK National Institute for Health Research.

Q30. Lindsay Pennington: Improving Speech Intelligibility in Developmental Dysarthria

What is the Speech Systems Approach to the assessment and differential diagnosis of, and intervention for developmental dysarthria? What are the key considerations for the SLP/SLT in selecting targets, setting, and attacking goals, and choosing appropriate procedures and activities while progressing through the therapy hierarchy? How would you advise explaining this approach to their MSD, and expected outcomes, to a child or young person engaged in the intervention, and to their parent(s) or primary caregiver(s)?

A30. Lindsay Pennington: Targeting Intelligibility with the Speech Systems Approach

Developmental dysarthria is common in cerebral palsy and following early acquired brain injury. It is caused by damage to or maldevelopment of the speech motor pathways in the central nervous system, which reduce voluntary control of the range, speed, strength, and consistency of movements of the vocal tract. Dysarthria in cerebral palsy and acquired brain injury usually affects the control and coordination of respiration, phonation, resonance, articulation, and prosody. Children's voices may sound weak, breathy, and monotonic; some may have sudden variations in pitch and loudness; many have difficulties sustaining breath supply, sometimes speaking on residual air, or taking a breath at unexpected places in a phrase. Their speech may be nasalized, and their phonemic repertoire reduced, particularly affecting corner vowels and obstruents that depend on a high degree of articulatory precision and air pressure (Lee et al., 2014; Levy et al., 2016; Schölderle et al., 2016; Workinger & Kent, 1991). These impairments can dramatically reduce speech intelligibility, and dysarthria can have substantial impacts on children's social participation and quality of life, as they struggle to make themselves heard or understood in everyday life.

What is the Speech Systems Approach?

The Speech Systems Approach is a motor learning intervention designed to be delivered 1-to-1, three times per week for 6 weeks. Its aim is to increase children's speech intelligibility by targeting speech intensity and rate. Children learn to generate and maintain sufficient air pressure to sustain clear voice across a phrase and to speak at a rate that promotes articulatory precision (Pennington et al., 2010; Pennington, Virella et al., 2013). Its efficacy has been tested with children and young people, aged 6–18 years, with spastic and dyskinetic motor disorders and has been delivered face to face and remotely via videoconferencing software (Pennington et al., 2019).

Assessment

When considering the suitability of the Speech Systems Approach, the SLP/SLT needs to confirm that dysarthria is present and that impairments in respiratory and phonatory control are contributing to intelligibility limitations.

A diagnosis of dysarthria is made on the observation of impaired neuromuscular control of the speech system. As the same musculature underpins eating, drinking, swallowing, saliva control, and airway maintenance and clearance, these functions should be observed for speed, control, and accuracy and their development explored in case histories. Oromotor control of individual nonspeech movements (e.g., blowing, tongue movements) can be screened using checklists such as that developed by Robbins and Klee (1987) and the Oromotor section of the *Diagnostic Evaluation of Articulation and Phonology* (DEAP) (Dodd et al., 2002).

The control of individual speech subsystems is then best assessed through observation of naturally occurring speech, prolonged vowels and tasks designed to stress one or more systems coupled with a standardized assessment of phonology. Lexical stress tasks include repeating phrases of increasing length on one breath; incrementally increasing and decreasing loudness when counting from one to five or more; increasing and reducing pitch in open vowels; and producing the same phrase with different stress patterns to change meaning (e.g., *You bought a puppy. You bought a puppy! You bought a puppy?* etc.). Each of these tasks allows the clinician to observe the impact of stressing the respiratory and/or phonatory system on the function of successive speech systems – resonance, articulation, prosody – and the effect on intelligibility. Diadochokinetic tasks, e.g., repeating /pʌ pʌ pʌ/, /pʌ tʌ kʌ/, can help in examining children's control when increasing speech rate. The *Mayo Clinic Dysarthria Studies* system for describing dysarthric speech can then be applied, to rate the perceptual characteristics of respiration, pitch, loudness, voice quality, resonance, prosody, and articulation on a five-point scale ranging from 0= normal to 4 = severely deviant (Duffy, 2012).

This assessment of perceptual characteristics enables SLPs/SLTs to ascertain the extent of children's voluntary control of individual speech systems and their coordination. Findings directly inform therapy, indicating whether working on rate control might be useful and whether the focus will be to increase intensity (loudness) or to reduce fluctuations in intensity. As the primary goal of dysarthria therapy is to increase the proportion of words listeners recognise in children's speech, clinicians must also assess intelligibility prior to and during intervention. Subjective ratings of intelligibility have been shown to lack reliability (Sakash et al., 2021), but the objective measurement of both single words and connected speech (to investigate the effect of breath group duration) by listeners selecting words they have heard, or orthographically transcribing speech are time consuming. Recording children speaking short phrases and asking familiar listeners (e.g., school staff) to identify key words usually works better in clinical practice (Ertmer, 2011).

Using the Approach

The Speech Systems Approach starts with finding the cue that helps children produce a clear open vowel. Guided by the perceptual assessments above, this cue is usually related to intensity e.g., 'big', 'loud', 'strong', though for children who start off with large amplitude movements and tail off rapidly or who have difficulty starting voluntary movements, a 'nice and easy' cue may work better.

Once a cue has been found and the target (loud, strong, big, etc.) voice can be achieved following a model in an open vowel, the target voice is practiced in words. When learning to produce the target voice there is an acquisition phase in which clinicians provide children with frequent knowledge of performance (KP) feedback on the sound of their voice (e.g., *'Well done, that was strong'*) and encouragement to pay attention to their internal feedback (*'How did it feel to make that loud voice?'* etc.) to achieve consistent production of the target voice (Maas et al., 2008). Sound pressure meters, available in several Apps, are useful tools for external feedback. When children achieve 8/10 correct with feedback from the clinician, feedback is faded in a retention phase, when children self-monitor and correct their performance (Schmidt et al., 2019). Knowledge of results (KR) feedback can be given at the end of a block of practice items–*'6 out of 10 were loud'*.

When the target voice is consistently achieved in single words without feedback from the clinician (8/10 correct), multisyllabic words and short phrases are introduced. At each increase in utterance length there is usually an acquisition phase and retention phase, the duration of which depends on children's motor control and memory for the task. For each length of utterance targeted, elicitation tasks increase in cognitive demand from repetition, to picture naming then answering questions. Once children can consistently produce their target voice in three to four-word phrases, length is not strictly controlled, and tasks become more conversation based. Children are encouraged to parse productions, taking breaths where necessary to sustain the target voice. Practice also includes a range of intonation patterns e.g., to contrast statements and questions.

In summary, children's 18 intervention sessions, across 6 weeks comprise open vowels to recalibrate the target voice, exercises in the hierarchy, random elicitation tasks, and practice of individually selected functional phrases that children use in daily life.

Explaining the Approach

The Speech Systems Approach is best explained to children and their parents by talking about listeners being able to hear children clearly – if children use a loud, clear voice, listeners will be able hear individual sounds that children are saying. As the approach is holistic, it is unnecessary to refer to individual parts of speech or speech characteristics.

Evaluating Impact

The goal of the Speech Systems Approach is improved intelligibility in daily life. Goal Attainment Scaling (GAS) is a useful tool for evaluating individuals' intelligibility outcomes (Schlosser, 2004; Steenbeek et al., 2007). Before intervention starts, children and their clinician discuss the environments in which their speech is clear and when listeners have difficulty hearing (understanding) their speech. Children, sometimes with their parents, then decide on one frequent interaction in which they specifically want to improve their intelligibility, such as when talking to their parent while travelling by car. Children's intelligibility (the proportion of times they are understood) in this interaction becomes the outcome measured in GAS. Children, parents, and the clinician set outcomes that would be expected (0); greater than expected (+1); much greater than expected (+2); less than expected (-1) and much less than expected outcome (-2) and evaluate outcome using the scale. For example, GAS scores for *answering questions in a whole class activity* would be [child's name] is understood:

- 4/10 = 0
- 6/10 = +1
- 8/10 = +2
- 2/10 = −1
- 0/10 = −2

What Next?

Outside the therapy sessions, people in children's support network (e.g., parents and classroom assistants) can help them to apply their new voice in daily life. Reminders and prompts can be the verbal the cue from therapy (e.g., *'use your strong voice'*); and nonverbal prompts that minimise intrusion (e.g., signing 'big' or opening the hand wide to indicate loud).

The Speech Systems Approach helps children control intensity and rate to maximise the clarity of their speech signal. Once children can use their target voice when they need to, therapy might move on, beyond the 6-weeks' timeframe, to target segmental aspects of speech, such as the articulation of individual phonemes or specific phonotactic features to incrementally increase intelligibility.

Integral Stimulation

Over 70 years ago, ASHA published a Monograph by Robert L. Milisen, archived at https://www.asha.org/publications/monographs. This learned treatise introduced a multi-layered program for articulation therapy involving imitation and auditory and visual models (Milisen, 1954). Milisen called the method integral stimulation, and it has shaped the treatment of functional articulation disorders, dysarthria, and acquired apraxia of speech. It utilizes hierarchical cueing procedures that begin with high levels of clinician support via simultaneous production of slowly spoken simple utterances, with visual and tactile cues. The cues are subtly, and expertly faded and amplified as required until, at the lowest level of support, they disappear, and the client produces delayed repetition of increasingly complex stimuli.

Research by Rosenbeck et al. (1973) and Strand and Debertine (2000) shows that the use of integral stimulation intervention with individuals with apraxia of speech is efficacious. Integral stimulation is widely used by SLPs/SLTs who treat children's speech and language difficulties, although they may be unaware of its origins or great longevity. It involves a familiar procedure whereby the clinician provides a model, and the child *imitates* it, while the clinician ensures that the child's attention is as focused as possible on *listening to* the model and *looking at* the clinician's face (watching the model, in fact).

Integral stimulation proceeds from bottom up, starting with simple phonetic segments and sequences and then short utterances, building in a hierarchy of difficulty to longer and more phonetically complex stimuli. It can be used alone when working with children with CAS, but it is thought to be more effectively applied in combination with tactile and gesture cues that shape the accuracy of articulatory gestures and prosodic cues (Strand, 1995, 2020; Strand et al., 2006). These cues might involve melodic intonation therapy techniques (Helfrich-Miller, 1983, 1984, 1994) or contrastive stress (Velleman, 2002). A prominent feature of the application of the integral-stimulation-combined-with-prosodic-cues approach with children with CAS is that syllable, word, and sentence stress are emphasized early in therapy – from its outset, and with young children *if possible*.

Dynamic Temporal and Tactile Cueing

For non-verbal children with sCAS, and children with severe CAS, for whom the method described above is too difficult, Strand developed and tested a variation of integral stimulation called *Dynamic Temporal and Tactile Cueing (DTTC) for Speech Motor Learning* (Strand A31; Strand, 2020; Strand et al., 2006; see also a conference presentation by Jakielski et al., 2006). Incorporating the principles of motor learning (PML), outlined above, it can be used with children who struggle fruitlessly with articulatory imitation and who, with fluky exceptions among many failed attempts, seem unable to achieve even the remotest approximation for consonants or vowels.

DTTC is an explicitly principled, modified version of the *Eight-Step Continuum for Treatment of Acquired Apraxia of Speech* (Rosenbeck et al., 1973), originally designed for adult clients with AOS. It allows for what Strand calls 'a continuous shaping of the movement gesture', to (1) improve motor planning and (2) program speech processing as speech and language acquisition progresses. The eight steps and essential adjustments of the therapy dance within DTTC have a familiar ring to many clinicians.

Step 1: Direct Imitation

In its implementation, DTTC begins with direct, immediate imitation of natural speech. This may seem like a big 'ask', but sometimes a child experiences success. If the child cannot imitate, the task is changed to the simplified, more 'supported' one of simultaneous production (Step 2). Steps two to five, inclusive, are a preparation for the integral stimulation method and Steps one, six, seven and eight are the integral stimulation method per se.

Step 2: Simultaneous production with prolonged vowels (most support)

At this easier level, the SLP/SLT says the utterance at normal volume *with* the child first, very slowly with the addition of touch cues and/or gesture cues as required, and as tolerated. Slowing the utterance by sustaining the *vowel* ([si::::] rather than [ssssi]), as explained in Chapter 7, helps the child, and at the same time lets the SLP/SLT run a visual check to see that the jaw and lip postures are correct. For example, the clinician can ensure that there is no jaw slide and that there is acceptable facial symmetry.

Step 3: Reduction of vowel length

As the simultaneous production phase of therapy advances the rate of stimuli production is increased. This is achieved by reducing vowel length, allowing the child's speech output to sound more natural.

Step 4: Gradual increase of rate to normal

Practice continues at this level to the point where the child synchronizes effortlessly with the therapist at normal rate, with normal movement gestures, and without extraneous movements such as silent posturing (groping).

Step 5: Reduction of therapist's vocal loudness, eventually miming

Using delicate timing, the SLP/SLT is then able to reduce his or her vocal volume, eventually reaching a point where the clinician is producing a mime (mouthing the utterance) as the child says it aloud. Because of the intellectual closeness within the dyad, this can be a tricky point in therapy, and some children will dutifully follow *exactly* what the adult is doing so that the two are miming at each other! 'Like a pair of goldfish' as one parent commented. This is obviously not the goal, and children may need explicit instruction to keep their voice or voice box 'turned on' even though the adult's is 'off'. Sometimes it is helpful to mime flipping or rotating an imaginary on-switch or volume control on the larynx if the child's voice drops away, and/or make an upward hand gesture to indicate that the volume needs to increase if they are too quiet. The other gesture and touch cues may still be needed at this point too and will almost certainly be necessary in the next step: the integral stimulation method proper.

Step 6: The Integral Stimulation Method: Direct imitation

Ensuring that the child is secure and comfortable with moving to this harder level, the SLP/SLT instructs the child to watch the adult's face (*Look at me for help*) while an auditory model is delivered. The child attempts to repeat the model and, if successful, does so many times. If unsuccessful, the therapist may backtrack, as far as is necessary, to the simultaneous model or silent mouthing level described above. Eventually all miming is faded, and the child directly imitates and 'repeats' targets numerous times before step 7 is introduced.

Step 7: Introduction of a one-or two-second S–R delay (least support)

Once the child is directly imitating the therapist's model with normal rate, with prosody he or she can vary, and with appropriate articulatory gestures, the therapist inserts a new requirement. This is in the form of a one- to two-second stimulus-response (S–R) delay before the child imitates, so that the child produces a *slightly* delayed response. To facilitate this for the children who find the delay difficult and want to 'jump in', miming while the child produces the delayed response can help.

Step 8: Spontaneous production

Finally, the SLP/SLT elicits short and long spontaneous utterances, for example, by asking the child, 'What is this called?' using cloze tasks like '*Twinkle, twinkle _____*', sentence completion like '*Mother elephant is very big, her baby is _____*', 'Three things I like about the beach are ___', engaging in story telling (e.g., with wordless picture books), picture and object description, running commentaries (e.g., while making a sandwich), narrative and role play.

Keys to Success

The keys to successful implementation of integral stimulation are the clinician's empathic, informed observations of and sensitivity to what the child is 'giving' by way of responses. The professional skill and flexibility involved in continually fine-tuning the hierarchy of stimuli *and* fine-tuning the amount of support provided to enable the child to imitate spontaneously, is critical. Auditory (including prosodic), visual, and tactile cues and the level of demand on the child are continually augmented and faded in each practice trial according to the child's responses.

The clinician's alertness to the child's responses is especially important with the CAS population, who have good and bad days with their speech-processing capabilities. The SLP/SLT must always be prepared to take the therapy 'down a notch' if required, and to explain to parents why this is happening.

What Distinguishes DTTC from Other SSD Interventions?

Specifically designed for children with CAS, DTTC differs from, or bears some similarities to, other evidence-based approaches to SSD in several important respects:

- Treatment centres on the movement gesture, rather than on individual consonants, clusters, syllables, or words, with no work on isolated phones. This distinguishes it from the 'brick wall' hierarchy of difficulty in the NDP3 (Williams, A33).
- Prosody is focused upon early in intervention with an emphasis on inflection and rhythm, highlighting vowel accuracy. In this respect it shows similarities to ReST (McCabe, A32) with its emphasis on stress assignment, syllable duration and speech rate, vocal intensity, pitch variation, and speech naturalness.
- Word targets are meaningful, relevant ('important' or 'powerful'), and individualized for each child, so that there are no predetermined wordlists or picture stimuli. The words chosen may include the names of people, places, and favoured toys and activities, and functional words, sometimes referred to as 'power words', that have the 'power' to make things happen in the child's life. Here, we see a characteristic in common with

Core Vocabulary Intervention for Inconsistent Speech Disorder (not CAS), described in Chapter 5. The difference is that the SLP/SLT selects the words not only relative to the child's needs, preferences, and interests, but also in relation to necessary movement goals.

- Unlike Cued Articulation, Cued Speech, and PROMPT, for example, there are no standardized tactile, visual, imagery or gestural cues or models. In DTTC, cues are kept as simple as possible and are retained in therapy sessions because the SLP/SLT considers them to be of most value to the individual child. No matter how 'helpful' they appear to be, they are faded (removed) as soon as possible to make way for independent effort and possibly self-cueing, with scope to reintroduce them if greater SLP/SLT support is deemed necessary.
- In common with many intervention approaches for SSD, in DTTC
  - Opportunities for maximal practice to optimise motor learning, and immediate, rapidly dispensed reinforcement, are provided in sessions to keep the child on-task, interested, and engaged.
  - The SLP/SLT strives to establish and maintain an enjoyable atmosphere in sessions that is upbeat and positive.

The evidence base for DTTC is compelling (Murray, McCabe, & Ballard, et al., 2015a) and there are numerous resources available to support its use, for example, a video featuring Dr. Edythe Strand: https://childapraxiatreatment.org/dttc on the informative Child Apraxia Treatment website https://childapraxiatreatment.org/ which warrants detailed exploration by interested SLPs/SLTs at all levels of experience, and students.

Dr. Edythe Strand is Emeritus Speech Pathologist, Department of Neurology, Mayo Clinic, and Emeritus Professor, Mayo College of Medicine. Dr. Strand's research has focused on developmental, acquired, and progressive apraxia of speech, as well as degenerative dysarthria. She is an ASHA Fellow and has been awarded Honors of the Association of the American Speech-Language and Hearing Association, as well as Honors of the Academy of Neurologic Communication Disorders and Sciences

Q31. Edythe Strand: The Importance of Dynamic Motor Speech Assessment

Why is a motor speech evaluation (MSE) an essential component in the differential diagnosis of CAS from other speech impairment, and why does it have to be a dynamic motor speech assessment (DMSA)? How do DEMMS test results contribute to short-term and long-term goal setting and treatment planning for children and young people with motor speech disorders, and how does it interface with DTTC and integral stimulation?

A31. Edythe Strand: Dynamic Assessment, DEMSS and DTTC

A MSE has long been known to be an essential part of assessment procedures in in the differential diagnosis of motor planning/programming difficulty in adults (Duffy, 2012. Historically, however, they have seldom been used in the assessment of speech sound disorders (SSD). A MSE is particularly important in the differential diagnosis of CAS in that it allows the clinician to observe specific characteristics frequently associated with that diagnosis across utterances that systematically vary programming demands.

Dynamic Assessment

A DMSA offers particular and important contributions to differentiating CAS from other speech sound disorders (SSD). First, DSMA facilitates eliciting behaviours that the clinician can then compare to accepted phenotypes for different types of SSD. DMSA also allows the clinician to make more accurate judgments of severity and prognosis by observing responses to cueing. In DA, multiple attempts at repeating a word may be elicited, with the clinician using different types of cues with scoring reflecting the child's change in performance. Researchers have studied the role of dynamic assessment in language disorders (e.g., Olswang & Bain, 1996); and phonological disorders (e.g., Glaspey & Stoel-Gammon, 2007), but until recently its role in childhood motor speech disorders has had little discussion.

The Role of DA in Differential Diagnosis

One of the biggest challenges for the SLP/SLT is determining whether *motor* speech impairment is contributing to the child's SSD. Because there are no biomarkers for CAS (or other SSDs) classification is typically made by observing characteristics associated with a particular label. There is now increasing consensus regarding the behavioural characteristics associated with CAS (e.g., Shriberg et al., 2011; Van der Merwe & Steyn, 2018) Strand (2017) lists some characteristics frequently present but not discriminative in that they are also common in other SSDs (e.g., sound omissions; reduced intelligibility) as well as those that are more discriminative (e.g., awkward movement from one articulatory configuration to another, presence of vowel and consonant distortions, prosodic errors, and intrusive schwa).

DA is important to differential diagnosis as it facilitates observations of these speech characteristics by offering the child support, through cueing, over several attempts. This contrasts with observations of spontaneous speech during which the child will often produce only approximations or utterances they can already say, without focused attempts at correct production. This limits observation of behaviours which may occur when trying a novel utterance.

What we see and hear produced spontaneously and in static testing is different from what we perceive when children actively *try* to correctly produce a new word or one that they typically mispronounce. The cueing involved in DA enables observations of what the child does while really attempting specific movement gestures. In the case of children

with suspected CAS, we can evaluate discrete characteristics associated with that label. For example, we may see groping that is not evident in spontaneous speech, but evident in when cues are used to encourage accurate imitation of an articulatory gesture. Inconsistency is likely more evident across repeated trials as cueing occurs, as is segmentation of syllables which may occur only when the child really concentrates on producing correct articulatory movement gestures.

Dynamic Evaluation of Motor Speech Skill (DEMSS)

To address the need for a DA for differential diagnosis of CAS, the Dynamic Evaluation of Motor Speech Skill (DEMSS) was developed and tested for reliability and validity (Strand et al., 2013; Strand & McCauley, 2019a, 2019b). It is designed specifically for younger children and/or those who have more severe SSD. It utilizes systematic, progressive cueing to facilitate imitative production of utterances that vary in length and phonetic complexity.

The Role of the DEMSS In Short- and Long-Term Goal Setting

The DEMSS may be an important resource for determining the severity of the child's motor speech disorder, as well as determining prognosis for improvement, both of which are essential when it comes to setting appropriate and realistic goals. The DEMSS is sensitive to changes that result from the child's *responses* to cueing, in other words, his or her *learning*.

Traditional standardized tests allow comparison of a child's performance on a task (e.g., articulation performance) with the performance of a normative group, at one point in time. While this may allow some idea of severity, it is quite conceivable that two children may exhibit the same standard score on a measure but have very different levels of severity and different prognoses for change (see

Flipsen Jr, A8). This is because most standardized tests do not provide the clinician with the opportunity to observe the child's responses to different types of cueing, or their potential to learn via such cueing.

Because it is dynamic, the DEMSS can more accurately determine the severity of the motor programming deficit as well as the likelihood of improvement and perhaps the rate of that improvement. The therapist provides different levels of support such as gestural and tactile cueing, visual attention to the clinician's face, having the child produce the response more slowly, and/or having the child produce the utterance simultaneously with the examiner. Observations of the child's response to cueing facilitates the clinician's judgments of how much cueing will be *needed* in early therapy, and how long it may take to achieve initial progress.

Prognostic decisions lead the clinician to short and long-term goal setting. Parents of non-verbal children often come with the question, 'Will my child ever talk?' If the child's responses to cueing and facilitation during the DEMSS indicate potential as a verbal communicator, then the long-term goal is to establish functional verbal communication. Short-term goals are also facilitated by the DEMSS, and they are closely tied to decisions about where to start. Rather than examining at what level (V vs. CV and VC vs. CVC, etc.) the child is successful, using binary scoring, the DEMSS allows observations of the level of cueing needed to improve production at varying levels of phonetic complexity. Consider a non-verbal child who exhibits numerous vowel distortions in isolation, syllables, and words, but improves production in all contexts when the clinician helps him or her achieve the initial articulatory position and stay in the steady state of (sustaining) the vowel for longer.

Logically, this would lead to the decision to work at *and beyond* the CV, VC and CVC levels. On the other hand, if a child cannot improve vowel production even with maximum cueing and slowed rate, the clinician would begin with a smaller stimulus set, and fewer vowel targets within CV and VC syllable shapes.

The Interface between the DEMSS and DTTC

DTTC (Strand, 2020), a treatment designed for severe CAS, uses auditory, visual, and tactile cueing. DTTC, however, emphasizes varying the temporal relationship between the stimulus and the response, maximizing cueing at first, then fading cues over continued practice. This variation in levels of cueing characterizes the similarity between DTTC and the DEMSS. In the DEMSS however, cues are progressively *added* to determine how *much* help the child needs to improve accuracy of movement gestures. In DTTC, cues are maximized at first for utterances the child cannot produce, and *then gradually faded* as improvement occurs. This strategy helps the child to take increasing responsibility for the planning/programming and execution of the movement gestures for the target utterance.

Case Example

Peter aged 4;2 came for speech and language evaluation due to his continued delayed speech acquisition. Since 2;6 he had received individual speech therapy utilizing traditional articulation therapy approaches which had evoked little speech progress. His parents' chief concern was whether he would ever talk. They were considering abandoning work on his speech to focus only on augmentative communication.

Peter's receptive language was in the normal range. He initiated communication readily, using sign and gestures, a few intelligible words, and many word approximations understood only by his mother. The DEMSS was administered, revealing numerous CAS characteristics including difficulty achieving initial articulatory configurations, with instances of groping and trial and error behaviour; frequent vowel distortions which varied with coarticulatory context; prosodic errors; and token-to-token inconsistency across trials. He was able to produce only 6 of the 68 items correctly in direct imitation without any cues (*do; up; mama; papa; boo-boo; and mom*). These results were consistent with his Goldman and Fristoe (2015) scores.

His DEMSS scores, however, also reflected *improvement* with visual attention to the clinician's face, tactile cueing, slowing down and simultaneously producing the movement gesture *with* the clinician. His performance improved with progressive cueing on over 65% of DEMSS utterances, and correct production after cues on 28% of incorrect items, although it usually took the maximum cues to achieve correct production. Because of his ability to benefit from cues focused on movement accuracy, a favourable prognosis for functional communication was determined. Because of the severity of his apraxia of speech, and therapy progress to date, intensive therapy was recommended.

Peter was seen for two daily 30-minute therapy sessions over six weeks, using DTTC. Initial goals focused on producing correct movement gestures for speech; improving his ability to produce the syllable shapes of CVC, VC and CV CVC (as in *hi Mom*); and improving accuracy for /i/ /æ/ and /aɪ/. Seven functional words and short phrases were chosen for the initial stimulus set to allow enough massed practice for attaining movement accuracy, yet some distributed practice to facilitate motor learning. By the end of the six weeks, he had mastered around 20 target utterances and had generalized them to spontaneous speech. He had mastered most vowels across co-articulatory contexts and was achieving accuracy for new words and phrases at a much more rapid pace.

This relatively rapid improvement likely occurred because of frequent therapy, an approach that focused on facilitating accurate movement for segmental and syllabic sequences, the clinician's knowledge of the speech sound system, *and* therapy that was based on the principles of motor learning, including judging when and how to provide feedback. We maximized the number of practice trials within sessions by using reinforcers that were quick and given only after several responses. Early in treatment feedback was frequent, immediate, and contained specific information regarding movement performance (KP feedback) to maximize movement accuracy. As therapy progressed, feedback was provided less frequently, with slightly longer delays, and with less specificity to maximise motor learning

(KR feedback). We varied rate of movement, starting with slow movement and prolonged vowels to achieve accuracy, gradually increasing rate to normal by reducing vowel length. We worked to vary prosody to avoid habituation of rote prosodic contours. As therapy continued, progress toward correct production of words and phrases became faster. He now has many functional words and phrases and continues in therapy.

Lexical Stress, Excessive And/or Equal Stress: EES, and CAS

Changes in duration, loudness and pitch across words and longer utterances that express linguistic and affective information are referred to collectively as prosody, and lexical stress is one aspect of it. Cutler and Carter (1987) determined that over 90% of English words exceed one syllable. So, children with typical speech and language capabilities who are learning English gain the ability to apply lexical stress to most of the words they speak. From studies of English-language learners with SSD, it appears that prosodic difficulties are a core deficit in CAS, and this includes difficulty with lexical stress (Shriberg et al., 2003). Affected children tend to apply excessive and/or equal stress (EES) impacting their speech acquisition, naturalness, and intelligibility.

While it occurs in English, the tendency towards EES is not attested in French (Brosseau-Lapré & Rvachew, 2017; Rvachew & Matthews, 2017), and there is emerging evidence that this also applies to Hebrew (Segal et al., 2022). This raises the prospect that children growing up with other, as yet unidentified, languages also escape the EES propensity. Just as we don't apply English norms such as speech sound acquisition criteria, to other languages we must not assume that so called core deficits, derived from English-speaking research participants, will necessarily apply cross linguistically. We must also recognise that the emphasis in assessment tasks and in intervention materials may differ sharply from language to language. In her update of the Rapid Syllable Transition Treatment (ReST) Tricia McCabe (A32) highlights this using Italian – with its different prosody, phonotactics and allophones, when compared to English – as an example.

Targeting the Core Diagnostic Features of CAS

The author of A32 and A34 is **Dr. Tricia McCabe**. Her research, teaching, and clinical practice focus on improving treatment outcomes for children and adults with severe or difficult to treat speech disorders, particularly those with Childhood Apraxia of Speech. She is the leader of the CAS Treatment Research Group at The University of Sydney and leads the research program which developed ReST.

Q32.   Tricia McCabe

Since the previous edition of this book, much has happened in the development and evaluation of the ReST treatment for childhood apraxia of speech and other motor speech disorders. Can you update readers, particularly in terms of implementing the approach with acceptable fidelity?

A32.   Patricia McCabe: Update on Rapid Syllable Transition Treatment (REST): A Treatment for Childhood Apraxia of Speech and Other Motor Speech Disorders

Rapid Syllable Transition Treatment, known as ReST, is an evidence-based treatment for children and young people with motor speech disorders, particularly childhood apraxia of speech (CAS) but there is also emerging evidence of ReST being an effective treatment for children with dysarthria. ReST (and the related TEMPO intervention; Miller et al., 2021) is designed to treat the ASHA (2007) three core diagnostic features of CAS: inconsistent articulation, errors in lexical stress, and difficulty moving from sound to sound or syllable to syllable within words. This goal is achieved by using multisyllabic nonwords as practice targets in a treatment regime designed around the principles of motor learning (Schmidt et al., 2019)

with high frequency, high intensity therapy and low frequency feedback. In ReST therapy, the three ASHA features are labelled as sounds (inconsistent articulation), beats (lexical stress) and smoothness (transition between sounds and syllables) and children are asked to repeat the nonwords accurately on all three features simultaneously. More information about the treatment and a range of free training and therapy resources can be found on the ReST website (https://rest.sydney.edu.au) and in a tutorial paper (McCabe et al., 2020).

As a treatment for CAS, ReST has been examined in two randomized control trials (Murray, McCabe & Ballard, 2015a; McCabe et al., submitted), six repeated single case experimental design studies (Ballard et al., 2010; Miller et al., 2021; McCabe et al., 2014; Thomas et al., 2014, 2017, 2016) and one unpublished quasi-experimental pilot study (Staples et al., 2008), all in English. Additionally, a single case experimental design paper reporting efficacy in Italian (Scarcella et al., 2021) along with quasi-experimental papers in Korean (Oh & Ha, 2021), Danish (Ostergaard, 2021) and Brazilian Portuguese (de Oliveira Silveira, 2021) have been published. Two studies have been conducted using ReST with children who had moderate dysarthria arising from cerebral palsy (Korkalainen et al., 2022; Korkalainen et al., submitted) and one with a single child who had a cerebellar dysarthria following brain cancer (Murray et al., 2011). Across the studies children have been aged 4–14 although ReST is not recommended for most 4-year-olds. Clinically, ReST is used with older adolescents with CAS and adults with acquired apraxia however the efficacy with these groups is not yet proven experimentally.

Over the 15 years since the first ReST study began, the main clinical questions about ReST have circled around treatment fidelity, particularly providing sufficient dose. Providing enough therapy is a challenge worldwide and in the case of ReST we have now tested weekly, and two-, three-, and four-times weekly treatment both in person and online. Thomas et al. (2022) showed that therapy once per week was less effective than any other frequency of treatment. We have however shown that a combination of two clinicians can share providing therapy (Thomas et al., 2016) and that older children can achieve the desired 100 practice trials in a shorter therapy session (McCabe et al., submitted). Because we have shown that parents find the treatment difficult (Thomas et al., 2017) and dislike being the clinician (Thomas et al., 2018), treatment must be provided by a clinician, who can be a qualified SLP/SLT or, as has been the case in most of the ReST studies, a trained and supervised SLP/SLT student.

Until recently, we had assumed that children with CAS who were older or those with milder difficulties would be most suitable for ReST (Murray, McCabe, Ballard et al., 2015a) but did not have evidence which supported this hypothesis. Ng et al. (2022) reported the results of an Individual Participant Data meta-analysis which pooled the data from seven of the ReST English language studies. This study showed that the best predictor of performance on the treated nonwords was a pre-treatment combination of higher expressive language standard scores and consonant accuracy on the Goldman Fristoe Test of Articulation (Goldman & Fristoe, 2000) with lower vowel accuracy and lower consistency. The best pre-treatment predictors of generalisation from the nonwords used in therapy to real words was performance on real words prior to treatment. Additionally, despite our clinical predictions, age, memory (e.g., digit span), and receptive language did not predict improvement in treatment. Importantly, all children across the studies showed some improvement in speech accuracy regardless of their individual characteristics or pre-treatment performance.

Providing ReST treatment to children who speak languages other than English initially appeared challenging. Each language has its own prosodic and phonotactic rules and therefore translating ReST as an intervention required understanding the new language. To give an example of what is required, to translate ReST to Italian and test it as an intervention, we needed to first consider the stress patterns of Italian which differ from those of English and in three syllable words, three patterns are equally likely in Italian–Strong- weak- weak (Sww); weak- Strong- weak (wSw); and weak- weak- Strong (wwS). The last pattern (wwS) is not accommodated in ReST in English and so we needed to adapt the stimuli used in Scarcella et al. (2021) to spread the 20 nonword stimuli across the three stress patterns; moving from two stress patterns with ten practice nonwords each to three stress patterns was achieved by reducing the number of exemplars of each nonword from ten to seven, giving 21 in total. The same process was then followed for other linguistic features including syllable structures and allophonic variations.

Further adaptations have been made to test ReST as an intervention for children aged 8–14 years with dysarthria associated with cerebral palsy (CP). Two studies have been conducted with this population, a single case experimental design study (Korkalainen et al., 2022), which was conducted face-to-face before the CO-VID-19 pandemic, and a randomized control trial (RCT; Korkalainen et al. submitted) comparing ReST to usual care which was conducted completely by Zoom teletherapy. Here the potential for physical fatigue in children with CP meant that rather than 12 one-hour long sessions spread over 6 weeks, we trialled 18 sessions of 45 minutes over the same period–3 shorter sessions per week with longer breaks between practice sets. This is slightly more time in therapy but seemed to be a reasonable adjustment and maintained the standard 1200 practice trials over the 18 sessions. Both studies show that providing ReST to older children with CP can be used to improve both speech accuracy and mean length of utterance, and the RCT showed a significant improvement in communicative participation as well.

As a treatment for motor speech disorders in children, ReST has good evidence for both a treatment effect and generalisation to real words and clinicians can use it with confidence where the child in their care matches the children in the research.

An Evolving and Versatile Treatment Approach

Readers should not be misled by the publication date associated with The Nuffield Dyspraxia Programme, Third Edition (Williams & Stephens, 2004). While the third edition was released some 20 years ago, the NDP3's photocopiable loose-leaf and ring binder format coupled with print-on-demand technology has facilitated regular updates since 2004. Once criticized for the inclusion of 35 pages on 'oromotor work' (NS-OME) introduced in the early stage of intervention, the authors responded to its slim-to-non-existent evidence based (Lof, A24) by replacing them in 2012 with 'speech motor skills' activities comprising 'sound and vocal play', and/or procedures to develop lip and tongue articulatory gestures (Williams, 2021, p. 452).

The picture stimuli in the NDP3 occupy three categories (Williams, 2021). They are: (i) single sounds – both consonants and vowels, (ii) words representing different phonotactic structures: CV, VC, CVCV, CVC, etc. and (iii) word combinations in phrases (e.g., *dirty car; watching the television*), clauses (e.g., *cow pushing, Bobby eating butter*), and sentences (e.g., *The diver is looking at the submarine*). Sample pages and cards are available at https://www.ndp3.org

The program has drawn unfavourable responses for the inclusion of single-sound (consonant) production drill at the lowest course of its bottom-up hierarchy of difficulty, likened to a brick wall by its British developers. For example, Brousseau-Lapré & Rvachew (2020, p. 205) comment: '*Typically, this [single sound focus] is not advised, however, because it is known that children with motor speech disorders and especially CAS have difficulty with co-articulation of adjacent segments within syllables. Furthermore, most theories of linguistic organization suggest that there is a mental store of syllable- sized motor plans for speech production (*Levelt et al., 1999*)*'. Similarly, the same authors (Rvachew & Brousseau-Lapré, 2018, p. 506) say the '*practice of teaching words as isolated parts and then building them back up leads the authors to caution against "schwa insertion," which must be*

difficult to avoid with many phonemes. In some cases, this intervention may lead to poor coarticulation and unusual prosody as unintended treatment effects.'

These reasoned criticisms are well founded. Breaking words into onset and coda (sh-oo /ʃ-u/ rather than shoo /ʃ u/ for *shoe*) does not leverage what we know about the existence of a mental *syllabary* of motor plans for speech production rather than a mental *phonetic* store (Kröger et al., 2022) and it is a practice that can create extra work for child and clinician. Many clinicians come to regret the decision, when working with children with CAS, and some children with articulation or phonological disorders, to introduce words like *bee, day*, and *go* with a segregated initial stop (b-ee, d-ay, g-oh) and words like *she, zoo*, and *shy* with a hiatus between onset and rime (sh-e, z-oo, sh-y). This is because they find they must then *unteach* epenthetic productions like [bəˈiː, bəʔˌiː. bʌʔ ˈi ː] for *bee*, and [ʃəˈiː, ʃəʔˌiː. ʃʌʔˈiː] for *she*, involving shwa or other vowel insertion, with or without glottal insertion.

I have had the privilege of spending time with several of the Nuffield SLTs – particularly Shula Burrows, Frances Ridgeway, Hilary Stephens, and Pam Williams – who are skilled veterans when it comes to understanding the range of difficulties children with CAS have and implementing the NDP3. My sense is that these experienced clinicians would typically pre-empt such disruptions to progress by noticing a child's tendency to insert vowels or glottal stops after onset consonants or between consonants in clusters (e.g., [pəleɪ] for *play*, [kəˈɹaʊn] for *crown*), and subtly changing tack in intervention before the unwanted 'extras' became established. It should be remembered that the copious materials in the NDP3 are there to give clinicians choice, and that there is no requirement to use all the activities provided for each level of the hierarchy. Furthermore, the NDP3 authors acknowledge these schwa and 'gap' difficulties.

'At this stage motor programs for consonants and vowels, established at single sound level and practised in C + V and V+ C sequences, are combined to form CV or VC syllables and

given linguistic meaning as CV or VC words. Making the transition from single sounds to CV syllables (C + V = CV) can be a very difficult process for children with developmental verbal dyspraxia as it involves the creation of new motor programs (i.e., the process of motor programming) – a core difficulty in dyspraxia. Combining motor programs, without the "gap" left earlier in sequencing tasks, involves modifying the two existing programs so that they join smoothly. Children may have difficulty combining sounds at all to begin with or may need help just with particular sounds or groups of sounds.

Therapy
Once the child can produce "artificial" C + V sequences, C+V=CV worksheets can be attempted. These should be modelled first by the therapist with demonstration/explanation that the two sounds are to be joined to make the word. Utilise the joining presentations e.g., two jigsaw pieces to explain this to the child. The child can then attempt this himself. If his production of the CV word reverts to his own motor program, nonsense syllables should be practised as an intermediate stage'.

(NDP3, p. 118)

Dr. Pam Williams, FRCSLT stepped down from her role as Consultant SLT at the Nuffield Hearing and Speech Centre in 2017, after more than 30 years' service. She was a contributor to the original 1985 *Nuffield Centre Dyspraxia Programme* and co-authored and edited the third edition's Therapy Manual (Williams & Stephens, 2004). Pam holds Honorary lectureships with University College London and University College London Hospitals NHS Foundation Trust. She has run in-person training courses for SLPs/SLTs on CAS/DVD and NDP3 for over 30 years and virtual training courses via Zoom on the same subjects since June 2020, in collaboration with Reeves Consultancy and Training Ltd. trading as Course Beetle.

Q33.   Pam Williams: The Nuffield Dyspraxia Programme Third Edition (NDP3)

Numerous readers in Britain, Ireland, Australia, New Zealand, Singapore, and South Africa are familiar with, and have used the NDP3. Can you explain, for students and practitioners who are unfamiliar with its history, development, theoretical underpinning, implementation and intervention outcomes and evidence-base, what it is all about?

A33.   Pam Williams: The NDP Approach to Childhood Apraxia of Speech

Publication of the first edition of NDP (Connery, 1985) was welcomed by practitioners in the UK, at a time when few commercial therapy products were available. This package of over 500 photocopiable line-drawn pictures and worksheets was developed from resources originally created by a team of British SLTs for their personal use with individual clients in a clinical department. A revised edition in 1992 generated interest from practitioners in other English-speaking nations, and acknowledged adaptations in Dutch (van der Meulen, 1994) and Swedish (Hellqvist, 2016 and associated resources) were published. A third edition, dubbed the NDP3 (Williams & Stephens, 2004) saw the necessary addition of a detailed therapy manual that explained the intervention approach within the Stackhouse and Wells (1997) psycholinguistic framework and model, and provided step by step guides to planning and implementing treatment. While there have been no further edition or version numbers assigned to newer iterations, the NDP3 picture resources, examples of which are displayed in Figures A33.8.1 to A33.8.5, and much of the text of the programme continues to evolve. A website, https://www.ndp3.org, managed by the publisher, Anthony Allison, provides information on current resources, including the software package *NDP3® Speech Builder* (Allison et al., 2011).

Theoretical Underpinning

The NDP3 is primarily a motor programming treatment approach, which aims to support children with CAS to build accurate motor programs (Stackhouse & Wells, 1997) for individual speech sounds, syllables, and words of varying phonotactic complexity. In the following description of the NDP3, the reader should note that when V is used, either to refer to a single sound or to a constituent of a phonotactic structure such as CV or CVC, it can represent diphthongs, as well as long and short monophthongs. The skills that children need to acquire are conceptualized metaphorically in the NDP3 as a 'brick wall', with consonants (C) and vowels (V), and CV syllables and words seen as the wall's foundations, with other word level skills built up in layers of bricks on top of the foundations: CVCV, CVC, CVCVC and multi-syllabic words, cluster words, word combinations of phrases and sentences, finally reaching the top layer of connected speech. Therapy proceeds in a hierarchy, with the ability to produce words with complex phonotactics, and word combinations considered to be dependent on mastery of single phones and simple phonotactic structures. Treatment involves a multi-level, multi-target approach, whereby the SLP/SLT works concurrently on several targets at a particular level *and* targets at two or more different levels. For example, a child might be working on producing /l/, /f/, /ɔ/, and /ɜ/ at single sound level, voicing contrasts for plosives (stops) at CV level, and CVCV words with /b, d, m, n/ in a variety of contexts. This horizontal goal attack strategy is thought to enhance motor learning and accords with the **principles of motor learning**: PML (Maas et al., 2008; Schmidt et al., 2019).

The NDP3 approach also incorporates other PML, such as breaking tasks down into smaller, achievable steps, many repetitions of sounds and words in therapy activities and frequent opportunities for practice of targets. Knowledge of Performance (KP) feedback (highlighting what the client did, or did not do correctly: e.g., 'that sounded really good as you remembered to round your lips when you said /u/' vs. 'you need to round your lips for /u/'), is particularly used to support the child. The KP feedback is often also combined with Knowledge of Results (KR) feedback (e.g., 'I really understood you that time'; 'That sounded great'; 'Good for you!' with no specific comment on *what* they did correctly). A variety of cues may also be used by the SLP/SLT, including verbal, tactile, gestural, manual, and orthographic cues, and particularly visual cues, using the NDP3 resources. These include pictures to represent words, sound cue pictures for individual consonant and vowel sounds (e.g., /b/ is represented by a picture of a ball; /aɪ/ is represented by a picture of an eye) and diagrammatic images, 'articulograms' (Stephens & Elton, 1986) as shown in Figure A33.8.1, which provide phonetic feature cues such as 'lips together' (place) and 'voice on'.

As speech is not only a complex motor skill, but also a linguistic medium, motor programs at each level of the 'brick wall' must be contrastive. Therefore, once new motor programs are created, they must be incorporated into the sets of sounds and/or words that the child can already produce, thus developing a contrastive system at each phonotactic level (CV, CVCV, CVC).

There are minimal pair worksheets (see, Figure A33.8.2, for example) in the NDP3 resources which support this learning. In this respect, NDP3 treatment combines motor and linguistic approaches. The materials can also be used to support the development of other phonological processing skills (Stackhouse & Wells, 1997), such as auditory discrimination, rhyme judgement and production, segmentation (by syllable, onset-rime and/or phoneme) and consonant-vowel blending.

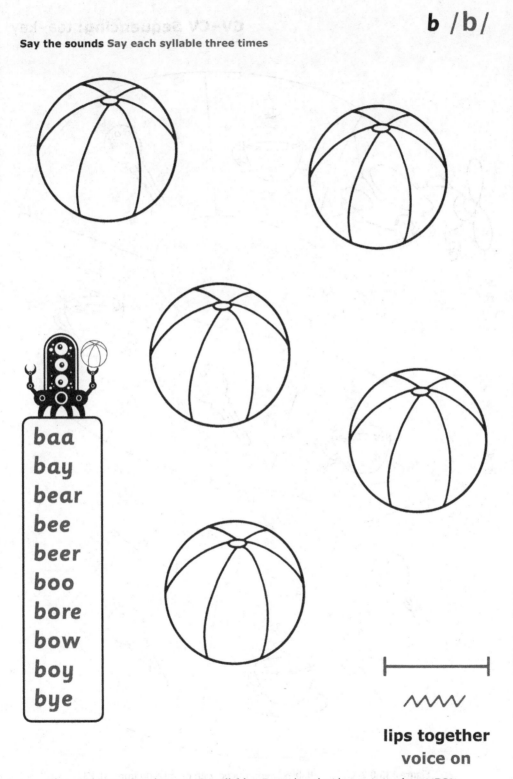

b /b/

Say the sounds Say each syllable three times

baa
bay
bear
bee
beer
boo
bore
bow
boy
bye

lips together
voice on

Figure A33.8.1 Articulograms: CV syllables. Reproduced with permission from NDP3.

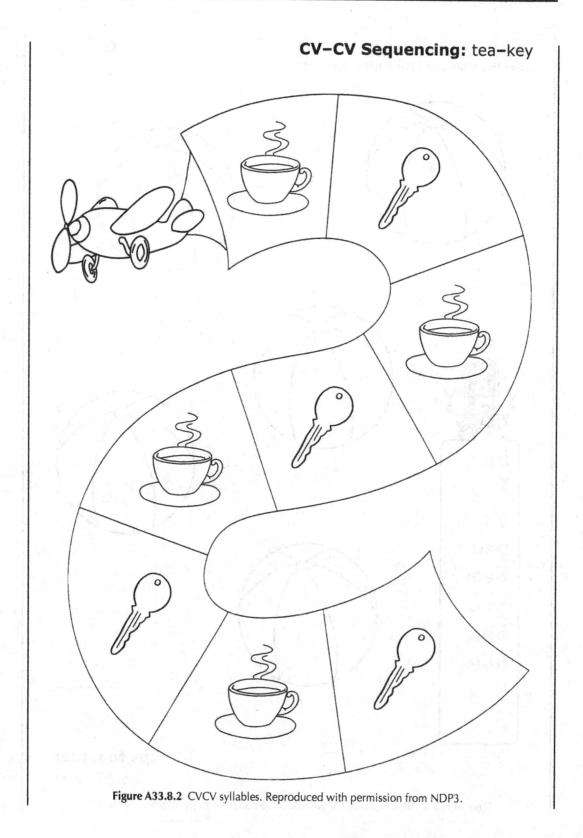

Figure A33.8.2 CVCV syllables. Reproduced with permission from NDP3.

Empirical Evidence

The NDP3 treatment approach was evaluated in randomized controlled trials (RCTs) published in 2015 and 2020. In the first ever RCT to test CAS interventions, Murray et al. (2015a) randomly assigned 26 children, aged 4–12 years, with mild to severe idiopathic CAS, to receive either NDP3 treatment or Rapid Syllable Transition Treatment (ReST). Intervention was delivered intensively (one hour a day, four days a week for three weeks) by trained student speech pathologists in a university clinic. NDP3 treatment followed the tenets of the published programme (Williams & Stephens, 2004), but was guided by an operationalized manual, devised for this study. Each child worked on three individually selected goals (segmental, structural, and prosodic) and received a combination of KP and KR feedback after each production. Post-treatment outcomes showed significant and large treatment effects for the 13 children who received NDP3 intervention, as well as moderate generalisation to untreated real words. Similar positive treatment effects were replicated in a second RCT (McKechnie et al., 2020), for 14 children, aged 4–10 years, with mild to severe idiopathic CAS, who all received NDP3 treatment, delivered by similar personnel over the same duration and intensity, as in the Murray et al., 2015a study. Therapy activities were presented using images on an android tablet, and the types and schedules of feedback given varied. Children were randomly assigned to receive either: (a) high frequency KP and KR feedback and cues in each treatment session (as in the Murray et al., 2015a study) or (b) high frequency KP and KR feedback and cues in one session a week, followed by three sessions, in the same week, with only KR feedback given. Only the children in group (a) showed immediate gains in accuracy, but over time both groups produced significant gains. McKechnie et al. pointed to the need for further research to understand more about the effects of different feedback schedules. Nonetheless, their RCT provides additional evidence of the effectiveness of NDP3 as a treatment approach for children with CAS, this time for four- to ten-year-olds rather than four to twelves.

Treatment Planning and Goal Setting

Clinicians frequently report that they find treatment planning and goal setting in NDP3 challenging, mainly because of the multi-level, multi-target aspect of the approach. This has therefore been a focus of the professional development workshops I have designed and delivered in the UK, Ireland, Europe, Australia and online, and my thinking has been supported by working collaboratively with Dr. Elizabeth Murray from the University of Sydney. It is recommended that SLPs/SLTs follow a step-by-step approach to NDP3 treatment planning and goal setting.

The **first step** involves administering the NDP3 assessment and analysing the phonetically transcribed data in detail, in accordance with advice in the NDP3 manual. Findings can be summarized under headings: single sounds (C and V, including diphthongs), CV, VC, CVCV, CVC, cluster and multisyllabic words, and phrases and sentences, thus producing a personalized case profile of strengths and weaknesses for an individual child. For a CVCV example, see, Figure A33.8.3 (CV+CV: toe – bee–Toby).

The **second step** involves relating this case profile to the four stages of treatment plans described in the NDP3 manual (Williams & Stephens, 2004, pp. 82–83), to help identify the most appropriate starting stage(s) for treatment: *stage one* targets single sounds and CV words; *stage two* continues with single sound and CV words, but also targets CVCV (e.g., Toby) and CVC words (as in Figure A33.8.4: boo + t = boot; bow + t = boat); *stage three* continues with stage two target areas but also targets cluster words, multisyllabic words and early phrase level work; and *stage four* consolidates all previous targets, but with a focus on extending the range and complexity of words, as well as the maintenance of accuracy in phrases and sentences. The SLP/SLT is advised to start at stage one and consider whether the child has immediate needs at each of the items listed, before doing similarly at stages two to four. It should be noted that voice, resonance, and prosody (stress, intonation, rhythm and/or rate) targets are included at all stages, along with sound and word targets.

Transition (CV + CV = CVCV): toe + bee = Toby

Figure A33.8.3 CV + CV = CVCV toe + bee = Toby. Reproduced with permission from NDP3.

Transition (CV + C = CVC): boo + t = boot **and** bow + t = boat

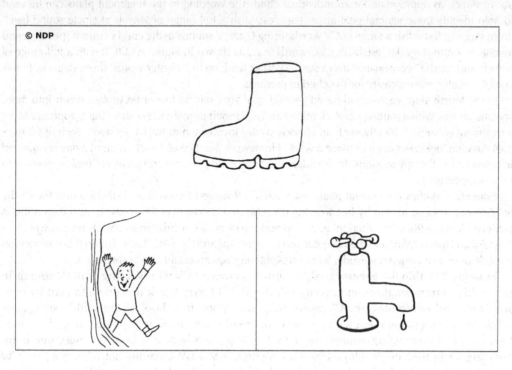

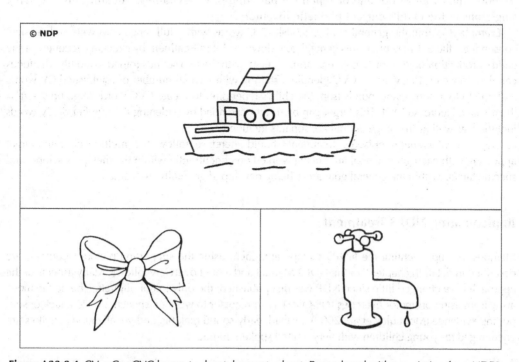

Figure A33.8.4 CV + C = CVC boo + t = boot, bow + t = boat. Reproduced with permission from NDP3.

The **third step** is for the SLP/SLT to select two to four general goal areas from one or more of the above stages, as appropriate for an individual child. The wording in the treatment plans can be used to help identify these general goal areas: e.g., 'establish a full range of vowels at single sound level' (from stage 1); 'establish a range of CV words, using C and V sounds in the child's current speech sound inventory' (from stage 1); 'establish CVC words (e.g., as shown in Figure A33.8.5) with a full range of vowels and "easier" consonants' (from stage 2); 'start work on first cluster words' (from stage 3). In this context, 'easier' means easier for the child to produce.

In the **fourth step**, each broad-based general goal area selected must be broken down into more specific targets, with a starting point identified and a planned progression of that target, appropriate for a treatment episode. Typically, such an episode would involve ten to twelve sessions, each of 60 minutes duration, delivered once or twice a week. Homework practice of 15–20 minutes a day is expected in between the therapy sessions. In the following three examples, general goals are broken down into more specific goals.

Example 1 Within the general goal, 'establish a full range of vowels at a single sound level', the SLP/SLT may choose to start by just working on achieving accuracy of long vowels; and then if this is achieved (using a 90–95% criterion) to also include work on the nearby short vowels on a vowel chart (e.g., /iː/ and then /ɪ/; /ɑː/ and then /æ/; /ɔː/ and then /ɒ/; /uː/ and then /ʊ/). Later, within this intervention episode or in a subsequent episode, work on diphthong vowels could also be included.

Example 2 Within the general goal, 'establish a range of CV words, using C and V sounds in the child's current single sound inventory', the SLP/SLT may break this down to start by consolidating and reinforcing any CV words (e.g., me, more, bee, boo, hi) the child can already produce by associating them with pictures, and then saying them in repetitive (e.g., bee, bee, bee, bee) and contrasting sequencing activities (e.g., bee-boo, bee-boo, bee-boo, bee-boo). This target can then be developed by working on C + V = CV blending activities e.g., /m/+/u/ = 'moo'; /n/ + /əʊ/ = 'no' and/or repetitive babbling of CV syllables, but still only involving singletons in the child's current phonetic inventory.

Example 3 Within the general goal 'establish CVC words with a full range of vowels and "easier" consonants', the SLT may break this general goal down and start treatment by checking accuracy of the child's production of VC words (e.g., eat, arm, in, egg), with the two sounds joined smoothly. The focus can then move on to CV + C = CVC blending, starting with a small number of established CV words and one to four consonant sounds from the child's repertoire, to create CVC words (e.g., bow + /t/ = 'boat') as in Figure A33.8.4. This target can be further extended by widening the number of CV words included, as well as the range of final consonants included.

Over an intervention episode, treatment should therefore follow the multi-level, multi-target approach, with each general goal area being worked on concurrently within the therapy sessions, and specific targets within the general goal areas being developed gradually over time.

Implementing NDP3 Treatment

Methods for implementing the NDP3 therapy approach, using the supporting picture resources, are described in detail in chapter 5 of the NDP3 Manual and a brief overview follows. Many aspects of the approach have changed little since NDP was first published; the only major difference being the move away from using oromotor exercises (NS-OME) as a precursor to work on speech, due to a lack of supporting evidence (McCauley et al., 2009). Instead, early sound making, and vocalization activities are encouraged for young children with very limited spoken output.

CV–CVC Sequencing: Lee-leaf

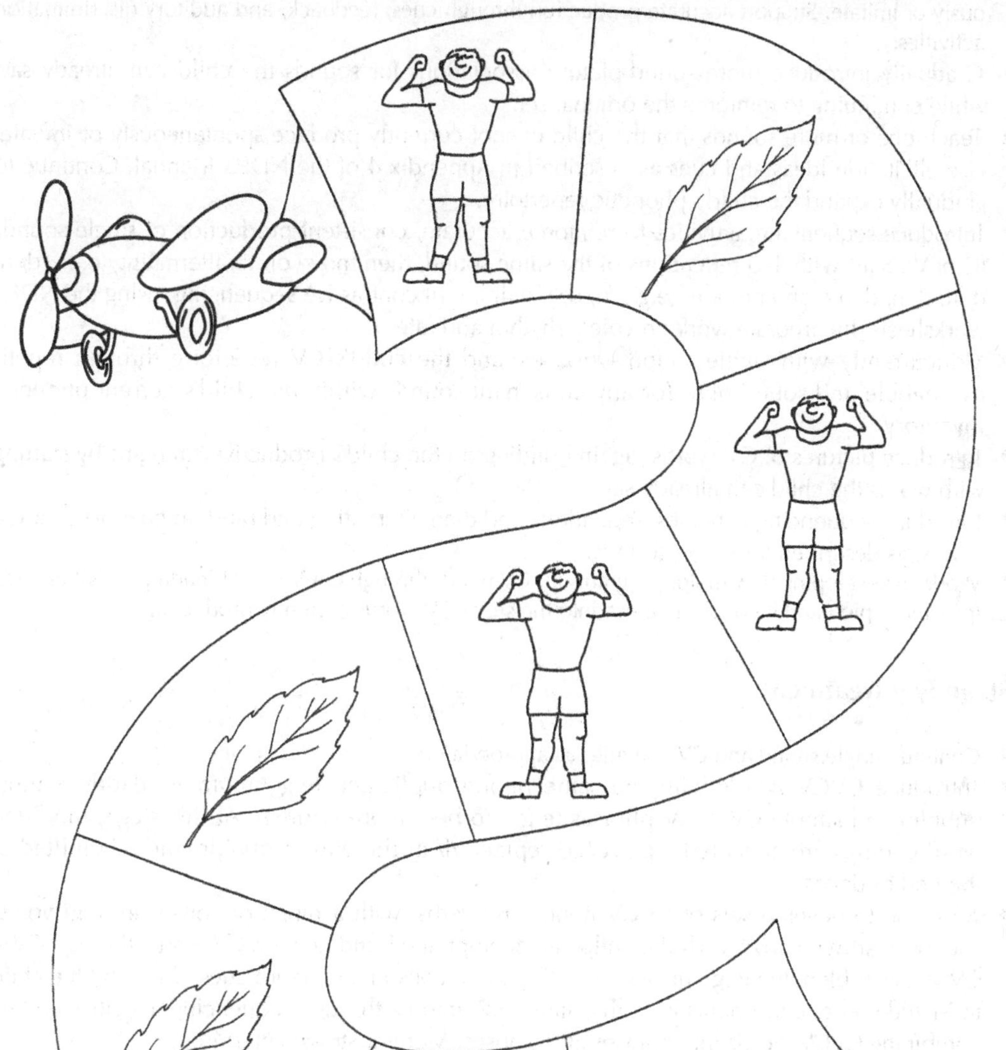

Figure A33.8.5 CV–CVC sequencing. Reproduced with permission from NDP3.

Stage One Treatment

- Introduce 4 to 6 NDP3 sound-cue pictures of Cs and Vs that the child can already produce spontaneously or imitate. Support accurate production through cues, feedback, and auditory discrimination activities.
- Gradually introduce more sound-picture associations for sounds the child can already say, while continuing to reinforce the original set.
- Teach one or more sounds that the child cannot currently produce spontaneously or imitate. Use elicitation ideas and cues as described in Appendix 4 of the NDP3 Manual. Continue to gradually expand the child's phonetic repertoire.
- Introduce sequencing activities to reinforce accurate, consistent production of single sounds (C or V). Start with 4–8 repetitions of the same sound, then move on to alternating (e.g., /d, n, d, n, d, n, d, n /) and random (e.g., /u, u, i, u, i, i, i, u) contrastive sequencing, using the NDP3 worksheets. Incorporate work on voice, rhythm and rate.
- Concurrently with single sound work, expand the child's CV repertoire through repetitive babble and sound play, for any consonant sounds within the child's current phonetic inventory.
- Introduce pictures of CV words, again building on the child's productive strengths by starting with words the child can already say.
- Introduce sequencing activities (repetitions and then alternating and random contrasts) for CV words, as described for single sounds.
- Work on developing new motor programs for CV words through C + V = CV blending activities (e.g., /p/ +/aɪ/ = 'pie') and incorporate these into the set of CV words currently produced.

Stage Two Treatment

- Continue single sound and CV activities as appropriate.
- Introduce CVCV words with the same phone duplicated (e.g., mummy, daddy, nanny, bubble) and simple CV + CV phrases (e.g., no bee, more door(s)). At this stage, modified word endings are accepted e.g., /ʊ/ to replace /l/ at the end of bubble and /s/ omitted at the end of doors.
- Move on to develop sets of CVCV nouns and verbs, with a range of consonant and vowel sounds. Start with any words the child can attempt and build new CVCV words through CV + CV = CVCV blending (e.g., tie + knee = tiny). Use consonant picture cues to remind the child to include onset consonants in both syllables. Reinforce through sequencing activities and by combining CVCV words into phrases and clauses. Monitor stress patterning.
- Introduce pictures for VC words that the child can already say and expand the range, through V + C = VC blending e.g., /i/ + /t/ = 'eat'.
- Move on to work on CVC words through CV + C = CVC blending activities e.g., boo + /t/ = 'boot'. Gradually widen the range of CVC words.
- Practise CVC sequencing activities, working towards CV/CVC contrasts e.g., 'boo-boot'; 'Lee-leaf'.

Treatment Stages Three and Four

- Continue work on single sounds, CV, CVCV and CVC words as appropriate.
- Start working on cluster words, through C+ CV(C) = CCV(C) blending (e.g., /s/ + tar = 'star') and working through to cluster/no cluster contrasts e.g., 'bed-bread', 'tar-star'.

- Introduce multisyllabic words, by breaking 3 syllable words into constituent syllables and then re-assembling. Expand the range of words gradually, monitor stress patterning and re-check once articulatory accuracy has been achieved.
- Continue to expand range and complexity of words of all phonotactic structures and work on maintenance of accurate, consistent production in phrases and sentences.

Summary

The NDP3 is a comprehensive, published intervention package which provides both a set of therapy procedures and techniques, and a flexible resource of pictorial materials, from which the SLP/SLT can select appropriate components to plan and implement treatment for individual children. Treatment planning can be challenging, but practitioners are advised to take a careful step-by-step approach and to follow the advice in the NDP3 Manual. The multi-level, multi-target NDP3 treatment approach has been evaluated in two RCTs, with positive treatment and generalization outcomes reported.

Long-term Consequences of CAS

So far, Chapter 8 has covered the early-warning signs of speech delay that become apparent in infancy and/or early childhood (Overby, A28); aspects of assessment of children with MSD (Skinder-Meredith, A28; Allison, A29); intervention for dysarthria in 6- to 18-year-olds applying the Speech Systems Approach (Pennington, A30); dynamic assessment of MSD with the DEMMS and dynamic intervention for CAS using DTTC (Strand, A31); and intervening with ReST (McCabe, A32) and NDP3 (Williams, A33). In the process, assessment, and intervention procedures with infants through to adolescents and young adults with MSD were surveyed.

Attention now turns to what might be in store for individuals who were diagnosed with CAS as children as they negotiate an adolescence and an adulthood impacted by the sequelae of CAS, and for some, concomitant and co-occurring issues. These can include language and literacy impairment and social anxiety, particularly speech-related anxiety. The author of A34, **Dr. Tricia McCabe** was introduced at the top of Q32 and A32, and readers will recall that she has a longstanding interest in speech development and disorders, leads the CAS Treatment Research Group at The University of Sydney and the research program that developed ReST.

Q34.   Tricia Mccabe

A long-awaited development in the study of Childhood Apraxia of Speech (CAS) is the current emergence of data around the long-term speech and psychological consequences of this motor speech disorder. What do we already know and what do we need to know next and into the future? Why are these data important, and how should we advise parents, as well as older adolescents and adults who were diagnosed with CAS in childhood, about, management and prognosis?

A34.   Patricia McCabe: Childhood Apraxia of Speech: An emerging image of a lifelong disorder

Current consensus is that Childhood Apraxia of Speech (CAS; previously developmental verbal dyspraxia: DVD) arises from difficulties with planning and programming the complex movement sequences required for accurate and intelligible speech (ASHA, 2007). Historically, CAS was thought of as an issue of early to middle childhood with limited data available about what happens to these children when they grow up. We might assume that clinicians and researchers believed that with sufficient, effective therapy, people with CAS would no longer have a speech disorder and therefore would also not suffer any long-term negative effects of their childhood speech disorder.

In recent years, it has become increasingly clear that this assumption is probably untrue, and in fact, children with CAS grow up to be adults with CAS. Indeed, there may be significant lifetime consequences for these people, extending beyond speech accuracy. This new perspective comes from three sources; case reports, cohort studies and surveys of adolescents and adults who were diagnosed with CAS as children.

Case Reports

The case literature includes three examples of adults with histories of CAS. First, BJ and his family who were described by Carrigg and colleagues (Carrigg et al., 2015, 2016). BJ was part of a large multigenerational family with CAS, where some of the family members had a known genetic cause for their CAS, a variant of the FoxP2 gene. As a young man, BJ was described as reluctant to talk with strangers, socially anxious. His reduced intelligibility led him to use AAC outside his home. The members of his broader family who had CAS experienced persistent anxiety when talking to unfamiliar listeners, distress and frustration when not understood, and self-consciousness about their speech. Family members reported avoiding certain words, speaking situations (e.g., work meetings) and sounds that were difficult to produce. The two in the family with the lowest intelligibility each had a diagnosed social anxiety disorder.

The only other formally reported case is of a 21-year-old woman described in Rusiewicz and Rivera (2017). While this study is focussed on treatment, the paper details CAS related speech errors persisting into adulthood and difficulties establishing correct /ɹ/ production. The young woman was also anecdotally

described as requiring literacy support with her college studies. An additional case is reported in Hill (2016), in a masters thesis. In this case, a 20-year-old college student is described as still having articulation and phonological errors, and difficulty with polysyllabic words and DDK type tasks. She reported having a small but close group of friends and making occupational decisions based on her speech history.

A Cohort Study

A single, longitudinal cohort study has followed some children with CAS since the 1990s as part of the Cleveland Family Speech and Reading study which enrolled children between the ages of 3 and 6 years and has since followed many of them into adulthood. This body of work by Barbara Lewis and colleagues (e.g., Miller et al., 2019; Lewis et al., 2021) has shown that as a group, adolescents with CAS or suspected CAS, are more likely than their peers with other speech sound disorders to have a range of ongoing issues including ongoing speech errors and reading difficulties, while some individuals are more likely to have social problems. Reading difficulties were more frequent in adolescents who also had difficulty with phonological awareness or co-morbid language impairment (Miller et al., 2019) while social difficulties were thought to be related to a higher rate of speech errors in adolescents with CAS than those with other speech sound disorders (Lewis et al., 2021). Importantly, nearly four in five participants still had measurable speech difficulties.

Survey Research

The final source of information about what happens in adulthood to people with CAS comes from survey research. Adults with a history of CAS report continuing to have speech difficulties and to avoid some speaking tasks such as using the telephone and speaking to strangers (Cassar et al., 2022; McCabe et al., 2017). Such self-reported behaviours are reminiscent of what we see with adults who stutter (e.g., James et al., 1999; Lowe et al., 2017). Some adults with CAS report 'speech recovery' but even they report difficulties with their speech when they are tired or stressed. Almost all adults with a history of CAS report still having difficulty with individual sounds or words. In addition to ongoing speech issues, Cassar et al. (2023) collected self-reported anxiety measures along with speech samples containing polysyllabic words, especially those with weak onsets (e.g., flamingo, gorilla, spaghetti) on their own, and sentences containing at least two of those poly-syllabic words (e.g., The flamingo went to the cinema). Adults with a history of CAS had more anxiety than would be expected in the general population and this anxiety correlated with speech accuracy. Finally, survey research has also shown that adults with a history of CAS self-report difficulties at school, especially with spelling and other literacy tasks (Cassar et al., 2023; P. J. McCabe et al., 2017).

Living with CAS in Adulthood

Putting it all together, it appears unlikely that most children with CAS will grow out of it but that for many adults, CAS will be present but masked in everyday speech. The described problems with speech motor planning and programming may be hidden as speech motor plans are stored and retained through deliber-ate practice, daily use, and therapy. Adults with a history of CAS report and have been shown to have more difficulty with new or complex words because these require a new speech motor plan and new learning.

It is possible that the reported long-term effects of CAS in adults are associated with *when* they became research participants. This may be the case because in the late twentieth century the professions' understanding of CAS, and particu-larly understanding of how it should be treated, was less developed. If this so, then as treatment improves, we may see a reduction in the long-term effects of CAS. On the other hand, given the reported persistence of CAS features, even in those who believe they have recovered, it is likely that

CAS is a lifetime disorder. This makes sense if the underlying genotype which includes diffi-culties creating, evaluating, modifying, stor-ing, and retrieving speech motor plans is at best partially remediated by therapy which addresses the surface presentation of the dis-order, or phenotype of disordered speech. The CAS phenotype includes inconsistent errors, difficulty with prosody, and difficulty transition-ing across speech units, among other surface features.

Assessing Adolescents and Adults with Histories of CAS

In considering assessment of adolescents and adults with a history of CAS, SLPs/SLTs need to account for the possible normalisation of less complex speech and provide more challeng-ing speech tasks to assess, diagnose and facil-itate selection of appropriate therapy goals. To address this issue, clinicians are encouraged to use a mixture of novel or made-up words, technical words, and polysyllabic words to stretch the speech motor planning capacity of the adolescent or adult with a childhood diag-nosis of CAS. An example of such is available from the ReST website https://www.rest.sydney.edu.au/resources

Impact on Phonological Awareness, Reading, and Spelling

As shown here, there is emerging evidence that difficulties in phonological awareness, reading and spelling are more frequent in children, adolescents, and adults with CAS. The science of reading suggests that literacy is acquired in part through deliberate, explicit phonics instruction (e.g., Hempenstall, 2019). In practice, phonics is often implemented by asking the child to understand phoneme-grapheme correspondence, convert graph-emes to phonemes, hold the phonemes in short term memory and finally verbally blend the resultant phonemes to read a word out loud. Children with CAS, who (by definition) have inconsistent speech, may be at a disadvantage with this approach. Further research on how to ensure children with CAS acquire age-appropriate literacy is required. In the meantime, non-verbal or input phonics may be an interim solution. In such an approach a young child would be asked to silently convert graphemes to phonemes, blend the sounds in their head and then select the picture that matches the written word (see for example, Pascoe et al., 2006).

Expanding Our (Research and Intervention) Horizons

Given the emerging association between residual or extended speech impairment and anxiety, we may need to consider multi-disciplinary practice for adults with a history of CAS. Importantly, most current treatment regimens are focussed on simpler and earlier acquired skills, with fewer than five participants older than 14 years in the entire literature (Preston et al., 2013; Rosenthal, 1994; Rusiewicz & Rivera, 2017). To date, no group or repeated single case design treatment studies have explored speech (or any other goal) treatment for adolescents and adults with a history of CAS. Research is urgently required to establish diagnostic criteria for CAS in adolescents and adults and to determine appropriate interventions for this population, both for their speech and for any concomitant disorders.

Talking to Families, Older Adolescents, and Adults About CAS Prognosis and Management

What should we tell parents about prognosis? The future is unknowable; but what we can say is that treatment has improved substantially since about 2008. We can also say, with confidence, that early multidisciplinary intervention that starts in the preschool years, not only aimed at improving speech, but also designed to target both psychological harm minimisation and effective literacy acquisition,

may provide their child with the best possible start.

What should we tell adolescents and adults about prognosis and management? To start, we must acknowledge (to them) the work they and their families have done since their early childhood, and what they accomplished. Then, we need to explore and recognise the specific issues they want to address rather than assuming their SLP/SLT need is essentially phoneme specific.

The current CAS literature in working with adolescents and adults is sparse, but we can generalise from other areas of SLP/SLT practice. For example, if anxiety is an issue, the stuttering literature reveals that speaking anxiety can be effectively managed through Cognitive Behavioural Therapy (CBT) so that logically, CBT may be an appropriate means of support. Finally, we can explain that short blocks of intensive treatment that follows the principles of neuroplasticity and motor learning should be more effective than weekly therapy for an indefinite period. Given the rate of change in treatment for younger children, the hope is that the profession takes up the challenge of research and practice with this lifelong disorder.

Early Days

Having considered MSD from various angles, and at different developmental ages and stages, we return to the first steps in the referral, diagnosis, and treatment journey. In the initial stages of assessment and intervention for children with CAS or suspected CAS (sCAS), parents face a huge learning trajectory and may feel swamped with information, emotion, and fatigue. Many parents experience uncertainty and grief, traversing stages of denial, anger, bargaining, depression, and ultimately, acceptance. It is also a time for hard work for parents as they adjust to their changed situation (Hennessy & Hennessy, 2013), keeping the child occupied with fun, relevant activities that match the child's needs and strengths. Guidelines from Hammer and Stoeckel (2001), outlined in bulleted lists below, remain helpful. Note that there is deliberate overlap between sections.

- **Early on it is important to help parents to**
  - work *with* the therapist or team, by encouraging the child's motivation, participation and cooperation in therapy sessions and in homework.
  - learn about CAS and relevant techniques to employ at home.
  - question anything not understood, or anything worrying, straight away.
  - be available at key times to participate in sessions, observations, or video viewing.
  - report openly about home practice frequency and the child's responses.
  - work within realistic parameters.
  - understand treatment limitations and prognostic indicators.
  - have high and reasonable expectations of the child.
- **Parents will do best if shown how to**
  - organise the environment to facilitate communication.
  - make some homework 'invisible' or 'indirect'.
  - make some of the homework visible and direct.
  - provide input without always insisting on a response from the child.
  - identify nursery rhymes, songs, and stories to use relative to targets.
  - use 'communicative temptations' (desired objects the child will request; favoured activities/games they will ask to do/play) that are visible but inaccessible.
  - employ modelling and recasting techniques optimally.
  - choose targets that will be functional and powerful to motivate the child to *try*.
  - use fun games, activities and drill-play.
- **Alert parents to potential pitfalls, such as**
  - over cueing; for example, providing exaggerated, distorted speech models.
  - initiating many new targets quickly: new content is best balanced with older content.
  - tackling targets that are too difficult for the child.
  - avoiding practising things that the child is 'good at' (it is not a waste of time!).
  - burnout of child, parents, and other helpers. Burnout is an issue that must be considered in relation to homework. Sometimes parents are so eager to do as much as they can that they

quickly kill off any good will on the child's part, and face exhaustion and thorny cooperation issues. In the early months, it may be helpful to limit the duration of speech focus at home, and then to expand it gradually if necessary so parents are not overwhelmed, and the child is not put off.

- **The clinician's responsibility**

In intervention, the clinician's paramount goal is for the child to become as fully functional a communicator as possible by teaching needed skills based on individual, on-going assessment, and collaboration with the child's parents. Parents must know that the clinician sees them as the most important members of the treatment team, and integral to any progress, and that he or she will

  - acknowledge and welcome their (parents' and child's) efforts and hard work.
  - educate them about CAS and its management.
  - provide information about networking options and available support (if wanted).
  - teach them specific strategies relative to their child's intervention needs.
  - be flexible with targets and strategies and programme implementation.
  - maximise production practice.
  - maximise *functional* communication goals.
  - maintain high and reasonable expectations of the child within their capabilities.
  - maintain high, reasonable expectations of the parent(s) within their capabilities.
- **To accomplish the above objectives, the SLP/ SLT must be able to**
  - explain goals in clear language and signal and explain changes in treatment strategies, particularly as changes may be misinterpreted as a sign of failure on the part of child, parent, or clinician.
  - genuinely welcome and value parents' why-questions.
  - ensure opportunities for participation, observation, and discussion.
  - work with parents to motivate and reinforce child's learning.
- **Parents have a responsibility to**
  - Choose (if choice is available) an SLP/SLT skilled with children in their child's age-group.

It does not have to be a CAS expert! Realistically, can one *be* a CAS expert?

- Understand that while it may be preferable to have an SLP/SLT who is experienced with CAS and other childhood speech and language disorders, there are advantages to having a newly qualified clinician. For example, they may be more familiar with current research and bring fresh energy and enthusiasm to intervention sessions. Moreover, in many instances their lack in experience may be offset by mentoring and advice from a knowledgeable, supportive colleague.
- Learn about CAS and the techniques the therapist uses.
- Be available for participation in, observations of, or video viewing of sessions.
- Report openly about home practice frequency and the child's responses.
- Understand treatment limitations, especially if there are complex negative prognostic indicators.
- Have high (and reasonable) expectations of their child. This includes avoiding underestimating what the child can do.
- Question anything not understood and to address worries straight away.
- **The child, older child or adult has a responsibility to**
  - Accept help from the parents and SLP/SLT in the process of learning to communicate more effectively.
  - Ultimately, as an older child or adult, with ongoing professional or nonprofessional support if wanted, to start taking responsibility for maintaining skills, using adaptive strategies and accepting that there will be communicative consequences when they do not.

Regarding the final two points on the list provided by Hammer and Stoeckel (2001), we – parents and clinician – must be aware that children and youth can tire of 'trying all the time' and many will effectively 'grow out of therapy'.

Andy: *'I was done with speech therapy.'*
Hennessy and Hennessy (2013, p. 148) write

I was in and out of therapy from the earliest time that I can remember and continued until just about the end of my eighth-grade year of *school. By that point in my life, I was sick of speech therapy. Skipping class had changed from being cool to being annoying ... I just wanted to be like the other kids. I wanted to go to all my classes ... So, I told my mother I was done with speech therapy.*

James: *'Do you think I'll always need to come and see you?'*

My client James, with CAS was referred at the age of 4;0 and came happily to once weekly, and at times twice-weekly 50-minute sessions with one or other parent and me until he was 6;0, making good progress with his speech and language. Then, his father took a diplomatic post in a country in which SLP/SLT services were usually unavailable. Fortuitously, a retired British expatriate SLT volunteered to help. She liaised with me via email and saw James once weekly for a year in school terms.

When James was 7;1 his father died suddenly, and he and his mother returned to Australia to live with her mother and sister. James, finding his life dominated by women – his mother, grandmother, aunt a series of female teachers, my SLP teammate and me – saw me for help with his speech, and my colleague for literacy intervention until he was 11;6. By that time he was fed up with it. The situation came to a head for him in a treatment session when, to his mother's horror, he told me exasperatedly to f-off. His mother had to agree that it was time for a break. James disdained my promise that my door would be open if he wanted to come back when he was older. But when he was 14 and wanting to ask a girl to a school social, he asked his mother if he could return. She agreed on condition that he must take responsibility for making and keeping appointments and complying with any programme. She also mentioned to him that I might not want to see him, as he had been rude to me at our last meeting!

He made an appointment and then attended weekly, working on a few late developing sounds with a strong focus on prosody and fluency, for about a year, primarily motivated by his wanting to 'talk to girls'. He returned for brief intervention–8 sessions – at 19, as a university student needing help with acute performance anxiety experienced when speaking is tutorials. James assumed that his sense of panic, elevated heartrate and shaky voice were due to having CAS. He was relieved and reassured when it was normalized as something many people, even actors and seasoned public speakers, experience, and heartened by reading Mark Twain's 'How I conquered stage fright' speech (Twain, 1910).

Still initiating contact, he returned at 22 as a new graduate in computer science, wanting to role-play a job interview at an IT company run by the brothers Wojciechowski [vɔɪˈtʃeˌhɒvˌskɪ]. Although James rehearsed it to perfection over two sessions, he remained apprehensive that he would, in his words, '*say their names wrong*', '*mix up the syllables*' and '*sound dumb*' on the day. Imagine his relief when the interviewers greeted him with, '*You must be James. I'm Tom, and this is my brother, Nick. Our other brother, Alex, will be here shortly*'. He got the job and eventually discovered that Tom, Nick, and Alex were short for Tomasz, Nicholas, and Aleksander Wojciechowski. The last time I saw James he was 25 needing help rehearsing his wedding speech. The speech was sounding good at the end of the second session, and James sat back in his seat and said, '*Do you think I'll always need to come and see you?*' One thing led to another, and I asked him if his fiancée ever remarked on his speech. He said that she did, and that he appreciated it when Hannah corrected his pronunciation or helped him say new or difficult words. He brought her along the following week, and it turned out that they had known since entering high school. She greeted me with, 'I've always wanted to meet *you*!'

I tell the story because we do not often see the positive effect of what we do as SLPs/SLTs quite so clearly from the perspective of someone close to an adult with CAS. Hannah had observed much of his progress, and he had filled out any missing details. How he had been a 4-year-old that none of the children or the teachers at his preschool could understand. How, as he saw it, his parents and I had taught him to speak intelligibly, but not perfectly. How they, as a family, had a thrilling overseas adventure that stopped abruptly with his father's death when James was seven years old. How my colleague and I had helped him, and been important to him, in pre-adolescence, and how he had been 'horribly rude' to me nonetheless; and how we had 'been there for him' intermittently ever since. The

way she told it, often quoting James, it was a moving and inspiring story, and a wonderful example of an adult maturely taking responsibility for his own communication needs. For completeness I should add that Hannah and I had three sessions alone to explore simple strategies she could employ to help James with problematic utterances and speaking situations, and a final session with the three of us working together.

Homework and the Homework Habit

No matter how 'in tune', creative, flexible, encouraging and motivating we, as clinicians, are in therapy sessions, the necessary carryover is unlikely without solid family support. So, homework – when recommended – must be understood and implemented properly, one-to-one in good listening and learning conditions, and often. It is essential to impress upon parents that we see this as a collaborative process, that they are not expected to do all the work or to perform miracles, and that their suggestions and feedback are welcome. As the people who know their child best, it is often parents who can tell us how to get things done without a battle, which rewards will be effective, which activities will appeal, and the signs we should look for that tell us that the child wants or needs us to 'back off' a little.

If parents can be encouraged to regard 'speech homework' as part of the family's normal routine, it can help enormously. If brief, regular 5- to 7-minute bursts of homework are as usual as mealtimes and bathing, and as non-negotiable as wearing a car seatbelt or looking both ways before crossing the road (and hopefully not just a job for *one* parent to do with the child), explicitly principled homework is not so difficult for most families to accomplish despite additional family commitments, work and other responsibilities and life-events.

Distributed, random bursts of practice with appropriate reinforcement, taken cumulatively, can contribute to significant change. Rehearsal of homework tasks during therapy sessions, and 'coaching' of parents by the clinician, is valuable as it helps parents build confidence in their skills, and it lets their child know that *their* parents genuinely are part of *their* treatment team. Parents can be engaged early as 'the homework experts' for their own child, compiling power word and phrase lists (words and phrases that are important to the child), collecting speech samples and making a 'brag book'.

Brag Book

A brag book is a small, durable album or picture book, owned by the child and devoted to what the child *can* do, even if it only contains a couple of signs and a few sound effects. It is not a collection of words the adults in the child's life would *like* him or her to say, or that they are trying to teach! There is no 'right way' to compile one of these books, but it is quite popular (with children) to start with a few pictures of the child, so that when asked 'Who's this?' they can point to indicate 'me' even if they cannot say it yet; or simply nod when asked 'Is this you?' if they are not yet able to respond with 'Mmm', 'Uh-huh' or 'Yes'. If the child has some signed or spoken verbs (e.g., *go, stop, eat*) or verbal approximations, these could follow, with photographs of the child engaged in the actions. Favourite toys or foods and drinks that they have a sign, iconic gesture, sound, or word for might come next, followed by important people (parents, siblings, and grandparents, perhaps), pets, places (e.g., *home, my house, my room, my bed*) and possessions (e.g., *my book* for the brag book). Next come all the words and approximations the child can say (including *poo, wee, bum,* etc. if they are in the repertoire) and the child's sound effects for vehicles, machines, animals, musical instruments, and appliances. For all the images in the brag book, it is important to print, in lower case, the intended word or sound effect (e.g., *ee-ee* or *ee ee* for mouse and not *EE-EE* or *EE EE*) and instructions for executing any signs or gestures, so that *anyone* who picks up the book knows how to enjoy it with the child. If touch cues, prompts and imagery are being used, include appropriate graphics and instructions. 'Favourite words' (e.g., *Bob*) or 'good words' (words or phrases that the child says well or is proud of, such as their age: *three, four* or *five,* etc.) can go in several times, making sure that there are some easy, fun words at the beginning of the book and again at the end, to finish on a positive note. Songs, rhymes,

rebus and cloze where the child *can* provide the punch line can add to the enjoyment. As the book grows, the pictures can be rearranged so that they are loosely organized by theme and initial sound, encouraging everyone to think in terms of patterns and prosody from early on.

The brag book can include a note or letter from the therapist in accessible, jargon-free language to let the family and significant others know that

- The emphasis should be on *meaningful* word production and syllable production (e.g., *bee, boo, moo, neigh, go, me too, no way, bye-bye, up*) and that isolated sounds are really only a goal if they carry meaning (e.g., *sh* for be-quiet, *ss* as a snake sound, *ee-ee* for a mouse sound effect, *mm* for yes and yum), and as a means to an end in stimulability therapy (Miccio, A23; Williams A33).
- Isolated sound production *may* be used briefly as a 'therapy step', but that *ba-ba-ba, bee-bee-bee, ta-ta-ta,* etc. are more desirable than practice drills comprising sequences such as [b-b-b-b-b-], [t-t-t-t-], [p-t-p-t-p-t-p-t-p-t-], [t-k-t-k-t-k-] etc.
- Suprasegmentals (rhythm, melody, stress, loudness, pitch, rate, resonance including nasal resonance, and intonation) should be emphasized from the start. This may promote more natural sounding speech ('speech naturalness') earlier, as opposed to the 'programmed' sound with odd prosody, and the excessive and equal stress (EES) characteristic of many English-speaking children who have been treated for CAS.
- The desired goal is *many* 'repeats' of therapy targets whether they are syllables, syllable sequences, single words or word sequences. The 'repeats' or 'practice trials' are needed to facilitate optimal, 'automatic' speech production.

Parents' ingenuity and input, particularly in the initial stages, are necessary to get therapy off to a good start, and we rely on them to help find activities and rewards that are beneficial and motivating and fun for toddlers and pre-schoolers. Parents can be reassured that, with appropriate support, most children will start to 'bring the homework to parents', understand what the therapy is for, and take some responsibility for their own practice needs.

10 Tips for Intervention for Young Children with Severe CAS

With children who are non-verbal or who have few word approximations, early goals are to:

1. Establish a 'core vocabulary'. This constitutes a selection of power-words or words to 'sign and say' like *no, more, go* and *me too*.
2. Select phonetic stimuli, favouring ones that are already spontaneously produced, most stimulable, and most visual.
3. Start with CV and VC and CVC combinations. Include isolated vowels, making them meaningful, if possible, but avoid isolated consonants unless they carry meaning.
4. Establish the most beneficial facilitators for the individual child (ask the parents or *tell* them!).
5. Establish an appropriate stimulus/response relationship. Parents need to know how many models to provide and how many trials (repeats) to expect, and to provide feedback for around 50% of correct responses.
6. Set criteria for subsequent changes in stimuli (How many correct trials?).
7. Choose reinforcers (rewards) carefully, knowing that achieving the necessary intensity of drill is difficult and that it is often hard to maintain the child's attention and cooperation. The aim here is to ensure enough responses within a practice session.
8. Be mindful of linguistic load. Keep it simple. Do not use complex carrier phrases or cloze, or awkward prosody.
9. Use alternative and augmentative communication (AAC), including sign and picture exchange to augment verbal attempts, to enhance language development and to reduce the child's frustration. Reassure parents that AAC will not stifle verbal communication.
10. Keep therapy fresh – sameness and boredom kill *everyone's* motivation.

Controversial Interventions

Bowen and Snow (2017) was published after the previous edition of this book, and its success drove the decision to write a plain-English companion book for families and teachers (Bowen & Snow, 2024). Both books were responses to the problem of widely available, popular but nonevidence-based interventions that abound for children and young people with developmental disorders, including those with SSD. As mentioned in the final paragraph of Chapter 3, in SSD, CAS and speech motor delay (SMD) associated with Down syndrome seem to spawn the most activity from those who develop and profit commercially from interventions with no, or at best, scant empirical support. In researching the books, we found a proliferation of non-evidenced assessments and interventions for children and young people with articulation, disorders, CAS, childhood dysarthria, dyslexia and specific learning disabilities in general, stuttering, and communication disorders associated with autism, and Down syndrome. They encompassed untested dietary regimens, nutritional supplements, mouth exercises, and SLP/SLT-like treatments, some of which are summarized below.

- **Diets and Nutritional Supplements.**
  These included the regimens proposed by Morris and Agin (2009) who 'revealed a new syndrome' comprising food allergies, gluten sensitivity, CAS, and nutrient malabsorption, alongside low muscle tone, poor coordination and abnormal sensory integration (and often, ASD). They, and their imitators who promote the so called 'Apraxia Diet', advocate Vitamin E and omega 3 fatty acid supplementation.
- **Non-Speech Oral Motor Exercises.**
  Exercises for the articulators, or Non-Speech Oral Motor Exercises: NSOME (Lof, A23; and see comments by Golding-Kushner, A16, and Ruscello, A38) have no place in the treatment of CAS, or any SSD. Thankfully, their use by SLPs/SLTs in many settings appears to be declining somewhat, probably in response to vigorous publication in peer reviewed journals, with Heather M. Clark, Karen Forrest, Megan M. Hodge, Alan G. Kamhi, Norman J. Lass, Gregory L. Lof, Rebecca J. McCauley, Mary Pannbacker, Thomas W. Powell, Dennis M. Ruscello, Edythe A. Strand, and Maggie M. Watson leading the charge. But, as Lof (A23) points out, thorough systematic reviews (Lee & Gibbon, 2015; McCauley et al., 2009; Ruscello & Vallino, 2020) have been unable to

unearth published data to show whether NSOME for speech aid in intervention for SSD or whether they do not, pinpointing a research-practice gap (Malamud et al., 2021).

But NSOME haven't gone away and are still promoted by SLPs/SLTs who work with children with SSD only, or children with SSD and other developmental disorders, such as Down syndrome (for representative examples see, Shukla, 2021; van Vuren, 2008), and autism (e.g., Griffith, 2022).

SLPs'/SLTs' use of NSOME have been surveyed in numerous countries and regions. For example, Baigorri et al. (2022) in Guatemala; Diepeveen et al. (2020) in the Netherlands; Hodge et al. (2005) in Canada; Joffe and Pring (2008) in the UK; Kamal (2021) in Jordan; Lof and Watson (2008) and Brumbaugh and Bosma Smit (2013) in the USA; Pratomo and Siswanto (2020) in Central Java, Indonesia; Rumbach et al. (2016, 2019) in Australia, and Thomas and Kaipa (2015) in India. Reviewing the percentages of clinicians who said they used NSOME for child speech intervention, the score card for the surveyed participants is Australia: 26% for articulation disorder, 6% for phonological disorder, 69% for childhood dysarthria, and 38% for CAS %; and for SSD generally, Canada 85%, Guatemala 66%, India 91%, Indonesia 85%, Jordan 74%, UK 71%; and USA 85%.

Baigorri et al. (2022) argue that SLPs/SLTs working in 'high income' countries (i.e., countries with high Gross National Income), where the profession has been established for a long time are more likely, historically to have adopted NSOME. By contrast, those in low- to middle income countries (e.g., Guatemala where the profession has existed for 50 years) where SLP/SLT and its academic programs are less well established, and access to relevant literature is difficult, may not be as likely to employ NSOME. They say insightfully, '*new programs may not need to follow certain trajectory, and missteps, that occurred in high-income countries as the field evolved over decades*', and the results of their small, qualitative survey bear this out.

It must be said, however, that doubtful and dissenting voices were heard very early in our history. Kanter (1948) who was an early champion of blowing exercises to strengthen the velopharyngeal mechanism in children with clefts, later criticized them, asserting that they are time wasting when the palate is short, and the velopharyngeal gap is large.

Agreeing with Kanter three years on in a literature review, McDonald and Baker (1951) counselled against their use, noting that there was scant evidence in their favour. They wrote, '*Clinical experience with over 200 patients has demonstrated that cleft palate patients can develop intelligible and, in many cases, near-normal speech without recourse to blowing exercises.*'

Still in the cleft palate-craniofacial domain, we do need to be careful not to throw the baby out with the bathwater when we eschew NSOME, e.g.:

> *It is important to point out that while we do not believe that simple blowing activities can strengthen muscles, we do agree with the 70% (63/90) of respondents in this study who indicated that simple blowing activities can heighten a child's awareness of oral air flow. This latter finding is consistent with recommendations provided by several authors who consider such activities (when used sparingly) helpful in the young toddler with cleft palate who does not understand that she/he can direct air orally following palatal surgery.*
>
> Hardin-Jones et al., 2020

- **Application Software (Apps).**
  NSOME published by SLPs/SLTs are available in the App Store and Google Play. These include for example, Barbara Fernandes' ('geek SLP') *Smart Oral Motor 4+: Oral Motor Activities* from Smarty Ears LLC. Some parents, especially home-schooling parents, buy these Apps with a view to 'going it alone', and some do so to augment their children's SLP/SLT programs.

- **NSOME Products: Books, Equipment (tools and toys), and Manuals.**
  Retailers of SLP/SLT assessment and intervention resources, including books and manuals, exhibit regularly at national, state, and regional professional conferences and meetings, and they often stock huge ranges of NSOME equipment. See for example, https://www.superduperinc.com/topics/oral-motor.html from Super Duper, and https://www.proedaust.com.au/motor-speech-and-oral-motor from Pro-Ed Australia.

- **Treatment Approaches.**
  'Invented' (Vashdi's word, not mine) by a physiotherapist with a master's in physical education and a doctorate in physical therapy, Apraxia

Verbal Motor Learning Method (VML) by Dr. Elad Vashdi, is an aspect of his Multi-Dimensional Therapy Method (MDT). Like MDT as an entity, VML falls squarely in four categories. one, it is atheoretical, two, it is non-evidence based, three it is purported to address an unlikely range of disorders in toddlers, children and adults, and four it does not appear in peer reviewed journals of good standing. Some details of VML are on the Yael Center site https://yaelcenter.com, with videos of it in action and a link to the associated Facebook page where there is more information and a free online assessment in English and Mandarin, 'for children with special needs'.

Misleading Claims

When parents ask about the method the clinician uses, it may be an indication that they believe a 'best method' exists, a favoured 'therapy package' can be accessed or there is a 'therapy kit' or manualized intervention tool that they should source.

Some families hear about interventions that lack empirical support via the Internet, and their questions may be fuelled by statements like: *'Therapists and parents have found OPT to be effective with a variety of populations and diagnoses, including but not limited to Down syndrome, Autism, Cerebral Palsy, Childhood Apraxia of Speech, Tethered Oral Tissue, cleft lip and palate and more.'* (https://talktools.com). Then there are these fulsome promises: *'Our clinically proven practice tools work nearly twice as fast and our speech therapists are the best in the nation. We back all of our speech solutions with a 100% guarantee.'* from https://www.speechbuddy.com Such statements mislead, by:

- Suggesting that the products are backed by evidence when they are not.
- Implying, or stating, a guarantee of effectiveness, setting up unrealistic expectations.
- Asserting that the products are effective with a variety of populations and diagnoses.
- Employing the weasel words (meaningless expression) 'clinically proven'.
- Making baseless claims, e.g., 'our speech therapists are the best in the nation'.

While such language may entice some families it will put others off. Parents with an appreciation of professionalism may well recoil from such elaborate assertions, forming a negative view of SLPs'/SLTs' advertising standards and ethicality (see Leitão A1). Other parents may already be convinced by or engaged in 'complementary' or 'alternative' (non-evidence based) interventions. They may attend an initial consultation, or a subsequent consultation if it takes them a while to trust their SLP/SLT with pamphlets and articles promoting various panaceas and nostrums. Among them may be auditory integration treatments, Cellfield, chiropractic, cranio-osteopathy, craniosacral therapy, Myomunchee, and sensory integration therapy, and more (Bowen & Snow, 2017; 2024). In general, they wish to determine whether the clinician will cooperate with, or at least not actively oppose, their 'alternative practitioners'.

Answering Questions about Controversial Interventions

When parents ask about controversial, 'experimental', pseudoscientific, or Complementary and Alternative (CAM) interventions a short talk by the clinician on E^3BP is rarely appropriate. My strategy has been to reframe their question as, 'What you are asking me is, *"is this treatment scientific?"*' and then inform the person that I am unaware of 'scientific evidence' in support of the intervention concerned, but that I will take another look to see if I am up to date with the available literature. If I find nothing, when I see the parent(s) again, I will tell them that, and follow up by saying *'I want* [child's name]*'s speech therapy to be based in the best science'*, explaining in straightforward terms that SLP/SLT is a science-based profession. If they have said that they like the CAM under discussion, and that they have investigated it, *'researched it'* or *'done their own research'* it provides an opening to say something like *'It sounds like you're interested in science?'*. Few people will say they are not, and this too can lead to, *'OK. Then let's look at the science. Bring me the evidence that convinced you in your research, and I'll see what I can find, and we'll compare notes next time, if you'd like that'*. I guard against being dismissive, criticizing the intervention, or leaving them feeling stupid or naïve. Rather, I approach the topic with interest, really listening respectfully to why they are attracted to the method (or repelled, or frightened by conventional, mainstream interventions) because adopting a respectful, considered stance is more likely to lead to a grown-up conversation.

Which Is the Best Method?

Families of children and young people with CAS, and other diagnoses such as ADHD, autism, cerebral palsy, cleft lip and palate, childhood dysarthria, and Down syndrome explore, atheoretical, non-evidenced interventions full of hope and with the best of motives. Some are advised in good faith, by well-intentioned people, to pursue assessment, with a view to treatment using this or that unscientific method or technique. Although the practitioner may lack relevant qualifications, and the methods and techniques are supported by neither theory nor evidence, they may be alluring because they are charismatic, or because they sound more exotic, interesting and exciting, and even more 'scientific' than mainstream SLP/SLT. Indeed, some clinicians seem to believe that a therapy that comes in a box has more appeal than one that comes in the form of a journal article.

A Good Method

It may be beneficial to counsel some parents and colleagues that not all treatments suit every child and that all treatments must be individually and expertly tailored in response to the child's needs, strengths, challenges, comorbidities, assessment and re-assessment outcomes, and response to intervention. In that sense, there is no 'best method'. A 'good method' or 'good approach' is one that is

- *Evidence based* and/or *theoretically sound.*
- *Adaptable* to short-term changes in the child, in terms of attention, behaviour, interest, motivation, and wellbeing 'on the day'.
- *Flexible* over time, as the child develops.
- *Adjustable* for different settings, e.g., clinic, home, pre-school and 'out'.

- *Modifiable* to suit different service delivery conditions, e.g., in a child-clinician dyad, a child-parent-clinician triad, and in a group.

The same applies to the target selection approaches and therapy techniques we select, and some of these are presented in Chapter 9.

References

Allison, A., Hadcroft, S., Williams, P., & Stephens, H. (2011). *NDP3® Speech builder*. Nuffield Centre Dyspraxia Programme Ltd.

Allison, K. M. (2020). Measuring speech intelligibility in children with motor speech disorders. *Perspectives of the ASHA Special Interest Groups, 5*(4), 809–820. https://doi.org/10.1044/2020_PERSP-19-00110

Allison, K. M., & Hustad, K. C. (2014). Impact of sentence length and phonetic complexity on intelligibility in 5 year old children with cerebral palsy. *International Journal of Speech-Language Pathology, 16*(4), 396–407. https://doi.org/10.3109/17549507.2013.876667

Allison, K. M., Yunusova, Y., & Green, J. R. (2019). Shorter sentence length maximizes intelligibility and speech motor performance in persons with dysarthria due to amyotrophic lateral sclerosis. *American Journal of Speech-Language Pathology, 28*(1), 96–107. https://doi.org/10.1044/2018_AJSLP-18-0049

American Speech-Language-Hearing Association. (2007). *Childhood apraxia of speech [Technical Report]*. www.asha.org/policy

Aziz, A., Shohdi, S., Osman, D., & Habib, E. (2010). Childhood apraxia of speech and multiple phonological disorders in Cairo-Egyptian Arabic speaking children: language, speech, and oro-motor differences. *International Journal of Pediatric Otorhinolaryngology, 74*(8), 578–585. https://doi.org/10.1016/j.ijporl.2010.02.003

Baigorri, G., Crowley, C. J., Sommer, C. L., Blackwell, A., Miranda, A. J., & Moya-Galé, G. (2022). Examining the prevalence of intervention approaches internationally: the use of nonspeech oral motor exercises in guatemala. *Perspectives of the ASHA Special Interest Groups, 7*(4), 1203–1210. https://doi.org/10.1044/2022_PERSP-21-00285

Ballard, K. J., Robin, D. A., McCabe, P., & McDonald, J. (2010). A treatment for dysprosody in childhood apraxia of speech. *Journal of Speech, Language, and Hearing Research*, *53*(5), 1227–1245. https://doi.org/10.1044/1092-4388(2010/09-0130)

Barefoot, S., Bochner, J., Johnson, B. A., & vom Eigen, B. A. (1993). Rating Deaf speakers' comprehensibility: An exploratory investigation. *American Journal of Speech-Language Pathology*, *2*(3), 31–35. https://doi.org/10.1044/1058-0360.0203.31

Benway, N. R., & Preston, J. L. (2020). Differences between school-age children with apraxia of speech and other speech sound disorders on multisyllable repetition. *Perspectives of the ASHA Special Interest Groups*, *5*(4), 794–808. https://doi.org/10.1044/2020_PERSP-19-00086

Boliek, C. A., & Fox, C. M. (2017). Therapeutic effects of intensive voice treatment (LSVT LOUD®) for children with spastic cerebral palsy and dysarthria: A phase I treatment validation study. *International Journal of Speech-Language Pathology*, *19*(6), 601–615. https://doi.org/10.1080/17549507.2016.1221451

Bowen, C., & Snow, P. (2017). *Making sense of interventions for children with developmental disorders*. J & R Press.

Bowen, C., & Snow, P. (2024). *The developmental disorders roadmap*. [Manuscript in preparation]. J & R Press.

Brosseau-Lapré, F., & Rvachew, S. (2017). Underlying manifestations of developmental phonological disorders in french-speaking preschoolers. *Journal of Child Language*, *44*(6), 1337–1361. https://doi.org/10.1017/S0305000916000556

Bruder, M. B. (2010). Early childhood intervention: A promise to children and families for their future. *Exceptional Children*, *76*(3), 339–355. https://doi.org/10.1177%2F001440291007600306

Brosseau-Lapré, F. & Rvachew, S. (2020). *Introduction to speech sound disorders*. Plural Publishing.

Brumbaugh, K. M., & Smit, A. B. (2013). Treating children ages 3-6 who have speech sound disorder: A survey. *Language, Speech, and Hearing Services in Schools*, *44*(3), 306–319. https://doi.org/10.1044/0161-1461(2013/12-0029)

Carrigg, B., Baker, E., Parry, L., & Ballard, K. J. (2015). Persistent speech sound disorder in a 22-year-old male: communication, educational, socio-emotional, and vocational outcomes. *Perspectives on School-Based Issues*, *16*(2), 37–49. https://doi.org/10.1044/sbi16.2.37

Carrigg, B., Parry, L., Baker, E., Shriberg, L. D., & Ballard, K. J. (2016). Cognitive, linguistic, and motor abilities in a multigenerational family with childhood apraxia of speech. *Archives of Clinical Neuropsychology*, *31*(8), 1006–1025. https://doi.org/10.1093/arclin/acw077

Caruso, A., & Strand, E. A. (1999). Motor speech disorders in children: Definitions, background, and a theoretical framework. In A. J. Caruso & E. A. Strand (Eds.), *Clinical management of motor speech disorders in children*. Thieme.

Cassar, C., McCabe, P., & Cumming, S. (2023). "I still have issues with pronunciation of words": A mixed methods investigation of the psychosocial and speech effects of childhood apraxia of speech in adults. *International Journal of Speech-Language Pathology*, *25*(2), 193–205. https://doi.org/10.1080/17549507.2021.2018496

Chan, J., Arnold, S., Webber, L., Riches, V., Parmenter, T., & Stancliffe, R. (2012). Is it time to drop the term 'challenging behaviour'? *Learning Disability Practice*, *15*(5), 36–38. https://doi.org/10.7748/ldp2012.06.15.5.36.c9131

Clark, E. L., Easton, C., & Verdon, S. (2021). The impact of linguistic bias upon speech-language pathologists' attitudes towards non-standard dialects of English. *Clinical Linguistics & Phonetics*, *35*(6), 542–559. https://doi.org/10.1080/02699206.2020.1803405

Cobo-Lewis, A., Oller, D. K., Lynch, M., & Levine, S. (1996). Relations of motor and vocal milestones in typically developing infants and infants with down syndrome. *American Journal of Mental Retardation*, *100*(5), 456–467.

Connery, V. (1985). *The Nuffield Centre Dyspraxia Programme*. RNTNE Hospital.

Cutler, A., & Carter, D. M. (1987). The predominance of strong initial syllables in the english vocabulary. *Computer Speech and Language*, *2*(3–4), 133–142. https://doi.org/10.1016/0885-2308(87)

Davis, B., Morrison, H., von Hapsburg, D., & Czyz, W. (2005). Early vocal patterns in infants with varied hearing levels. *The Volta Review*, *105*(1), 7–27.

de Oliveira Silveira, B. (2021). *Translation and cultural and linguistic adaptation of the therapeutic intervention method ReST- rapid syllable transition treatment into Brazilian Portuguese*. Unpublished Thesis (Graduate in Speech Therapy) - Federal University of Santa Catarina. Brazil.

Diepeveen, S., van Haaften, L., Terband, H., de Swart, B., & Maassen, B. (2020). Clinical reasoning for speech sound disorders: Diagnosis and intervention in speech-language pathologists' daily practice. *American Journal of Speech-Language Pathology*, *29*(3), 1529–1549. https://doi.org/10.1044/2020_AJSLP-19-00040

Dodd, B., Zhu, H., Crosbie, S., Holm, A., & Ozanne, A. (2002). *Diagnostic evaluation of articulation and phonology*. The Psychological Corporation.

Duchow, H., Lindsay, A., Roth, K., Schell, S., Allen, D., & Boliek, C. A. (2019). The co-occurrence of possible developmental coordination disorder and suspected childhood apraxia of speech. *Canadian Journal of Speech-Language Pathology & Audiology*, *43*(2), 81–93. https://cjslpa.ca/files/2019_CJSLPA_Vol_43/No_2/CJSLPA_Vol_43_No_2_2019_MS_1159.pdf

Duffy, J. R. (2012). *Motor speech disorders: Substrates, differential diagnosis, and management* (3rd ed.). Elsevier Mosby.

Easton, C., & Verdon, S. (2021). The influence of linguistic bias upon speech-language pathologists' attitudes toward clinical scenarios involving nonstandard dialects of English. *American Journal of Speech-Language Pathology*, *30*(5), 1973–1989. https://doi.org/10.1044/2021_AJSLP-20-00382

Eilers, R., Oller, D. K., Levine, S., Basinger, D., Lynch, M., & Urbano, R. (1993). The role of prematurity and socioeconomic status in the onset of canonical babbling in infants. *Infant Behavior and Development*, *16*, 297–315. https://doi.org/10.1016/0163-6383(93)80037-9

Ertmer, D. J. (2011). Assessing speech intelligibility in children with hearing loss: Toward revitalizing a valuable clinical tool. *Language, Speech & Hearing Services in the Schools*, *42*(1), 52–58. https://doi.org/10.1044/0161-1461(2010/09-0081)

Flipsen, J. P. (1995). Speaker-listener familiarity: parents as judges of delayed speech intelligibility. *Journal of Communication Disorders*, *28*(1), 3–19. https://doi.org/10.1016/0021-9924(94)00015-r

Flipsen, J. P. (2006). Measuring the intelligibility of conversational speech in children. *Clinical Linguistics & Phonetics*, *20*(4), 303–312. https://doi.org/10.1080/02699200400024863

Garcia, J. M., & Cannito, M. P. (1996). Influence of verbal and nonverbal contexts on the sentence intelligibility of a speaker with dysarthria. *Journal of Speech, Language, and Hearing Research*, *39*(4), 750–760. https://doi.org/10.1044/jshr.3904.750

Gillon, G. T., & McNeill, B. C. (2007). *Integrated phonological intervention*. University of Canterbury. https://tinyurl.com/IPAintegratedApraxia

Gillon, G. T., & Moriarty, B. C. (2007). Childhood apraxia of speech: Children at risk for persistent reading and spelling disorder. *Seminars in Speech & Language*, *28*(1), 48–57. https://doi.org/10.1055/s-2007-967929

Glaspey, A., & Stoel-Gammon, C. (2007). A dynamic approach to phonological assessment. *Advances in Speech Language Pathology*, *9*(4), 286–296. https://doi.org/10.1080/14417040701435418

Goldman, R., & Fristoe, M. (2000). *Goldman-Fristoe Test of Articulation-2 (GFTA-2)*. American Guidance Service.

Goldman, R., & Fristoe, M. (2015). *Goldman-Fristoe Test of Articulation-3 (GFTA-3)*. PsychCorp.

Griffith, M. (2022 January 14). *Oral motor exercises for children with autism*. Autism Parenting Magazine Limited.

Guenther, F., Hampson, M., & Johnson, D. (1998). A theoretical investigation of reference frames for the planning of speech movements. *Psychological Review*, *105*, 611–633. https://doi.org/10.1037/0033-295X.105.4.611-633

Hall, N. E. (2007). Fluency in childhood apraxia of speech. *Perspectives on Fluency & Fluency Disorders*, *17*(2), 9–14. https://doi.org/10.1044/ffd17.2.9

Hall, P. K., Hardy, J. C., & La Velle, W. E. (1990). A child with signs of developmental apraxia of speech with whom a palatal lift prosthesis was used to manage palatal dysfunction. *Journal of Speech and Hearing Disorders*, *55*(3), 454–460. https://doi.org/10.1044/jshd.5503.454

Hammen, V. L., Yorkston, K. M., & Dowden, P. A. (1991). Index of contextual intelligibility I: Impact of semantic context in dysarthria. In C. Moore, K. M. Yorkston, & D. R. Beukelman (Eds.), *Dysarthria and apraxia of speech: Perspectives on intervention*. Paul H. Brookes.

Hammer, D., & Stoeckel, R. (2001). Teaching and talking together: Building a treatment team. *Presentation at the Annual Convention of the American Speech-Language Hearing Association*, New Orleans, Louisiana, ASHA.

Hardin-Jones, M., Jones, D. L., & Dolezal, R. C. (2020). Opinions of speech-language pathologists regarding speech management for children with cleft lip and palate. *The Cleft Palate-Craniofacial Journal*, *57*(1), 55–64. https://doi.org/10.1177/1055665619857000

Hawthorne, K., & Fischer, S. (2020). Speech-language pathologists and prosody: Clinical practices and barriers. *Journal of Communication Disorders*, *87*(Sep-Oct), 106024. https://doi.org/10.1016/j.jcomdis.2020.106024

Helfrich-Miller, K. R. (1983). The use of melodic intonation therapy with developmentally apractic children: A clinical perspective. *Journal of the Pennsylvania Speech-Language-Hearing Association*, 11–15.

Helfrich-Miller, K. R. (1984). Melodic intonation therapy with developmentally apraxic children. *Seminars in Speech and Language*, 5(2), 119–125. https://doi.org/10.1055/s-0028-1082518

Helfrich-Miller, K. R. (1994). Clinical perspective: melodic intonation therapy for developmental apraxia. *Clinics in Communication Disorders*, 4(3), 175–182. PMID: 7994292.

Hellqvist, B. (2016). *Praxis helt paket*. Studentlitteratur.

Hempenstall, K. (2019). *Read about it: Scientific evidence for effective teaching of reading*. Multilit Pty Ltd. https://fivefromfive.com.au/publications

Hennessy, K., & Hennessy, K. (2013). *Anything but silent: Our family's journey through childhood apraxia of speech*. Word Association Publishers.

Highman, C., Hennessey, N. W., Leitão, S., & Piek, J. P. (2013). Early development in infants at risk of childhood apraxia of speech: A longitudinal investigation. *Developmental Neuropsychology*, 38(3), 197–210. https://doi:10.1080/87565641.2013.774405

Highman, C., Hennessey, N. W., Sherwood, M., & Leitão, S. (2008). Retrospective parent report of early vocal behaviors in children with suspected childhood apraxia of speech (CAS). *Child Language Teaching and Therapy*, 24(3), 285–306. https://doi.org/10.1177/0265659008096294

Highman, C., Leitão, S., Hennessey, N., & Piek, J. (2012). Prelinguistic communication development in children with childhood apraxia of speech: A retrospective analysis. *International Journal of Speech-Language Pathology*, 14(1), 35–47. https://doi:10.3109/17549507.2011.596221

Hill, N. (2016). *Social functioning characteristics of a young adult with a history of childhood apraxia of speech*. (Doctoral dissertation, Duquesne University).

Hodge, M., Salonka, R., & Kollias, S. (2005, November). Use of nonspeech oral-motor exercises in children's speech therapy. *Poster Presented at the Annual Meeting of the American Speech-Language-Hearing Association*, San Diego, CA, ASHA.

Hodge, M. M., Brown, C., & Kuzyk, T. (2013). Predicting intelligibility scores of children with dysarthria and cerebral palsy from phonetic measures of speech accuracy. *Journal of Medical Speech-Language Pathology*, 20(4), 41–46. https://

go.gale.com/ps/i.do?p=HRCA&u=anon~d269ea58&id=GALE|A328852879&v=2.1&it=r&sid=googleScholar&asid=a678bf93

Hodge, M. M., Daniels, J., & Gotzke, C. L. (2007). *TOCS+ intelligibility measures*. University of Alberta. http://www.tocs.plus.ualberta.ca/software_Intelligibility.html

Hodge, M. M., & Gotzke, C. L. (2014). Construct-related validity of the TOCS measures: Comparison of intelligibility and speaking rate scores in children with and without speech disorders. *Journal of Communication Disorders*, 51, 51–63. https://doi.org/10.1016/j.jcomdis.2014.06.007

Hustad, K. C. (2012). Speech intelligibility in children with speech disorders. *Perspectives on Language Learning and Education*, 19(1), 7–11. https://doi.org/10.1044/lle19.1.7

Hustad, K. C., Oakes, A., & Allison, K. M. (2015). Variability, stability, and diagnostic accuracy of speech intelligibility scores in children. *Journal of Speech, Language & Hearing Research*, 58(6), 1695–1707. https://doi.org/10.1044/2015_JSLHR-S-14-0365

Hustad, K. C., Sakash, A., Broman, A. T., & Rathouz, P. J. (2019). Differentiating typical from atypical speech production in 5-year-old children with cerebral palsy: a comparative analysis. *American Journal of Speech-Language Pathology*, 28(2S), 807–817. https://doi.org/10.1044/2018_AJSLP-MSC18-18-0108

Hustad, K. C., Sakash, A., Natzke, P., Broman, A. T., & Rathouz, P. J. (2019). Longitudinal growth in single word intelligibility among children with cerebral palsy from 24 to 96 months of age: Predicting later outcomes from early speech production. *Journal of Speech, Language & Hearing Research*, 63(1), 1599–1613. https://doi.org/10.1044/2019_JSLHR-19-00033

Hustad, K. C., Schueler, B., Schultz, L., & DuHadway, C. (2012). Intelligibility of 4-year-old children with and without cerebral palsy. *Journal of Speech, Language and Hearing Research*, 55(4), 1177–1189. https://doi.org/10.1044/1092-4388(2011/11-0083)

Iuzzini-Seigel, J. (2019). Motor performance in children with childhood apraxia of speech and speech sound disorders. *Journal of Speech Language, and Hearing Research*, 62(9), 3220–3233. https://doi.org/10.1044/2019_JSLHR-S-18-0380

Iuzzini-Seigel, J., Hogan, T., & Green, J. (2017). Speech inconsistency in children with childhood apraxia of speech, language impairment and speech delay: Depends on the stimuli. *Journal of Speech Language and Hearing Research, 60*(5), 1194–1210. https://doi.org/10.1044/2016_JSLHR-S-15-0184

Iuzzini-Seigel, J., & Murray, E. (2017). Speech assessment in children with childhood apraxia of speech. *Perspectives of the ASHA Special Interest Groups, 2*(2), 47–60. https://doi.org/10.1044/persp2.SIG2.47

Iyer, S., & Oller, D. K. (2008). Prelinguistic vocal development in infants with typical hearing and infants with severe-to-profound hearing loss. *The Volta Review, 108*(2), 115–138.

Jakielski, K. J., Kostner, T. L., & Webb, C. E. (2006, June). Results of integral stimulation intervention in three children. *Paper Presented at the 5th International Conference on Speech Motor Control.* Nijmegen: the Netherlands.

James, D. G. H. (2006). *Hippopotamus is so hard to say: Children's acquisition of polysyllabic words.* Unpublished PhD thesis, University of Sydney. http://hdl.handle.net/2123/1638

James, S. E., Brumfitt, S. M., & Cudd, P. A. (1999). Communicating by telephone: Views of a group of people with stuttering impairment. *Journal of Fluency Disorders, 24*(4), 299–317. https://doi.org/10.1016/S0094-730X(99)

Joffe, V., & Pring, T. (2008). Children with phonological problems: A survey of clinical practice. *International Journal of Language & Communication Disorders, 43*(2), 154–164. https://doi.org/10.1080/13682820701660259

Kalikow, D. N., Stevens, K. N., & Elliott, L. L. (1977). Development of a test of speech intelligibility in noise using sentence materials with controlled word predictability. *The Journal of the Acoustical Society of America, 61*(5), 1337–1351. https://doi.org/10.1121/1.381436

Kamal, S. (2021). The use of oral motor exercises among speech language pathologists in Jordan. *Journal of Language Teaching and Research, 12*(1), 99–103. https://doi.org/10.17507/jltr.1201.10

Kanter, C. E. (1948). Diagnosis and prognosis in cleft palate speech. *Journal of Speech & Hearing Disorders, 13*(3), 211–222. https://doi.org/10.1044/jshd.1303.211

Kent, R., Miolo, G., & Bloedel, S. (1994). The intelligibility of children's speech: A review of evaluation procedures. *American Journal of Speech-Language Pathology, 3*(2), 81–95. https://doi.org/10.1044/1058-0360.0302.81

Kiesewalter, J., Vincent, V., & Lefebvre, P. (2017). Wee words: A parent-focused group program for young

children with suspected motor speech difficulties. *Canadian Journal of Speech-Language Pathology and Audiology, 41*(1), 58–70. https://cjslpa.ca/files/2017_CJSLPA_Vol_41/No_01/CJSLPA_Vol_41_No_1_2017_1-142.pdf

Kopera, H. C., & Grigos, M. I. (2020). Lexical stress in childhood apraxia of speech: Acoustic and kinematic findings. *International Journal of Speech-Language Pathology, 22*(1), 12–23. https://doi.org/10.1080/17549507.2019.1568571

Korkalainen, M. J., McCabe, P., Smidt, A., & Morgan, C. (2022). Outcomes of a novel single case study incorporating rapid syllable transition treatment, AAC and blended intervention in children with cerebral palsy: A pilot study. *Disability and Rehabilitation: Assistive Technology.* https://doi.org/10.1080/17483107.2022.2071488

Korkalainen, M. J., McCabe, P., Smidt, A., & Morgan, C. (submitted). *The effectiveness of rapid syllable transition treatment in improving communication in children with cerebral palsy: A randomized controlled trial.*

Kröger, B. J., Bekolay, T., & Cao, M. (2022, May). On the emergence of phonological knowledge and on motor planning and motor programming in a developmental model of speech production. *Frontiers in Human Neuroscience, 16.* https://doi.org/10.3389/fnhum.2022.844529

Kwiatkowski, J., & Shriberg, L. D. (1992). Intelligibility assessment in developmental phonological disorders: Accuracy of caregiver gloss. *Journal of Speech-Language and Hearing Research, 35*(5), 1095–1104. https://doi.org/10.1044/jshr.3505.1095

Lang, S., Bartl-Pokorny, K. D., Pokorny, F. B., Garrido, D., Mani, N., Fox-Boyer, A. V., Zhang, D., & Marschik, P. B. (2019). Canonical babbling: A marker for earlier identification of late detected developmental disorders? *Current Developmental Disorders Reports, 6*(3), 111–118. https://doi:10.1007/s40474-019-00166-w

Lee, A. S. Y., & Gibbon, F. E. (2015). Non-speech oral motor treatment for children with developmental speech sound disorders. *Cochrane Database of Systematic Reviews, 2015*(3), CD009383. https://doi.org/10.1002/14651858.CD009383.pub2

Lee, J., Hustad, K. C., & Weismer, G. (2014). Predicting speech intelligibility with a multiple speech subsystems approach in children with cerebral palsy. *Journal of Speech, Language, and Hearing Research, 57*(5), 1666–1678. https://doi.org/10.1044/2014_JSLHR-S-13-0292

Lee, L., Stemple, J. C., Glaze, L., & Kelchner, L. N. (2004). Quick screen for voice and supplementary documents for identifying pediatric voice disorders. *Language, Speech, and Hearing Services in Schools, 35*(4), 308–319. https://doi.org/10.1044/0161-1461(2004/030

Levelt, W. J., Roelofs, A., & Meyer, A. S. (1999). A theory of lexical access in speech production. *The Behavioral and Brain Sciences, 22*(1), 1–75. https://doi.org/10.1017/s0140525x99001776

Levy, E. S., Chang, Y. M., Hwang, K. H., & McAuliffe, M. J. (2020). Perceptual and acoustic effects of dual-focus speech treatment in children with dysarthria. *Journal of Speech, Language, and Hearing Research, 64*(6S), 2301–2316. https://doi.org/10.1044/2020_JSLHR-20-00301

Levy, E. S., Leone, D., Moya-Gale, G., Hsu, S.-C., Chen, W., & Ramig, L. O. (2016). Vowel intelligibility in children with and without dysarthria: An exploratory study. *Communication Disorders Quarterly, 37*(3), 171–179. https://doi.org/10.1177%2F1525740115618917

Lewis, B. A., Benchek, P., Tag, J., Miller, G., Freebairn, L., Taylor, H. G., Iyengar, S. K., & Stein, C. M. (2021). Psychosocial comorbidities in adolescents with histories of childhood apraxia of speech. *American Journal of Speech-Language Pathology, 30*(6), 2572–2588. https://doi.org/10.1044/2021_AJSLP-21-00035

Lewis, B. A., Freebairn, L. A., Hansen, A. J., Iyengar, S. K., & Taylor, H. G. (2004). School-age follow-up of children with childhood apraxia of speech. *Language, Speech & Hearing Services in Schools, 35*(2), 122–140. https://doi.org/10.1080/17549507.2019.1568571

Lof, G. L., & Watson, M. (2008). A nationwide survey of nonspeech oral motor exercise use: Implications for evidence-based practice. *Language, Speech, and Hearing Services in Schools, 39*(3), 392–407. https://doi.org/10.1044/0161-1461(2008/037)

Lowe, R., Helgadottir, F., Menzies, R., Heard, R., O'Brian, S., Packman, A., & Onslow, M. (2017). Safety behaviors and stuttering. *Journal of Speech, Language, and Hearing Research, 60*(5), 1246–1253. https://doi.org/10.1044/2016_JSLHR-S-16-0055

Maas, E., Robin, D. A., Austermann Hula, S. N., Freedman, S. E., Wulf, G., Ballard, K. J., & Schmidt, R. A. (2008). Principles of motor learning in treatment of motor speech disorders. *American Journal of Speech-Language Pathology, 17*(3), 277–298. https://doi.org/10.1044

Maassen, B. (2002). Issues contrasting adult acquired versus developmental apraxia of speech. *Seminars in Speech and Language, 23,* 257–266. https://doi:10.1055/s-2002-35804

Malamud, H., McDaniel, J., Krimm, H., & Schuele, M. (2021, April). Understanding the research-practice gap for speech-language intervention via SLPs' endorsement of myths. *Poster Presented at the Gatlinburg Conference on Research and Theory in Intellectual and Developmental Disabilities.* Gatlinburg Conference.

Masso, S., McLeod, S., & Baker, E. (2018). Tutorial: Assessment and analysis of polysyllables in young children. *Language, Speech, and Hearing Services in Schools, 49*(1), 42–58. https://doi.org/10.1044/2017_LSHSS-16-0047

McCabe, P., Macdonald-D'Silva, A. G., van Rees, L. J., Ballard, K. J., & Arciuli, J. (2014). Orthographically sensitive treatment for dysprosody in children with childhood apraxia of speech using ReST intervention. *Developmental Neurorehabilitation, 17*(2), 137–145. https://doi.org/10.3109/17518423.2014.906002

McCabe, P., Preston, J., Evans, P., & Heard, R. (submitted). *A Pilot Randomized Control Trial of motor-based treatments for childhood apraxia of speech: ReST and Ultrasound Biofeedback.*

McCabe, P., Thomas, D. C., & Murray, E. (2020). Rapid syllable transition treatment–A treatment for childhood apraxia of speech and other pediatric motor speech disorders. *Perspectives of the ASHA Special Interest Groups, 5*(4), 821–830. https://doi.org/10.1044/2020_PERSP-19-00165

McCabe, P. J., Preston, J., Murray, E., Bricker, G., & Morgan, A. (2017). What happens when they group up: A survey of adults who had childhood apraxia of speech. *Stem-, Spraal-en Taalpathologie, 22,* 130.

McCauley, R. J., Strand, E., Lof, G. L., Schooling, T., & Frymark, T. (2009). Evidence- based systematic review: Effects of nonspeech oral motor exercises on speech. *American Journal of Speech-Language Pathology, 18*(4), 343–360. https://doi.org/10.1044/1058-0360(2009/09-0006)

McCune, L., & Vihman, M. (2001). Early phonetic and lexical development: A productivity approach. *Journal of Speech, Language, and Hearing Research, 44,* 670–684. https://doi.org/10.1044/1092-4388(2001/054)

McDonald, E. T., & Baker, H. K. (1951). Cleft palate speech: an integration of research and clinical observation. *Journal of Speech and Hearing Disorders, 16*(1), 9–20. https://doi.org/10.1044/jshd.1601.09

McKechnie, J., Ahmed, B., Gutierrez-Osuna, R., Murray, E., McCabe, P., & Ballard, K. J. (2020). The influence of type of feedback during tablet-based delivery of intensive treatment for childhood apraxia of speech. *Journal of Communication Disorders*, *87*, 106026. https://doi.org/10.1016/j.jcomdis.2020.106026

McLeod, S. (2020). Intelligibility in context scale: Cross-linguistic use, validity, and reliability. *Speech, Language and Hearing*, *23*(1), 9–16. https://doi.org/10.1080/2050571X.2020.1718837

McLeod, S., & Baker, E. (2017). *Children's speech: An evidence-based approach to assessment and intervention*. Pearson.

McLeod, S., Harrison, L. J., & McCormack, J. (2012). The intelligibility in context scale: Validity and reliability of a subjective intelligibility measure. *Journal of Speech-Language-Hearing Research*, *55*(2), 648–656. https://doi.org/10.1044/1092-4388(2011/10-0130)

Milisen, R. (1954). A rationale for articulation disorders. *Journal of Speech and Hearing Disorders*, (Monograph supplement) *4*, 6–17. https://www.asha.org/siteassets/publications/monographs4.pdf

Miller, G. J., Lewis, B., Benchek, P., Freebairn, L., Tag, J., Budge, K., Iynger, S. K., Voss-Hoynes, H., Taylor, H. G., & Stein, C. (2019). Reading outcomes for individuals with histories of suspected childhood apraxia of speech. *American Journal of Speech-Language Pathology*, *28*(4), 1432–1447. https://doi.org/10.1044/2019_AJSLP-18-0132

Miller, H. E., Ballard, K. J., Campbell, J., Smith, M., Plante, A. S., Aytur, S. A., & Robin, D. A. (2021). Improvements in speech of children with apraxia: The efficacy of Treatment for Establishing Motor Program Organization (TEMPO[SM]). *Developmental Neurorehabilitation*, *24*(7), 494–509. https://doi.org/10.1080/17518423.2021.1916113

Moeller, M. P., Hoover, B., Putman, C., Arbataitis, K., Bohnenkamp, G., Peterson, B., Wood, S., Lewis, D., Pittman, A., & Stelmachowicz, P. (2007). Vocalizations of infants with hearing loss compared with infants with normal hearing: Part I – phonetic development. *Ear and Hearing*, *28*(5), 605–627. https://doi:10.1097/AUD.0b013e31812564ab

Moriarty, B. C., & Gillon, G. T. (2006). Phonological awareness intervention for children with childhood apraxia of speech. *International Journal of Language & Communication Disorders*, *41*(6), 713–734. https://doi.org/10.1080/13682820600623960

Morris, C. R., & Agin, M. C. (2009). Syndrome of allergy, apraxia, and malabsorption: Characterization of a neurodevelopmental phenotype that responds to omega 3 and vitamin E supplementation. *Alternative Therapies in Health and Medicine*, *15*(4), 34–43.

Murray, E., Iuzzini-Seigel, J., Maas, E., Terband, H., & Ballard, K. (2021). Differential diagnosis of childhood apraxia of speech compared to other speech sound disorders: A systematic review. *American Journal of Speech-Language Pathology*, *30*(1), 279–300. https://doi.org/10.1044/2020_AJSLP-20-00063

Murray, E., McCabe, P., & Ballard, K. (2011). Using ReST intervention for paediatric cerebellar ataxia: A pilot study. *Stem-, Spraal-en Taalpathologie*, *17*, S55.

Murray, E., McCabe, P., & Ballard, K. J. (2015a). A randomized controlled trial for children with childhood apraxia of speech comparing rapid syllable transition treatment and the Nuffield Dyspraxia Programme (3rd edition). *Journal of Speech, Language & Hearing Research*, *58*(3), 669–686. https://doi.org/10.1044/2015_JSLHR-S-13-0179

Murray, E., McCabe, P., Heard, R., & Ballard, K. J. (2015b). Differential diagnosis of children with suspected childhood apraxia of speech. *Journal of Speech, Language & Hearing Research*, *58*(1), 43–60. https://doi.org/10.1044/2014_JSLHR-S-12-0358

Nathani, S., Oller, D. K., & Neal, R. (2007). On the robustness of vocal development: An examination of infants with moderate-to-severe hearing loss and additional risk factors. *Journal of Speech, Language, and Hearing Research*, *50*(6), 1425–1444. https://doi.org/10.1044/1092-4388(2007/099)

Newman, R., Rowe, M., & Ratner, N. (2016). Input and uptake at 7 months predicts toddler vocabulary: The role of child-directed speech and infant processing skills in language development. *Journal of Child Language*, *43*, 1158–1173. https://doi.org/10.1017/S0305000915000446

Ng, W. L., McCabe, P., Heard, R., Park, V., Murray, E., & Thomas, D. (2022). Predicting treatment outcomes in rapid syllable transition treatment: An individual participant data meta-analysis. *Journal of Speech, Language, and Hearing Research*, *65*(5). https://doi.org/1784-1799.10.1044/2022_JSLHR-21-00617

Oetting, J. B., Gregory, K. D., & Rivière, A. M. (2016). Changing how speech-language pathologists think and talk about dialect variation. *Perspectives of the ASHA Special Interest Groups*, *1*(SIG 16), 28–37. https://doi.org/10.1044/persp1.SIG16.28

Oh, D. H., & Ha, J. W. (2021). Development and clinical application of Korean-version nonword intervention to improve speech motor programming. *Phonetics and Speech Sciences*, *13*(2), 77–90. https://doi.org/10.13064/KSSS.2021.13.2.077

Oller, D. K., Eilers, R., Neal, A. R., & Schwartz, H. (1999). Precursors to speech in infancy: The prediction of speech and language disorders. *Journal of Communication Disorders*, *32*, 223–245. https://doi.org/10.1016/S0021-9924(99)00013-1

Oller, D. K., Eilers, R., Neal, R., & Cobo-Lewis, A. (1998). Late onset canonical babbling: A possible early marker of abnormal development. *American Journal on Mental Retardation*, *103*(3), 249–263. https://doi.org/10.1352/0895-8017(1998)103%3C0249:LOCBAP%3E2.0.CO;2

Oller, D. K., & Eilers, R. E. (1988). The role of audition in infant babbling. *Child Development*, *59*, 441–449. https://doi.org/10.2307/1130323

Olswang, L., & Bain, B. (1996). Assessment information for predicting upcoming change in language production. *Journal of Speech and Hearing Research*, *39*(2), 414–423. https://doi.org/10.1044/jshr.3902.414

Ostergaard, G. (2021). "Så kan jeg bedre kontrollere det med min hjerne, så det ikke kun er munden, der siger det" [Translation from Danish: Then I can better control it with my brain, so it's not just the mouth that says it]. *Dansk Audiolopædi*, *3*, 15–20. https://issuu.com/danskaudiologopaedi/docs/dansk_audiologop_di_3_2021

Overby, M., Belardi, K., & Schreiber, J. (2019). A retrospective video analysis of canonical babbling and volubility in infants later diagnosed with childhood apraxia of speech. *Clinical Linguistics & Phonetics*, *34*(7), 634–651. https://doi.org/10.1080/02699206.2019.1683231

Overby, M., & Caspari, S. (2015). Volubility, consonant, and syllable characteristics in infants and toddlers later diagnosed with childhood apraxia of speech: A pilot study. *Journal of Communication Disorders*, *55*, 44–62. https://doi.org/10.1016/j.jcomdis.2015.04.001

Overby, M., Caspari, S., & Schreiber, J. (2019). Volubility, consonant emergence, and syllabic structure in infants and toddlers later diagnosed with CAS, SSD, and typical development: A retrospective video analysis. *Journal of Speech, Language, and Hearing Research*, *62*(6), 1657–1675. https://doi.org/10.1044/2019_JSLHR-S-18-0046

Overby, M., Moorer, L., Belardi, K., & Schreiber, J. (2020). Retrospective video analysis of the early speech sound development of infants and toddlers later diagnosed with lateralization errors. *International Journal of Speech-Language Pathology*, *22*(2), 196–205. https://doi.org/10.1080/17549507.2019.1645884

Pascoe, M., Stackhouse, J., & Wells, B. (2006). *Persisting speech difficulties in children: Children's speech and literacy difficulties*. John Wiley & Sons.

Patel, R., & Connaghan, K. (2014). Park Play: A picture description task for assessing childhood motor speech disorders. *International Journal of Speech-Language Pathology*, *16*(4), 337–343. https://doi.org/10.3109/17549507.2014.894124

Pennington, L., & Hustad, K. C. (2019). Construct validity of the viking speech scale. *Folia Phoniatrica Et Logopaedica*, *71*(5–6), 228–237. https://doi.org/10.1159/000499926

Pennington, L., Miller, N., & Robson, S. (2009). Speech therapy for children with dysarthria acquired before three years of age. *Cochrane Database of Systematic Reviews*. https://doi.org/10.1002/14651858.CD006937.pub2

Pennington, L., Miller, N., Robson, S., & Steen, N. (2010). Intensive speech and language therapy for older children with cerebral palsy: A systems approach. *Developmental Medicine & Child Neurology*, *52*(4), 337–344. https://doi.org/10.1111/j.1469-8749.2009.03366.x

Pennington, L., Parker, N. K., Kelly, H., & Miller, N. (2016). Speech therapy for children with dysarthria acquired before three years of age. *Cochrane Database of Systematic Reviews*. https://doi.org/10.1002/14651858.CD006937.pub3

Pennington, L., Roelant, E., Thompson, V., Robson, S., Steen, N., & Miller, N. (2013). Intensive dysarthria therapy for younger children with cerebral palsy. *Developmental Medicine & Child Neurology*, *55*(5), 464–471. https://doi.org/10.1111/dmcn.12098

Pennington, L., Stamp, E., Smith, J., Kelly, H., Parker, N., Stockwell, K., ... Vale, L. (2019). Internet delivery of intensive speech and language therapy for children with cerebral palsy: A pilot randomised controlled trial. *BMJ Open*, *9*(1), *BMJ Open*. http://dx.doi.org/10.1136/bmjopen-2018-024233

Pennington, L., Virella, D., Mjøen, T., da Graça Andrada, M., Murray, J., Colver, A., Himmelmann, K., Rackauskaite, G., Greitane, A., Prasauskiene, A., Andersen, G., & de la Cruz, J. (2013). Development of the viking speech scale to classify the speech of children with cerebral palsy. *Research in Developmental Disabilities*, *34*(10), 3202–3210. https://doi.org/10.1016/j.ridd.2013.06.035

Persson, A., Al-Khatib, D., & Flynn, T. (2020). Hearing aid use, auditory development, and auditory functional performance in Swedish children with moderate hearing loss during the first 3 years. *American Journal of Audiology*, *29*(3), 436–449. https://doi.org/10.1044/2020_AJA-19-00092

Peter, B., Potter, N., Davis, J., Donenfeld-Peled, I., Finestack, L., Stoel-Gammon, C., Lien, K., Bruce, L., Vose, C., Eng, L., Yokoyama, H., Olds, D., & VanDam, M. (2020). Toward a paradigm shift from deficit-based to proactive speech and language treatment: Randomized pilot trial of the Babble Boot Camp in infants with classic galactosemia. *F1000Research*, *8*, 271 https://doi.org/10.12688/f1000research.18062.5

Pratomo, H. G. A., & Siswanto, A. (2020). Penggunaan non speech oral motor treatment (NSOMT) Sebagai Pendekatan Intervensi Gangguan Bunyi Bicara. *Jurnal Keterapian Fisik*, *5*(2), 109–121. https://doi.org/10.37341/jkf.v5i2.213

Preston, J. L., Hull, M., & Edwards, M. L. (2013). Preschool speech error patterns predict articulation and phonological awareness outcomes in children with histories of speech sound disorders. *American journal of speech-language pathology*, *22*(2), 173–184. https://doi.org/10.1044/1058-0360(2012/12-0022)

Robbins, J., & Klee, T. (1987). Clinical assessment of oropharyngeal motor development in young children. *Journal of Speech and Hearing Disorders*, *52*(3), 271–277. https://doi.org/10.1044/jshd.5203.271

Roberts, M., & Hampton, L. (2018). Exploring cascading effects of multimodal communication skills in infants with hearing loss. *Journal of Deaf Studies and Deaf Education*, *23*(1), 95–105. https://doi.org/10.1093/deafed/enx041

Roche, L., Zhang, D., Bartl-Pokorny, K., Pokorny, F., Schuller, B., Esposito, G., Bolte, S., Roeyers, H., Poustka, L., Gugatschka, M., Waddington, H., Vollmann, R., Einspieler, C., & Marschik, P. (2018). Early vocal development in autism spectrum disorder, rett syndrome, and fragile X syndrome: Insights from studies using retrospective video analysis. *Advances in Neurodevelopmental Disorders*, *2*, 49–61. https://doi.org/10.1007/s41252-017-0051-3

Rosenbeck, J. C., Lemme, M. L., Ahern, M. B., Harris, E. H., & Wertz, R. T. (1973). A treatment for apraxia of speech in adults. *Journal of Speech and Hearing Disorders*, *38*(4), 462–472. https://doi.org/10.1044/jshd.3804.462

Rosenthal, J. B. (1994). Rate control therapy for developmental apraxia of speech. *Clinics in Communication Disorders*, *4*(3), 190–200. PMID: 7994294

Rumbach, A. F., Rose, T. A., & Cheah, M. (2019). Exploring Australian speech-language pathologists' use and perceptions of non-speech oral motor exercises. *Disability and Rehabilitation*, *41*(12), 1463–1474. https://doi.org/10.1080/09638288.2018.1431694

Rumbach, A., Rose, T., & Bomford, C. (2016). Analysis of speech-language pathology students' knowledge regarding the use of non-speech oral motor exercises (NSOMEs) in clinical practice: An exploratory pilot study. *Speech, Language and Hearing*, *19*(1), 46–54. https://doi.org/10.1080/2050571X.2015.1116730

Ruscello, D. M., & Vallino, L. D. (2020). The use of nonspeech oral motor exercises in the treatment of children with cleft palate: A re-examination of available evidence. *American Journal of Speech-Language Pathology*, *29*(4), 1811–1820. https://doi.org/10.1044/2020_AJSLP-20-00087

Rusiewicz, H. L., Maize, K., & Ptakowski, T. (2018). Parental experiences and perceptions related to childhood apraxia of speech: Focus on functional implications. *International Journal of Speech-Language Pathology*, *20*(5), 569–580. https://doi.org/10.1080/17549507.2017.1359333

Rusiewicz, H. L., & Rivera, J. L. (2017). The effect of hand gesture cues within the treatment of /r/ for a college-aged adult with persisting childhood apraxia of speech. *American Journal of Speech-Language Pathology*, *26*(4), 1236–1243. https://doi.org/10.1044/2017_AJSLP-15-0172

Rvachew, S., & Brosseau-Lapréro, F. (2018). *Developmental phonological disorders: Foundations of clinical practice* (2nd ed.). Plural Publishing, Inc.

Rvachew, S., Hodge, M., & Ohberg, A. (2005). Obtaining and interpreting maximum performance tasks for children: A tutorial. *Journal of Speech-Language Pathology and Audiology*, *29*(4), 146–157.

Rvachew, S., & Matthews, T. (2017). Using the syllable repetition task to reveal underlying speech processes in childhood apraxia of speech: A tutorial. *Canadian Journal of Speech-Language Pathology and*

Audiology, 41(1), 106–126. http://www.cjslpa.ca/detail.php?ID=1207&lang=en

Sacrey, L.-A. R., Bryson, S., Zwaigenbaum, L., Brian, J., Smith, I. M., Roberts, W., Szatmari, P., Vaillancourt, T., Roncadin, C., & Garon, N. (2018). The autism parent screen for infants: Predicting risk of autism spectrum disorder based on parent-reported behavior observed at 6-24 months of age. *Autism: The International Journal of Research and Practice, 22*(3), 322–334. https://doi.org/10.1177/1362361316675120

Sacrey, L. A. R., Zwaigenbaum, L., Bryson, S., Brian, J., Smith, I. M., Roberts, W., Szatmari, P., Vaillancourt, T., Roncadin, C., & Garon, N. (2021). Screening for behavioral signs of autism spectrum disorder in 9-month-old infant siblings. *Journal of Autism Developmental Disorders, 51*(3), 839–848. https://doi.org/10.1007/s10803-020-04371-0

Sakash, A., Mahr, T., & Hustad, K. C. (2021). Validity of parent ratings of speech intelligibility for children with cerebral palsy. *Developmental Neurorehabilitation, 24*(2), 98–106. https://doi.org/10.1080/17518423.2020.1830447

Scarcella, I., Michelazzo, L., & McCabe, P. (2021). A pilot single-case experimental design study of rapid syllable transition treatment for italian children with childhood apraxia of speech. *American Journal of Speech-Language Pathology, 30*(3S), 1496–1510. https://doi.org/10.1044/2021_AJSLP-20-00133

Schlosser, R. W. (2004). Goal attainment scaling as a clinical measurement technique in communication disorders: A critical review. *Journal of Communication Disorders, 37*(3), 217–239. https://doi.org/10.1016/j.jcomdis.2003.09.003

Schmidt, R. A., & Lee, T. D. (2011). *Motor control and learning: A behavioral emphasis* (5th ed.). Human Kinetics.

Schmidt, R. A., Lee, T. D., Winstein, C. J., Wulf, G., & Zelaznik, H. N. (2019). *Motor control and learning: A behavioral emphasis* (6th ed.). Human Kinetics Europe Ltd.

Schölderle, T., Staiger, A., Lampe, R., Strecker, K., & Ziegler, W. (2016). Dysarthria in adults with cerebral palsy: Clinical presentation and impacts on communication. *Journal of Speech, Language, and Hearing Research, 59*(2), 216–229. https://doi.org/10.1044/2015_JSLHR-S-15-0086

Sealey, L. R., & Giddens, C. L. (2010). Aerodynamic indices of velopharyngeal function in childhood apraxia of speech. *Clinical Linguistics & Phonetics, 24*(6), 417–430. https://doi.org/10.3109/02699200903447947

Segal, O., Tubi, R., & Ben-David, A. (2022, November). Lexical stress in Hebrew-speaking children with and without childhood apraxia of speech. *Paper Presented at the American Speech, Language, Hearing Association Convention*, New Orleans, LA, ASHA.

Shriberg, L. D., Austin, D., Lewis, B. A., McSweeny, J. L., & Wilson, D. L. (1997). The percentage of consonants correct (PCC) metric: Extensions and reliability data. *Journal of Speech, Language and Hearing Research, 40*(4), 708–722. https://doi.org/10.1044/jslhr.4004.708

Shriberg, L.D., Campbell, T.F., Karlsson, H.B., McSweeney, J.L., Nadler, C.J. (2003). A diagnostic marker for childhood apraxia of speech: The lexical stress ratio. *Clinical Linguistics & Phonetics, 17*(7), 549–574. https://doi.org/10.1080/026992003100013812

Shriberg, L. D., Kwiatkowski, J., Best, S., & Terselic-Weber, B. (1986). Characteristics of children with phonological disorders of unknown origin. *Journal of Speech and Hearing Disorders, 51*(2), 140–161. https://doi.org/10.1044/jshd.5102.140

Shriberg, L. D., Kwiatkowski, J., & Mabie, H. L. (2019). Estimates of the prevalence of motor speech disorders in children with idiopathic speech delay. *Clinical Linguistics & Phonetics, 33*(8), 679–706. https://doi.org/10.1080/02699206.2019.1595731

Shriberg, L. D., Potter, N. L., & Strand, E. A. (2011). Prevalence and phenotype of childhood apraxia of speech in youth with galactosemia. *Journal of Speech, Language, and Hearing Research, 54*(2), 487–519. https://doi.org/10.1044/1092-4388(2010/10-0068)

Shriberg, L. D., Strand, E. A., Fourakis, M., Jakielski, K. J., Hall, S. D., Karlsson, H. B., Mabie, H., McSweeney, J. L., Tilkens, C. M., & Wilson, D. L. (2017). A diagnostic marker to discriminate childhood apraxia of speech from speech delay: I. Development and description of the pause marker. *Journal of Speech, Language & Hearing Research, 60*(4). https://doi.org/10.1044/2016_JSLHR-S-15-0296

Shukla, S. (2021, April 8). *Oral motor exercises for Down's syndrome*. 1SpecialPlace, https://1specialplace.com/2021/04/08/oral-motor-exercises-for-downs-syndrome

Skinder, A. (2000). *The relationship of prosodic and articulatory errors produced by children with developmental apraxia*. University of Washington, Unpublished Doctoral Dissertation.

Skinder-Meredith, A., Carkowski, S., & Graff, N. (2004, December 15). *Comparison of nasalance* measures in children with childhood apraxia of speech and repaired cleft palate, to their typically developing peers. SpeechPathology.Com. https://www.speechpathology.com/articles/comparison-nasality-measures-between-children-1460

Skinder-Meredith, A. E. (2015). Speech characteristics rating form. In C. Bowen (Ed.), *Children's speech sound disorders* (2nd ed., pp. 312–318). Wiley-Blackwell.

Stackhouse, J., & Wells, B. (1997). *Children's speech and literacy difficulties: A psycholinguistic framework*. Whurr Publishers.

Staples, T., McCabe, P., Ballard, K. J., & Robin, D. A. (2008). Childhood apraxia of speech: Treatment outcomes at 6 months of an intervention incorporating principles of motor learning. *Paper Presented at the Joint New Zealand Speech-Language Therapy Association/Speech Pathology Australia Conference*, May 2008, Auckland, New Zealand.

Steenbeek, D., Ketelaar, M., Lindeman, E., Galama, K., & Gorter, J. W. (2007). Interrater reliability of goal attainment scaling in rehabilitation of children with cerebral palsy. *Archives of Physical Medicine and Rehabilitation*, *91*(3), 429–435. https://doi.org/10.1016/j.apmr.2009.10.013

Stephens, H., & Elton, M. (1986, December). Description of systematic use of articulograms. *Bulletin, College of Speech and Language Therapists*.

Stipancic, K. L., Yunusova, Y., Berry, J. D., & Green, J. R. (2018). Minimally detectable change and minimal clinically important difference of a decline in sentence intelligibility and speaking rate for individuals with amyotrophic lateral sclerosis. *Journal of Speech Language and Hearing Research*, *61*(11), 2757–2771. https://doi.org/10.1044/2018_JSLHR-S-17-0366

Stoel-Gammon, C. (1991). Normal and disordered phonology in two year olds. *Topics in Language Disorders*, *11*(4), 21–32. https://doi.org/10.1097/00011363-199111040-00005

Stoel-Gammon, C., & Cooper, J. (1984). Patterns of early lexical and phonological development. *Journal of Child Language*, *11*(2), 247–271. https://doi.org/10.1017/S0305000900005766

Strand, E. (1995). Treatment of motor speech disorders in children. *Seminars in Speech and Language*, *16*(2), 126–139. https://doi.org/10.1055/s-2008-1064115

Strand, E. A. (2020). Dynamic temporal and tactile cueing: a treatment strategy for childhood apraxia of speech. *American Journal of Speech Language Pathology*, *29*(1), 30–48. https://doi.org/10.1044/2019_AJSLP-19-0005

Strand, E., Stoeckel, R., & Baas, B. (2006). Treatment of severe childhood apraxia of speech: Treatment efficacy study. *Journal of Medical Speech Pathology*, *14*(4), 297–307.

Strand, E. A. (2017). Appraising apraxia: When a speech-sound disorder is severe, how do you know if it's childhood apraxia of speech? *The ASHA Leader*, *22*, 50–58. https://doi.org/10.1044/leader.FTR2.22032017.50

Strand, E. A., & Debertine, P. (2000). The efficacy of integral stimulation with developmental apraxia of speech. *Journal of Medical Speech-Language Pathology*, *8*(4), 295–300.

Strand, E. A., & McCauley, R. J. (2019a). *Dynamic evaluation of motor speech skill*. Paul Brookes Publishing Co. https://bit.ly/DEMSS

Strand, E. A., & McCauley, R. J. (2019b). *Dynamic evaluation of motor speech skill (DEMSS) manual*. Paul Brookes.

Strand, E. A., McCauley, R. J., Weigand, S. D., Stoeckel, R. E., & Baas, B. S. (2013). A motor speech assessment for children with severe speech disorders: Reliability and validity evidence. *Journal of Speech, Language, and Hearing Research*, *56*(2), 505–520. https://doi.org/10.1044/1092-4388(2012/12-0094)

Terband, H., Namasivayam, A., Maas, E., van Brenk, F., Mailend, M.-L., Diepeveen, S., van Lieshout, P., & Maassen, B. (2019). Assessment of childhood apraxia of speech: A review/tutorial of objective measurement techniques. *Journal of Speech, Language & Hearing Research*, *62*(8S), 2999–3032 https://doi.org/10.1044/2019_JSLHR-S-CSMC7-19-0214

Teverovsky, E. G., Bickel, J. O., & Feldman, H. M. (2009). Functional characteristics of children diagnosed with childhood apraxia of speech. *Disability and Rehabilitation*, *31*(2), 94–102. https://doi.org/10.1080/09638280701795030

Thomas, D. C., McCabe, P., & Ballard, K. J. (2014). Rapid Syllable Transitions (ReST) Treatment for childhood apraxia of speech: The effect of lower dose-frequency. *Journal of Communication Disorders*, *51*, 29–42. https://doi.org/https://dx.doi.org/10.1016/j.jcomdis.2014.06.004

Thomas, D. C., McCabe, P., & Ballard, K. J. (2017). Combined clinician-parent delivery of rapid syllable transition (ReST) treatment for childhood apraxia of speech. *International Journal of*

Speech-Language Pathology, *20*(7), 683–698. https://doi.org/10.1080/17549507.2017.1316423

Thomas, D. C., McCabe, P., Ballard, K. J., & Bricker-Katz, G. (2018). Parent experiences of variations in service delivery of Rapid Syllable Transition (ReST) treatment for childhood apraxia of speech. *Developmental Neurorehabilitation*, *21*(6), 391–401. https://doi.org/10.1080/17518423.2017.1323971

Thomas, D. C., McCabe, P., Ballard, K. J., & Lincoln, M. (2016). Telehealth delivery of Rapid Syllable Transitions (ReST) treatment for childhood apraxia of speech. *International Journal of Language & Communication Disorders*, *51*(6), 654–671. https://doi.org/10.1111/1460-6984.12238

Thomas, D. C., Murray, E., Przulj, M., & McCabe, P. (2022). Less frequent is less good: A single case experimental design study of once weekly reST therapy. *Paper Presented at the Apraxia-Kids Research Symposium*, Las Vegas, July 2022. CASANA.

Thomas, R. M., & Kaipa, R. (2015). The use of non-speech oral-motor exercises among Indian speech-language pathologists to treat speech disorders: An online survey. *The South African Journal of Communication Disorders.*, *62*(1), 1–12. https://doi.org/10.4102/sajcd.v62i1.82

Twain, M. (1910). How I conquered stage fright. *Published as "Mark Twain's First Appearance" in Mark Twain's Speeches*. Harper & Brothers.

Van der Merwe, A., & Steyn, M. (2018). Model driven treatment of childhood apraxia of speech: positive effects of the speech motor learning approach. *American Journal of Speech-Language Pathology*, *27*(1), 37–51. https://doi.org/10.1044/2017_AJSLP-15-0193

van der Meulen, S. (1994). *Dyspraxieprogramma 1*. Uitgever Pearson.

van Vuren, M. (2008 January 1). *Oral motor exercises for down syndrome – devising your own oral motor home programme*. PediaStaff. https://www.pediastaff.com/blog/slp/oral-motor-exercises-for-down-syndrome-devising-your-own-oral-motor-home-programme-19059

Velleman, S. (2002). Phonotactic therapy. *Seminars in Speech and Language*, *23*(1), 43–57. https://doi.org/10.1055/s-2002-23510

Velleman, S., & Shriberg, L. (1999). Metrical analysis of the speech of children with suspected developmental apraxia of speech. *Journal of Speech, Language & Hearing Research*, *42*(6), 1444–1460. https://doi.org/10.1044/jslhr.4206.1444

von Hapsburg, D., & Davis, B. (2006). Auditory sensitivity and the prelinguistic vocalizations of early-amplified infants. *Journal of Speech, Language, and Hearing Research*, *49*(4), 809–822. https://doi.org/10.1044/1092-4388(2006/057)

Williams, A. L., & Elbert, M. (2003). A prospective longitudinal study of phonological development in late talkers. *Language, Speech, and Hearing Services in Schools*, *34*(2), 138–153. https://doi.org/10.1044/0161-1461(2003/012)

Williams, P. (2021). The Nuffield Centre Dyspraxia Programme. In A. L. Williams, S. McLeod, & R. J. McCauley (Eds.), *Interventions for speech sound disorders in children* (2nd ed., pp. 447–475). Paul H. Brookes.

Williams, P., & Stephens, H. (Eds.). (2004). *The nuffield centre dyspraxia programme* (3rd ed.). Nuffield Centre Dyspraxia Programme Ltd.

Workinger, M. S., & Kent, R. D. (1991). Perceptual analysis of the dysarthrias in children with athetoid and spastic cerebral palsy. In C. A. Moore, K. M. Yorkston, & D. R. Beukelman (Eds.), *Dysarthria and apraxia of speech: Perspectives on management* (pp. 109–126). Paul Brookes.

Yorkston, K. M., & Beukelman, D. R. (1981). Communication efficiency of dysarthric speakers as measured by sentence intelligibility and speaking rate. *Journal of Speech and Hearing Disorders*, *46*(3), 296–301. https://doi.org/10.1044/jshd.4603.296

Yorkston, K. M., Strand, E. A., & Kennedy, M. R. T. (1996). Comprehensibility of dysarthric speech: Implications for assessment and treatment planning. *American Journal of Speech-Language Pathology*, *5*(1), 55–65. https://doi.org/10.1044/1058-0360.0501.55

Zwaigenbaum, L., Bryson, S., & Garon, N. (2013). Early identification of autism spectrum disorders. *Behavioural Brain Research*, *251*, 133–146. https://doi.org/10.1016/j.bbr.2013.04.004

Chapter 9
Treatment Targets and Strategies

In 1949, Hollywood cameraman John Alton wrote the first edition of the first book on cinematography, calling it *Painting with Light* (Alton, 1995). The title may have inspired *The Publicity Photograph* (Galton & Simpson, 1958), a BBC radio sketch for *Hancock's Half Hour*. Persuaded by Miss Pugh (Hattie Jacques), Bill (Kerr) and Sid (James) that he needs to update his image, Hancock (Tony Hancock) and Sid consult glitzy theatrical photographer Hilary St. Clair (Kenneth Williams, he of the soaring triphthongs). When Sid tells St. Clair, *'I want you to take some snaps'*, he is outraged! *'Snaps*, Sidney? I don't take *snaps*; I *paint* with *light!'*

The topic of therapy tips, tricks and ideas arises frequently in social media and at professional development events. When it does, there can be an impulse to mount one's high horse and emulate St. Clair. *'Tips? Tips? I don't do tips! I put solid theory and evidence into practice!'* or whatever the SLP/SLT equivalent of painting with light might be.

Seasoned interventionists know, however, that therapy breakthroughs often come when, without forsaking E³BP, we play educated clinical hunches, intuit what will best motivate a particular child, have a good idea, or apply brainwaves shared by mentors and colleagues. Sometimes we just do something different, or implement a tip, trick or idea from our repertoire that has previously made our jobs as scientific clinicians easier, especially with complex clients. Chapter 9 offers many such strategies that may help in SSD assessment, target selection, and intervention, and pointers to where to find more.

Phonological Disorder Diagnostic Signs

There is a list in Box 7.1 of four diagnostic signs accompanying the six characteristics of phonological disorder: (1) the puzzle phenomenon, (2) unusual errors, (3) marking, and (4) relatively ready stimulability compared with stimulability in CAS. The signs may assist in establishing whether a child's speech difficulties, or *some* of them, are phonological in nature. We should consider the possibility of phonological disorder and a phonological intervention approach if the puzzle phenomenon is evident, if there is a pattern of unusual errors, if the child is marking contrasts 'oddly' or subtly, and if error sounds are relatively readily stimulable. Two of the giveaway signs, the puzzle phenomenon (Macken, 1980; Schwartz & Leonard, 1982) and marking, can be difficult to 'pick' unless clinicians deliberately seek them out.

1. The puzzle phenomenon

The puzzle phenomenon occurs when a child consistently mispronounces sounds where they should occur but uses them as substitutes where they should not! A 'demonstration' (to me) by Dane, father of Quentin, 6;1, exemplifies this.

Dane: Show her how you say *thumb*.
Quentin: *Fum*.
Dane: Now say *sum*.
Quentin: *Thum*.
Dane: If he can say *thumb* when he means *sum*, how come he says *fum* when he means *thumb*? I think he's just lazy.

Andrew, 4;6 provides a second example of the puzzle phenomenon. It is intriguing to see what happened, prior to intervention, with his approximants (/ɹ/, /j/, and /l/) in *yellow, glove, brother, globe,* and *rabbit,* and his fricatives in *then, those, glove, breathe, snooze, brother, some, thumb,* and *zoo*. For example, the /ð/ in *then* and *those* was realized as [d]; in *breathe* it became [v]; and in *brother* it was /z/; whereas the /ð/ occurred twice in *snooze* [ðuð] replacing /s/ in the cluster and /z/ SFWF, and again in *zoo* [ðu]. Thus, for Andrew /ð/ sometimes matched the adult target, but never in the right position, and it could be replaced by [d], [v]. and [z]. It was interesting then to look at /v/ and /z/. The /v/ became [b] in *glove,* and /z/ was correct in *those* but was [ð] SFWF in *snooze* and [ð] SIWI in *zoo*.

yellow	[lɛloʊ]	brother	[bwʌzə]
then	[dɛn]	globe	[bloʊb]
those	[doʊz]	rabbit	[bɹæbɪt]
glove	[gwʌb]	some	[θʌm]
breathe	[bwiv]	thumb	[sʌm]
snooze	[ðuð]	zoo	[ðu]

2. Unusual errors

Unusual errors are generally obvious to SLPs/SLTs. For example, Sam 4;1, had no clusters, prevalent final consonant deletion, and an idiosyncratic pattern of replacing SIWI and SIWW stops with /f/

or /v/. The following example is in the symbols proposed by Harrington et al. (1997) for transcribing Australian English vowels. Sam spoke what they called General Australian English.

'Where did my black car go? I put it on the bed in a safe place.'
[ˈweː ˌvɪ mɑe ˈvæ ˈveː vəʉ ‖ ɑe fʊ ɪt ɔn ðə ve ɪnə ˌsæɪf ˈfæɪs]

3. Marking

Some of the errors that children make deceive our trained ears; but when we listen closely, we may find that the errors provide subtle hints that a child knows more than they can produce, and that their difficulties are phonological and not phonetic. Children drop these hints unconsciously by 'marking' the presence of the correct sound, with nasality and/or vowel length. Note that 'marking' has nothing to do with 'markedness', and the concept that some consonants are 'marked'. Markedness, discussed later in this chapter, is a term used in the study of the sound systems of all natural languages and is a phenomenon that applies to a relationship between two or more words.

Marking with Nasality: Uzzia

Uzzia, 5;1, with extensive final consonant deletion, talked about going to [bɛ] (*bed*) and referred to her brother as [bɛ̃] (*Ben*). Although it was easy to hear these as homonyms, it was apparent that Uzzia was *marking* the presence of the /n/ in *Ben* by nasalizing the preceding vowel. This trace of a nasal final consonant was consistent with what happens normally; vowels preceding nasal consonants are usually nasalized.

Marking with Vowel Length: Owen

Like Uzzia, Owen, 4;3 exhibited final consonant deletion, producing bus as [bʌ] and Buzz Lightyear's name as [bʌː], and again these two productions, [bʌ] with a short vowel and [bʌː] with the vowel produced with a longer duration, were readily mistaken for homonyms. But when we recall that vowels are typically longer before voiced consonants, we would be reasonably safe to assume that

Owen's lengthening of the short vowel /ʌ/ to [ʌː] meant that he 'knew' (underlyingly) the difference between /s/ and /z/ but was not yet able to produce them SFWF.

I wanted to know whether [bʌ] and [bʌː] for *bus* and *Buzz* was an isolated example of marking with vowel length in Owen's speech output, so presented him with five pictured minimal pairs, one pair at a time, and asked him to '*Listen to me say these two words. Now you say them to me. Make them sound different from each other*'. The pairs were: *bus Buzz; ice eyes; sauce saws; fleece fleas;* and *price prize*. His responses were [bʌ] [bʌː] (as expected); [aɪ] [aɪː]; [sɔ] [sɔː]; [fwi] [fwiː]; and [pwaɪ] [pwaɪː]. QED!

4. Relatively ready stimulability in comparison with CAS

In earlier editions of *Children's Speech Sound Disorders*, the fourth sign of phonological disorder read 'Error sounds are readily stimulable'. The wording has changed because, to my consternation, some CPD participants took 'readily' to mean that stimulability would be achieved in a flash (mea culpa). To correct the record, *some* children with articulation disorder and/or phonological disorders struggle with phonetic placement and stimulability, including those who take a long time to acquire velar stops (Unicomb et al., 2019), voiceless fricatives /s, ʃ, θ/ (Howson & Redford, 2022), and /ɹ, ɚ, ɝ/ (Ball et al., 2013; Flipsen Jr. A37).

Individualized Education Programs or Plans

The aim of Individualized Education Programs (IEP), Individualized Education Plans (IEP), or Individual Learning Plans (ILP) is to assist students who need 'supports' or additional help with their education. The term IEP is typically used to refer to a written statement detailing the adjustments, goals and strategies that are in place to meet a student's educational needs with a view to their reaching their potential. The document is written collaboratively by an IEP team which includes the student if they are old enough and parent(s) or guardian(s), as well as school personnel: a classroom teacher, a special

educator, a representative of the school authority or district, a psychologist or school counsellor, and specialist service providers such as SLPs/SLTs. Specialist providers, external to the school, may be invited by the child's parents, who let the team know in advance, and who may have to explain why their presence is desirable. The role of IEP planning meetings, or case conferences, held at least twice a year, is to discuss and document teaching and learning adjustments for the child and the goals the child's school team will pursue for an agreed period, usually 3 to 6 months. Often, the IEP is provided to parent(s) in advance of the meeting in good time for them to request any changes they want. When everyone meets, the team is encouraged to collaborate in tweaking, clarifying, adding, or subtracting any parts of the plan.

Expressing IEP Goals for Children with Articulation Disorder

IEPs for articulation therapy tend to be like Alison's, below. She was 7;1 and had /s/ as a phonetic target.

Alison's IEP goals
Long-Term Goal: Alison will produce /s/ with 90% mastery.
Short-Term Objectives

1. Alison will produce /s/ in isolation with 90% accuracy.
2. Alison will produce /s/ in syllables with 90% accuracy.
3. Alison will produce /s/ in all positions of words with 90% accuracy.
4. Alison will produce /s/ in sentences with 90% accuracy.
5. Alison will produce /s/ in oral reading tasks with 90% accuracy.
6. Alison will produce /s/ in structured conversation with 90% accuracy.
7. Alison will produce /s/ in spontaneous speech with 90% accuracy.
8. Alison will improve self-monitoring skills for /s/ with 90% accuracy.
9. Alison will produce /s/ outside of the therapy setting with 90% accuracy.

Expressing IEP Goals for Children with Phonological Disorder and/or CAS

Chapter 7 contains an exploration of the six-shared characteristics of phonological disorders and childhood apraxia of speech (CAS) (see Tables 7.1, 7.2 and 7.3 and associated discussion) and 14 goals in common. The six characteristics that are seen in both SSDs are: (1) Consonant inventory constraints; vowel inventory constraints; phonotactic inventory constraints. (2) Omissions of consonants, vowels and syllable shapes that are already in the child's inventory. (3) Vowel errors. (4) Altered suprasegmentals. (5) More errors with longer and/or more complex utterances, including the so-called 'SODA' errors of substitution, omission, distortion, and addition. (6) Use of simple, but not complex, syllable shapes and word shapes.

The 14-shared goals are: (1) Consonant inventory expansion. (2) Vowel inventory expansion. (3) Phonotactic inventory expansion. (4) Syllable shape inventory expansion. (5) Word shape inventory expansion. (6) Increased accuracy of production of target structures. (7) More complete vowel repertoire. (8) More accurate vowel production. (9) Production of strong and weak syllables. (10) Differentiation of strong and weak syllables. (11) Generalization of new consonants and vowels, syllable structures, and word structures, to more challenging contexts. (12) More complete phonotactic repertoire. (13) More varied use of phonotactic range within syllables and words. (14) Improved accuracy.

Clearly, when goal setting and writing IEPs for children with phonological disorder and/or CAS these 14 goals cannot be expressed similarly to articulation goals, in terms of 'mastery' criteria and percentages. So, what follows is a suggested guide for wording IEP goals, based on the six characteristics common to both diagnoses, and the 14 common treatment goals. Then follows an IEP for Tad, 5;3 who had CAS *and* significant phonological issues. Tad's IEP goals encompassed 1, 2, 4 and 8, asterisked (*) in the following guide.

Guide: IEP Goals for Children with Phonological Disorder and CAS

1. Expanding the consonant inventory; promoting more accurate consonant production*.
2. Expanding the vowel inventory; promoting more accurate vowel production*.
3. Expanding the syllable shape inventory; promoting more accurate syllable shapes.
4. Expanding the word shape inventory; promoting more accurate word structures*.
5. Expanding the capacity to produce/differentiate accurate strong and weak syllables.
6. Promoting more varied and accurate use of phonotactics in syllables and words.
7. Promoting more effective accurate suprasegmental use and more typical prosody.
8. Promoting generalization of accurate new: segments, syllable structures, word structures and prosodic features – to more challenging contexts*.

Tad's IEP Goals

1. **Expanding the consonant inventory; promoting more accurate consonant production.**

   Long-Term Goal: **Tad will produce the stops /p b t d k g/ and the fricatives /f s ʃ/ or close approximations in CV and VC syllable and word contexts.**
   Short-Term Objectives
   1. Tad will perceive and produce /p b t d/ in CV and VC words.
   2. Tad will perceive and produce /k g/ in isolation and CV and VC syllables.
   3. Tad will perceive and produce /k g/ in CV and VC words.
   4. Tad will perceive and produce / f s ʃ / in CV and VC words

2. **Expanding the vowel inventory; promoting more accurate vowel production.**

   Long-Term Goal: **Tad will produce all vowels and diphthongs in CV and VC syllable and word contexts.**

Short-Term Objectives

1. Tad will discriminate /ɜ/ from /ɔ/ in single word contexts.
2. Tad will discriminate /ɜ/ from /ɔ/ in short sentences.
3. Tad will produce /ɜ/ and /ɔ/ in isolation.
4. Tad will produce /ɜ/ in CV and VC nonwords and words.

Expanding the word shape inventory; promoting more accurate word structures

Long-Term Goal: **Tad will produce the clusters /pl bl kl and gl/ or close approximations in CCV and CCVC word contexts.**

Short-Term Objectives

1. Tad will produce /pl bl kl and gl/, or close approximations, in CCV words.
2. Tad will produce /pl bl kl and gl/, or close approximations, in CCVC words.
3. Tad will produce /pl bl kl and gl/, or close approximations, in CCV and CCVC words, in short utterances.

Promoting generalization of accurate new: segments, syllable structures, word structures and prosodic features – to more challenging contexts.
Long-Term Goal: **Tad will produce segmentally correct trochaic sequences, with appropriate prosody (stress and intonation), in word and sentence contexts.**

Short-Term Objectives

1. Tad will produce two-syllable trochaic words with Strong-Weak stress (e.g., super).
2. Tad will produce four-syllable trochaic sequences with Strong-Weak-Strong-Weak stress (e.g., superhero, helicopter, birthday party, station wagon).

Target Selection

A tradition is a ritual, belief or object passed down within a society, maintained in the present, with origins in the past. A scientist embarking on a research trend inherits the tradition of preceding scientists, along with their conclusions and critical discussion. A sense of such a crucial inheritance of tradition is what sets apart the best scientists; those who change their fields through their embrasure [widening] of tradition. Thomas Kuhn, in a 1977 lecture.

In the left column of Table 9.1 is a list of eight traditional target selection criteria that are not strongly based, if at all, in either evidence or solid theory. In the right column are eight newer criteria with stronger linguistic underpinnings and

Table 9.1 Traditional and newer criteria for treatment target selection.

Traditional Criteria	Newer Criteria
These are associated with little or no evidence, and are based on logic, intuition, experience, and hunches	These tend to be evidence-based, linguistically driven, and theoretically sound
1. Work in typical developmental sequence	9. Work on later developing sounds and syllable structures first
2. Choose socially important targets	10. Work on marked consonants first
3. Work on phonemes that are stimulable (especially at first)	11. Work on non-stimulable phonemes first
4. Use minimal feature contrasts in minimal pairs treatment	12. Use maximal or multiple feature contrasts in minimal pairs treatment
5. Select, as targets, unfamiliar words	13. Use a systemic approach to analyse the child's rules
6. Work on sounds that are inconsistently erred	14. Apply the sonority sequencing principle
7. Target sounds that are most destructive of intelligibility	15. Prioritise least knowledge sounds in treatment
8. Target non-developmental errors (especially at first)	16. Consider lexical properties of 'therapy words'

empirical support. The implication here is *not* 'out with the old, and in with the new(ish)'! We can combine these criteria selectively to bring the evidence, theory and critical discussion of science, and the wisdom of tradition, to the same table while, in the spirit of E³BP, respecting the characteristics and preferences of the child, the family and the clinician, and the child's intervention needs.

Traditional Target Selection Criteria

1. Work in typical developmental sequence

Working on sound targets in the typical sequence of acquisition rests on the logical assumption that earlier developing sounds are easier for a child to learn first, less frustrating for the child to attempt, or easier for the clinician to teach (Hodson, 2007, 2010; Prezas et al., 2021; Van Riper & Irwin, 1958). A clinician using this strategy might prioritise intervention targets by following the age and order of acquisition data displayed in Tables 1.2, 1.3, and 3.1. Table 3.1 is duplicated under item 9 on this list for ease of reference. These normative data are explained by McLeod and Crowe (A42) in Chapter 10, where they draw on Crowe and McLeod (2020) and McLeod and Crowe (2018) as well as McLeod (2020) regarding intelligibility expectations.

2. Choose socially important targets

The notion of 'social importance' usually implies a target that is significant for the child and/or parents in terms of how the child is perceived, and may relate to avoiding hurt, ridicule, or embarrassment, as in the following examples. Stoel-Gammon (A7) describes Brett, 4;9, who was teased for saying *Bwett*. Tired of the hilarity it generated, the Ayres family were anxious for Gerri, 5;3, to stop calling herself [dɛɹiɛːz] (example used by permission); and Shaun, 4;9, was eager to work on /ʃ/ because he was taunted for saying his name [dɔn] (example used by permission). Many SLPs/SLTs are asked by parents if the word *truck* might be considered as a target in children who pronounce /tɹ/ as in *tree* as [f].

3. Work on phonemes that are stimulable

Prioritizing for intervention the child's stimulable, 'most knowledge' sounds (see Table 9.4) is based on the interwoven ideas of developmental readiness, ease of learning, and early success as a motivator (Hodson, 2007, 2010) for the child, and ease of teaching (for the clinician). Traditionally, 'stimulable' has meant that a consonant or vowel can be said in isolation by the child, in direct imitation of an auditory and visual model with or without instructions, cues, imagery, feedback, and encouragement. For example, a clinician might elicit /f/ by modelling it and providing placement cues such as, *bite your lip and blow*.

Table 3.1 (duplicated) Developmental schedules in the USA (1993; 2020), and internationally (2018).

Order of acquisition* Shriberg, 1993 USA children	Order of acquisition** Crowe & McLeod, 2020 USA children ***	Order of acquisition* McLeod & Crowe, 2018 English-speaking children***
Early 8	Early 2;0–3;11	Early 2;0–3;11
m n j b w d p h	b, n, m, p, h, w, d, g, k, f, t, ŋ, j	p, b, m, d, n, h, t, k, g, w, ŋ, f, j
Middle 8	Middle 4;0–4;11	Middle 4;0–4;11
t ŋ k g v tʃ dʒ	v, dʒ, s, tʃ, l, ʃ, z	l, dʒ, tʃ, s, v, ʃ, z
Late 8	Late 5;0–6;11	Late 5;0–6;11
ʃ ʒ l ɹ s z ð θ	ɹ, ð, ʒ, θ	ɹ, ʒ, ð, θ

*Data source: monosyllabic words in conversational speech samples
**Data source: single words; 90%–100% acquisition criteria averaged across eight studies
***McLeod & Crowe list consonants in age of acquisition order, from youngest to oldest

4. Use minimal feature contrasts in treatment

Meaningful minimal word-pairs, that is two real words, contrasted with each other, can be maximally opposed, like *sick-wick*, which differs in place, voice, manner and major class (and markedness); 'nearly maximally opposed', like *big-jig*, which cuts across many featural dimensions but shares the voicing feature; or minimally opposed, like *pat-bat* differing in voice, *tip-sip* differing in manner, and *cap-tap* differing in place of articulation.

Targeting error phonemes, or error patterns, using *minimally* opposed words is done on the understanding that it is the most direct way of demonstrating (his or her own) homophony to a child (Dean et al., 1995; Grunwell, 1989). So, in choosing treatment words for a child exhibiting voiced velar fronting SFWF, word contrasts such as *bug-bud*, *bag-bad*, and *beg-bed* would be selected, with just one feature difference (in place) between error and target.

In constructing minimal pair sets, the clinician would attempt to find phonetically appropriate picturable words representing age-appropriate vocabulary that lend themselves to activities for pre-readers, and in most instances would include printed captions, in lower case, on picture cards and worksheets. For example, *peel* would be printed 'peel', not 'PEEL' or 'Peel' and *Paul* would be printed 'Paul' not 'PAUL' or 'paul', to be consistent with the way early literacy instruction is commonly delivered.

Note that a near minimal pair is formed with the addition or removal of a sound, changing the syllable structure, as in *nail-snail* and *block-lock* (CVC-CCVC) and *net-nest* and *sink-sing* (CVCC-CVC). Bound morphemes used to mark inflection can be used to generate morphosyntactic minimal pairs (e.g., *jumps-jumped*, *drags-dragged*) and morphosyntactic near minimal pairs (e.g., *book-books*, *run-runs*).

5. Choose unfamiliar words as targets

Choosing unfamiliar words or low-frequency words (in terms of their frequency of occurrence in everyday speech) for treatment stimuli is based on the premise that a child's error production of seldom-spoken or novel words (like *yowie*, *yeti*, and *yen*) will not be as habituated as

familiar words (such as *yes*, *you* and *yet*), or entrenched frozen (fossilized) forms like /ˈlɛloʊ/ for *yellow* and /ˈbakˌsɪt/ or /ˈbatˌsɪt/ for *basket*.

6. Work on inconsistently erred sounds

The principle governing the selection of sounds that are sometimes erred, and sometimes pronounced correctly is that, because the child demonstrates *some* knowledge of an inconsistently erred target, it will be easier to learn and teach than a sound for which a child has less (or no) knowledge. For example, following the developmental trend, a child receiving intervention might have acquired velar stops word finally in words like *shake* and *big*, but not in other syllable contexts, encouraging the clinician to target /k/ and /g/ pre-vocalically, inter-vocalically, and in clusters, perhaps using facilitative contexts containing final velars (see Backward Chaining, and Backward Build-ups in Chapter 7).

Similarly, a child might be producing the /k/ and /g/ in /kl/ and /gl/ clusters but not /k/ and /g/ as singletons (e.g., producing *clock* as [klɒt] and *clog* as as [klɒd]), as can happen in typical acquisition. This might prompt the construction of near minimal pairs, such as *clap-cap*, *club-cub*; *glow-go*, *glue-goo*, to facilitate velar stops SIWI.

Again, a child might only produce the voiceless affricate in words ending with /ntʃ/, suggesting that practising words such *bunch*, *bench*, *launch*, *lunch*, *punch*, *pinch*, etc. (see https://www.speech-language-therapy.com/pdf/cluster-sNCHsfwf.pdf) coupled with auditory input activities around pairs like *pinch-pitch*, *crunch-crutch*, *hunch-hutch*, *inch-itch*, *winch-witch*, and *paunch-porch* might be facilitative.

7. Target sounds most destructive of intelligibility

Sometimes an error has such a pervasive, negative impact on intelligibility that it compels consideration as a high treatment priority (Grunwell, 1989). For example, my client Yoshi, 4;2, with English as his first language (L1), and Japanese as his second language (L2) had a PCC below 30% in both languages. His mother's L1 was German, her L2 was Japanese (Nihongo), and her L3 English. His father's language was English, and he spoke some German with better comprehension than expression, and (he said) 'terrible pronunciation'. Yoshi's Japanese au pair communicated with him in her L1, Japanese and fluent German. In English, Yoshi had widespread glottal insertion before and after utterances and pre- and post-vocalically (as in typical Nihongo). Yoshi's phonology was unusual, exhibiting no glottal *replacement*, only glottal *insertion*. This, coupled with an absence of voiced stops, had a profound effect on his intelligibility. Early treatment goals included achieving stimulability of /b d g/ to two-syllable positions and elimination of glottal insertion.

Sam, 4;1, discussed above in terms of 'unusual errors'; had no consonant clusters and widespread final consonant deletion. He also the unusual pattern of replacing stops with /f/ or /v/, a substitution error that I saw only twice in 42 years of clinical practice. His word productions included for example, *boo* → [vu]; *blue* → [vu]; *Pooh* → [fu]; *do* → [vu]; *coo* → [fu]; *goo* → [vu] with consistent application of voiced-voiceless cognate correspondences. The effect of these idiosyncratic errors was the create widespread homophony and meant that stops and clusters virtually *had* to be early targets for him.

8. Target non-developmental errors

Phonological Patterns / Phonological Processes

Flipsen Jr. and Parker (2008) scrutinized Dodd and Iacono (1989), Edwards and Shriberg (1983) and Khan and Lewis (1983) to list non-developmental and developmental phonological patterns, based on the 1983 and 1989 authors' classifications.

They listed the **non-developmental patterns** as: initial consonant deletion; within word consonant deletion (SIWW and SFWW); deletion of unmarked elements of clusters; within word consonant replacement (SIWW and SFWW); errors of insertion and addition (e.g., schwa insertion or addition; vowel addition word finally) and intrusive consonants; backing of stops, fricatives, and affricates; denasalization; devoicing of stops; idiosyncratic systematic sound preferences; and non-dialectal glottal replacement.

The **developmental phonological patterns** were final consonant deletion; reduplication; weak syllable deletion; cluster reduction; context-sensitive voicing; depalatalization; fronting of fricatives, affricates, and velars; alveolarization of stops and fricatives; labialization of stops; stopping of fricatives and affricates; gliding of fricatives and liquids; deaffrication; epenthesis; metathesis; migration; and vocalization.

Grunwell (1989) recommended that patterns that 'deviated most from normal development' (i.e., non-developmental phonological patterns) should be given priority as treatment targets, particularly initial consonant deletion, which is not attested in normal development in English, and non-dialectal glottal replacement. These non-developmental patterns often beg to be eliminated because they can sound 'odd' even to the untrained ear, and they can disrupt prosody and affect intelligibility.

Phonetic Errors (Articulation Errors)

Non-developmental phonetic errors are also often given priority. These include the lateralization errors with the sibilant fricatives /s, ʃ, z, ʒ/ and the affricates /tʃ, dʒ/ (Overby et al., 2022), ingressive fricatives, phoneme specific nasality and vowel errors.

Vowel Errors

Prevalent or inconsistent vowel errors are a diagnostic marker for CAS. Children with CAS and those with moderate through to severe phonological disorder frequently experience difficulties producing vowels, and indeed, vowel errors may occur in as many as 50% of children with these diagnoses (Eisenson & Ogilvie, 1963; Pollock & Berni, 2003). Depending which study is consulted, 24%–65% typically developing children below 35 months have a high incidence of vowel errors. This is a wide range, and hard to interpret. A more meaningful, useful piece of information for clinicians' guidance is that by 35 months vowel errors are far less prevalent, ranging from zero to 4% (Pollock & Berni, 2003). Note that Idiopathic Speech Motor Delay (SMD) is a prevalent clinical entity (Shriberg, Kwiatkowski et al., 2019, p. 699) that may be misidentified and treated as CAS, because CAS and MSD share certain speech, prosody, and voice features – notably, *vowel distortions*, as well as slow rate, inappropriate stress, and voice quality deficits.

Newer Target Selection Criteria

9. **Work on later developing sounds and structures first**

Some research suggests selecting *later developing sounds* (see Table 3.1 duplicated above (or, on page 431) for convenience); and/or *complex targets* including *clusters* (Krueger A35); and/or *nonstimulable sounds*, otherwise known as the client's least knowledge sounds (see the knowledge 'types' from most to least displayed in Table 9.4) as early treatment targets. The rationale for these choices is that training them will result in greater system-wide change (Gierut et al., 1996).

It is anticipated that there will be variation in the order of acquisition norms clinicians choose to consult, with some adhering to a 'what we always do' philosophy. This reflects the logical fallacy called 'appeal to common practice' discussed in Chapter 6. Looking at various options, some SLPs/SLTs, particularly in Australia, may wish to apply Kilminster and Laird (1978), shown in Table 1.2, perhaps because their norms are familiar. Some others, in the USA and around the world, may prefer the Early-8, Middle-8, and Late-8 acquired sounds (Shriberg, 1993) as they have been used by many since the early 90s. Some may even turn to the once ground-breaking norms compiled by Dr. Mildred Templin (1913–2008). Templin (1957) examined the consonants (only) in single word productions by 480 US three-to-eight-year-olds to establish age expectations for consonant acquisition (see, Sander, 1972 for an interesting discussion of Templin's analysis).

It is desirable, however, that most SLPs/SLTs working with children with English as their L1 will adopt the Early 2;0–3;11, Middle 4;0–4;11, and Late 5;0–6;11 for English-speaking children (McLeod & Crowe, 2018) or for USA children (Crowe & McLeod, 2020). The case for adopting the 2018–2020 norms can be presented to administrators, if necessary, in terms of their being current, superseding previous systems, and in

terms of their supporting best practice among SLPs/SLTs engaged in speech assessment, and making clinical decisions on children's eligibility for apposite services.

Preliminary Evidence for Targeting Word-final Clusters

Most research into the generalization effects of targeting clusters has concerned word-initial clusters (e.g., /sn-/ in snail) focusing on phonology alone, without considering grammatical morphemes. Potapova et al. (2023) however, conducted initial investigations via case studies of two monolingual English-speakers, Anna (3;7) and David (4;1), with phonological disorder, in which verbs with /-ks/ word-finally were targeted. The children were seen in 45-minute sessions conducted three times weekly over 18 sessions, with high cumulative intervention intensity, namely, mean attempts at producing the target cluster per session = 165; SD = 36.83. Treatment followed a drill and drill-play format in the first, imitative phase, and play and shared reading in the second, spontaneous phase, with the clinician maximizing target-production opportunities, and delivering feedback, via verbal, visual, tactile, and gestural cues throughout.

The authors reasoned that treatment words that combined, simultaneously, both phonological and morphological complexity would facilitate generalization. Before treatment, both children had 0% accuracy for word-final clusters. For word-final singletons Anna's accuracy was 46% and David's 62%.

In choosing treatment words, the researchers focused on what they called 'word-final morphology' (personal correspondence, Potapova September 2022). For example, while the word *unbox* is bimorphemic, and the word *unpacks* is trimorphemic, they classified the [-ks] in in *box* and *unbox* as monomorphemic, and the [-ks] in *packs* and *unpacks* as bimorphemic. Accordingly, Anna's targets were morphologically simple comprising the monomorphemic verbs *mix, max, wax, nix, fix* and *unbox*, whereas David's were morphologically complex comprising the bimorphemic verbs *kicks, knocks, packs, unpacks, locks,* and *unlocks*, inflected with third-person singular (e.g., *she locks, he kicks*).

When their intervention ended, Anna and David had high target production accuracy, were more intelligible, and were producing more word-final consonant clusters, with David demonstrating further generalization across multiple measures. Importantly, generalization of /-ks/ to untreated words was evident. These encouraging results spur further research into the effects on phonology and morphology of choosing complex word-final clusters and grammatical morphemes.

10. Work on marked consonants first

A distinctive feature, or 'feature', is an acoustic or articulatory parameter whose presence or absence defines a phonetic category, distinguishing it from another phonetic category (Chomsky & Halle, 1968). Targeting the marked properties (features) of phonemes is prioritized on the basis that it may facilitate acquisition of unmarked aspects of the system.

Markedness is a concept from the study of the sound systems of all natural languages. A marked feature in a language *implies* the necessary presence of another feature, hence the term *'implicational* relationship'. There are languages, like English, that have stops *and* fricatives. There are languages that have stops, but *no* fricatives. But no language has fricatives and no stops. This means that fricatives are a marked class of sounds because the presence of fricatives necessarily implies the presence of stops in a particular language. Thus, it is said that there is an *implicational relationship* between the fricatives /f v θ ð s z ʃ ʒ h/ and stops (Elbert et al., 1984).

Another way of putting this is to say that the fricatives, /f v θ ð s z ʃ ʒ h/, are marked because they imply stops. Similarly, the voiceless stops that occur in /s/ clusters (/p t k/) are marked because they imply voiced stops: /b d g/. Furthermore, according to this interesting but somewhat controversial body of research, consonants imply vowels (Robb et al., 1999); affricates /tʃ/ and /dʒ/ imply fricatives (Schmidt & Meyers, 1995); clusters (except for the adjuncts, /sp, st, sk/) imply affricates (Gierut & O'Connor, 2002); and true clusters with small sonority differences imply true clusters with larger sonority differences (Gierut, 1999).

David Ingram (personal correspondence, May 2011) notes that Jakobson discussed the voiceless stops /p/, /t/ and /k/ as unmarked, and that this opinion is common in the linguistics literature (e.g., Dinnsen, 2019). It is also common in the SLP/SLT literature, e.g., Gierut (2007; Gierut & Hulse, 2010), McReynolds and Jetzke (1986), Stoel-Gammon (2019), and Storkel (2018a, 2018b) who say voiced obstruents imply voiceless obstruents.

In clinical practice, I have deferred to Ingram with respect to the unmarked status of voiced stops. Ingram says that the general claim that voiced stops are the marked ones is based on languages where the voiceless stops are unaspirated and have roughly a zero (0) voice-onset-time (VOT). English-speaking children start out with stops that are characterized by 0 VOT, but English-speaking parents (including researchers) hear and often transcribe these as voiced because they are within the VOT boundaries for English voiced stops. So, the unmarked stop for L1 English-speaking children is neither the English voiced nor voiceless aspirated stop, but those stops that occur after 's' in clusters (i.e., the /t/, /p/, and /k/ that occur in /st/, /sp/ and /sk/ respectively). Based on judgements of accuracy, the *voiced stops* in English *are* acquired before the voiceless ones and can be interpreted as the *unmarked* ones.

Interestingly, the opposite occurs in Spanish where the voiceless stops have 0 VOT and the voiced stops are pre-voiced. Spanish children start out doing well with voiceless stops, which are perceived by Spanish speakers as voiceless, and have errors with the voiced ones, sometimes making them as fricatives, something rarely if ever seen in children with English as their first language (L1). So, the markedness of stops must be viewed in relation to whether a language has one, two or even three series of stops, and in relation to their VOT values.

In summary then, some research suggests we should target the *marked* consonants and clusters, particularly those with small sonority differences (see point 14 below), to facilitate the acquisition of unmarked ones. Clinicians interested in applying these ideas in intervention can be guided as follows:

Fricatives imply **Stops** (e.g., Elbert et al., 1984)
    Target fricatives to promote functional generalization to (other) fricatives and stops.

Voiceless Stops that occur in /s/ clusters (adjuncts) imply **Voiced Stops**
    Target voiceless stops to promote functional generalization to voiced and voiceless stops (Williams, 2003 p. 13). Note that opinions differ and see the brief explanation above of David Ingram's view. You might choose, instead, to follow Dinnsen, 2019; Gierut, 2007; McReynolds & Jetzke, 1986; Stoel-Gammon, 2019; and Storkel, 2018a, 2018b, by giving priority to voiced stops in the expectation that that will generalise to voiced and voiceless stops.

Affricates imply **Fricatives** (e.g., Schmidt & Meyers, 1995)
    Target affricates to promote functional generalization to affricates and fricatives.

Clusters imply **Singletons** (e.g., Gierut & O'Connor, 2002)
    Target clusters to promote functional generalization clusters and singletons.

Other implicational relationships that may be of interest regarding generalization are

- **Consonants** imply **Vowels** (e.g., Robb et al., 1999)
- **Liquids** imply **Nasals** (e.g., Gierut et al., 1994)
- **True clusters** with small sonority differences imply **True clusters** with large sonority differences (e.g., Gierut, 1999)
- **Velars** imply **Coronals** (e.g., Bernhardt & Stoel-Gammon, 1996)Velars: /k, g, ŋ/ Coronals: /θ, ð, t, d, s. z, n, l, ʃ, ʒ, tʃ, dʒ, ɹ/
- **Voiced obstruents** imply **Voiceless obstruents** (e.g., McReynolds & Jetzke, 1986)

11. **Work on non-stimulable phonemes first**
    Since the mid-1990s, sections of the research world have encouraged clinicians to target non-stimulable sounds because if a sound *is* stimulable, or if it *becomes* stimulable (e.g., as a product of SLP/SLT intervention), it is likely to be added to a child's inventory, even without direct treatment (Miccio, A17; Miccio et al., 1999). As sounds that are *not* stimulable have poorer short-term prognosis than those

that are, treatment outcomes are likely to be enhanced when SLPs/SLTs use their unique skills to address the production of those non-stimulable sounds – to *make* them stimulable. Once the sounds are stimulable, in two-syllable positions (e.g., /f/ SIWI and SFWF in *fie* and *off*, respectively; or /f/ SIWI and SIWW in *far* and *tofu*, respectively; or /f/ SIWW and SFWF in *muffin* and *woof* respectively), they are likely to progress and become established in the child's productive repertoire even if not targeted directly for treatment beyond that level.

This has strong implications for clinicians who, for whatever reason, can only see a child with significant inventory constraints infrequently. The available time to provide intervention in such circumstances may be best spent doing stimulability therapy, something we are uniquely qualified to do, rather than expect an inexpert non-SLP/SLT, perhaps armed with a 'home program', to teach sounds absent from the child's repertoire.

Targeting stimulable sounds yields short-term but limited gains, in terms of generalization (Powell & Miccio, 1996), whereas targeting *non-stimulable* sounds via stimulability therapy (Miccio, A17), exploratory sound play, and phonetic placement techniques increases the probability of generalization, once stimulability is achieved (Rvachew et al., 1999). Rvachew & Nowak (2001) determined that clinicians can be reasonably confident that provided child has relatively greater productive phonological knowledge for them (i.e., the child is stimulable for them), developmentally earlier targets will be easier for pre-schoolers to acquire than target phonemes that are *both* non-stimulable *and* late developing.

12. **Use maximal feature contrasts in treatment**
    The rationale for using maximally opposed, non-proportional contrasts (Gierut, 1992) is that the heightened perceptual saliency of the contrasts so formed increases learnability, facilitating phonemic change. This is discussed under *Maximal Oppositions and Empty Set* in Chapter 4 with examples of treatment targets for Xing-Fu, 4;5, and Vaughan, 5;8, and elaborated by Krueger (A35).

Table 9.2 'Place-voice-manner chart' for PVM analysis, Adapted from Hanson,1983.

English phonemes

MANNER		Labial		Coronal			Palatal	Dorsal	
NOTE cognate pairs: voiceless on the left		Bilabial	Labiodental	Interdental	Alveolar	Palato-alveolar	Palatal	Velar	Glottal
Obstruents	Stop	p b			t d			k g	ʔ
	Fricative		f v	θ ð	s z	ʃ ʒ			h
	Affricate					tʃ dʒ			
Sonorants	Nasal	m			n			ŋ	
	liquid				l		ɹ		
	Glide	w					j	w	

Maximal oppositions cross many featural dimensions. For example, the PVM Charts in Figure 2.1, or Table 9.2, or the Full Chart of the IPA (https://www.internationalphoneticas sociation.org/IPAcharts/IPA_chart_orig/pdfs/ IPA_Kiel_2020_full.pdf) show that the contrast between /b/ and /s/ in the word pair *bun-sun* is in place (labial is distinct from coronal), manner (stop is distinct from fricative) and voice (/b/ is voiced and /s/ is voiceless). *Fat-gnat* also differs in place, manner, and voice, *and* there is a major class distinction between sonorant /f/ and obstruent /n/.

13. Use a systemic approach to analyse the child's rules

Williams (2010) and Williams and Sugden (2021) describe a non-traditional approach to target selection, based on analysis of the function of the sound in the child's own system, as having maximal impact on phonological restructuring. This is explained with examples in Chapter 4 under the heading *Minimal Pair Approaches: Multiple Oppositions*, and by Lynn Williams in A19.

14. Apply the sonority sequencing principle

Sonority is determined by the amount of 'sound' (loudness or intensity) in a consonant or vowel; the amount of 'stricture' of the vocal tract during its production; and the extent to which the consonant or vowel can be prolonged. Linguists Davenport and Hannahs (2020, p. 79) say 'the more sonorant a sound, the louder, more sustainable, and more open it is'.

There is a way of representing sonority numerically in a scale, from zero to seven, called the 'sonority hierarchy' (Steriade, 1990). Steriade's scale runs from most to least sonorous (or most to least sonorant if you prefer). Vowels, with a sonority value of zero (=0) are the most sonorous, followed by glides (=1), liquids (=2), nasals (=3), voiced fricatives (=4), voiceless fricatives (=5), voiced stops (=6) and finally voiceless stops (=7), the least sonorous.

Markedness data tell us that consonant clusters are more marked than singletons (see point 10 above). Sonority theory adds to the picture by ranking two-element consonant clusters (note: *just* the two-element ones) in terms of markedness, according to their sonority difference scores (Ohala, 1999), as displayed in Table 9.3. For example, /kl/ (7 minus 1 in Steriade's hierarchy, because /k/=7 and /l/=1) has a sonority difference score of 6, whereas /fɹ/ (5 minus 2) scores 3.

Clusters with *small* sonority differences of 3 (like /sl/ and /ʃɹ/) or 4 (like /gl/ and /sw/), *and* the three-element clusters under certain conditions, may promote generalized change to singletons *and* clusters more efficiently than other two-element clusters (Gierut, 1999; Gierut & Champion, 2001; Morrisette, 2021). The 'certain conditions' for the three-element clusters (/spɹ/ /stɹ/ /skɹ/ /spl/ and /skw/) are that

Table 9.3 Sonority difference scores.

Most Complex			Sonority Difference
⬍	Voiceless fricative+nasal	sm sn	2
	Voiceless fricative+liquid	fl fɹ θɹ sl ʃɹ	3
	Voiced stop+liquid or voiceless fricative +glide	bl bɹ dɹ gl gɹ sw	4
⬍	Voiceless stop+liquid	pl pɹ tɹ kl kɹ	5
	Voiceless stop+glide	tw kw	6
Least Complex			

they should only be targeted if the child already has the relevant stop (/p/, /t/ or /k/) *and* the relevant liquid (/l/) or glide (/w/) present in his or her phonemic inventory. For example, before targeting /skw/ ensure that the child has productive knowledge of /k/ and /w/, noting that they do not need to have productive knowledge of /s/.

Consider targeting three-element clusters, and two-element clusters with smaller sonority differences 2 or 3 or 4.
Note that Gierut and O'Connor (2002) and Morrisette et al. (2006) count the initial /s/ + stop combinations (/sp/, /st/, and /k/) as adjuncts and not 'true clusters', asserting that targeting them is unlikely to evoke the same generalization expected when true clusters are targeted.

It has been observed clinically that by working on /sp/, or /st/ or /sk/, the child 'learns' the target, but that there is little or no generalization to clusters in general, or to other fricatives, or to other stops. Applying clinical reasoning however, SLPs/SLTs sometimes target initial /sp/, /st/ or /sk/ to give a child 'the idea' of a 2-step sound (see Table 4.1), noting that it is comparatively easy to find child-friendly picture stimuli for them, and that the child can *see* both elements of /st/ and /sp/, but not /sk/, when the clinician models them. Children can also view their own correct production of /st/ and /sp/ in a mirror.

15. **Prioritise least knowledge sounds in treatment**
Some research suggests selecting sounds for which the child has 'least knowledge' in terms of the 'knowledge types' described in

Table 9.4, because they will be easier to learn (Barlow & Gierut, 2002; Gierut, 2001; Williams, 1991). Applying learnability theory, Gierut (2007) provides support for the position that, for efficient learning to occur, we should teach phonologically impaired children complex aspects of the target system, outside of what they have learned already.

16. **Consider the lexical properties of 'therapy words'**
We can consider word properties when we choose words to use in intervention. In this respect we have the choice of selecting words that are either of '*high frequency*' in the language, or words with '*low neighbourhood density*'.

High-frequency Words

These are words that occur often in the language (Storkel, 2013). They are recognized (comprehended) faster *by children* than low-frequency words.

High Neighbourhood Density Words

These words are similar phonetically to many other words. Children recognise and repeat high-density words slower and with less accuracy than low-density words. As well, children name high-density words more accurately than low-density words, suggesting

Table 9.4 Knowledge types. Reproduced with permission from the American Speech-Language-Hearing Association.

Description	Examples	
Type-1 knowledge – Most knowledge	sun [sʌn]	
A child displaying type-1 knowledge of target /s/ would produce this sound correctly in all word positions and for all morphemes; /s/ would never be produced incorrectly.	soup [sup] messy [mesi] missing [mɪsɪŋ] miss [mɪs]	
Type-2 knowledge	sun [sʌn]	<u>BUT</u>
A child displaying type-2 knowledge of target /s/ would produce this sound correctly for all morphemes and positions. However, a phonological rule would apply to account for observed alternations between, for example, /s/ and /t/ in morpheme final position.	soup [sup] messy [mesi] ice [aɪs]	miss [mɪt] kiss [kɪt]
Type-3 knowledge	sun [sʌn]	<u>BUT</u>
A child displaying type-3 knowledge of target /s/ would produce this sound correctly in all positions. However, certain morphemes that were presumably acquired early and acquired incorrectly 'fossilized' would always be produced in error.	messy [mesi] miss[mɪs]	Santa [næntə] juice [wu]
Type-4 knowledge	sun [sʌn]	<u>BUT</u>
A child displaying type-4 knowledge of target /s/ would produce this sound for all morphemes, in, for example, initial position. However, production of /s/ would be incorrect in within-word and word final positions.	soup [sup]	messy [meti] missing /[ɪtɪŋ] miss [mɪt] kiss [kɪt]
Type-5 knowledge	sun [sʌn]	<u>BUT</u>
A child displaying type-5 knowledge of target /s/ would produce this sound correctly in, for example, initial position. However, only some morphemes in this position would be produced correctly. All /s/ morphemes in post-vocalic positions would be produced incorrectly.	soup [sup]	soap [təup] sock [sɔk] messy [meti] kiss [kɪt]
Type-6 knowledge – Least knowledge	sun [tʌn]	
A child displaying type-6 knowledge of target /s/ would produce this sound incorrectly in all word positions and for all morphemes; /s/ would never be produced correctly.	soup [tup] missing [mɪtɪŋ] miss [mɪt] kiss [kɪt]	

that lexical processing in children entails a high-density disadvantage in recognition and a high-density advantage in production (Storkel et al., 2006).

Five Target-word Selection Criteria Based on Lexical Properties

In view of this, in choosing stimulus words, or 'treatment words', the clinician might consider those that fit any one of the following five criteria Storkel (2018a, 2018b)

1. high-frequency *and* high-density, or
2. low-frequency *and* high-density, or
3. high-frequency *and* mixed density, or
4. low-frequency *and* late-acquired, or
5. nonwords.

Examples: High-frequency Words

Table 9.5 contains selected high-frequency words with /s/ SIWI and SFWF. These words, pictured, are at https://speech-language-therapy.com/pdf/SwordsHF.pdf

Table 9.5 Selected, picturable, 'child friendly' high-frequency words for /s/.

/s/ SIWI				/s/ SFWF				
cell	sat	summer	seam	audience	face	miss	police	space
city	saw	seven	sun	case	force	office	press	us
say	scene	six	sent	class	house	peace	price	voice
same	season	small	science	close	less	place	race	yes

Examples: Low Neighbourhood Density Words

High-density words are similar phonetically to many other words and have 11 or more neighbours. The words residing in a neighbourhood are based on one sound substitution, e.g., *sat* to *pat*, one sound deletion, e.g., *sat* to *at* or one sound addition, e.g., *sat* to *scat*. The word *bat* is in a dense neighbourhood of 40, and its 39 neighbours are: *back bad badge bag baht bait ban bang bash bass bast batch bath batteau batten batter battle beat bet bight bit boat boot bought bout brat but cat chat fat gnat hat mat pat rat sat tat that* and *vat*.

If a Wordle player, aiming for a 5-letter-word solution in six or fewer attempts, were to enter STAKE as a first guess, achieving S T A ☐ E, neighbourhood density dictates that they *would* solve the puzzle with one of five close neighbours: STAVE, STAGE, STALE, STARE, or STATE

It is interesting to consider words with /dʒ/ word initially in terms of neighbourhood density. The easy-to-illustrate (picturable) words *gym, jack, jam, jet, jig, jog, juice, joke, and jug* are often chosen as stimulus items. They are readily available in apps, on flashcards, and in games and other media from publishers and retailers such as LessonPix, Pro-Ed, Smart Kids, and Super Duper, and from enterprising SLPs/SLTs who create and sell such materials. If we want to let *low* neighbourhood densities inform our target selection choices, however, we will think twice about including these words in the mix because *jog* and *joke* have 11 neighbours, *juice* has 13, *gym* has 14, *jam* and *jug* have 16, *jack* and *jig* have 17, and *jet* has 20. We might opt instead for words with fewer than 11 neighbours such as *germ* (7), *giant* (0), *jaguar* (0), *jalopy* (0), *jester* (1), *jazz* (7), *jeans* (4), *jelly* (5), *jetty* (4), *jewel* (6), *joey* (0),

joust (5), *judo* (1), *jump* (8), and *junk* (9). It unnecessary to give preference to words with the lowest possible numbers, aiming for zeros, ones, and twos, provided the word is in a sparse neighbourhood of 10 or fewer other words.

A picture and word worksheet that includes the low-density /dʒ/ SIWI words *germ jaguar jalopy jazz jelly jetty jewel judo jump* and *junk*, is available at https://speech-language-therapy.com/pdf/dg-siwi.pdf

Picturable, Child Friendly Low Neighbourhood Density Verbs

blink block blow bounce bring broke brush bump camp carve change chirp clean climb clip cough count crawl crush cry dance dream dress drill drink drip drive drop dry faint film flap flip frown fry gasp give grab grow growl help honk hunt iron jive join judge jump love march pinch plant point push quack scan scold scream shrug ski skid skip smash smell smile snap sneeze snooze snore snort speak speed spell spend spill spit splash splat spray spread spy squash squawk squeak squeal stand start stay steal step stir stitch stomp stop surf sweat sweep swish swoop thank throw trim trot waltz want wash watch whoosh woof zoom

Picturable, Child Friendly Low Neighbourhood Density Nouns

ant arch ark arm axe bench blade blind block blood blouse branch breath bridge brooch broom brush bulb bump bunch bush champ child chimp church clamp clasp claw clay cliff clog cloth clove clown club couch crab craft cream crop crow crowd crown crumb crust crutch cube desk dial disc disk dog drain drawer dress drill drum farm fence five flag flake flame flash flask fleece flex flock flood floor flower fluff flute fog foot frame fridge friend fringe frog front frost froth fruit fudge geese germ gift glass glove glue golf gown grouch knife ground group grub harp hinge hoist ink jazz jewel junk lion lounge lump lunch lamp mask milk month moth mouth mulch mumps noise nurse palm plan plane plant plough plug plum plus pond porch pouch pram prawn price prince print pulse queen quiche quilt choir ramp ranch scab scar scarf school scone scoop score screen screw shark shelf shield shrub chef silk skin skirt skull skunk sky sleeve slice slime slug smock smog smoke snack snail snake snow salt spa space spark speech spice spire sport spring sprout spud square squid staff stag stage stalk stamp star steam steel stem stilt store stork storm stove straw stream street string stripe stump stunt sty swag swamp swan swarm swatch thatch thief thong thread three throat throne thud thump torch towel track tram trap trash treat tree troll trout trowel truck trunk tube tusk twig twin view voice wasp watch web whale wharf wheat wheel whip wolf world worm yolk zinc

Picturable, Child Friendly Low Neighbourhood Density Adjectives

black brave brown clean crisp cross cute damp dark flash fresh glad good grey huge large old proud quick real sharp short smart small soft strong sweet white

Researching Phonological Complexity

Many SLPs/SLTs, clinical phonologists and other linguists have developed research interests around phonological complexity and the impact of selecting complex treatment targets – including the 'treatment words' we choose – upon phonological generalization (e.g., Baker, 2015; Gierut, 2007; Morrisette, 2021; Rvachew & Nowak, 2001; Storkel, 2018a, 2018b).

Dr. Breanna Krueger is one such scholar (see Krueger & Storkel, 2022). She is an Assistant

Professor in the Division of Communication Disorders at the University of Wyoming. Her research interests include the development of speech sounds and words in typically developing and disordered populations, and the social impact of SSD (Krueger, 2019). She is particularly interested in the impact of variability in the speech signal on word and sound learning; specifically, she is interested in how children learn words from their peers despite variability in their productions, such as misarticulations and dialectal variation. Breanna believes that through advancing our understanding of the development of the sound system, treatment efficacy and efficiency may be improved.

Q35. Breanna Krueger: Identifying Target Words Within a Complexity Approach

Emergent evidence supports the use of various combinations of lexical characteristics within 'treatment words' in intervention for phonological disorder (Storkel, 2018b), on the understanding that the word-stimuli an SLP/SLT selects are among the 'active ingredients' in intervention. For example, the therapist can choose, with reasonable optimism, to target (1) high-frequency *and* high-density words, (2) low-frequency *and* high-density words, (3) high-frequency *and* mixed density words, (4) low-frequency *and* late-acquired words and (5) nonwords.

What are the potential benefits, for a child with phonological disorder, if the clinician adopts a complexity approach (Morrisette, 2021) to treatment target selection while considering lexical properties? In identifying suitable candidates for a complexity approach, what aspects of the child's language development (e.g., receptive, and expressive vocabulary) are considered? What challenges and facilitators exist for SLP/SLT clinicians and researchers wanting to apply lexical properties in clinical practice and/or investigate them empirically?

A35.   Breanna Krueger: Selecting Treatment Words for a Complexity Approach to Phonological Intervention

The goal of phonological treatment is to broaden a child's access to the phonological system of their language. There are several lexical features to consider when selecting treatment words for phonological disorders. If the appropriate features are selected, treatment is expected to result in significant change in a child's phonological system through improving accuracy of treatment sounds' production and generalization to untreated sounds and sound classes. These lexical features include **word frequency**, **phonological neighbourhood density**, and **age of acquisition** (AoA) of words. Storkel (2018b) referred to these items as 'active ingredients' in intervention because research demonstrates that these features play a role in the development and acquisition of speech sounds in children with phonological disorders (e.g., Gierut et al., 1999; Gierut & Morrisette, 2012b).

Lexical Properties of Words

Word frequency is one feature to consider in selecting stimuli for treatment, and words can be categorized as either 'high' or 'low' frequency. Frequency values are calculated by identifying the number of times a word appears in a corpus of spoken and/or written language (e.g., Kučera & Francis, 1967). Applying this method, high frequency words are those commonly used by people in day-to-day speech. As 'treatment words', high frequency words promote learning of treatment sounds as well as promoting generalization to untreated sounds (Gierut et al., 1999; Morrisette & Gierut, 2002). The improved learning observed in these studies is theorized to be due to reduced linguistic processing time. That is, when a child can rapidly access a word in the lexicon, they can focus more attention to the treatment tasks.

Phonological neighbourhood density of words is the phonological similarity of words and their relationship to one another in the lexicon. Words can be categorized as high density (i.e., many phonologically similar forms) or low density (i.e., very few phonologically similar forms). For example, a word like *log* ([lɑg] in my variety of English) has phonological neighbours such as *hog* and *dog* [hɑg] and [dɑg] because they are minimal pairs. A word with a high neighbourhood density is *red*, while a word with low neighbourhood density is *orange*. There is a significant body of evidence suggesting that words are connected to one another in the lexicon based on shared phonemes (e.g., Morrisette & Gierut, 2002).

Phonological neighbourhood density is often investigated alongside word frequency because they are related to one another in terms of their influence in changing the lexicon. Research indicates that words with many neighbours (i.e., high density words) promote change in the phonological system resulting in more widespread generalization to untreated sounds than do low density words (Bellon-Harn et al., 2013; Gierut & Morrisette, 2012b). According to Gierut (2016), when many words belong to the same neighbourhood, the lexical representations of these neighbours are required to be in rich enough detail to differentiate between sounds.

Age of acquisition may also influence treatment efficacy for phonological disorders. AoA is the age at which children generally acquire words. Words can be categorized as early acquired or late acquired; however, there is variability from child to child regarding when words are learned. Early words tend to be concrete nouns that are highly familiar to a child based on daily experience. Since early acquired words are more familiar and practiced, it is thought that their representations are more stable than those of late-acquired words that are in the beginning stage of lexical representation formation. The research on AoA in the context of other lexical features (e.g., neighbourhood density, frequency) is limited (Storkel, 2018a). In one study investigating AoA in phonological treatment, the researchers found that the use of late-acquired words as treatment stimuli promoted the most change in both treated and untreated error sounds (Gierut & Morrisette, 2012a). Possibly, since late-acquired words have less complete lexical representations – or may be unknown to the child – they may be less stable, with more flexible phonological representations that are amenable to treatment (Storkel, 2018b).

The hypothesis about the lexical status of late-acquired words may also apply to the use of nonwords in treatment. For example, since nonwords – by definition – are devoid of semantic representation in the lexicon, they provide an opportunity to focus exclusively on phonological targets. Using nonwords in treatment is an alternative approach to using real words as stimuli, and their use is effective in the treatment of phonological disorders (Cummings & Barlow, 2011; Gierut et al., 2010). In these studies, the investigators examined treatment with nonwords versus real words. They found that children attained a higher level of accuracy in fewer sessions on treatment sounds in nonwords than children treated with real words. It is important to note, however, that children treated with sounds in real words eventually attained a similar level of progress to the nonword treatment group. One benefit of employing nonwords is that the frequency, density and AoA of words can be controlled, using tools such as the online database developed by Storkel (2013).

Lexical Features and the Complexity Approach

Each of the lexical features can be used in conjunction with a complexity approach to treatment target selection. A complexity approach involves selecting treatment targets that are more phonetically complex than other sounds, that are not present in the phonological system, less frequent, and nonstimulable (Gierut, 2001). This contrasts with other approaches (e.g., Prezas et al., 2021; A5) that have focused on using treatment targets based on developmental normative data. Several studies suggest that complexity approaches to target selection result in generalization to untreated sounds (e.g., Gierut, 2001; Gierut & Champion, 2001; Kamhi, 2007; Morrisette, 2021). When combined with the word-level features discussed here, or nonwords, children may experience a variety of ben-

efits. First, treatment is more advantageous to the entire system because children experience generalization of complex treatment targets across multiple sounds and sound classes. Second, treatment is more efficient and may require less time, potentially reducing missed classroom time and social opportunities. Finally, the reduction of treatment time may, in turn, reduce the likelihood that children experience social stigma and negative academic and literacy outcomes (Bernhardt & Major, 2005; Feeney et al., 2012; Lewis et al., 2015).

Client Suitability for a Complexity Approach

Complexity approaches to treatment target selection were designed to foment broad, system-wide change across sound classes. It is particularly applicable to children who have many sounds in error across feature classes (e.g., a moderate to severe level of involvement in terms of clinical judgment) because they are likely to experience significant growth across the phonological system. In determining whether a complexity approach is suitable for a child, it is important to consider receptive and expressive language abilities since phonological disorders are linguistic in nature. What a child understands (receptive language) and their spoken linguistic ability (expressive language) both may influence the course of treatment. According to some estimates, approximately 50–75% of children, between the ages of 3 and 11, who have phonological disorders also have more widespread difficulty with language, suggesting frequent interactivity between phonological and other language difficulties (Shriberg & Kwiatkowski, 1994). Due to the possibility of interaction due to concomitant language disorder (see McCauley, A15; Stoeckel, A14), children with language disorders were excluded from the complexity research. Therefore, it is unclear whether those children will respond to lexical features in treatment in the same way as children with a discrete diagnosis of phonological disorder.

Challenges and Facilitators

SLPs/SLTs intending to use a complexity approach to treatment target selection while considering lexical features may encounter facilitators and challenges. The clear benefit to using these features and complexity is to reap the benefits of efficient treatment and to improve children's speech production and intelligibility. Furthermore, if using nonwords, lexical variables are easily controlled to promote acquisition of treatment sounds and generalization to untreated sounds. While employing lexical features provides benefits to children with phonological disorder, there are challenges to initiating this as a treatment strategy. First, development of treatment stimuli involves seeking out those features of words or nonwords and finding enough words for each child's treatment sounds can be time consuming.

Developing stimuli with all the desired lexical properties within a treatment target can be challenging too, but the burden of locating them is greatly reduced through various resources available publicly at https://kuscholarworks.ku.edu/handle/1808/24767 through Creative Commons licenses (Storkel, 2018b). Due to the overall benefits for children with phonological disorders, the initial effort required to design stimuli becomes a worthwhile endeavour.

Phonetic Placement or Sound Elicitation

Chapter 4 contains a description of sound elicitation or phonetic placement techniques including *imitation* and *shaping*, with the inclusion of *visual, auditory, motor-kinaesthetic, touch,* and *metalinguistic cues* (see Table 4.1 for the latter). These techniques are individually tailored for children across the SSD range, whether they present with articulation disorder, phonological disorder, CAS, developmental dysarthria, a structurally based SSD – or some combination of these, with or without auditory perceptual difficulties (Hearnshaw et al., 2018, 2019). It all sounds quite straightforward – and often is – until you engage with a child who, for example, struggles to achieve placement for velar stops (Unicomb et al., 2019), or who experiences

coarticulation resistance with the voiceless fricatives /s, ʃ, θ/ (Howson & Redford, 2022).

In the next three contributions, Kenneth Bleile, Peter Flipsen Jr., and Dennis Ruscello discuss potential difficulties that an SLP/SLT can encounter when working with a child on their production of fricatives and affricates (A36), /ɹ/ as an articulatory target (A37), and compensatory errors in the presence of repaired cleft lip and palate (A38).

Dr. Kenneth Bleile is a university professor and an ASHA Fellow. He served twice as Associate Editor of the *American Journal of Speech-Language Pathology* and is the former Chair of ASHA's International Issues Board. Dr. Bleile is a recipient of the association's Multicultural Board's Diversity Champion Award and was awarded the State of Iowa's Regents Scholar Award for excellence in teaching and scholarship.

Q36.   Kenneth Bleile: Targeting Fricatives and Affricates

The fricatives, particularly /s/ and /z/, and affricates pose difficulties for many SLP/SLT clients. Can you define for readers what is meant by phonetic placement and shaping techniques, explain how they differ from nonspeech oral motor exercises (NS-OME), and provide examples of how they are applied when working on typical and atypical perception and production errors with these troublesome groups of sounds?

A36.   Kenneth Bleile: Phonemic Placement and Shaping and Targeting Fricatives and Affricates

Phonetic placement and shaping are techniques to teach speech sounds. Phonetic placement involves instructing a student on how to place their articulators. A simple example of a phonetic placement technique is to instruct a student 'Place your tongue tip behind your upper front teeth'. Shaping entails converting a sound a student already produces into one a clinician is teaching. To illustrate, a clinician might convert /g/ to [k] by instructing the student to 'Say /g/, but turn off your voice box', resulting in [k].

Non-Speech Oral Motor Exercises (NS-OME)

Phonetic placement and shaping are sometimes confused with NS-OME. The two differ both in theory and practice. Phonetic placement and shaping are based on clinical phonetics and phonology, components of the linguistic study of speech. As consonant charts reveal, speech sounds share phonetic similarities and differences. SLPs/SLTs can take advantage of these similarities and differences when they employ phonetic placement and shaping techniques. To illustrate, a shaping technique converting /g/ into /k/ relies on a shared velar place of production and a voicing contrast. NS-OME, on the other hand, is based on non-evidenced theories or atheoretical 'beliefs' that practice with non-speech exercises benefit the production of speech. To illustrate, a clinician using NS-OME might have a student practice blowing bubbles, puffing their cheeks, or touching their tongue to their nose to increase the range, strength and flexibility of the speech mechanism, the benefits of which (the theory of NS-OME contends) help a student achieve articulatory accuracy. Many studies document that NS-OME activities do not improve speech (Clark, 2003; Forrest, 2002; Forrest & Iuzzini, 2008; Lass & Pannbacker, 2008; Lof, 2009; Muttiah et al., 2011; Ruscello, 2008c; Ruscello & Vallino, 2020). As the collective evidence demonstrates, the reasons NS-OME are ineffective include that speech uses oral structures differently from non-speech activities, the strength requirements for speech differ from those for non-speech exercises, and speech uses different brain areas from non-speech exercises (Maas, 2017).Clinical Populations

Years ago, speech treatment entailed teaching phonetic placement and shaping to students with speech errors affecting individual phones. Knowledge and use of these techniques decreased as our scope of practice grew to include younger children as well as persons of all ages with a wider range of cognitive abilities. Today in the United States, phonetic placement and shaping receive the greatest use among clinicians whose caseloads include students for whom the techniques were chiefly developed (ASHA, 2018): school children who have challenges with individual consonants that tend to be acquired late in typical development. Simpler phonetic placement and shaping techniques are also useful when working with preschool aged children from the age of 3;6. Furthermore, phonetic placement and shaping may also be useful with multilingual populations and additional language learners.

Clinical Uses

Phonetic placement and shaping remain in the clinical toolbox because they provide ways to teach sounds that may largely be unteachable by other means. In essence, they help a clinician convert unstimulable sounds into stimulable sounds. Once stimulable, the sound is treated as any other stimulable sound.

Examples

Phonetic placement and shaping offer practical applications of clinical phonetics. The techniques were developed by clever clinicians and communicated from one generation to the next through books, conference presentations, and clinician-to-clinician word of mouth. Many such techniques exist for late acquired fricatives and affricates. The following examples illustrate their use for seven fricatives /v θ ð s z ʃ ʒ/, but not /f/ and /h/ and the affricates /tʃ dʒ/, with special attention given to /s/. The examples are adapted slightly from Bleile, 2017, 2019, which contain over one hundred such techniques. Because of length limitations, I have selected simpler examples with fewer steps. Voiceless consonants are presented first, followed by techniques to teach voicing.

Targeting /θ/

The dental consonants /θ ð/ pose significant challenges to some students. Also, because such consonants are relatively rare across the world's languages, they may present special difficulties for non-native English speakers. While they are designated 'dental' in an IPA Consonant Chart, these cognates are often described as 'interdental' (see the PVM Chart in Table 9.1 above) although in connected speech the tongue only protrudes between the teeth sometimes. It is helpful, though, to start with frankly interdental placement.

Phonetic Placement: First, demonstrate placing the tongue between the upper and lower front teeth. Next, place a feather or small piece of paper in front of the student's mouth, and instruct the student to blow air through the teeth to make the object move.

Shaping /f/ to [θ]: Begin by modelling the difference in places of production for labiodental /f/, and /θ/. Next, while the student says [f], with a gloved finger or a tongue depressor move their tongue to lie between the upper and lower front teeth, one of the positions for /θ/, and have them gently breathe out.

Targeting /s/

The human articulatory system is flexible, allowing speakers to produce a 'good ess' either with alveolar placement with the tongue tip up behind the upper front teeth or down behind the lower front teeth. Both are acceptable. A little experimentation usually is sufficient to determine which variety a student may prefer. If, after trial therapy, it turns out you may have picked the wrong placement for /s/ for a particular student, consider trying the other place of articulation. Here are examples of differing complexity for the techniques.

Phonetic Placement (tongue tip up or down): With a gloved hand, carefully place a Q-Tip (cotton bud), a piece of candy (a Lifesaver often works well) behind the student's front teeth (upper teeth or lower teeth, depending on the /s/ placement you are teaching). Ask the student to hold the object in place with their tongue tip. Next, carefully remove the object and ask the student to breathe out.

Phonetic Placement (tongue tip up or down): Place a tongue depressor or the dull end of a pencil (not the pointed end!) against the lower edges of the student's upper teeth, for a 'tongue-up ess' or the upper edges of the student's lower teeth for a 'tongue-down ess'. Next, ask the student to place their tongue on 'the shelf' (for tongue-up) or under 'the shelf' (for tongue-down). Raise or lower 'the shelf' to place the student's tongue tip in the position for /s/ and ask them to breath out through their mouth.

Shaping /ʃ/ to [s]: Ask the student to say a long [ʃ]. Then, while the student still is saying /ʃ/, ask them to smile, which often results in something amazingly ess-like. The change from /ʃ/ to [s] occurs because the smile spreads the lips (as occurs in /s/) while pulling the tongue forward (as also occurs in /s/). Which goes to show, sometimes all you need to succeed is a smile.

Shaping 'lateral-ess' to [s]: The 2015 'ex-tIPA symbols for disordered speech' (Ball et al., 2018) phonetic symbols for 'lateral ess' and 'lateral-zee' (zed) are /ls/ and /lz/ respectively. Begin by helping the student contrast the difference between lateral airflow (air over the sides of the tongue) and central air flow (air over the centre of the tongue). A traditional means to teach this contrast is to have the student practice central air flow by gently blowing through a straw placed over the centre of the tongue, and then contrast this with lateral airflow when the student gently blows through straws placed at the side of the mouth, one at each corner. Placing a paper flower or other light object in front of the straw may help the student see the results when blowing through the straw. Next, remove the straw and ask the student to keep the tongue in the same position and to breathe in. When the straw is placed over the centre of the tongue, the student should feel cool air over the centre of the tongue when they inhale air. Similarly, when the straws are placed in the corners of the mouth, the student should feel cool air over the sides (lateral) part of the tongue when inhaling. To heighten the lesson, ask the student to suck on a mint Lifesaver before the straw work, which intensifies the cool feeling when breathing in. Lastly, have the student practice moving the paper flower when placed in front of the mouth, resulting in central air flow.

Targeting /ʃ/

This postalveolar fricative is made behind the alveolar ridge. The tongue blade is raised, and the lips are rounded.

Phonetic Placement: To begin, have the student sit before a mirror and ask them to open their mouth and stick out their tongue. With a tongue depressor or another appropriate and clean object, touch the student's tongue just behind the tongue tip. Next, ask the student to move the place you touched just behind the 'bumpy part' on the roof of the mouth. Ask the student to lower the tongue slightly, pucker the lips slightly, and to gently breathe out through the mouth.

Shaping /s/ to [ʃ]: Ask the student to say /s/, to pucker the lips slightly, and to draw the tongue back a little.

Targeting /tʃ/

In phonology, an affricate comprises an intimate combination of a stop with a fricative of the same position or in a very close position. For the English affricates / tʃ dʒ/, alveolar /t d/ and postalveolar /ʃ ʒ/ have adjacent places of articulation. The place of articulation for /tʃ dʒ/ is just behind the alveolar ridge with the lips slightly puckered.

Phonetic Placement: Ask the student to pucker the lips slightly and to make the tongue tip touch 'the bump' behind the two upper front teeth. Next, ask the student to make the sneezing sound ('choo!') while keeping the lips slightly puckered and the tongue tip on the alveolar ridge. If the result is [ts], instruct the student to move the tongue tip back slightly while maintaining contact with the roof of the mouth.

Shaping /ʃ/ to [tʃ]: Ask the student to say a quick /ʃ/ with the tongue tip touching 'the bump' behind the upper front teeth, resulting in [tʃ].

Targeting Voicing

The voiced fricatives covered here are /v ð z ʒ/ but not /h/ and the voiced affricate. /dʒ/. Three methods to teach voicing are covered below.

First technique Focus a student's awareness of voicing by having them listen to and identify the difference between a voiceless and voiced /ɑ/ or between /h/ and /ɑ/. To illustrate, ask the student to say /ɑ/ 'with the motor on' and then, keeping the mouth in the same position, say it 'with the motor off', (without voicing), focusing their attention on the difference between the two pronunciations. Alternatively, you can achieve the same awareness by asking the student to listen to the difference between /h/ (voiceless, 'motor off') and /ɑ/ (voiced, 'motor on').

Second technique Ask a student to place their hands over their ears and to hum, which heightens the sensation of vocal cord vibration. You might also contrast the hum with a voiceless sound, such as /h/ or a voiceless fricative.

Third technique Practice the voicing of fricatives by including activities in which a student covers their ears while saying voiced and voiceless fricatives.

Saying 'ARR' Like a Pirate

Dr. Peter Flipsen Jr. was introduced at the top of Q8 where he talked about measuring the severity of speech sound disorders. He is a widely published Professor of Speech-Language Pathology in the School of Communication Sciences and Disorders at Pacific University, in Forest Grove, Oregon. His book *Remediation of /r/ for SLPs* (Flipsen Jr, 2022) was the inspiration for the next question.

Q37.   Peter Flipsen Jr.: R-Trouble

Probably, most SLPs/SLTs agree that treating difficulties with 'R' can be more problematic than targeting other consonants. From deciding whether to transcribe it as voiced trilled alveolar approximant /r/, or as a voiced alveolar approximant /ɹ/ (International Phonetic Association, 2005), or a palatal, postalveolar, or alveolar approximant /ɹ/ (Shriberg, Kent et al., 2018), to the experience of treating a child with a persistent R-error that does not want to budge, this consonant can often be bothersome. But why? Why is it so difficult for some children and adults to talk like a pirate?

A37.   Peter Flipsen Jr.: Why Is /ɹ/ Such a Challenge for SLPs/SLTs?

Let me start by saying that my answer here relates only to the voiced, palatal alveolar or postalveolar approximant /ɹ/. Any consideration of the trill (/r/) which is seen in some English dialects like Scottish English, or in Spanish I will leave to others who are more qualified. I really haven't looked at it much at all.

That said, many clinicians report difficulties remediating /ɹ/. This concern is not new. As early as 1882 Potter called it '… the most difficult sound …' (p. 34). It appears to me that there are many interrelated factors involved. These factors don't all apply in each case, but each situation likely involves several of these factors operating at the same time. For ease of discussion, we can group the factors in three categories: those related to /ɹ/ itself, those related to us as clinicians, and those related to the therapy process.

A Sound Unlike Most Others

As to /ɹ/ itself, Potter (1882) wasn't kidding when he said that /ɹ/ is difficult. Unlike most speech sounds which require one or possibly two constrictions to be made in the vocal tract, /ɹ/ actually requires three (lips, palate, pharynx). Thus, a great deal more coordination is required among the articulators for /ɹ/ than is required for most other speech sounds. And as if that weren't bad enough, two different parts of the tongue (blade/dorsum and root) must be moved in different ways at the same time. In 2007, Gick and colleagues (Gick et al., 2007) argued that the common /w/ for /ɹ/ substitution pattern may represent an attempt to replace those two independent movements of the tongue with one (i.e., just moving the tongue dorsum toward the velum). Of course, /w/ does have two places of articulation (lips and velum) but only one general movement of the tongue is required, and many speakers may be so focused on their lips that they don't realize their tongue is doing anything.

A second reason for the difficulty of /ɹ/ production is that this is a sound that doesn't involve much physical contact between the tongue and the rest of the vocal tract. Hence, many texts refer to /ɹ/ as an 'approximant', or a sound which only involves a general narrowing of the vocal tract (i.e., it approximates a constriction). Some recent studies (e.g., Gick et al., 2013) have suggested that as with most speech sounds during production of /ɹ/ there is some amount of bracing of the tongue against the back teeth. However, I would argue that the available feedback is likely minimal and may vary depending on the specific way in which /ɹ/ is produced (more on that coming up next). The net result is that during production attempts most speakers receive only minimal tactile feedback which limits our ability to self-monitor our ongoing productions.

A third reason that /ɹ/ is difficult to produce is that it can be produced multiple different ways and each of them results in the same acoustically normal /ɹ/ (i.e., they all sound like equally valid productions). Several studies (e.g., Delattre & Freeman, 1968; Hagiwara, 1995; Westbury et al., 1998) have suggested multiple tongue shapes for /ɹ/. It is not clear whether they all have clinical relevance but at least two of these (retroflex, bunched) likely do. Both may need to be tried by the clinician.

Four Clinician Related Factors

Which brings us to the clinician related factors. I apologize in advance if this comes across as clinician bashing, but we must acknowledge that sometimes we seem to get in our own way. This is likely not any different for /ɹ/. The first of these reasons follows from the last point. There is more than one way to make it, but there is a tendency to fixate on one of them, the retroflex shape. Although good data are lacking, a 'bunched' tongue shape may be used at least as often as a retroflex shape, and both should at least be tried.

A second clinician-related reason for difficulty with /ɹ/ is that we have long tended to ignore the pharyngeal constriction. When we give our clients feedback about how to change their productions the focus has been almost exclusively on what to do with the body and front portion of the tongue (with an occasional mention of the lips). Only rarely does feedback or instruction involve doing *anything* with the **tongue root** or the **pharynx**. In fairness, until recently studies of normal /ɹ/ production have largely ignored the pharynx, so most clinicians know little about what should be happening there. Even if we did, none of us really knows what sort of feedback to provide in that area to help our clients change what they are doing.

The recent application of ultrasound to correcting /ɹ/ errors is beginning to offer some insights.

A third reason for difficulty with remediating /ɹ/ that relates to the clinician is an old concept known as categorical perception. As competent users of the language, there is a strong natural tendency to want to put the speaker's production into a specific phonemic category in the language. In the case of American English /ɹ/ when judging their productions, we want to call it either /ɹ/ or /w/. Unfortunately, many of our clients (particularly those above age 7 years) produce neither. They produce a distortion that is part-way in between. Speakers are quite capable an almost infinite number of versions of /ɹ/ that are at some point along the continuum between /ɹ/ and /w/. With distorted productions, many of us struggle with how to provide appropriate feedback. Do we say it was correct? Incorrect? A bigger program may be that we may not be very consistent with our judgements about those distortions leading to equally inconsistent feedback. Dare I say we need to consider acoustic analysis more seriously?

A fourth clinician-related reason is that we have been ignoring speech perception. This remains a challenge for much of speech sound intervention. I am one who, like a few others including Barbara Hodson and Susan Rvachew (A18), has long felt that speech perception generally has been ignored at our peril. There has long been a tendency to jump right into production training. It is certainly true that general problems of speech perception are rarely an issue for children with speech sound disorders, but there is mounting evidence that some of the production errors that some children produce may be, at least in part, the result of an underlying perceptual problem. Perhaps there are having difficulty hearing the difference between what they say and what they are supposed to say for that specific sound. Given the limited intra-oral feedback discussed above, it should not be a surprise that some of the /ɹ/ errors we are treating as production errors may need to also be treated concurrently as problems based in perception.

Intervention-Related Factors

Finally, there are two therapy-related factors. The first of these is a problem that is not limited to /ɹ/, but when most clinicians – in the US, at any rate – begin working on this sound at age 7–8 years, the error has been practiced many, many times. That production form has become habitual because of that practice frequency. It has also been effectively reinforced many, many times by the rest of the world because distortions don't compromise intelligibility. The intended message is being understood. The result is a highly ingrained habit which can be difficult to break. Trying to do so with only a brief therapy period each week may be a fool's errand.

The Motor Theory of Speech Perception

I've left the one remaining reason to the end because it is based largely on some theoretical speculation on my part. I call this reason the problem of *demographic dynamics*. Most SLPs/SLTs are female. And /ɹ/ errors are more common in males (incidentally, /s/ errors are more common in females). Why does that matter? It requires invoking something called the *motor theory of speech perception*. This theory holds that when listeners hear others speaking, they are (on some deep level) imagining a set of vocal tract shapes that produced the sounds they are hearing. If this is true, during speech acquisition children are basing their production attempts on what they think the vocal tract shape is supposed to look and feel like. But you may recall from anatomy class that male and female vocal tracts are organized a bit differently. For females, the length of the oral cavity is about the same length as the height of the pharyngeal cavity. But for males, the two cavities are different sizes: the oral cavity is shorter than the pharyngeal cavity is tall. Hagiwara (1995) has suggested that this means that males and females must create both the oral and pharyngeal constrictions for /ɹ/ at relatively different locations to achieve the same acoustic output. So, it is possible that some male clients may struggle to reproduce a good /ɹ/ if their only models in therapy are from females. The model they are hearing reflects a vocal tract that is organized differently from the one they are using to try to generate the sound. At the very least, it suggests that if we have a client whose problem with /ɹ/ is partly one of perception, it may be crucial to provide a variety of different speaker models (i.e., including both males and females) to improve both perception and production.

So, are you surprised now that /ɹ/ is so difficult to remediate? I'm not. I'm surprised it gets sorted out as often as it does.

Orofacial Clefting

Orofacial clefts are commonly associated with SSD (Nachmani et al., 2022). Ideally, children with clefts are managed by a multidisciplinary team (Golding-Kushner A17), whether they have unilateral or bilateral cleft palate, unilateral or bilateral cleft lip, overt or occult submucous cleft palate, or craniofacial anomalies affecting other facial and jaw structures. Individualized care, in the industrialized world, may include early and often ongoing surgeries to correct or modify structural anomalies, with professional services from clinical audiologists, general and paediatric dentists and orthodontists, psychologists, SLPs/SLTs, and other health providers. With appropriate surgical and other intervention by the cleft lip and palate team, intelligible and acceptable speech is the outcome for most, but not all children with craniofacial anomalies (Alighieri et al., 2021; Sand et al., 2022).

In comparison with the non-cleft population, children with cleft lip and palate frequently have atypical nasal airflow while speaking, including nasal emission ('nasal air escape') and/or nasal turbulence; compensatory (active) and/or obligatory (passive) speech characteristics (Nachmani et al., 2022; Ruscello A38); delay in the transition from babbling to the onset of first words; excessive nasal resonance (hypernasality); slower early vocabulary acquisition; smaller consonant inventories particularly involving missing or aberrant high-pressure consonants; and voice disorder often characterized by distinctive nasal resonance.

The children's limited intraoral pressure may result in abnormal nasal airflow and nasalized voiced stops and fricatives (Sweeney & Sell, 2008). Active, **compensatory speech characteristics** occur when certain articulatory gestures replace target consonants, i.e., glottal replacement, atypical backing, and velar distortions (Harding & Grunwell, 1998). Passive, **obligatory speech characteristics** involve audible nasal (air) emission in the production of some or all high-pressure consonants – the stops, fricatives, and affricates (Harding & Grunwell, 1998).

There are frequent comments in the literature about generalist SLPs'/SLTs' lack of competence, know-how and agency in assessing and treating children with clefts and counselling their families. For example, Alighieri et al. (2021) write:

The community SLPs are lacking professional confidence when treating children with a CP±L. They put themselves in a subordinate position towards the cleft team SLPs and expect the latter to provide ready-made answers to problems and questions. This expectation can perhaps be explained by their fear of making mistakes during therapy preventing treatment progress. If they handle in accordance with the experts' advice, they cannot blame themselves in cases where no treatment progress is seen. Educational programmes need to pay more attention to gaining professional confidence (in the search for the most optimal treatment approach for each individual patient) rather than merely focusing on competency-based learning tools.

Their article was entitled *From excitement to self-doubt and insecurity: Speech–language pathologists' perceptions and experiences when treating children with a cleft palate* and it probably did little to lift the readership's morale. Luckily, in A38 Dennis Ruscello shares practical, straightforward treatment strategies, in company with the why and how of choosing strategies that best suit individual clients.

Dr. Dennis Ruscello is Professor Emeritus of Communication Sciences and Disorders at West Virginia University. His major interests are the assessment and treatment of children with SSD, particularly those with structurally based deficits. His research and teaching have focused primarily on this population. He holds the Certificate of Clinical Competence in Speech-Language Pathology and was awarded the Honors of ASHA. Dr. Ruscello's recent publications deal with the assessment and treatment of children with craniofacial anomalies (Ruscello, 2017; Vallino et al., 2019).

Q38. Dennis M. Ruscello: Compensatory Errors and Cleft Lip and Palate

Many generalists in paediatric SLPs/SLTs rarely encounter children with speech and resonance disorders secondary to cleft palate, craniofacial anomalies, and velopharyngeal dysfunction (VPD). Terms like pressure-sensitive consonants, nasal rustle (turbulence), compensatory articulations, prosthetic management, phoneme-specific nasal emission, glottal substitutions, and the like may be only dimly understood. Can you share with the non-specialist reader the practical techniques they should know about when approaching this population, and the therapy tools they should have to hand, and dispel some of the myths surrounding VPD and its management?

A38. Dennis Ruscello: Treating Compensatory Errors in the Cleft Palate Population: Some Treatment Techniques

Before discussing treatment, it is important to emphasise several points. First, these children have structurally based problems that can manifest in different resonance and speech sound disorders. Practitioners must be cognizant of this because it will dictate the type of treatment. Second, many SLPs/SLTs see such clients infrequently and have limited content knowledge and clinical skills. Third, these children exhibit heterogeneous speech production errors that include developmental, obligatory, and/or compensatory error types.

Developmental variation occurs in the speech of children acquiring the sound system(s) of their language(s) (Bernthal et al., 2022; Cronin et al., 2020). These errors are unrelated to structural problems and may be outgrown or persist requiring treatment. **Obligatory errors** result from structural differences, which negatively influence the physiologic movement(s) requisite to correct sound produc-

tion (Golding-Kushner, 2001; Peterson-Falzone et al., 2009). Generally, obligatory errors are identified as sound distortions and typically resolve spontaneously once structural defects are corrected (Kummer et al., 1989; Moller, 1994). Finally, **compensatory errors** are learned and involve substitution of individual sounds or sound classes and found in children with VPD (Golding-Kushner, 2001; Kummer, 2020a). They include glottal stops, nasal snorts, velar fricatives, pharyngeal fricatives, pharyngeal stops, and pharyngeal affricatives. Identification and classification of the different errors is accomplished through comprehensive phonetic/phonemic assessment (Cronin et al., 2020; Vallino et al., 2019).

Hardin-Jones and Jones (2005) examined the incidence of resonance and compensatory errors in children with repaired cleft palate. Of 212 preschool children, 78 participants (approximately 37%) had moderate to severe hypernasality, while fifty-three (25% of the group) had compensatory errors. Collectively, studies conducted to date show similar findings with glottal and pharyngeal articulations identified in 20% to 25% of children studied (Hardin-Jones et al., 2020).

Treatment Techniques for Compensatory Errors

The treatment of hypernasality generally requires surgical or prosthetic intervention, while treatment of compensatory errors is the responsibility of the SLP/SLT. Treatment is important since research shows elimination of compensatory errors positively influences velopharyngeal movement (Henningsson & Isberg, 1986; Peterson-Falzone et al., 2009). Treatment techniques for compensatory errors have been described in various publications (e.g., Golding-Kushner, 2001; Kummer, 2020b; Peterson-Falzone et al., 2009, 2017; Ruscello, 2008a; Trost-Cardamone, 2009; Zajac & Vallino-Napoli, 2017). The techniques are based primarily on judicious clinical decision-making and a modicum of treatment efficacy research (Baker & McLeod, 2004). Comprehensive reviews by

Bessell et al. (2013) and Peterson-Falzone et al. (2009) support the efficacy of treatment with both a traditional motor-phonetic approach and a linguistic-phonological (phonemic) approach. A more recent study (Alighieri et al., 2020) also found support for both, but an advantage for a phonemically motivated treatment using a modified *Metaphon* approach (Dean et al., 1995; and see Chapter 5).

A limitation with all treatment studies is that they provide scant information on techniques for modifying compensatory errors. I use the following treatment techniques differentially in a motor-phonetic paradigm. Each has a specific purpose and rationale, tied to the research literature. They comprise acquisition techniques directed to attaining correct conscious production of a target sound; automatization techniques aimed at establishing correct spontaneous production; and techniques that may be used in both phases via a motor learning model (Mass et al., 2008; Ruscello, 2017; Ruscello & Vallino, 2014). When picture stimuli are used, so that there is no requirement for the client to read, the acquisition techniques are suitable for pre-schoolers as young as 3;0. The automatization tasks are appropriate for school-aged children from 6;0 and beyond. Self-monitoring incorporates acquisition and automatization activities for children aged 3;0 upwards.

Acquisition

Imitative Modelling

Imitative modelling is important in early treatment. Stimuli should be presented with normal loudness because excessive loudness or overstimulation may cause children to produce their practice-stimuli loudly too, thereby distorting target sounds. More particularly, this is best avoided, since children with cleft palate are at risk for hyperfunctional voice disorders (Peterson-Falzone et al., 2017), and undue loudness may mask the SLP's/SLT's assessment of target productions.

Non-Speech Sound Stimulation and Nonce Words

Producing a target 'pressure sound' (obstruent) can be very difficult for some children because they revert to their customary substitution during sound stimulation trials or, if they are backing, produce another posterior-based articulation (i.e., a non-target glottal or velar production). Accordingly, it is helpful to begin with the sound in *isolation* for target fricatives. Stops and affricates are elicited in CV contexts, since they are produced with vocal tract closure prior to adjacent vowel release. I have also found it useful to incorporate nonspeech sounds, to reduce error sound interference (Ruscello, 2008a). For example, I may ask children to whistle with their tongue for /s/, which of course they say they cannot! I then instruct regarding tongue placement and lip position. I follow this with a whistle sound made with the tongue tip. Sometimes, the child's imitative token is judged to be /s/ in isolation. The child receives positive verbal feedback (Kim et al., 2012), continuing to practice until the target is elicited with the verbal cue alone ('Make the whistle sound'.). After /s/ production has stabilized through practice, I inform the child that the 'whistle sound' is really /s/.

Another approach to reducing contextual interference is the use of nonce words. A nonce item is a sound combination that is not a free morpheme, with or without a permissible phonological structure. It is generally paired with a picture or line drawing, for example, ⊕, to assign meaning to it. 'Billy, this is a sud'. (the clinician proffers ⊕) 'Say sud'. In this way the child rehearses a 'word unit', absent from her or his lexicon to reduce error interference.

Nasal Occlusion

During practice trials at the isolation, nonce, and word levels, I have children gently pinch their nostrils with their thumb and forefinger (Golding-Kushner, 2001). I emulate this while producing the stimuli, to cue them. Since the children have obligatory VPD, nasal occlusion helps them generate and sustain adequate oral air pressure for obstruent target production. It also provides auditory and tactile feedback for the child (Kummer, 2020b).

Imagery

Imagery helps some children distinguish between target sound(s) and their substitution error(s). Since many compensatory errors preserve manner of articulation but change place to a more posterior point of articulation (Trost-Cardamone, 2009), a place distinction can be made. For example, if a child substituted glottal [ʔ] or velar [k] or [g], for /t/ and /d/, a place-based distinction between 'throaties' and 'tippies' respectively can be made (Klein, 1996). Introductory identification trials contrast glottal or velar versus alveolar target(s), with the child required to make the appropriate auditory distinction. Once able to make the distinction, children are queried periodically during practice trials. 'Billy, did you make the tippy sound or the throaty sound?'

Automatization

The term 'automatization' refers to the establishment of an automatic process. A process that is 'automatic' (e.g., an established error production) is typified by a high level of speed and accuracy, is performed unconsciously, makes negligible demands on attention, and while it can be changed with considerable effort and practice, is difficult to suppress, or influence.

Speed Drills

Speed drills can assist in the automatization of a target sound (Ruscello, 1993). The child practises the target in context, while the SLP/SLT manipulates speaking rate to transition to automatic production. The goal is to increase rate of production, while maintaining response accuracy. Speed drills consist of practice sets with a gradual reduction in the time necessary to produce a practice set. For instance, the clinician may present 20 phrases, to be read or 'picture-read' citation-naming style. The child must read (or 'read') aloud the phrases using the target sound correctly. The time needed to produce the stimuli and the accuracy-rate are recorded and shared with the child. The child is then instructed to read the phrases taking less time, while maintaining the accuracy-rate. Time and accuracy-rate are taken (measured), and the results discussed with the client. Speed drills may also be performed with words or sentences, at the therapist's discretion. Variations include practice lists that contain the target only (Blocked Practice) or interspersed with non-target items (Random Practice) (Preston et al., 2019). Speed drills can be spread throughout treatment, randomly, as supplementary activities. If the child's performance deteriorates, the SLP/SLT should withdraw the drills, re-introducing when the child appears ready (applying clinical judgement).

Auditory Masking

Manning et al. (1976) developed auditory masking for the purpose of *assessing* the automatic use of a target sound. The authors reasoned that a client relies on auditory information during the automatization phase of treatment and limiting auditory information provides an indication of automatic use. The following is a potentially effective treatment variation I employ. The child reads or picture-reads a list of words, phrases or sentences containing the target, and an accuracy rate is established. The child is then instructed that s/he will read the material again, wearing a headset. Masking noise from an audiometer is digitized and the signal played through a headset, while the child produces the practice material. Comparative accuracy rates between the masking and non-masking conditions are then reviewed with the child.

Acquisition/Automatization

Self-Monitoring

Self-monitoring tasks are used in several treatments (Bernthal et al., 2022; Shriberg & Kwiatkowski, 1987), and the author has found that self-monitoring can be useful for children with cleft palate. Tasks include the client:

1. monitoring correct and incorrect productions of targets in production practice,
2. identifying, discriminating, and/or monitoring the production of another speaker such as the clinician or caregiver, and
3. assessing the accuracy of her or his productions in more spontaneous treatment activities, such as conversation.

My preference is to employ self-monitoring in conversation or during other automatization tasks. Initially, a topic is introduced, and the child is instructed that 'one idea at a time' will be discussed and to be sure to make the 'new sound' correctly. The use of limited spontaneous speech is intended to lessen potential frustration for the child without diminishing spontaneity. When the conversation ends, the child is queried regarding a word or words containing the target sound. The child identifies words containing the target sound, indicating the accuracy of those productions. As the child's self-monitoring skills improve, conversations grow longer, and the dialogues approximate actual interchanges.

Motor Learning Model

Preston and his associates (Preston et al., 2019) have developed an instructional program based on motor learning principles known as Speech Motor Chaining. It allows the SLP/SLT to work through the stages of acquisition and automatization, while controlling the instructional variables of stimuli presentation and difficulty, types and rates of feedback, treatment dose and performance evaluation. It provides an excellent structure for phonetic treatment that is based on both clinical and research evidence.

Caregiver Involvement

Ideally, caregivers are involved in their children's treatment, but the type of involvement varies as most SLPs/SLTs can attest (Ruscello, 2008a). I meet with the caregiver, discuss the child's speech and any coexisting communication disorders, and the proposed treatment, answering their questions. Stressing the importance of careful monitoring of hearing acuity, considering the high incidence of conductive hearing loss in this population (Vallino et al., 2019), I ask caregivers to provide verbal feedback to the child regarding speech progress, and to project a positive attitude to treatment. If a caregiver is willing to take a more active role, I involve the person in the treatment process, encouraging observation of some treatment sessions,

and providing home activities that offer additional opportunities for practice. A brief written contract that succinctly describes the parent's (or parents') responsibilities is prepared. Crucially, the actively involved caregiver must first be trained to discriminate between correct and incorrect responses, because the child must receive reliable feedback. I recommend that the caregiver carry out short practice sessions of approximately 8 to 10 minutes daily, recording the accuracy of the child's responses. These data are discussed each week with the caregiver and modifications to practice sessions made.

Nonspeech Oral Motor Treatment (NS-OME)

One treatment technique not recommended is nonspeech oral motor exercises (Ruscello, 2008b; Ruscello & Vallino, 2020). The overwhelming majority of children with cleft palate and speech disorders in general do not have muscle weakness or muscle tone problems, and even if they did, NS-OME divorced from speech production activities would not be appropriate (Golding-Kushner, 2001; Potter et al., 2019). Nonspeech oral motor treatment techniques, such as blowing, sucking or specific resistance exercises to 'improve' lip, tongue, or palate strength are not indicated and lack an evidence base (McCauley et al., 2009). Moreover, studies designed to improve velopharyngeal function for speech through nonspeech oral motor treatment have largely been unsuccessful (Ruscello, 2008b; Tomes et al., 2004). The clinician (and parent) should avoid non-speech oral motor exercises.

Summary

The techniques described herein are used by the author in the treatment of children who present with compensatory errors. Most are based on research, but readers must be mindful that large-scale RCT treatment studies have not occurred to validate the treatment efficacy of each. Thus, it is important for the SLP/SLT to measure the client's performance, so that the efficacy of the techniques can be assessed empirically, and necessary changes made.

Targeting Speech Perception

There is ample evidence to show that a large component of the SSD population has more difficulty with speech perception than their peers with age-typical speech (Rvachew A18). In an individual client, it is possible that one or more errors are due to the child's inability to hear the difference between their usual production and the target correctly produced, but this difficulty may not be readily apparent.

Locke's (1980) procedure takes the guesswork out of trying to decide whether a child can hear the difference between error and target, at word level, when an adult says them. The form displayed in

Table 9.6a allows testing for two different discrimination errors (or to test and re-test one), and instructions for the task are in Table 9.6b. For a discussion of perceptually based interventions, see Rvachew, A25.

Words and Pictures

Words familiar to children in one linguistic milieu may be unfamiliar in another. For example, the luggage compartment of a car is called a *trunk* in the United States and a *boot* in Australia; a *jersey* or *pullover* in the United Kingdom is called a *sweater* in the

Table 9.6a Locke's speech perception task.

Date:		Date:	
Task 1		**Task 2**	
/ / →/ /		/ / →/ /	
Target / / Error / / Control / /		**Target / / Error / / Control / /**	
Stimulus –Class	**Response**	**Stimulus –Class**	**Response**
1. / / -Control	yes -NO	1. / / -Target	YES -no
2. / /-Error	yes -NO	2. / /-Control	yes -NO
3. / / -Target	YES -no	3. / / -Target	YES -no
4. / / -Target	YES -no	4. / / -Control	yes -NO
5. / / -Error	yes -NO	5. / / -Error	yes -NO
6. / /-Control	yes -NO	6. / /-Error	yes -NO
7. / / -Control	yes -NO	7. / / -Target	YES -no
8. / / -Target	YES -no	8. / / -Error	yes -NO
9. / /-Error	yes -NO	9. / /-Target	YES-no
10. / / -Target	YES -no	10. / / -Control	yes -NO
11. / / -Error	yes -NO	11. / / -Control	yes -NO
12. / / -Control	yes -NO	12. / / -Error	yes -NO
13. / /-Error	yes -NO	13. / / -Target	YES -no
14. / / -Target	YES -no	14. / / -Control	yes -NO
15. / /-Control	yes -NO	15. / / -Error	yes -NO
16. / /-Error	yes -NO	16. / / -Target	YES -no
17. / / -Target	YES -no	17. / /-Error	yes -NO
18. / /-Control	yes -NO	18. / / -Control	yes -NO
Mistakes: Error Control Target		Mistakes: Error Control Target	

Table 9.6b Instructions for Locke's speech perception task.

1. Under 'Task', enter the target word and the substitution. For example, if the child said /fʌm/ for *thumb*, enter thumb→/fʌm/, or /θʌm/→/fʌm/

2. Indicate the target sound in the space marked Target /θ/ in the above example, the substituted sound in the space marked Error /f/ in the above example, and a related sound as a control in the space marked Control. /s/ might be chosen for this example with the word *sum*. So the three contrasting words will be thumb (the target), Fum (the error, represented by an imaginary character) and sum (the control item).

3. In each of the 18 spots under 'Stimulus – Class' fill in the appropriate sounds from #2 above depending on which item is listed. For example if the item says Target, write /θ/, if it says Error write /f/, and if it says Control write /s/. This creates the stimuli for the test. Now familiarise the child with the three pictures and word before proceeding to step 4.

4. To administer the test, *only* show the child the picture of the target (thumb). Ask the speaker to judge whether or not you said the right word. For example:

   1. Is this *fum*?

   2. Is this *sum*?

   3. Is this *thumb*?

   4. Is this *thumb*?

   5. Is this *fum*? ... etc

   If the speaker says 'yes', circle yes next to the item. If the speaker says 'no' circle no. **'YES'** and **'NO'** indicate correct answers; **'yes'** and **'no'** indicate incorrect responses.

5. Count the mistakes 'yes' and 'no' in each category Target, Error, Control.

6. The speaker is said to have a problem with perception if 3 or more mistakes in perception are noted in response to the Error stimuli out of 6 Error stimuli. 3/6 indicates that at least half the child's responses are incorrect indicating that the child may have trouble distinguishing their customary production from the adult target.

7. Repeat the process for each erred sound suspected to have a perceptual basis. The column headed Task 2 can be used to re-test, or to test another error sound.

United States and a *jumper* in Australia and New Zealand; a *pacifier* in the United States is a *dummy* in the United Kingdom, Australia, and New Zealand. Depending on where you are, a *dumpster* is a *skip*, a *lorry* a *truck*, an *elevator* a *lift*, a *queue* is a *line*, a *quay* is a *wharf*, and a *courgette* is a *zucchini*.

Because of these semantic differences, vowel variation between varieties of English, and other difficulties associated with commercially available picture resources (e.g., cost, sharp edges or pointy corners on cards, and poor durability in some instances), clinicians often elect to create 'homemade' materials that are linguistically, developmentally, and culturally suited to their clients.

At www.speech-language-therapy.com readers will find – or judging by the millions of hits received monthly – may *already* have found, free, homemade worksheets. They include worksheets for singleton consonants, consonant clusters, vowels and vowel contrasts, minimal pairs and near minimal pairs,

facilitative contexts and complexity principles, and self-monitoring (the fixed-up-one routine). They can be located by clicking on the RESOURCES tab at the top of every page of the site. Also on the RESOURCES tab are links to Assessment Resources, Forms, Handouts, Slideshows and Word Lists, a Reference list, and a Glossary.

Most of the vocabulary used in these resources represents non-rhotic Australian English pronunciation, and although most of the words and minimal pairs will 'work' in other varieties of English, users may need to discard some. The resources were made using the insert table feature in Microsoft Word and PowerPoint, with original photographs, and royalty-free pictures from the legacy 1998–2014 Microsoft Images collection. Some of the free images are still available and readers can search Bing (https://www.bing.com) for 'free clipart' or go to https://tinyurl.com/bej347x3.

The Word documents were converted into portable document files (pdf) using Adobe software within Office 365 for Mac. Colleagues are free to save them to their own computers and customise them to suit individual clients and service delivery models and share them with clients and colleagues. Copyright information is on the ABOUT tab which is on www.speech-language-therapy.com. The resource pages that attract the most downloads are the consonants, clusters, and vowels, minimal pairs, and the near minimal pairs pages, described and discussed in the next three sections.

Consonants, Clusters and Vowels

There is a page on the site devoted to consonants, consonant clusters, and vowels. The consonant pictures are organized by major class: Obstruents: Stops, Fricative and Affricates; and Sonorants: Nasals, Liquids and Glides. There is a selection of cluster worksheets with consonant clusters SIWI and SFWF, and vowel worksheets. There are also worksheets for working with facilitative contexts such as the aspiration trick for voiceless fricatives and stops, chaining for /k/, /f/, /s/, /n/ and /ɹ/, and additional facilitative contexts for /s/, /tʃ/, /ɹ/ and /l/, and a collection of 'long words' of two syllables of more.

Minimal Pairs

The quest for picture pairs with age-appropriate vocabulary can be disappointing. Many of the published cards and worksheets intended for child speech intervention involve words selected because an artist can represent them pictorially. In fact, it often appears that word-choices may have been *decided* by an artist, a publisher, or by someone minimally acquainted with child phonology. It is rare to encounter materials that take account of the necessary linguistic and developmental criteria. Consequently, clinicians often need to discard minimal word pairs because they are too challenging. For example, picturable word-pairs like *kite-tight*, *coat-tote*, *cart-tart*, *can-tan*, *Ken-ten*, *corn-torn*, *code-toad* are usually unsuitable in the early stages of work on voiceless velar fronting because the assimilatory effects of the alveolars /t, d, n/ will likely lead to productions like [taɪt] for *kite* and [tɛn] for *Ken*.

Velar Consonants

There are few picturable English CVCs for the voiced velar–alveolar opposition SFWF to select from without resorting to abbreviated proper nouns and slang (e.g., *Ed-egg*, *Doug-dud*, *jug-Judd*) and fictional words, such as the names of aliens, monsters, and creatures (e.g., *Zig-Zid*).

The picturable real word pairs are *big-bid*, *bag-bad*, *bug-bud*, *cog-cod*, *beg-bed*, *mug-mud*, *leg-lead*, *hag-had*, *rig-rid*, *dig-did*, *rogue-road*, *sag-sad*, available at www.speech-language-therapy.com/pdf/ mpDvsGsfwf.pdf, and not many more. Of these, *dig-did* probably must be rejected because *did* may feed the tendency for *dig* to be pronounced [dɪd]; *bag-bad*, *hag-had* and *rogue-road* will be unsuitable if clinicians or parents regard *bad*, *hag* and *rogue* as scary, pejorative, or politically incorrect. Some children don't like pictures of *sad* because they makes them feel sad, so *sag-sad* may be unacceptable; and *big-bid*, *cog-cod*, *beg-bed*, *leg-lead*, *hag-had*, *rig-rid*, *dig-did*, *rogue-road* and *sag-sad* are likely to be problematic because *bid*, *did* and *rid* are difficult conceptually, and *cod*, *cog*, *lead* (/lɛd/), *hag* and *rogue* may be unfamiliar to the child. That leaves three potential pairs, which may be enough (Elbert et al., 1991): *bug-bud*, *beg-bed*, and *mug-mud*. A similar process of elimination may be necessary with minimal pairs for the voiced velar – alveolar contrast SIWI (www.speech-language-therapy.com/pdf/ mpDvsGsiwi.pdf). The word pairs are *go-dough*, *gown-down*, *game-dame*, *got-dot*, *gull-dull*, *guy-dye*, *gear-deer*, *ghee-D*, *guide-died*, and SLPs/SLTs will quickly realise that *gig-dig*, *gown-down*, *got-dot*, *guide-died* may promote unwanted assimilation.

Near Minimal Pairs

A minimal pair is formed when two words differ by one sound, as in *tap-tip*, *bed-Ted*, and *limb-lip*. A near minimal pair is formed when adding or removing a sound, as in *tap-trap*, *tip-trip*, *bed-bread*, *Ted-tread*, *limb-limp* and *limb-slim*, changes the structure of the syllable. Near minimal pairs are often used to work on cluster reduction, and by clinicians interested in complexity approaches (e.g., applying markedness theory and the sonority sequencing principle discussed above) and who employ them in the expectation of facilitating widespread generalization.

Long Words

The page entitled *Long words* contains a collection of polysyllabic words that can be used in ReST with children with Childhood Apraxia of Speech: CAS (McCabe A32) for assessment purposes and follow-up probe assessments. The words are *aeroplane, ambulance, animals, banana, broccoli, bulldozer, butterfly, capsicum, computer, crocodile, cucumber, dinosaur, echidna, elephant, hamburger, hospital, kangaroo, koala, medicine, microwave, mosquito, motorbike, octopus, platypus, policeman, potato, pyjamas, rectangle, sausages, spaghetti, stethoscope, tomato, triangle, umbrella, Vegemite, vegetables, zucchini, avocado, caterpillar, cauliflower, escalator, helicopter, Pinocchio, rhinoceros, television, thermometer, vacuum cleaner, washing machine, watermelon*, and *hippopotamus*.

They are available is several formats. Each one has the words captioned orthographically.

- Version 1 (https://www.speech-language-therapy.com/images/ReSTpsw1.pdf) has the words transcribed in Mitchell and Delbridge (1965) vowel phonetic symbols for Australian English.
- Version 2 (https://www.speech-language-therapy.com/images/ReSTpsw2.pdf) has no phonetic symbols so that speakers of other English varieties can add their own.
- Version 3 (https://www.speech-language-therapy.com/images/ReSTpsw3.pdf) also has Mitchell and Delbridge vowels, with spaces under each word to transcribe the client's production.
- Version 4 (https://www.speech-language-therapy.com/images/ReSTpsw4.pdf) has Harrington et al. (1997) vowel symbols and spaces to record the client's production, and a Record Form with the same symbols (https://www.speech-language-therapy.com/images/ReSTpolysyllabicwordsrecordform.pdf).

The Long words page also contains 15 collections of polysyllables, for example https://www.speech-language-therapy.com/pdf/poly10.pdf; iambic words, https://www.speech-language-therapy.com/images/

poly15_compressed.pdf, four sets of trochaic words, e.g., http://speech-language-therapy.com/pdf/metre/trochees1.pdf; two sets of words with /ə/ SFWF http://speech-language-therapy.com/pdf/vowels-schwa_WF1.pdf reflecting non-rhotic English production; five worksheets with two-element and three-element clusters SIWI and low sonority differences e.g., https://www.speech-language-therapy.com/pdf/clpoly2.pdf; two sets with Long words starting with /pl/, /pɹ/, /tɹ/, /kl/, /kɹ/, /tw/, and /kw/SFWF; e.g., https://www.speech-language-therapy.com/pdf/clpoly6.pdf; and one set of polysyllabic words with adjuncts SIWI: https://www.speech-language-therapy.com/pdf/clpoly8.pdf.

Alliterative Stories and Activities

Frustrated in 2013 by the dearth of therapy materials for 'experimenting with' and developing a feel for complexity approaches to intervention, with the help of my colleague Helen Rippon a UK-based SLT and Illustrator, I wrote a resource pack for Black Sheep Press entitled: *Consonant Clusters: Alliterative Stories and Activities for Phonological Intervention* (PW12).

Sample pages from PW12 are in Figures 9.1, 9.2, 9.3, 9.4 and 9.5. The PW12 pack (Bowen & Rippon, 2013) contains an explanations of the theoretical background for the materials; information about target selection; homework guidelines for families; a reference list; a *Cluster Screener: Monosyllabic-Word Imitation Task*; and illustrated activities for the more marked, or more complex clusters: namely, /spɹ/, /stɹ/, /skɹ/, /spl/ and /skw/, and /sm/, /sn/, /fl/, /fɹ/, /θɹ/, /sl/, /ʃɹ/, /bl/, /bɹ/, /dɹ/, /gl/, /gɹ/ and /sw/ – eighteen in all. There are five pages for each cluster.

1. A Story or Verse

First, there is an illustrated alliterative story, for example, Grass Karting displayed in Figure 9.1, which has /sl/ 21 times. It is suggested that when a new target is introduced the clinician starts by reading the story or verse to the child, preferably in a parent's presence. Then, the clinician talks about the story or verse, weaving in additional repetitious input, and involving parent and child, fuelling their interest and creativity, triggering language play (Crystal, 1996; Read et al., 2018).

/sl/

Grass Karting

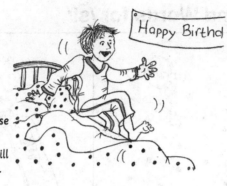

Time seemed to pass very slowly for Ike
while he waited for his ninth birthday.
Turning nine was important to him because
at that age he would be old enough to go
grass karting. Grass karts are off-road thrill
machines with four-wheel steering, shock-
absorbing pump-up tyres, and friction
brakes. In bed at night, before he went to sleep, Ike imagined what it would be like to sling
on a long-sleeved grass karting jacket, slide into the driver's seat of one of those karts and
slowly gather speed as his kart slammed its way downhill through the short grass that
covered the long, gradual slope. He imagined himself avoiding slippery moss and slimy mud
patches and turning the wheel slightly in order to slosh through a puddle, slicing through
piles of white sand and sliding slickly to a standstill at the end of the run. But Ike had to
wait.

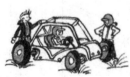

Finally the big day came. On his ninth birthday Ike and two
of his friends went grass karting. It was the best fun! They slid
and sliced their way down the slippery surface of the sloping
run, coming to a slick standstill at the bottom. There they
attached their karts to a mechanical lift and were pulled slowly
back up to the top in grand style, ready to zoom down the
inviting slope again.

Figure 9.1 Alliterative story for /sl/

2. **Pictures and words**

There are six pictures and words for each
cluster. For example, sleep, sleeve, slope, slip,
slime, slow for /sl/, (Figure 9.2). They are used
for input activities such as listening and judgement of correctness, and output activities
including production practice.

3. **Talk about**

Next, there is a Talk About picture, for
example, A Slippery Slope for /sl/ (Figure 9.3)
with a suggested 'script' for guidance for clinicians and for parents who do not find it easy, or
who do not wish to extemporise. Just as an aside,
sometimes parents are given tasks to perform that

Pictures and Words for /sl/

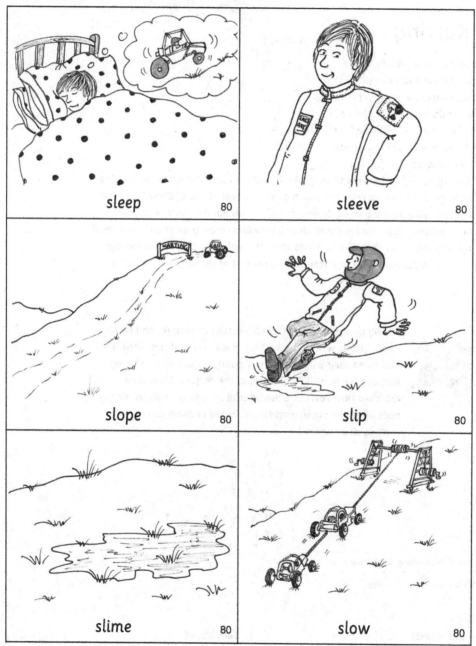

sleep 80

sleeve 80

slope 80

slip 80

slime 80

slow 80

Figure 9.2 Pictures and words for /sl/

/sl/ Talk about the picture using the following text as a guide.
The aim is for the child to hear (but not say) the /sl/ words many times.

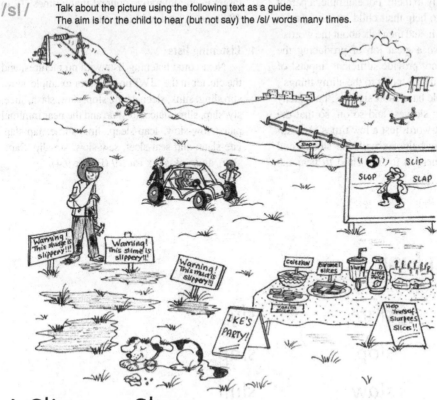

A Slippery Slope

This sleepy dog is called Slim. He looks sleepy, but he doesn't look very slim, does he?

A grass karter has hurt his arm and it is in a sling. He can't manage the slippery slope with his arm in a sling, so he is just looking sadly at the sludge and slime in the muddy spot. What do these warning signs say? 'This sludge is slippery!' 'This slime is slippery!' 'This mud is slippery!'

On the slate it says, 'Ike's party' and here are Ike and his two friends at the bottom of the slippery slope. There is a Slip! Slop! Slap! poster to remind everyone about slipping on long-sleeved clothes, slopping on sunscreen and slapping on hats, and a small sign pointing to the slow lift on the slope. There are lots of sl-things on Ike's party table: slaw, slices and Slurpees™. But what's this? It's lime juice. Maybe it is supposed to be slime juice to go with all the other sl-things. Can you think of a good recipe for slime juice, full of slimy things? We could look in The Slimy Book for ideas.

Figure 9.3 'Talk About' picture for /sl/ with a 'script' for guidance

do not come easily to them. For example, a parent might be asked to help their child 'make a poster with sl-words on it, and then talk about the words'. They might make a great job of producing the poster, but then not provide sufficient 'inputs' of the words, resorting to 'point to the slimy things', 'how many people have short sleeves', how many people have long sleeves' and so on, so that the child hears the sl-words just a few times. A script for guidance may help. As with the stories and verses the idea here is for the child to hear the target in an alliterative context many times (12 to 18 times, at least, within a minute).

4. **Listening lists**

Next come listening lists with no pictures, and the cluster in the SIWI position, for example, slow, slip sling, slink, sleep, slam, slop, slaw, slash, slice, sly, slap, slim, slate and slide and the near minimal pairs: low-slow, leap-sleep, lime-slime, lap-slap, late-slate; and seat-sleet, sew-slow, sip-slip, Sam-slam, and sink-slink for /sl/ (Figure 9.4).

/sl/

Listening List

slow	slam	sly
slip	slop	slap
sling	slaw	slim
slink	slash	slate
sleep	slice	slide

Near Minimal Pairs

low - slow	seat - sleet
leap - sleep	sew - slow
lime - slime	sip - slip
lap - slap	Sam - slam
late - slate	sink - slink

Figure 9.4 Listening list and near minimal pairs for /sl/

5. **Word pairs**

Finally, there are pictured word-pairs (e.g., low-slow, leap-sleep and lime-slime for /sl/) (Figure 9.5). Only a few word-pairs are provided for each cluster, bearing in mind the findings of Elbert et al. (1991) who determined that as few as three to five minimal pairs were all that were necessary for generalization to occur. It should be

Word Pairs for /sl/

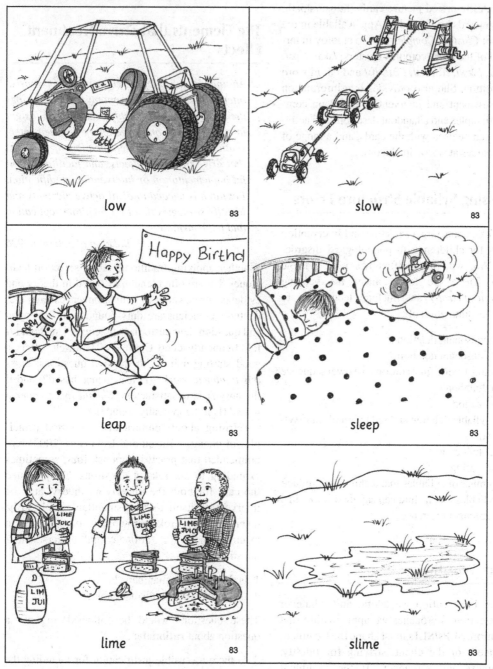

low

slow

leap

sleep

lime

slime

Figure 9.5 Word-pairs for /sl/

noted that in order to maintain a child's interest, clinicians might sometimes want to use more than five word-pairs and these are available from various sources including Black Sheep Press and www.speech-language-therapy.com.

In similar vein, Taps Richard has developed a set of 88 modestly priced picture cards (https://slpath.com/clustercards.html), and an App available in the App Store: *Clusters Complex Pro*, to employ in targeting 10 of the more complex clusters: /skɹ/, /spɹ/, /stɹ/, /spl/, /skw/, /fl/, /fɹ/, / θɹ/, /ʃɹ/ and /sl/ in word initial position. She also provides free information about assessment and intervention based on complexity principles and a handout describing 25 activities that can be used with the cards, and a range of other resources at www.slpath.com.

Addressing Syllable Structure Errors

Chapter 7 contains target selection and intervention strategies for children with phonological disorder and/or CAS, who have difficulties with syllable structure. These are found under the heading *Phonotactic therapy* and include techniques to address the elimination of

- Initial consonant deletion
- Initial consonant deletion
- Replacing a word-final consonant-vowel sequence with a diphthong
- Reduplication
- Weak syllable deletion and reduction of multisyllabic words
- Cluster reduction …
  and increasing
- The number of syllables that a child can produce
- The syllables that a child can say intelligibly in a word or longer utterance

Bells 'n' Whistles

Whatever intervention we adopt, and whatever target selection approaches we apply within that intervention, SLPs/SLTs must shape the treatment to the needs of the client, striving for fidelity, effectiveness and efficiency. If the treatment

sessions were to groan with extraneous activities or functionally trivial bells and whistles – perhaps introduced to make the therapy more 'interesting' – they would detract from any active ingredients present, and efficiency would be compromised.

The Elements that Drive Treatment Effects

An understanding of the elements that comprise interventions and a taxonomy that describes their structural relationships can provide insight into similarities and differences between interventions, help in the identification of elements that drive treatment effects, and facilitate faithful implementation or intervention modification. Research is needed to distil active elements and identify strategies that best facilitate replication and implementation.

Baker et al., 2018, p. 906

Whether applying traditional target selection techniques that are often tenuously based in theory and evidence, or newer ones with stronger research credentials, clinicians are duty-bound to reflect upon and question their customary practices. The thoughtful, frequently cited Clark (2003) article offers a good starting-point with the two questions: *Does this treatment work?* (Is it evidence-based?) and if the answer is unsatisfactory, *Should this treatment work?* (Is it theoretically sound?).

Writing about 'empirically supported principles of change', Rosen and Davidson (2003) recommended that practitioners ask four, sometimes extending to six related questions. They argued the case for both the underlying theory, and the intervention itself to be dismantlable; able to be taken apart or broken down into components to examine them for rationale and effects. Their questions were:

1. Is the theory dismantlable?
2. Is the intervention dismantlable?

These questions would be followed up with a question about **rationale**:

3. Is there a sensible justification for including the component?

Then a question about **effects**:

4. Is the component an 'active ingredient' in effecting change?

Alternatively:

5. Is there another reason the component is there?
6. Is it a valid reason, and can I explain the contribution it makes?

References

Alighieri, C., Bettens, K., Bruneel, L., D'haeseleer, E., Van Gaever, E., & Van Lierde, K. (2020). Effectiveness of speech intervention in patients with a cleft palate: Comparison of motor-phonetic versus linguistic-phonological speech approaches. *Journal of Speech, Language, and Hearing Research, 63*(12), 3909–3933. https://doi:10.1044/2020_JSLHR-20-00129

Alighieri, C., Van Lierde, K., De Caesemaeker, A. S., Demuynck, K., Bruneel, L., D'haeseleer, E., & Bettens, K. (2021). Is high-intensity speech intervention better? A comparison of high-intensity intervention versus low-intensity intervention in children with a cleft palate. *Journal of Speech, Language, and Hearing Research, 64*(9), 3398–3415. https://doi.org/10.1044/2021_JSLHR-21-00189

Alton, J. (1995). *Painting with light* (4th ed.). University of California Press.

American Speech-Language-Hearing Association. (2018). Schools survey report: SLP caseload characteristics trends 2000–2018. www.asha.org/Research/memberdata/Schools-Survey

Baker, E. (2015). The why and how of prioritizing complex targets for intervention. In C. Bowen, *Children's speech sound disorders* (2nd ed., pp. 106–111). Wiley-Blackwell. https://doi.org/10.1002/9781119180418

Baker, E., & McLeod, S. (2004). Evidence-based management of phonological impairment in children. *Child Language Teaching and Therapy, 20*(3), 261–285. https://doi.org/10.1191/026565900 4ct275oa

Baker, E., Williams, A. L., McLeod, S., & McCauley, R. (2018). Elements of phonological interventions for children with speech sound disorders: The development of a taxonomy. *American Journal of Speech-Language Pathology, 27*(3), 906–935. https://doi.org/10.1044/2018_AJSLP-17-0127

Ball, M., Howard, S., & Miller, K. (2018). Revisions to the extIPA chart. *Journal of the International Phonetic Association, 48*(2), 155–164. https://doi.org/10.1017/S0025100317000147

Ball, M. J., Muller, N., & Granese, A. M. (2013). Towards an evidence-base for /r/ therapy in English. *Journal of Clinical Speech and Language Studies, 20*(1), 1–23. http://dx.doi.org/10.3233/ACS-2013-20104

Barlow, J. A., & Gierut, J. A. (2002). Minimal pair approaches to phonological remediation. *Seminars in Speech and Language, 23*(1), 57–67. https://doi.org/10.1055/s-2002-24969

Bellon-Harn, M. L., Credeur-Pampolina, M. E., & LeBoeuf, L. (2013). Scaffolded-language intervention. *Communication Disorders Quarterly, 34*(2), 120–132. https://doi.org/10.1177/1525740111425086

Bernhardt, B., & Major, E. (2005). Speech, language and literacy skills 3 years later: A follow-up study of early phonological and metaphonological intervention. *International Journal of Language and Communication Disorders, 40*(1), 1–27. https://doi.org/10.1080/13682820410001686004

Bernhardt, B., & Stoel-Gammon, C. (1996). Underspecification and markedness in normal and disordered phonological development. In C. E. Johnson & J. H. V. Gilbert (Eds.), *Children's language* (Vol. 9, pp. 33–54). Lawrence Erlbaum Associates.

Bernthal, J. E., Bankson, N. W., & Flipsen, P., Jr. (2022). *Speech sound disorders: Articulation and phonological disorders in children* (9th ed.). Paul H. Brookes Publishing.

Bessell, A., Sell, D., Whiting, P., Roulstone, S., Albery, L., & Persson, M. (2013). Speech and language therapy interventions for children with cleft palate: A systematic review. *The Cleft Palate-Craniofacial Journal, 50*(1), e1–e17. https://doi.org/10.1597/11-202

Bleile, K. M. (2017). *The late eight* (3rd ed.). Plural Publishing.

Bleile, K. M. (2019). *Speech sound disorders: For class and clinic* (4th ed.). Plural Publishing.

Bowen, C., & Rippon, H. (2013). *Consonant clusters: Alliterative stories and activities for phonological intervention*. Black Sheep Press.

Chomsky, N., & Halle, M. (1968). *The sound pattern of English*. Harper and Row.

Clark, H. M. (2003). Neuromuscular treatments for speech and swallowing: A Tutorial. *American Journal of Speech-Language Pathology, 12*(4), 400–415. https://doi.org/10.1044/1058-0360(2003/086)

Cronin, A., McLeod, S., & Verdon, S. (2020). Holistic communication assessment for young children with cleft palate using the International Classification of Functioning, Disability and Health: Children and Youth. *Language, Speech, and Hearing Services in Schools*, *51*(4), 914–938. https://doi.org/10.1044/2020_LSHSS-19-00122

Crowe, K., & McLeod, S. (2020). Children's English consonant acquisition in the United States: A review. *American Journal of Speech-Language Pathology*, *29*(4), 2155–2169. https://doi.org/10.1044/2020_AJSLP-19-00168

Crystal, D. (1996). Language play and linguistic intervention. *Child Language Teaching and Therapy*, *12*(3), 328–344. https://doi.org/10.1177/026565909601200307

Cummings, A. E., & Barlow, J. A. (2011). A comparison of word lexicality in the treatment of speech sound disorders. *Clinical Linguistics & Phonetics*, *25*(4), 265–286. https://doi.org/10.3109/02699206.2010.528822

Davenport, M., & Hannahs, S. J. (2020). *Introducing phonetics and phonology* (4th ed.). Routledge.

Dean, E. C., Howell, J., Waters, D., & Reid, J. (1995). Metaphon: A metalinguistic approach to the treatment of phonological disorder in children. *Clinical Linguistics & Phonetics*, *9*(1), 1–19. https://doi.org/10.3109/02699209508985318

Delattre, P., & Freeman, D. (1968). A dialect study of American r's by x-ray motion picture. *Linguistics*, *44*, 29–68. https://doi.org/10.1515/ling.1968.6.44.29

Dinnsen, D. A. (2019). Phonology. In J. S. Damico & M. J. Ball (Eds.), *The SAGE Encyclopedia of human communication sciences and disorders* (pp. 1391–1396). Sage Publications

Dodd, B., & Iacono, T. (1989). Phonological disorders in children: Changes in phonological process use during treatment. *British Journal of Disorders of Communication*, *24*(3), 333–352. https://doi.org/10.3109/13682828909019894

Edwards, M. L., & Shriberg, L. D. (1983). *Phonology: Applications in communicative disorders*. College-Hill Press.

Eisenson, J., & Ogilvie, M. (1963). *Speech correction in the schools*. Macmillan.

Elbert, M., Dinnsen, D., & Powell, T. (1984). On the prediction of phonological generalisation learning patterns. *Journal of Speech and Hearing Disorders*, *49*(3), 309–317. https://doi.org/10.1044/jshd.4903.309

Elbert, M., Powell, T. W., & Swartzlander, P. (1991). Toward a technology of generalization: How many exemplars are sufficient? *Journal of Speech and Hearing Research*, *34*(1), 81–87. https://doi.org/10.1044/jshr.3401.81

Feeney, R., Desha, L., Ziviani, J., & Nicholson, J. M. (2012). Health-related quality-of-life of children with speech and language difficulties: A review of the literature. *International Journal of Speech-Language Pathology*, *14*(1), 59–72. https://doi.org/10.3109/17549507.2011.604791

Flipsen, P., Jr. (2022). *Remediation of /r/ for SLPs*. Plural Publishing, Inc.

Flipsen, P., Jr., & Parker, R. G. (2008). Phonological patterns in the speech of children with cochlear implants. *Journal of Communication Disorders*, *41*(4), 337–357. https://doi.org/10.1016/j.jcomdis.2008.01.003

Forrest, K. (2002). Are oral-motor exercises useful in the treatment of phonological/articulatory disorders? *Seminars in Speech and Language*, *23*(1), 15–26. https://doi.org/10.1055/s-2002-23508

Forrest, K., & Iuzzini, J. (2008). A comparison of oral motor and production training for children with speech sound disorders. *Seminars in Speech and Language*, *29*(4), 304–311. https://doi.org/10.1055/s-0028-1103394

Galton, R., & Simpson, A. (1958). *The publicity photograph*. Hancock's Half Hour, BBC, https://www.youtube.com/watch?v=aoFR0gYVsyA

Gick, B., Allen, B., Stavness, I., & Wilson, I. (2013). Speaking tongues are always braced. *Journal of the Acoustical Society of America*, *134*(5), 4204. http://dx.doi.org/10.1121/1.4831431

Gick, B., Bacsfalvi, P., Bernhardt, B. M., Oh, S., Stolar, S., & Wilson, I. (2007). A motor differentiation model for liquid substitutions: English /r/ variants in normal and disordered acquisition. *Proceedings of Meetings on Acoustics*, *1*, 060003, 2–9. http://doi.org/10.1121/1.2951481, https://scholars.cityu.edu.hk/files/21693879/A_Motor_Differentiation_Model_for_Liquid_Substitutions_in_Children_s_speech.pdf

Gierut, J. A. (1992). The conditions and course of clinically induced phonological change. *Journal of Speech and Hearing Research*, *35*(5), 1049–1063. https://doi.org/10.1044/jshr.3505.1049

Gierut, J. A. (1999). Syllable onsets: Clusters and adjuncts in acquisition. *Journal of Speech, Language, and Hearing Research*, *42*(3), 708–726. https://doi.org/10.1044/jslhr.4203.708

Gierut, J. A. (2001). Complexity in phonological treatment. *Language Speech and Hearing*

Services in Schools, *32*(4), 229. https://doi.org/10.1044/0161-1461(2001/021)

Gierut, J. A. (2007). Phonological complexity and language learnability. *American Journal of Speech-language Pathology*, *16*(1), 6–17. https://doi.org/10.1044/1058-0360(2007/003)

Gierut, J. A. (2016). Nexus to lexis: Phonological disorders in children. *Seminars in Speech and Language*, *37*(4), 280–290. https://doi.org/10.1055/s-0036-1587704

Gierut, J. A., & Champion, A. H. (2001). Syllable onsets II: Three-element clusters in phonological treatment. *Journal of Speech, Language, and Hearing Research*, *44*(1–4), 886–904. https://doi.org/10.1044/1092-4388(2001/071)

Gierut, J. A., & Hulse, L. E. (2010). Evidence-based practice: A matrix for predicting phonological generalization. *Clinical Linguistics & Phonetics*, *24*(4–5), 323–334. https://doi.org/10.3109/02699200903532490

Gierut, J. A., & Morrisette, M. L. (2012a). Age of word acquisition effects in treatment of children with phonological delays. *Applied Psycholinguistics*, *33*(01), 121–144. https://doi.org/10.1017/s0142716411000294

Gierut, J. A., & Morrisette, M. L. (2012b). Density, frequency and the expressive phonology of children with phonological delay. *Journal of Child Language*, *39*(4), 804–834. https://doi.org/10.1017/S0305000911000304

Gierut, J. A., Morrisette, M. L., & Champion, A. H. (1999). Lexical constraints in phonological acquisition. *Journal of Child Language*, *26*(2), 261–294. https://doi.org/10.1017/S0305000999003797

Gierut, J. A., Morrisette, M. L., Hughes, M. T., & Rowland, S. (1996). Phonological treatment efficacy and developmental norms. *Language, Speech and Hearing Services in Schools*, *27*(3), 215–230. https://doi.org/10.1044/0161-1461.2703.215

Gierut, J. A., Morrisette, M. L., & Ziemer, S. M. (2010). Nonwords and generalization in children with phonological disorders. *American Journal of Speech-Language Pathology*, *19*(2), 167–177. https://doi.org/10.1044/1058-0360(2009/09-0020)

Gierut, J. A., & O'Connor, K. M. (2002). Precursors to onset clusters in acquisition. *Journal of Child Language*, *29*(3), 495–517. https://doi.org/10.1017/s0305000902005238

Gierut, J. A., Simmerman, C. L., & Neumann, H. J. (1994). Phonemic structures of delayed phonological systems. *Journal of Child Language*, *21*(2), 291–316. https://doi.org/10.1017/s0305000900009284

Golding-Kushner, K. J. (2001). *Therapy techniques for cleft palate speech and related disorders*. Singular.

Grunwell, P. (1989). Developmental phonological disorders and normal speech development: A review and illustration. *Child Language Teaching and Therapy*, *5*(3), 304–319. https://doi.org/10.1177/026565908900500305

Hagiwara, R. E. (1995). Acoustic realizations of American /R/ as produced by women and men. *UCLA Working Papers in Phonetics*, *90*, 1–187. https://escholarship.org/uc/item/8779b7gq

Hanson, M. L. (1983). *Articulation*. W. B. Saunders Co.

Harding, A., & Grunwell, P. (1998). Active versus passive cleft-type speech characteristics. *International Journal of Language & Communication Disorders*, *33*(3), 329–352. https://doi.org/10.1080/136828298247776

Hardin-Jones, M., Jones, D. L., & Dolezal, R. C. (2020). Opinions of speech-language pathologists regarding speech management for children with cleft lip and palate. *Cleft Palate-Craniofacial Journal*, *57*(1), 55–64. https://doi.org/10.1177/1055665619857000

Hardin-Jones, M. A., & Jones, D. L. (2005). Speech production of preschoolers with cleft palate. *The Cleft Palate-Craniofacial Journal*, *42*(1), 7–13. https://doi.org/10.1597/03-134.1

Harrington, J., Cox, F., & Evans, Z. (1997). An acoustic study of broad, general, and cultivated Australian English vowels. *Australian Journal of Linguistics*, *17*(2), 155–184. https://doi.org/10.1080/07268609708599550

Hearnshaw, S., Baker, E., & Munro, N. (2018). The speech perception skills of children with and without speech sound disorder. *Journal of Communication Disorders*, *71*(Jan-Feb), 61–71. https://doi.org/10.1016/j.jcomdis.2017.12.004

Hearnshaw, S., Baker, E., & Munro, N. (2019). Speech perception skills of children with speech sound disorders: A systematic review and meta-analysis. *Journal of Speech and Hearing Research*, *62*(10), 3771–3789. https://doi.org/10.1044/2019_JSLHR-S-18-0519

Henningsson, G. E., & Isberg, A. M. (1986). Velopharyngeal movements in patients alternating between oral and glottal articulation: A clinical and cineradiographical study. *Cleft Palate Journal*, *23*(1), 1–9. PMID: 3455897

Hodson, B. (2007, 2010). *Evaluating and enhancing children's phonological systems: Research and theory to practice*. PhonoComp Publishers.

Howson, P. J., & Redford, M. A. (2022). A cross-sectional age group study of coarticulatory resistance: The case of late-acquired voiceless fricatives in English. *Journal of Speech, Language, and Hearing Research, 65*(9), 3316–3336. https://doi.org/10.1044/2022_JSLHR-21-00450

International Phonetic Association. (2005). *International phonetic alphabet chart*. https://www.internationalphoneticassociation.org/content/full-ipa-chart

Kamhi, A. G. (2007). Treatment decisions for children with speech–sound disorders. *Language, Speech, and Hearing Services in Schools, 37*(4), 271–279. https://doi.org/10.1044/0161-1461(2006/031)

Khan, L., & Lewis, N. (1983). *Khan–Lewis phonological analysis*. AGS.

Kilminster, M. G. E., & Laird, E. M. (1978). Articulation development in children aged three to nine years. *Australian Journal of Human Communication Disorders, 6*(1), 23–30. https://doi.org/10.3109/asl2.1978.6.issue-1.04

Kim, I., LaPointe, L. L., & Stierwalt, J. A. G. (2012). The effect of feedback and practice on the acquisition of novel behaviors. *American Journal of Speech-Language Pathology, 21*(2), 89–100. https://doi.org/10.1044/1058-0360(2011/09-0082)

Klein, E. S. (1996). Phonological/traditional approaches to articulation therapy: A retrospective group comparison. *Language, Speech, and Hearing Services in Schools, 27*(4), 314–323. https://doi.org/10.1044/0161-1461.2704.314

Krueger, B. I. (2019). Eligibility and speech sound disorders: Assessment of social impact. *Perspectives of the ASHA Special Interest Groups, 4*(1), 85–90. https://doi.org/10.1044/2018_PERS-SIG1-2018-0016

Krueger, B. I., & Storkel, H. L. (2022). The impact of age on the treatment of late-acquired sounds in children with speech sound disorders. *Clinical linguistics & phonetics*, 1–19. Advance online publication. https://doi.org/10.1080/02699206.2022.2093130

Kučera, H., & Francis, W. N. (1967). *Computational analysis of present-day American English*. Brown University Press.

Kummer, A. W. (2020a). Speech and resonance assessment. In A. W. Kummer (Ed.), *Cleft palate and craniofacial conditions* (4th ed., pp. 297–324). Jones & Bartlett Learning.

Kummer, A. W. (2020b). Speech therapy. In A. W. Kummer (Ed.), *Cleft palate and craniofacial conditions* (4th ed., pp. 515–548). Jones & Bartlett Learning.

Kummer, A. W., Strife, J. L., Grau, W. H., Creaghead, N. A., & Lee, L. (1989). The effects of Le Fort I osteotomy with maxillary advancement on articulation, resonance, and velopharyngeal function. *Cleft Palate Journal, 26*(3), 193–199. PMID: 2758671

Lass, N., & Pannbacker, M. (2008). The application of evidence-based practice to nonspeech oral motor treatments. *Language, Speech, and Hearing Services in the Schools, 39*(3), 408–421. https://doi.org/10.1044/0161-1461(2008/038)

Lewis, B. A., Freebairn, L., Tag, J., Ciesla, A. A., Iyengar, S. K., Stein, C. M., & Taylor, H. G. (2015). Adolescent outcomes of children with early speech sound disorders with and without language impairment. *American Journal of Speech-Language Pathology, 24*(2), 150–163. https://doi.org/10.1044/2014_AJSLP-14-0075

Locke, J. L. (1980). The inference of speech perception in the phonologically disordered child. Part II: Some clinically novel procedures, their use, some findings. *Journal of Speech and Hearing Disorders, 45*(4), 445–468. https://doi.org/10.1044/jshd.4504.445

Lof, G. L. (2009). The nonspeech-oral motor exercise phenomenon in speech pathology practice. In C. Bowen, *Children's speech sound disorders* (1st ed., pp. 181–184). Wiley-Blackwell.

Maas, E. (2017). Speech and nonspeech: What are we talking about? *International Journal of Speech-Language Pathology, 19*(4), 345–359. https://doi.org/10.1080/17549507.2016.1221995

Macken, M. A. (1980). The child's lexical representation: The '*puzzle-puddle-pickle*' evidence. *Journal of Linguistics, 16*(1), 1–17. https://doi.org/10.1017/S0022226700006307

Manning, W. H., Keappock, N. E., & Stick, S. L. (1976). The use of auditory masking to estimate automatization of correct articulatory production. *Journal of Speech and Hearing Disorders, 41*(2), 143–149. https://doi.org/10.1044/jshd.4102.143

Mass, E., Robin, D. A., Hula, S. N., Freedman, S. E., Wulf, G., Ballard, K. J., & Schmidt, R. A. (2008). Principles of motor learning in treatment of motor speech disorders. *American Journal of Speech-Language Pathology, 17*(3), 277–298. https://doi.org/10.1044/1058-0360(2008/025)

McCauley, R. J., Strand, E., Lof, G. L., Schooling, T., & Frymark, T. (2009). Evidence-based systematic review: Effects of nonspeech oral motor exercises on speech. *American Journal of Speech-Language Pathology, 18*(4), 343–360. https://doi.org/10.1044/1058-0360(2009/09-0006)

McLeod, S. (2020). Intelligibility in context scale: Cross-linguistic use, validity, and reliability. *Speech, Language and Hearing*, *23*(1), 9–16. https://doi.org/10.1080/2050571X.2020.1718837

McLeod, S., & Crowe, K. (2018). Children's consonant acquisition in 27 languages: A cross-linguistic review. *American Journal of Speech-Language Pathology*, *27*(4), 1546–1571. https://doi.org/10.1044/2018_AJSLP-17-0100

McReynolds, L., & Jetzke, E. (1986). Articulation generalization of voiced-voiceless sounds in hearing-impaired children. *Journal of Speech and Hearing Disorders*, *51*(4), 348–355. https://doi.org/10.1044/jshd.5104.348

Miccio, A. W., Elbert, M., & Forrest, K. (1999). The relationship between stimulability and phonological acquisition in children with normally developing and disordered phonologies. *American Journal of Speech-Language Pathology*, *8*(4), 347–363. https://doi.org/10.1044/1058-0360.0804.347

Mitchell, A. G., & Delbridge, A. (1965). *The pronunciation of English in Australia* (Revised ed.). Angus & Robinson.

Moller, K. T. (1994). Dental-occlusal and other oral conditions and speech. In J. Bernthal & N. Bankson (Eds.), *Child phonology: Characteristics, assessment, and intervention with special populations* (pp. 3–28). Thieme Medical Publishers.

Morrisette, M. L. (2021). Complexity approach. In A. L. Williams, S. McLeod, & R. McCauley (Eds.), *Interventions for speech sound disorders in children* (pp. 91–110). Paul H. Brookes Publishing.

Morrisette, M. L., Farris, A. W., & Gierut, J. A. (2006). Applications of learnability theory to clinical phonology. *International Journal of Speech-Language Pathology*, *8*(3), 207–219. https://doi.org/10.1080/14417040600823284

Morrisette, M. L., & Gierut, J. A. (2002). Lexical organization and phonological change in treatment. *Journal of Speech, Language, and Hearing Research*, *45*(1), 143–159. https://doi.org/10.1044/1092-4388(2002/011)

Muttiah, N., Georges, K., & Brackenbury, T. (2011). Clinical and research perspectives on nonspeech oral motor treatments and evidence-based practice. *American Journal of Speech-Language Pathology*, *20*(1), 47–59. https://doi.org/10.1044/1058-0360(2010/09-0106)

Nachmani, A., Masalha, M., & Kassem, F. (2022). Phonological profile of patients with velopharyngeal dysfunction and palatal anomalies. *Journal of Speech, Language, and Hearing Research*, *64*(12), 4649–4663. https://doi.org/10.1044/2021_JSLHR-20-00652

Ohala, D. K. (1999). The influence of sonority on children's cluster reductions. *Journal of Communication Disorders*, *32*(6), 397–422. https://doi.org/10.1016/s0021-9924(99)00018-0

Overby, M. S., Mezeika, S., DiFazio, M., Ioli, J., Birch, K., & Devorace, L. (2022). Clinicians' perspectives of treatment for lateralization errors: A quantitative and qualitative study. *Language, Speech, and Hearing Services in Schools*, *53*(3), 749–767. https://doi.org/10.1044/2022_lshss-21-00109

Peterson-Falzone, S. J., Hardin-Jones, M. A., & Karnell, M. (2009). *Cleft palate speech* (4th ed.). Mosby.

Peterson-Falzone, S. J., Trost-Cardamone, J. E., Karnell, M., & Hardin-Jones, M. A. (2017). *The clinician's guide to treating cleft palate speech*. Mosby.

Pollock, K. E., & Berni, M. C. (2003). Incidence of non-rhotic vowel errors in children: Data from the Memphis Vowel Project. *Clinical Linguistics & Phonetics*, *17*(4–5), 393–401. https://doi.org/10.1080/0269920031000079949

Potapova, I., Combiths, P., Pruitt-Lord, S., & Barlow, J. (2023). Word-final complexity in speech sound intervention: Two case studies. *Clinical Linguistics & Phonetics*, *37*(4–6), 363–384.

Potter, N. L., Nievergelt, Y., & VanDam, M. (2019). Tongue strength in children with and without speech sound disorders. *American Journal of Speech-Language Pathology*, *28*(2), 612–622. https://doi.org/10.1044/2018_AJSLP-18-0023

Potter, S. O. L. (1882). *Speech and its defects*. P. Blakiston, Son & Co.

Powell, T. W., & Miccio, A. W. (1996). Stimulability: A useful clinical tool. *Journal of Communication Disorders*, *29*(4), 237–253. https://doi.org/10.1016/0021-9924(96)00012-3

Preston, J., Leece, M. C., & Stortoa, J. (2019). Speech motor chaining treatment for school-age children with speech sound disorders. *Language, Speech, and Hearing Services in Schools*, *50*(3), 343–355. https://doi.org/10.1044/2018_LSHSS-18-0081

Prezas, R. F., Magnus, L., & Hodson, B. W. (2021). The cycles phonological remediation approach. In A. L. Williams, S. McLeod, & R. J. McCauley (Eds.), *Interventions for speech sound disorders in children* (pp. 251–278). Brookes Publishing Co.

Read, K., James, S., & Weaver, A. (2018). Pie, fry, why: Language play in 3- to 5-year-old children. *Journal of Early Childhood Research, 16*(2), 121–135. https://doi.org/10.1177/1476718X16664556

Robb, M. P., Bleile, K. M., & Yee, S. S. L. (1999). A phonetic analysis of vowel errors during the course of treatment. *Clinical Linguistics & Phonetics, 13*(4), 309–321. https://doi.org/10.1080/026992099299103

Rosen, G. M., & Davidson, G. C. (2003). Psychology should list empirically supported principles of change (ESPs) and not credential trademarked therapies or other treatment packages. *Behavior Modification, 27*(3), 300–312. https://doi.org/10.1177%2F0145445503027003003

Ruscello, D. M. (1993). A motor skill learning treatment program for sound system disorders. *Seminars in Speech and Language, 14*(2), 106–118. https://doi.org/10.1055/s-2008-1064163

Ruscello, D. M. (2008a). *Treating articulation and phonological disorders in children*. Mosby.

Ruscello, D. M. (2008b). An examination of nonspeech oral motor exercises for children with VPI. *Seminars in Speech and Language, 29*(4), 294–303. https://doi.org/10.1055/s-0028-1103393

Ruscello, D. M. (2008c). Nonspeech oral motor treatment issues in children with developmental speech sound disorders. *Language, Speech, and Hearing Services in Schools, 39*(3), 380–391. https://doi.org/10.1044/0161-1461(2008/036)

Ruscello, D. M. (2017). School-based intervention: Roles and responsibilities of the speech-language pathologist. In D. Zajac & L. Vallino-Napoli (Eds.), *Evaluation and management of individuals with cleft lip and palate: A developmental perspective* (pp. 281–318). Plural Publishing.

Ruscello, D. M., & Vallino, L. D. (2014). The application of motor learning concepts to the treatment of children with compensatory speech sound errors. *Perspectives, SIG 5, Speech Science and Orofacial Disorders, 24*(2), 39–47. https://doi.org/10.1044/ssod24.2.39

Ruscello, D. M., & Vallino, L. D. (2020). The use of nonspeech oral motor exercises in the treatment of children with cleft palate: A re-examination of available evidence. *American Journal of Speech Language Pathology, 29*(4), 1811–1820. https://doi.org/10.1044/2020_AJSLP-20-00087

Rvachew, S., & Nowak, M. (2001). The effect of target-selection strategy of phonological learning. *Journal of Speech, Language and Hearing Research, 44*(3), 610–623. https://doi.org/10.1044/1092-4388(2001/050)

Rvachew, S., Rafaat, S., & Martin, M. (1999). Stimulability, speech perception and the treatment of phonological disorders. *American Journal of Speech-Language Pathology, 8*(1), 33–43. https://doi.org/10.1044/1058-0360.0801.33

Sand, A., Hagberg, E., & Lohmander, A. (2022). On the benefits of speech-language therapy for individuals born with cleft palate: A systematic review and meta-analysis of individual participant data. *Journal of Speech, Language, and Hearing Research, 65*(2), 555–573. https://doi.org/10.1044/2021_JSLHR-21-00367

Sander, E. K. (1972). When are speech sounds learned? *Journal of Speech and Hearing Disorders, 37*(1), 55–63. https://doi.org/10.1044/jshd.3701.55

Schmidt, A. M., & Meyers, K. A. (1995). Traditional and phonological treatment for teaching English fricatives and affricates to Koreans. *Journal of Speech and Hearing Research, 38*(4), 828–838. https://doi.org/10.1044/jshr.3804.828

Schwartz, R., & Leonard, L. (1982). Do children pick and choose? an examination of phonological selection and avoidance in early lexical acquisition. *Journal of Child Language, 9*(2), 319–336. https://doi.org/10.1017/S0305000900004748

Shriberg, L. D. (1993). Four new speech and prosody-voice measures for genetics research and other studies in developmental phonological disorders. *Journal of Speech and Hearing Research, 36*(1), 105–140. https://doi.org/10.1044/jshr.3601.105

Shriberg, L., & Kwiatkowski, J. (1987). A retrospective study of spontaneous generalization in speech-delayed children. *Language, Speech, and Hearing Services in Schools, 18*(2), 144–157. https://doi.org/10.1044/0161-1461.1802.144

Shriberg, L. D., Kent, R. D., McAllister, T., & Preston, J. L. (2018). *Clinical phonetics* (5th ed.). Pearson.

Shriberg, L. D., & Kwiatkowski, J. (1994). Developmental phonological disorders I. *Journal of Speech, Language, and Hearing Research, 37*(5), 1100–1126. https://doi.org/10.1044/jshr.3705.1100

Shriberg, L. D., Kwiatkowski, J., & Mabie, H. L. (2019). Estimates of the prevalence of motor speech disorders in children with idiopathic speech delay. *Clinical Linguistics & Phonetics, 33*(8), 679–706. https://doi.org/10.1080/02699206.2019.1595731

Steriade, D. (1990). Greek prosodies and the nature of syllabification (Doctoral dissertation, Massachusetts Institute of Technology, 1982). https://dspace.mit.edu/bitstream/handle/1721.1/15653/10583995-MIT.pdf?sequence=2&isAllowed=y

Stoel-Gammon, C. (2019). Markedness. In J. S. Damico & M. J. Ball (Eds.), *The SAGE encyclopedia of human communication sciences and disorders* (pp. 1130–1131). Sage Publications.

Storkel, H. L. (2013). A corpus of consonant-vowel-consonant real words and nonwords: Comparison of phonotactic probability, neighborhood density, and consonant age of acquisition. *Behavior Research Methods*, *45*(4), 1159–1167. https://doi.org/10.3758/s13428-012-0309-7

Storkel, H. L. (2018a). Implementing evidence-based practice: Selecting treatment words to boost phonological learning. *Language, Speech, and Hearing Services in Schools*, *49*(3), 482–496. https://doi.org/10.1044/2017_LSHSS-17-0080

Storkel, H. L. (2018b). The complexity approach to phonological treatment: How to select treatment targets. *Language, Speech, and Hearing Services in Schools*, *49*(3), 463–481. https://doi.org/10.1044/2017_LSHSS-17-0082

Storkel, H. L., Armbrüster, J., & Hogan, T. P. (2006). Differentiating phonotactic probability and neighborhood density in adult word learning. *Journal of Speech, Language, and Hearing Research*, *49*(6), 1175–1192. https://doi.org/10.1044/1092-4388(2006/085)

Sweeney, T., & Sell, D. (2008). Relationship between perceptual ratings of nasality and nasometry in children/adolescents with cleft palate and/or velopharyngeal dysfunction. *International Journal of Language & Communication Disorders*, *43*(3), 265–282. https://doi.org/10.1080/13682820701438177

Templin, M. C. (1957). *Certain language skills in children: Their development and interrelationships* (NED-New ed., Vol. *26*). University of Minnesota Press. http://www.jstor.org/stable/10.5749/j.ctttv2st.

Tomes, L. A., Kuehn, D. P., & Peterson-Falzone, S. J. (2004). Research considerations for behavioral treatments of velopharyngeal impairment. In K. Bzoch (Ed.), *Communicative disorders related to cleft lip and palate* (5th ed., pp. 797–846). Pro-Ed.

Trost-Cardamone, J. E. (2009). Articulation and phonologic assessment procedures and treatment decisions. In K. T. Moller & L. E. Glaze (Eds.), *Cleft lip and palate: Interdisciplinary issues and treatment* (2nd ed., pp. 377–414). Pro-Ed.

Unicomb, R., Walters, J., Pullin, J., & Bowen, C. (2019). Listening to SLPs. How helpful are Australian-English acquisition norms for velar stops to the child speech evaluation process? *Journal of Clinical Practice in Speech-Language Pathology*, *21*(2), 87–93. https://speechpathologyaustralia.cld.bz/JCPSLP-Vol-21-No-2-2019-DIGITAL-Edition/41

Vallino, L., Ruscello, D. M., & Zajac, D. (2019). *Cleft palate speech and resonance*. Plural Publishing.

Van Riper, C., & Irwin, J. V. (1958). *Voice and articulation*. Prentice Hall.

Westbury, J. R., Hashi, M., & Lindstrom, M. J. (1998). Differences among speakers in lingual articulation for American English /ɹ/. *Speech Communication*, *26*, 203–226. https://doi.org/10.1016/S0167-6393(98)00058-2

Williams, A. L. (1991). Generalization patterns associated with training least phonological knowledge. *Journal of Speech and Hearing Research*, *34*(4), 722–733. https://doi.org/10.1044/jshr.3404.733

Williams, A. L. (2003). Target selection and treatment outcomes. *Perspectives on Language Learning and Education*, *10*(1), 12–16. https://doi.org/10.1044/lle10.1.12

Williams, A. L. (2010). Multiple oppositions intervention. In A. L. Williams, S. McLeod, & R. J. McCauley (Eds.), *Interventions for speech sound disorders in children* (pp. 73–94). Paul H. Brookes Publishing Co.

Williams, A. L., & Sugden, E. (2021). Multiple oppositions Intervention. In A. L. Williams, S. McLeod, & R. J. McCauley (Eds.), *Interventions for speech sound disorders in children* (2nd ed., pp. 61–89). Paul H. Brookes Publishing Co.

Zajac, D., & Vallino-Napoli, L. (2017). *Evaluation and management of individuals with cleft lip and palate: A developmental perspective*. Plural Publishing.

Chapter 10

Multilingualism and Language Variation

The contributions to Chapter 10 span four continents and five countries. The geographic mix includes authors in South Africa (Michelle Pascoe A39), the USA (Benjamin Munson and Alayo Tripp A40; and Brian Goldstein A47), Australia (Sharynne McLeod and Kathryn Crowe A42), Hungary (Krisztina Zajdó A43), and Canada (Karen Pollock A44; and Barbara May Bernhardt, Daniel Bérubé and Glenda Mason A48). They cover the topics of linguistic diversity (A39), social factors in phonological acquisition (A40), clinical services for multilingual children with speech sound disorders (A47), crosslinguistic knowledge about speech acquisition (A42 and A48), serious myth busting around children who are growing up speaking more than one language (A43), and the good oil on internationally adopted children learning English as a second first language (A44).

Linguistic Diversity

Preserving indigenous languages is such an urgent priority that the United Nations Educational, Scientific and Cultural Organisation (UNESCO) declared the years 2022 to 2032 as the International Decade of Indigenous Languages. Linguistic diversity is not simply about cultural heritage, language is not just an artefact. Investing in African languages contributes to increasing the potential for innovation because "language enables the delivery of information and knowledge coded in different socio-cultural, political, and economic contexts", according to UNESCO.

Karabo Kgoleng, 2022

Dr. Michelle Pascoe is a speech and language therapist and associate professor in the Division of Communication Sciences and Disorders at the University of Cape Town, South Africa. Her research focuses on speech and language acquisition in the languages of Southern Africa, multilingualism, and ways to support families from a range of language and cultural backgrounds.

Q39.   Michelle Pascoe: Culturally and Linguistically Appropriate Speech Assessments for South Africa

Since the previous editions of this book, there have been significant shifts in your research and publications output towards developing speech assessments, normative data and interventions for children acquiring the languages of Southern Africa. Can you describe what you have produced so far? What excites you about these massive topics (Khoza-Shangase & Mophosho, 2021; Mdlalo et al., 2019; Southwood & van Dulm, 2015), and what are the implications of this work for practice within South Africa?

A39. Michelle Pascoe: Towards the Development of Speech Assessments, Normative Data and Interventions for Children Acquiring the Languages of Southern Africa

In 2007, I was a new lecturer teaching a second-year class of undergraduate speech language therapy (SLT) students at the University of Cape Town. I taught the students about children's speech development and phonological processes, and there were opportunities to analyse data from children and practice transcription skills. The course texts included Stackhouse and Wells (2002), Dodd (2005), and Kamhi and Pollock (2005). At the end of the lecture, a small group of students waited behind to chat further with me.

These future SLTs were excited about what they had been learning but wanted to know where they could find similar information on languages other than English: where were the speech assessments, lists of phonological processes, and books on children's speech acquisition for their languages? The students were first-language speakers of indigenous South African languages: Setswana, SiSwati, and isiXhosa. Shamefacedly, I had to admit to them that there was very little or no information available about children's speech acquisition or published speech assessments in these languages. I wasn't surprised by the students' question: I was already painfully aware of, and ashamed about the lack of such tools and basic information about acquisition of many of the local languages. Moreover, I realized with increasing discomfort that I would be standing there the next year, and the year after, still feeling inadequate, if I did not use my

knowledge and position to attempt to change the status quo. From that point on, my research agenda was to advance knowledge of children's speech development in the indigenous languages of Southern Africa.

Research is always a team effort. In my case, the team was especially important as my ability to speak and understand indigenous South African languages is limited, which meant a heavy reliance on first language speakers: colleagues and students (Pascoe, et al., 2020). South Africa is a richly diverse country with many official (and unofficial) languages and a great variety of cultures. It is also one of the most unequal societies in the world (Mukong et al., 2017) and the country's history of apartheid (1948–1994) resulted in lost opportunities for many – individuals, families, and generations – with the long-term impact still felt decades later. Back in 2007, I therefore had few black colleagues who were fluent speakers of local indigenous languages; there were also few qualified SLTs whose first language was not English or Afrikaans, and although the student demographic in our classes was changing, the classes were still dominated by white monolingual English-speaking females. When I spoke with the group of mother-tongue indigenous language speaking students that day in 2007 I told them that together we would have to change things and that they would be intrinsic to the process. Motivated and true to their words, both Olebeng Mahura and Zinhle Maphalala returned to the university for postgraduate studies after qualifying as SLTs. Together, we embarked on a journey to better understand and document children's speech development in isiXhosa (e.g., Maphalala et al., 2014; Pascoe et al., 2018 and Setswana (e.g., Mahura & Pascoe, 2016) with many other students, clinicians, and colleagues (and their languages) joining in along the way. The focus of our work is on children's speech acquisition in South Africa and is driven by a need to develop reliable and valid clinical assessments of children's speech. These tools are needed to collect data about speech acquisition supported by an understanding of what typical development is like and how best to intervene to support children and families.

isiXhosa is one of the main languages spoken in the Western Cape region of South Africa where I live and work, and therefore the need to develop a clinical tool for SLTs in this language was immediate and pressing. Working with Zinhle Maphalala and the linguist Mantoa Motinyane (then Mantoa Smouse), we developed a speech assessment entitled '*Masincokoleni*' (Let's chat), together with a small set of preliminary normative data for preschool-children acquiring isiXhosa (Maphalala et al., 2014; Pascoe & Smouse, 2012). This small-scale project was exciting because for the first-time clinicians had a tool to use that was underpinned by normative data and theoretical knowledge. Furthermore, in my lectures I was now able to give examples of phonological processes in isiXhosa and outline the stages of consonant acquisition in that language. That preliminary project meant that we could now start to investigate bilingual English-isiXhosa acquisition (Pascoe, Mahura et al., 2018; Pascoe, Rossouw et al., 2018), speech processing in younger children (Pascoe et al., 2016) and intervention for isiXhosa-speaking children with speech difficulties (Pascoe, Rossouw et al., 2018; Rossouw & Pascoe, 2018). isiXhosa is closely related to isiZulu, the most widely spoken indigenous language in South Africa, and Zenia Jeggo's work (Pascoe & Jeggo, 2019) on isiZulu led to development of an isiZulu speech assessment for pre-schoolers and a preliminary set of norms for that language.

Meanwhile, over the past decade, Olebeng Mahura documented children's Setswana speech acquisition in South Africa in a meticulous and comprehensive way (Mahura & Pascoe, 2016). Her work includes both segmental and suprasegmental aspects of the language, and clinicians working in Southern Africa today can use her speech assessment to understand whether a Setswana-speaking child is following the expected course of typical development (in multiple dialects) or showing signs of difficulties that require further investigation.

Our adaptations of *The Intelligibility in Context Scale* into all South Africa's eleven official languages were a first for South African SLTs; again, filling a gap for researchers and clinicians (Pascoe & McLeod, 2016) and for the first time enabling clinicians working with families who speak any of the official languages to obtain essential information about the impact of a child's speech difficulty on those with whom they interact. More recent work

has seen us considering the overlaps between speech and lexical acquisition. As part of the Southern African CDI project developing CDIs for all the official languages (Southwood et al., 2021), we now have access to large datasets for languages like isiXhosa and Setswana which we can use to answer questions about both lexical and phonological aspects of early word acquisition.

It is exciting and heartening to be able to support families and clinicians in South Africa by providing materials and information about speech acquisition in languages such as isiXhosa and Setswana. When training students, we can use this information and the associated resources to make the teaching more relevant and context-specific for our classes (Pascoe & Jeggo, 2019) and to better prepare students for their clinical practice with a diverse clientele. Of course, that does not mean we no longer refer to key texts like Dodd, and Stackhouse and Wells, and Kamhi and Pollock as these are important to the field irrespective of languages spoken. Rather, we are now able to provide our students with more diverse and representative sets of materials and readings. I always hope to inspire students in my classes to see the gaps that remain in our professorial repertoires and to be aware that they can help fill these gaps through their research, often drawing on their own first language and culture.

Speech and language clinicians and researchers in South Africa are still not well equipped to serve all the population and much work remains to be done. There are many ways to contribute to changing the status quo and our specific focus on advancing knowledge of children's speech is just one way of eliciting change. For our group, it has provided the opportunity to ask (and hopefully answer) some theoretical questions about children's speech development, together with practical opportunities to support clinicians and researchers with some new (albeit imperfect) tools to respond to needs in the local situation, redress imbalances in the country and empower the next generation of SLTs and researchers. Nelson Mandela famously noted that 'If you talk to a *man* in a *language* he understands, that goes to his head. If you talk to him in his *language*, that goes to his heart.' These words continue to motivate our research and teaching.

Sociophonetics, Language Variation, and Change

The study of sociophonetics resides at the interface between sociolinguistics and phonetics. It uses modern phonetic methodologies, including instrumentation, to conduct sociophonetics research; carry out quantitative variationist analyses; measure language attitudes; quantify individual differences; conduct conversational analysis; and explore (language group) membership categorization analysis. Rather than being a discipline in its own right (yet) sociophonetics is a methodological approach that contributes to scholarship around the nature of language variation and change.

Mx. Benjamin Munson, PhD studies psycholinguistic and sociolinguistic aspects of speech sound development and disorders. In the 20+ years of his career so far, he has studied topics as diverse as relationships between vocabulary learning and speech sound learning in children with communication impairments, and phonological development across languages. In his current work he endeavours to understand how children navigate the task of simultaneously learning to speak intelligibly to all of those around them, and to speak in phonetically distinctive ways that convey attributes like their nascent gender identity. He is particularly interested in how these drives play out in clinical speech-sound learning, in which there might be mismatches between the social attributes of the speech produced by SLPs/SLTs and the attributes the child wishes to convey. Dr. Munson is Professor and Chair of the Department of Speech-Language-Hearing Sciences at the University of Minnesota, Twin Cities.

Dr. Alayo Tripp (they/them) is a linguist and cognitive scientist with a focus in sociophonetics and computational psycholinguistics. Their work explores the relationship between social knowledge and the perception of speech sounds throughout the lifespan. They earned their PhD in Linguistics from the University of Maryland in 2019. Their dissertation, entitled *An Affiliative Model of Early Lexical Learning*, uses computational methods to reanalyse findings in early phonological development, drawing on findings in developmental psychology to theorize how language users may rely on social information to interpret variation in speech. Dr. Tripp is currently a postdoctoral fellow in Speech-Language-Hearing Sciences at the University of Minnesota, Twin Cities.

Q40.   Benjamin Munson and Alayo Tripp: Linguistic Variation

The importance of SLPs/SLTs having informed views of linguistic variation, enabling them to distinguish genuine pathology from natural non-standard variation, cannot be overstated, and this is an area where sociophonetics can help. What are the methods of enquiry in this emerging area of study? Can you explore for the interested clinician or clinical researcher the likely impact of, and clinically relevant research areas in children's SSDs for, sociophonetics as its literature base mushrooms and interfaces with clinical phonology? More broadly, how do the literature and knowledge base around 'epistemic trust' relate to children's speech learning?

A40.   Benjamin Munson and Alayo Tripp: Social Factors in Phonological Acquisition: Sociophonetics and Social Identification

The language that we encounter in our daily lives is highly variable. This observation is familiar to SLPs/SLTs. Variability occurs at all levels of linguistic structure, including pronunciation. Imagine all the variation that might exist in the production of the word *last*. The pronunciation of that word varies considerably within individuals, as a function of things like lexical status (whether it is an example of the verb *to last*, the adjective, the noun, or the adverb *last*) and prosodic structure (i.e., whether the word received narrow-focus emphasis, as in the sentence *they weren't merely late to arrive, they were the very last to arrive*). The pronunciation might also differ across groups of speakers. For example, individuals who were born in the US cities surrounding the Great Lakes might produce the vowel in this word differently from those born in Southern

California, reflecting differences in regional dialect (Labov et al., 2008). This work is well known to SLPs/SLTs, in part because unfamiliar dialects may be difficult to perceive (Harte et al., 2016). But how is this kind of speech variation learned, and what should we presume about its relationship to phonological knowledge?

One example of variation between speaker groups is that associated with contrasts between speaking varieties of Mainstream American English (MAE) and African American English (AAE, e.g., a local Black or African American [Vernacular] English). Individuals who speak AAE might pronounce the word *last* as [læs], while their peers who speak varieties of MAE might pronounce last as [læst] (Thomas & Bailey, 2015). For the AAE speaker, this reflects normal learning of the target language. However, for a child acquiring MAE, this same pronunciation may be evidence of an underlying difficulty in producing sequences of consonants – the very topic of this book.

Much of the attention that SLPs/SLTs have given to variation in speech has focused on cases like this, in which it has been critical to differentiate between differences among language varieties, and disorders within a particular variety. AAE has attracted considerable attention because of the disproportionately high representation of Black individuals receiving speech and language services (Strand & Lindsay, 2009). Understanding the impact of SLPs'/SLTs' perception of AAE use on the diagnosis and treatment of those individuals is key to understanding and mitigating that overrepresentation. The ability of SLPs/SLTs to distinguish between dialect differences and disordered speech patterns improves with instruction (Blackburn, 2012).

Sociolinguistic Investigation and Variationist Approaches

SLP/SLT has benefitted from work in sociolinguistics, the branch of linguistics focused on studying the causes and consequences of socially meaningful variation in language. Sociolinguistic investigations traditionally examine the broader socio-political context of language variation by positing that these kinds of speech variation are involuntary products of natural linguistic learning (Chambers, 2007). However, variationist approaches emphasise a significant role for *social agency* in determining the behaviour of language users (Eckert, 2008). For example, the emergence of racialized variants of language in the contexts of endemically racist societies does not only reflect consequences of exposure to linguistic variation, but necessarily also variation in linguistic ideology.

Variationist sociolinguistics, which seeks to simultaneously validate all speech variation as meaningful human expression while appropriately locating social identities and speech behaviours in historical contexts of social inequity, provides an important and needed challenge to the power-neutral view of variation that characterizes much of the existing work in SLP/SLT.

SLPs'/SLTs' focus on dialect variation – both related to regional dialects and racialized dialects – gives the impression that speech variation in children arises primarily because of relative exposure to various kinds of talkers. Children would be presumed to learn a way of pronouncing the word *last* because they emulated the pronunciations of the people who they encountered during language acquisition, whether it was in Manhattan Beach, CA or Buffalo, NY, and whether it was speakers of the local mainstream variety or speakers of the local AAE variety. Indeed, some of the variation that is observed is due to the acquisition of distinct codes used by different speaker groups.

Acquisition of Gendered Pronunciation

However, this cannot describe the entire picture of acquiring socially meaningful variation. To illustrate, we focus on the acquisition of *gendered* pronunciation. The phonetic characteristics of men and women's speech differ. One hypothesis is that this is because of physical dimorphism, or cisgender (cis). A cisgender individual is one whose gender identity matches the sex assigned to them at birth. Adult cis men and women have different sized, different-shaped vocal tracts and vocal folds. Cis men's longer, thicker vocal folds and longer vocal tracts predispose them to produce speech with a lower average fundamental frequency and lower resonant frequencies than cis women (Munson & Babel, 2019). Indeed, men's and women's speech does differ in these ways, as is shown in large-scale normative studies of speech acoustics. However, male-female differences can also be traced to the performance of gender roles. Both adults and children can manipulate f0 and overall scaling of formant frequencies volitionally and do so when providing renditions of stereotypically masculine or feminine speech. Hence, while vocal tract and laryngeal morphology may impose limits on variation in f0 and formant frequencies, they do not dictate the absolute values that individuals use. Moreover, in some studies, researchers have found seemingly arbitrary phonetic variation between men and women. Sociolinguistic studies of variation in one distinctive, salient, and stereotyped feature of Tyneside English reveal that while both men and women produced glottalized variants of intervocalic /t/, women produced it at slightly lower rates than men (Foulkes et al., 2005). This is also illustrated in sociophonetic studies of variation in /s/. Numerous studies have shown that men and women produce different variants of /s/, with women producing a hypercorrect /s/, that is, an /s/ with an especially high peak frequency and a compact spectrum. Those characteristics resemble the characteristics of /s/ produced in a clear-speech style (e.g., Julien & Munson, 2012), and are not easily traced to sex dimorphism in vocal tract or laryngeal morphology; but may be connected to a socialized desire to perform hypercorrect speech. Moreover, male-female differences in /s/ are not uniform within populations, as would be predicted if these differences were solely because of sex dimorphism (Stuart-Smith, 2007).

The acquisition of gendered speech provides a model for answering the question of how children learn to produce socially meaningful variation. Research suggests that gendered speech is learned early in life. Munson et al. (2019) presented, to adult listeners, single-word productions by 55 children assigned male at birth (AMAB) and 55 children assigned female at birth (AFAB). The adults were asked to rate the talker on a continuous rating scale anchored by the text

as 'definitely a boy' at one end and 'definitely a girl' at the other. The 110 child speakers had participated in a longitudinal study of language development, and adults rated productions from both an earlier time-point, when they were aged 2;6–3;6 (years;months), and again at e 4;6–5;6. Different ratings were provided for AMAB and AFAB children at both time-points: the AFAB children were rated closer to the 'definitely a girl' end and the AMAB children closer to the 'definitely a boy' end. Moreover, the phonetic characteristics of the words that predicted the ratings included features that are clearly not the consequence of sex dimorphism, like attributes of /s/. Munson et al.'s findings are consistent with other studies on the topic, including Perry et al. (2001) and Fung et al. (2021).

One very unlikely scenario is that children learn gendered speech by growing up in uniform-gender communities; in only the most exceptional cases do children learn language from only men or only women. The acquisition of gendered speech represents a case of *selective learning*, in which children model their speech on only a subset of the individuals whom they encounter during language acquisition. How might variation be selectively adopted? Foulkes et al. (2005) examined glottalization of medial /t/ in child-directed speech (CDS) in Tyneside English and found that mothers of girls used this variant far less frequently in their CDS than mothers of boys. That is, the mothers were implicitly socializing the boys and girls to produce different variants of /t/, mirroring the distribution between adult men and women in the Tyneside variety. However, the relationship between CDS and children's acquisition in Foulkes et al., while statistically significant, was modest-sized, and it is unlikely that gender-specific CDS explains gendered speech acquisition entirely. In what follows, we use gender as an example to review several other mechanisms potentially implicated in the acquisition and production of socially meaningful linguistic variation.

Epistemic Trust

In developmental psychology, investigation into *epistemic trust,* or how children use their experience to assess the relative value of informants, has shown that familiarity and evidence of reliability have different impacts on the responses of children of different ages. Koenig and Harris (2005) exposed 3- and 4-year-old children to an adult speaker who labelled familiar objects accurately, and to another speaker either named them inaccurately, or said that they didn't know the object's name. Those same two adults then provided different names for novel objects. Four-year-old children were more likely to endorse the labels given to the novel objects by the adult who had labelled the known object correctly, and to say that they would ask the reliable adult about the names of other unknown objects.

Koenig and Harris's findings are powerful evidence that children's language learning is socially selective. In Koenig and Harris's study, this selectivity was based on epistemic trust, but we could imagine that children also might focus their language learning on individuals whom they identified as sharing attributes with them. Gendered speech might be acquired by a child learning a way of pronouncing /t/ or /s/ from adults whom they recognized as sharing the same gender identity.

A related possibility is that children learn the social meanings associated with certain pronunciations. Eckert (2008) argued that different pronunciations (like the different types of /s/ and /t/, described earlier) carry different social meanings about the person who produces them. For example, a talker might convey a particular attitude by producing a hypercorrect /s/. Children might learn gendered ways of speaking by emulating pronunciations whose social meanings convey states or traits that they see in themselves. Indeed, there is evidence of the early learning of gendered phonetics: the acoustic characteristics of the tokens of /s/ in the stimuli used by Munson et al. (2019) differed between the AFAB and AMAB children. AFAB children produced /s/ with a higher peak frequency than AMAB children, mirroring differences between adult women and men.

Koenig and Harris's work has inspired a re-evaluation of some classic findings in the language development literature relating to children's perceptions of adults who produce phonologically variable speech, including, potentially, SLPs/SLTs who produce words differently in an intervention session to illustrate correct and incorrect pronunciations. Tripp et al. (2021) argued that findings on children's perception of phonologically variable speech are best understood if we assume that children assign distinct social value to speech variation in accordance with beliefs about relative social value. The proffered mechanism describes children as having metalinguistic awareness of congruency between social group membership, social evaluations, and speech patterns, which they may leverage to selectively acquire socially meaningful variation.

The potential processes by which gendered speech is learned, presented here, are just a few of potentially many mechanisms that contribute to learning gendered speech. All are relevant to SLPs/SLTs. SLPs/SLTs should be aware that children's learning is potentially guided by their sociolinguistic knowledge and social preferences. Imagine a female SLP/SLT modelling a hyper-correct /s/ to a boy who has already learned the distribution of /s/ variants across adult men and women, and the different social meanings associated with /s/. The SLP/SLT cannot then assume that a child's failure to learn this sound is due entirely to cognitive, linguistic, perceptual, or motor factors. The failure may be due to the misalignment between the identity that the child is developing and the identity that is suggested by the variant of /s/ produced by the clinician. Much future research is needed to better understand how these social factors might affect speech-sound learning in clinical settings, and the literature reviewed in this section provides an ideal jumping-off point for these investigations.

Children Learning More than One Language

The publication of a position paper on *Multilingual children with speech sound disorders* (International Expert Panel on Multilingual Children's Speech, 2012) marked the culmination of a huge collaborative effort, described by McLeod et al. (2013), and the launch of further work in this fascinating area. The panel's position statement (p. 1) reads: '*The International Expert Panel on Multilingual Children's Speech recommends that:*

1. Children are supported to communicate effectively and intelligibly in the languages spoken within their families and communities, in the context of developing their cultural identities.
2. Children are entitled to professional speech and language assessment and intervention ser- vices that acknowledge and respect their existing competencies, cultural heritage, and histories. Such assessment and intervention should be based on the best available evidence.
3. SLPs aspire to be culturally competent and to work in culturally safe ways.
4. SLPs aspire to develop partnerships with families, communities, interpreters, and other health and education professionals to promote strong and supportive communicative environments.
5. SLPs generate and share knowledge, resources, and evidence nationally and internationally to facilitate the understanding of cultural and linguistic diversity that will support multilingual children's speech acquisition and communicative competency.
6. Governments, policy makers, and employers acknowledge and support the need for culturally competent and safe practices and equip SLPs with additional time, funding, and resources to provide equitable services for multilingual children.'

The 57 members of the International Expert Panel on Multilingual Children's Speech had worked in the following 31 countries: Australia, Austria, Brazil, Canada, China, Ecuador, Finland, France, Germany, Greece, Hong Kong, Hungary, Ireland, Israel, Jamaica, Japan, Korea, Malta, New Zealand, Paraguay, Peru, Russia, Slovakia, Singapore, South Africa, Sweden, Switzerland, Turkey, United Kingdom, United States of America, and Vietnam. The members used the following 26 languages in a professional capacity: Afrikaans, Arabic, Australian Sign Language (Auslan), Bulgarian, Cantonese, Danish, Dutch, English, Finnish, French, German, Greek, Hebrew, Hungarian, Icelandic, Italian, Jamaican, Korean, Mandarin, Portuguese, Russian, Spanish, Swedish, Turkish, Yiddish and Welsh plus many other languages in non-professional capacities.

The panel included several of the contributors to *Children's Speech Sound Disorders, Third Edition*:

Elise Baker (A26), Martin Ball (A3), B. May Bernhardt (A45), Daniel Bérubé (A45), Kathryn Crowe (A42), Brian Goldstein (A41), David Ingram (A4, A10), Glenda Mason (A45), Sharynne McLeod (A2, A42), Benjamin Munson (A51), Michelle Pascoe (A39), Susan Rvachew (A9, A18), Carol Stoel-Gammon (A7), A. Lynn Williams (A19), and Krisztina Zajdó (A43). Readers will see that the author of the next essay, Brian Goldstein, is on this list.

Dr. Brian Goldstein is Chief Academic Officer and Executive Dean University of St. Augustine for Health Sciences, San Marcos, CA, USA. Dr. Goldstein is well-published in the area of communication development and disorders in Latino children focusing on speech sound development and disorders in monolingual Spanish and Spanish-English bilingual children. He is the former editor of *Language, Speech, and Hearing Services in Schools*, is a Fellow of the American Speech-Language-Hearing Association (ASHA) and received the Certificate of Recognition for Special Contribution in Multicultural Affairs from ASHA.

Q41. Brian Goldstein: Children with Speech Sound Disorders Who are Multilingual

SLPs/SLTs who work with culturally and linguistically diverse families field an unending array of frequently asked questions about normative expectations, and when and why to refer a child growing up bilingual for speech assessment. For example, should all bilingual preschoolers be assessed 'just in case'; should a child hear one language or two if he or she has speech and language difficulties; do multilingual children acquire speech differently from monolingual peers; are they typically 'behind' in both languages for a period; do some combinations of languages pose more difficulties in acquisition than others; what significant speech characteristics should parents and teachers be alert to as a child who is to grow up multilingual acquires speech; and should the family seek out a multilingual clinician? Can you guide the reader as to expected developmental pathways for speech acquisition; suggest appropriate screening and assessment procedures and describe suitable intervention methodologies for multilingual children with speech sound disorders, and ways of managing homework. Certain concerns can arise in cases of bilingualism in families where the language(s) other than English are indigenous, perceived as low-status, unusual or endangered. Can you comment on this and reflect on the potential impact upon service delivery of attitudes, preconceptions, and beliefs, held by the clinician, and how a clinician might enhance his or her cultural competence in clinic and education settings.

A41.   Brian Goldstein: Providing Clinical Services for Multilingual Children with Speech Sound Disorders

Many parents who are raising multilingual children question the rate and quality of their children's speech and language development. They do so, in part, because they are concerned that the acquisition of more than one language will 'confuse' their children and result in delayed, or at least slowed, language development in both languages. SLPs/SLTs also might hold this view, especially if they do not believe they have the requisite knowledge and skills to provide services to those who are culturally and linguistically diverse (Guiberson & Atkins, 2012), particularly if they are multilingual (e.g., Williams & McLeod, 2012).

The literature on speech and language development unambiguously reports that multilingual children are not at-risk for speech sound disorders (SSD) simply because they are multilingual or because of the constellation of languages they are acquiring (Kohnert et al., 2020 for a comprehensive review). That is, from an acquisition perspective, no one language is more difficult to acquire than another, if children have significant opportunity to hear and speak each language.

That said, it is critical to know that language development, in general, and particularly

speech development, is not the same as it is for monolingual children. Multilinguals will exhibit similar and dissimilar speech sound skills/phonological patterns across languages (Fabiano-Smith & Barlow, 2010; Goldstein & McLeod, 2012; McLeod & Crowe, 2018). For example, multilingual children likely will exhibit similar rates of cluster reduction in both languages if the same clusters are common in each. Additionally, a child acquiring English and Italian will demonstrate a higher frequency of final consonant deletion in English than in Italian because of the phonotactic (structural) properties of English compared to Italian, which has many more words that end with a vowel or 'open syllable'. Thus, clinicians should not expect to see errors/patterns in one language duplicated in the other(s) in either multilinguals with speech sound disorders or those who are typically developing.

Speech Sound Development in Typically Developing Multilinguals

Speech sound development in multilinguals results in rates of acquisition which are similar and dissimilar to monolinguals (McLeod & Goldstein, 2012). Speech sound development can occur at a faster rate in multilinguals than in monolinguals. For example, Grech and Dodd (2008) examined speech sound skills in 2- to 6-year-old Maltese and English speakers, finding that their bilingual participants exhibited more advanced skills compared to monolingual speakers as exemplified by consonant accuracy, consistency of production, and fewer error patterns. Several other studies have shown that speech sound skills were not significantly different in multilinguals compare with monolinguals (e.g., Goldstein & Bunta, 2012). So, children acquiring multiple languages can maintain speech sound skills that are within normal limits relative to monolinguals.

Speech sound skills in multilinguals also develop at a slower rate than in monolinguals. Studies have indicated that the phonetic inventories in bilingual children were not age-appropriate compared to monolinguals (Holm & Dodd, 2006), that multilinguals exhibited lower accuracy and a higher number of errors than did monolinguals, and that multilingual children made more errors and produced more uncommon error patterns than monolinguals (Gildersleeve-Neumann et al., 2008). Importantly, over time, typically developing multilingual children achieve speech skills commensurate with those of monolinguals (e.g., Holm & Dodd, 2006).

Speech Development in Multilinguals with SSD

Not all multilinguals develop speech sound skills typically. Multilingual children will exhibit SSD, but SSD in this population do *not* result from *being multilingual*. Studies of SSD in multilingual children indicate the following characteristics (Dodd et al., 1997; Holm & Dodd, 1999a; Holm et al., 1998):

- Low intelligibility to family and non-family members.
- Low consonant accuracy in *both* languages.
- Similar, although not identical, phonological skills to monolinguals with SSD.
- Similar and dissimilar phonological patterns in both languages.
- Phonetic inventories consisting of mainly early developing sounds, although some later developing phones will occur as well.
- Numerous substitution errors in both languages when cross-linguistic effects and dialectal features are considered during scoring.
- Substitutions for both early developing and later developing phonemes in all languages.

Assessing Speech Sound Skills in Multilinguals

Best practices in providing clinical services to children with SSD are invariable regardless of the number of languages a child is acquiring. Moreover, clinical services should conform to the International Classification of Function-

ing, Disability and Health: Children and Youth Version (ICF-CY) (World Health Organization (WHO), 2007).

Regardless of the constellation of languages the child speaks, or the perceived status of the languages by the larger community, intervention emanates from comprehensive assessment (B. A. Goldstein & Fabiano, 2007) that takes all of them into account. Similarly, all languages spoken by the child need to be accounted for in the intervention processes. A monolingual approach to either assessment or intervention is untenable. As Kohnert (2008, 2020) has noted, a disorder in bilinguals is not caused by bilingualism or cured by monolingualism.

Ideally, assessment is performed by a clinician who speaks all the child's languages, but typically, this is not feasible. Most clinicians will need the help of support personnel such as interpreters and translators (Langdon & Saenz, 2015), in a comprehensive assessment (McLeod, 2020; McLeod et al., 2017).

Assessment begins with a case history that encompasses questions added about language history, language use, and language proficiency: dimensions that change over time and affect speech sound skills in multilinguals (e.g., Goldstein et al., 2010). The clinician then obtains single word and connected speech samples in all languages using tools designed for that population (International Expert Panel on Multilingual Children's Speech, 2012; McLeod, 2020). Assessments for languages other than English are listed in McLeod and Goldstein (2012), McLeod (2007) and on the www.csu.edu.au/research/multilingual-speech/speech-assessments page. Sampling all languages is paramount because multilingual children exhibit discrepant skills, errors, and error patterns that are distributed across their languages (e.g., Goldstein et al., 2005). Thus, measuring skills in only one language provides an incomplete picture of the child's phonological *system*. The samples are subjected to independent and relational analyses. In independent analyses, the child's speech sound system is examined without reference to the adult targets. Clinicians should create a phonetic inventory in each language consisting of, for example, singleton consonants, clusters, syllable types, syllable shapes, word length, and tones where applicable. Then, relational analyses (referencing the child's productions against the adult target system) should be completed. Common relational analyses include consonant accuracy, vowel accuracy, whole word accuracy (e.g., Ingram, 2002), and phonological patterns (e.g., final consonant deletion, velar fronting, unstressed syllable deletion). For multilingual children, also examine accuracy of shared elements (i.e., those common to all languages, such as /m/ between Italian and English) and unshared elements (i.e., unique to each language, such as the trill /r/, which occurs in Spanish (e.g., Fabiano-Smith & Goldstein, 2010) but not in most 'Englishes'. The exceptions include the voiced alveolar trill /r/ in Scottish-English and the voiceless trill /r̥/ in Welsh-influenced English Finally, complete an error analysis, examining for substitution and syllable structure errors.

In each analysis, it is vital to account for both cross-linguistic effects (using an element specific to one language in the production of the other language: for example, a child producing the Spanish trill /r/ in the production of an English word containing /ɹ/) and dialect features (Goldstein & Iglesias, 2001). Neither cross-linguistic effects nor dialect features should be scored as errors or considered to be appropriate intervention targets.

Providing Intervention to Multilinguals with Ssd

Clinicians base their intervention decisions on literature supporting approaches and techniques that are reliable and valid. Doing so for multilingual children with SSD is difficult given the paucity of relevant intervention studies. The available few include Holm and Dodd (1999b), Holm et al. (1997), Holm et al. (1998), and Ray (2002) in which only English was utilized as the language of intervention. Their results indicate that intervention in English generally positively influences speech sound skills in the other language. Thus, speech sound skills in all languages should be monitored throughout intervention in order to track cross-linguistic generalization flowing from interdependence between the two languages (e.g., Paradis, 2001).

Clinicians, with little evidence to guide them, often mistakenly believe that the first treatment decision for multilingual should be focused on the language of intervention (or the language of instruction, at school). They should really be asking themselves, 'When do I treat in each of the two languages?' (Goldstein, 2006). Answering this clinical question begins with a broad and deep understanding of the child's phonological system in each language. Determining initial goals can be completed through a Bilingual Approach and a Cross-Linguistic Approach (e.g., Kohnert & Derr, 2012; Kohnert et al., 2005). In a **Bilingual Approach** speech sound skills, errors, or error patterns common to all the languages spoken by the child (e.g., stopping of fricatives) should be targeted initially because, theoretically, this may promote cross-linguistic generalization from one language to the other language(s) (Yavaş & Goldstein, 1998). Once speech sound skills, errors, or error patterns common to all languages have been targeted, the clinician would introduce a **Cross-Linguistic Approach** to focus on speech sound skills, errors, or error patterns that occur in only one of the child's languages. This approach is adopted because, for example, Language A will contain a phoneme such as the palatal nasal /ɲ/ in Amharic that does not exist in the other language (English). Additionally, clinicians might target errors or error patterns that are exhibited with unequal frequency in each language. For example, unlike English, Korean does not contain word-initial clusters (Kim & Pae, 2007). Thus, remediation of cluster errors could occur only for English and in English.

Once the approach is chosen, the goal attack strategy can be determined. Fey (1986) outlined three goal attack strategies: vertical, horizontal, and cyclical. A vertical strategy focuses on one goal until a specified criterion is reached. The multilingual correlate would be focusing on a goal that is specific to one language but also measuring how it generalizes to the other language(s). For example, /s/ would be remediated in English and monitored in Cantonese. A horizontal strategy is one in which more than one goal is addressed in each session. The bilingual correlate is to target one goal in Language A and one goal in Language B within the same session, although the targets would be divergent. For example, the clinician might target final consonants in English and aspirated affricates in Hmong. In a cyclical strategy several goals are addressed in rotation, but only one goal is incorporated at a time within a session. The bilingual correlate would be to alternate both targets *and* languages. For example, in cycle 1, the clinician might target /s/ in Language A and clusters in Language B; in cycle 2, the clinician might focus on clusters in Language A and /s/ in Language B.

The language of intervention will probably be determined during the process of choosing the intervention approach goals, and goal attack strategy. There might be, however, additional factors to consider in deciding the language of intervention such as language history, language use, language proficiency, and the family's goals (Goldstein, 2006).

Summary and Conclusions

The number of multilingual children appears to be increasing making it more likely that clinicians will have to provide services to this population. Doing so might necessitate changed perspectives, enhanced cultural competence, and a need for updated information and knowledge.

SLPs/SLT clinicians are grounded in phonetics and phonology so that they can bring that knowledge to bear in the assessment and intervention of children with SSD, regardless of the type and number of languages they are acquiring. That knowledge can be reviewed, upgraded, or acquired to assess and treat multilingual children with SSD.

Providing clinical services to multilingual children with SSD can be daunting because of a general lack of research with this population, little to no pre-service training, and scant resources. Despite these limitations, it is possible to provide reliable, valid clinical services to multilingual children with SSD by keeping an open mind, knowing what you do not know, doing your homework at the pre-referral and pre-assessment stages, reaching out to others (interpreters, translators, cultural brokers), completing a comprehensive assessment in all languages, providing intervention based on bilingual and cross-linguistic approaches, and monitoring cross-linguistic generalization. Finally, remember to do the 'right' thing as 'this will gratify some and astonish the rest' (Mark Twain).

Crosslinguistic Prspectives on Consonant Acquisition

As SLPs increasingly assess and treat children from varying linguistic backgrounds, knowledge of typical acquisition must expand beyond descriptions of developmental milestones based predominantly on studies of English.

Davis, 2007, p. 51

When assessing the speech of any child with a suspected SSD or conducting ongoing assessment for a child engaged in intervention, familiarity with, and understanding of typical developmental profiles provides an SLP/SLT with a crucial aspect of the basic background information necessary for appropriate reporting, treatment planning, and in some instances, referral. The authors of A42 have contributed mightily to expanding this knowledge base with McLeod and Crowe (2018) and Crowe and McLeod (2020).

Crosslinguistic Knowledge about Children's Speech Acquisition

Readers met **Dr. Sharynne McLeod** at the top of A2 and will recall her longstanding interest and expertise in speech acquisition and speech sound disorders as they relate to children who are multilingual. Her co-author here is **Dr. Kathryn Crowe**. Dr. Crowe is a postdoctoral researcher at the University of Iceland and holds adjunct positions at the Center for Education Research Partnerships (National Technical Institute for the Deaf, Rochester Institute of Technology) and Charles Sturt University, Australia. She has worked as a speech pathologist, academic, and researcher and holds a Bachelor of Speech Pathology and Bachelor of Arts, Master of Special Education (Sensory Disability), and a PhD, as well as Diploma in Auslan/English interpreting. She is a member of the International Expert Panel on Multilingual Children's Speech and assisted in the development of Speech Pathology Australia's 'Working in a Culturally and Linguistically Diverse Society' position paper and clinical guidelines. Kathryn's research has focused on cultural and linguistic diversity in children, particularly children with hearing loss, their families, and the professionals who work with them. She is passionate about using evidence to inform practice when working with learners with hearing loss and making available evidence accessible to parents, professionals, and service providers.

Q42.   Sharynne Mcleod and Kathryn Crowe: Normative Expectations for Speech Acquisition across Languages

Many readers will be familiar with your, and your collaborators' extensive work on multilingual children's speech development and disorders and the associated web pages at www.csu.edu.au/research/multilingual-speech. Some, however, will be seeking information, advice, and answers about developmental expectations for the first child ever referred to them who is growing up with two or more languages and rich cultural exposure. Drawing on your research, how would you guide monolingual clinicians, and multilingual SLPs/SLTs who do not speak the same languages as their client, on their journey of discovery?

A42.   Sharynne McLeod and Kathryn Crowe: Crosslinguistic Knowledge about Children's Speech Acquisition

An important role undertaken by SLPs/SLTs is to determine whether children's speech is typical compared with others within their community. This decision-making occurs at the time of assessment, throughout intervention, and finally when determining whether intervention goals have been achieved. Decision-making requires consideration of many different factors including children's '(a) production of consonants, vowels, consonant clusters, polysyllables, and prosody, (b) perception, (c) phonology, (d) intelligibility, (e) stimulability, (f) phonological awareness, spelling, and reading, (g) academic and social impact, and

(h) insights from children and significant others in children's lives' (Ireland et al., 2020, p. 333).

A challenge for SLPs/SLTs is to access information about typical speech acquisition in all the languages and dialects spoken by the children they work with. While there are over 7,000 languages in the world, information is available about children's speech acquisition for fewer than 100 of them, including English, and mostly covers the production of consonants only. Free information is available at https://www.csu.edu.au/research/multilingual-speech and https://phonodevelopment.sites.olt.ubc.ca (see Bernhardt et al., A45).

Recently, three cross-linguistic reviews have been undertaken of studies of 49,000 children's consonant acquisition (Crowe & McLeod, 2020; McLeod & Crowe, 2018) and intelligibility (McLeod & Crowe, 2018). These reviews provide guidance to inform expectations about typically developing children's speech.

1.   Cross-linguistic Review of Speech Acquisition in 27 Languages

The first cross-linguistic review presented an analysis of consonant acquisition of 26,007 children speaking 27 languages (McLeod & Crowe, 2018). In the review, the authors considered 64 studies documented in 60 papers that described 10 or more typically developing participants and were identified via a systematic database search and input from members of the International Expert Panel on Multilingual Children's Speech (McLeod & Goldstein, 2012). Speech acquisition was described for 27 languages: Afrikaans, Arabic, Cantonese, Danish, Dutch, English, French, German, Greek, Haitian Creole, Hebrew, Hungarian, Icelandic, Italian, Jamaican Creole, Japanese, Korean, Malay, Maltese, Mandarin (Putonghua), Portuguese, Setswana (Tswana), Slovenian, Spanish, Swahili, Turkish, and Xhosa.

On average, by 5;0 children produced at least 93 per cent of consonants and 98% of vowels correctly. Fricatives, affricates, trills, and flaps were acquired later than nasals and plosives. Consonants with anterior tongue placement were acquired later than most labial, pharyngeal, and posterior lingual consonants; however, there was an interaction between place and manner. Across languages, the average age of acquisition for pulmonic consonants using the 90–100% criteria (across 37 studies) is displayed below.

- 1;10 –2;11 years: /ʨ, ʨʰ, ʄ, ʦ̢, ɫ, c, ʋ, p, m, t/
- 3;0–3;11 years: /pf, n, ʔ, cɕ, ʦʰ, k, ʁ, b, j, ŋ, h, pʰ, ɥ, d, tʰ, ʝz, f, cʰ, x, g, w, ɸ, ʂ, ɟ, kʰ, l, ɦ, kʷ, q, ɕ, bː, tːʕʰ, qː, ðʕ, χː, v, ɲ, ʧ/
- 4;0–4;11 years: /ɣ, ʝj, ç, ʤ, ʎ, kʷʰ, ʦ, s, ʦʰ, ð, ħ, ɾ, z, ʃ, tʕ/
- 5;0–5;11 years: /ʒ, cç, ɹ, χ, r, θ/
- 6;0–6;11 years: /β/
- 7;6 years: /ʍ/

Non-pulmonic consonants (e.g., clicks) generally were acquired early. The average age of acquisition for non-pulmonic consonants (e.g., ejectives, clicks) using the 75–85% criteria across 3 studies (of Setswana and Xhosa) was:

- 1;10–2;11 years: /p', t', c', k', ɓ, ǀ, ǃ/
- 3;0–3;11 years: /tʷ', kʷ', tsʷ', ǀʰ, ǁʰ, ts', kx', ǁ/
- 4;0–4;11 years: /ǃʰ, ʧ'/

The review by McLeod and Crowe (2018) included case studies of the acquisition of different languages that showed minor differences in acquisition, possibly because of consonant frequency and the comparative complexity of the syllable and consonant inventory. For example, the average age of acquisition for English consonants using the 90–100% criteria across eight studies follows:

- 2;0–3;11 = /p, b, m, d, n, h, t, k, g, w, ŋ, f, j/
- 4;0–4;11 = /l, ʤ, ʧ, s, v, ʃ, z/
- 5;0–6;11 = /ɹ, ʒ, ð, θ/

The average age of acquisition for Japanese consonants using the 90–100% criteria across five studies was:

- 3;0–3;11 = /m, t, j, cɕ, p, g, k, ʝz, d, n, b, w, ɸ, h/
- 4;0–4;11 = /ç, ɾ, ɕ, s, ts/
- 5;0–5;11 = /z/

In contrast, the average age of acquisition for Spanish consonants using the 90–100% criteria across four studies is as listed below:

- 3;0–3;11 = /p, t, m, k, j, ɲ, l, ʧ/
- 4;0–4;11 = /ŋ, ʒ, ʤ, g, n, b, d, f, x, ð, w, ɾ/
- 5;0–6;11 = /r, s, β/

Since the review was published there have been additional studies of speech acquisition. They related to Icelandic (Másdóttir et al., 2021), Persian (Zarifian & Fotuhi, 2020), Vietnamese (Phạm & McLeod, 2019) and isiZulu (Pascoe & Jeggo, 2019); however, the general principles of speech acquisition remain. By 5 years of age typically developing children can produce most of the consonants within their home language. It is important to note that most of these studies of children's speech acquisition examined monolingual speech acquisition. Multilingual speech acquisition is more difficult to summarise due to the wide variety in personal and environmental contexts.

2. Review of English Speech Acquisition in the US

The second review presented an analysis of consonant acquisition of 18,907 children speaking English in the United States (Crowe & McLeod, 2020). It was motivated by the social media discussion about McLeod and Crowe (2018) that 'broke the SLP internet'. The discussion was initiated by some people in the US who indicated that the age of 5 was much younger than the benchmark age they had been using for eligibility and access to SLP services for children with SSD. They indicated that their benchmark had been informed by Smit et al. (1990) who provided 'Recommended ages of acquisition for phonemes and clusters, based generally on 90% levels of acquisition' (p. 795). Specifically, Smit et al. indicated that consonants such as /s, z, ʃ, ʧ, ʤ, s, ɹ, ð, θ/ were acquired between 6;0 and 9;0 years of age. Consequently, the review by Crowe and McLeod (2020) considered 15 studies described in 6 papers and nine articulation/ phonology/ speech tests/ assessments. Across 15 studies of 18,907 children learning English in the US, the majority of consonants were acquired by 5;0 years, with none of the studies providing PCC data. The average age of acquisition for using the 90% criteria across 10 studies of typical English speech acquisition in the US (ordered by mean age of acquisition) was found to be:

- 2;0–3;11: /b, p, n, m, d, h, w, t, k, g, ŋ, f, j/ (all plosives, nasals and glides)
- 4;0–4;11: /v, ʤ, l, s, ʧ, s, ʃ, z/
- 5;0–6;11: /ʒ, ɹ, ð, θ/

These findings were almost the same as for English acquisition across the world (McLeod & Crowe, 2018). Importantly, on average across all studies of English consonant acquisition only four consonants were not acquired by 4;11 /ʒ, ɹ, ð, θ/. However, on average, children in the US review learned some consonants earlier (at 2 years); whereas in the analysis of English acquisition data in McLeod and Crowe (2018) only /p/ was acquired by 2 years.

To summarise, consonant acquisition is gradual as demonstrated by data being available using 50–75-90% criteria. Milestones are expectations for growth and shouldn't necessarily be used for eligibility for services. To make clinical and eligibility decisions consider the whole child assess more than simple single words including consonant clusters, polysyllables, and intelligibility.

3. **Cross-linguistic Review of Intelligibility in 14 Languages**

The third cross-linguistic review presented an analysis of intelligibility of 4,235 children speaking 14 languages: Cantonese, Croatian, Dutch, English, Fijian (Standard or dialects), Fiji-Hindi, German, Italian, Jamaican Creole, Korean, Portuguese, Slovenian, Swedish, Vietnamese. (McLeod, 2020). The review considered 18 studies that used the parent-reported Intelligibility in Context Scale (ICS, McLeod et al., 2012) which is available, free of charge, in over 60 languages http://www.csu.edu.au/research/multilingual-speech/ics. Across a range of languages, it was found that 4- to 5-year-old children are 'usually' to 'always' intelligible when talking with others, including strangers. Children were most intelligible to their parents and families, and least intelligible to strangers. There was cross-linguistic evidence regarding the validity and reliability of the ICS providing support for use of the ICS as a primary screening tool to identify which children require additional assessment.

To summarise information from these three studies. Across languages, 5-year-old children can produce ≈93% of consonants and 98% of vowels correctly and are usually-always intelligible, even to strangers. Five-year-old children can pronounce almost all consonants correctly; however, there may be a few language-dependent consonants that are difficult. The reviewed studies of consonant acquisition mostly assessed monolingual children, but the reviewed studies of intelligibility found no significant difference between scores for monolingual or multilingual children. Therefore, SLPs/SLTs can use these guidelines to inform their practice and to acknowledge that across the world young children learn to pronounce the speech sounds of their home languages at a young age.

Multilingualism Myth-busting

The widely read American journalist Elizabeth Meriwether Gilmer (1861–1951), was better known by the pen name Dorothy Dix. So popular were her life-advice columns that she became the highest paid female journalist of her day, with her advice on marriage syndicated in newspapers around the world. She was reputed to compose 'readers' questions' herself, closely followed by meticulously crafted answers. This practice sparked the mildly derogatory term 'Dorothy Dixer' which, in Australian politics, is a rehearsed or planted question put to a government minister by a backbencher from the same political party during Parliamentary Question Time. This enables the minister to make an announcement in the form of a reply.

Before writing Q43, a web search for 'multilingualism myths' yielded a staggering volume of returns, so I confess that the second part of the question to Krisztina Zajdó, *'do certain myths and misconceptions about this client group persist?'*

was a blatant Dorothy Dixer. The myths that prolif-erated on the web, all based on no convincing evi-dence, were along the lines of:

- Exposing children to multiple languages can cause delays in speech development.
- Exposure to more than one language may cause language disorder.
- Learning two languages will confuse your child and block other learning.
- Multilingual children will have academic prob-lems once they start school.
- Children will be confused if parents speak to them in two languages.
- If your paediatrician advises against two lan-guages, use the dominant one only.

By contrast, and as befits this book, the myths Dr. Zajdó rebuffs have more of a child speech acquisition focus and are backed by high quality research evidence.

Krisztina Zajdó, PhD is a linguist and speech scientist in Hungary, where she currently works as an associate professor in Special Education/Speech-Language Pathology at Széchenyi István University/University of Győr (SIU/UG). Her primary research interests are the acquisition of vowels in children and developmental changes in children's speech timing patterns crosslinguistically. She also studies phonetic differences between adult directed and child-directed speech. After returning from the US to her native Hungary in 2008, she directed the development of a new speech-language pathology program at SIU/UG. Recently, she developed an interest in studying speech, language, and cognitive development in children with mild intellectual disability being reared in both segregated and integrated learning environments.

Q43.   Krisztina Zajdó: Cross-linguistic Speech Acquisition and Multilingual Myths

The term 'multilingualism' incorporates bilingualism and multilingualism. Children who are multilingual can comprehend and/or produce, orally, manually or in writing, two or more languages. At a minimum, they exhibit a basic level of functional proficiency or use, irrespective of the age at which their languages were learned (McLeod et al., 2013). There are differences in the speech acquisition process between children who are monolingual and children who are multilin-gual, and between children learning English and children learning one or more languages other than English (LOTE). How does cross-linguistic research on vowel, consonant and phonotactic development guide SLPs'/SLTs' work with multilingual children with SSD, and do certain myths and misconceptions about this client group persist?

A43.   Krisztina Zajdó: It's Time to Say Goodbye: Applying Cross-linguistic Research Evidence to Debunk Unhelpful Myths about Speech Acquisition

With notable exceptions (e.g., McLeod & Baker, 2017, pp. 175–219) many studies, textbooks and long-established websites published since the 1990s centre on elucidating speech acquisition in English, or English and Spanish (see American Speech-Language-Hearing Association, n.d). Even today, introductory texts (e.g., Fogle, 2020; Owens & Farinella, 2019) and long-established websites (e.g., Williamson, 2008–2021) generally contain speech acquisition norms established by monolingual English SLPs/SLTs studying monolin-gual English-speaking participants (Williamson, 2015). Clinical phonetics texts typically contain limited or no information on non-English speech sound production (e.g., Ball, 2021; Shriberg et al., 2019), and volumes with an intervention focus hold scant information on treating SSD in multi-linguals (e.g., Williams et al., 2021). It is pleasing to see however, a gradual increase in the empha-sis afforded to understanding speech acquisition in non-English speaking language communities and multilinguals speaking languages other than English (LOTE) (e.g., Bauman-Waengler, 2020; Bleile, 2020; Jakielski & Gildersleeve-Neumann, 2018; McLeod, 2007; McLeod et al., 2017; Weismer & Brown, 2021; Yavaş, 2020).

Data are scarce on speech acquisition in children acquiring LOTE. An additional difficulty is that studies of LOTE apply diverse research methodologies. Thus, normative data must be reviewed and interpreted with caution.

Reconsidering OLD, Widely Held Beliefs

Research has uncovered new evidence about speech acquisition in various language environments, extending our understanding of speech acquisition. Crosslinguistic studies shed light both on universal and more restricted tendencies in speech sound acquisition. 'Facts' and observations based solely on data from monolingual English-speaking children, are being replaced by observations that are valid for specific language milieus rather than being constituent representatives of universal trends.

Myth 1: Vowels are Acquired Early

There is a persistent belief in the universal 'early' acquisition of vowels (Smith, 1973; Templin, 1957) summarized by Donegan (2013). In the contemporary literature, Owens and Farinella (2019) and Fogle (2020) assert that vowels are typically acquired by 3;0 (years; months). But we have known for some time that Cantonese-speaking children between 2;0 and 2;5 exhibit a percentage of vowels correct (PVC) is 98.8% (So & Dodd, 1995), and in the same age-range the PVC for Putonghua (Modern Standard Chinese) learners is 82.4% (Hua & Dodd, 2000). Hungarian-speaking children's vowel accuracy is at 85.2% at 2;0 (Zajdó, 2002).

Crosslinguistic research shows that in some languages rhotic and non-rhotic vowel acquisition takes considerably longer than once believed. For example, Van Haaften et al. (2020) found that, while children acquiring Dutch have PVCs of 90% at around 2;7, children aged 6;6-to-6;11 still produce vowel errors. In Hungarian, vowel errors persist in single word productions at 7;11-to-8;0, particularly for front rounded vowels /ø:/ and /y(:)/ (Nagy, 1980). Importantly, *crosslinguistic data demonstrate that accurate vowel production poses more challenges (and therefore takes longer) for children than once thought* (Zajdó, 2013).

Myth 2: The Order of Vowel Acquisition Is Uniform

Crosslinguistic results for children's speech acquisition call into question the order of acquisition of vowels, in categories, as posited by Jakobson (1941/1968). Building on the ideas of N. S. Trubetzkoy, Jakobson proposed that front vowels were produced with better accuracy earlier than back ones. He also speculated that unrounded vowels are acquired first, then back rounded ones and finally front rounded vowels, claiming, 'relative chronological order of development remains everywhere and at all times the same' (p. 46). Clark (2016) challenged the popular interpretation of Jakobson's influential theory, arguing that Jakobson only proposed a theory of *contrasts* between sounds, not a theory about order of acquisition of vowels and consonants. Interpretations of Jakobson's theory vary considerably, but in a longitudinal account of Putonghua vowel acquisition (Hua & Dodd, 2006), the central low /a/ and the back high /u/ were mastered earliest, while Hua (2002) showed that in Putonghua the front rounded /y/ is acquired before the back rounded /o/. In these examples, *crosslinguistic data contradict the 'language (speech) universals' concept proposed by Jakobson.*

Myth 3: Complex Vowel Inventories Take Longer to Acquire

Crosslinguistic findings show that Danish-speaking children's language development is slower than it is for L1 speakers of other Nordic languages (e.g., Icelandic, Norwegian and Swedish). Researchers (e.g., Bleses et al., 2011; Trecca et al., 2020) have proposed that the phonetic structure of Danish, with its large, complex vowel inventory, is responsible. Their proposal implies that a larger vowel inventory takes longer to acquire. Conversely, Clausen and Fox-Boyer (2017) demonstrate that children learning Danish do not lag behind children learning a language with smaller, simpler vowel inventories. They reported lower vowel accuracy values from 2;6-to-2;11 but not for children aged 3;0-to-4;11. *Thus, larger more complex vowel inventories do not necessarily take longer to develop.*

Myth 4: All Consonants are Acquired by School Age

This myth is relevant for SLPs/SLTs who inform parents and others – formally in assessment reports, informally in conversation, and in print and online 'information sheets' – about criteria for children's school readiness and/or reading readiness. Unfortunately, these distinct but related types of 'readiness' are sometimes conflated and discussed as one and the same thing. **School readiness** (National Academies of Sciences, Engineering and Medicine NASEM, 2016; UNICEF, 2012) is often used to describe how well-equipped children are, personally, socially, linguistically, physically, and intellectually – in their unique family and school circumstances – to transition to formal schooling. Here, 'linguistically' implies that it is desirable for children's speech be intelligible to adults and peers, but not necessarily adult-like, when they start school. Confusion arises because this is often referred to, in advice to parents, as 'clear speech' and interpreted by some as 'perfect speech'. This misunderstanding is exacerbated when over-simplified definitions of clear speech are provided, such as 'the ability to clearly pronounce sounds in words' to be found on an SLP/SLT website. In typical development, children are intelligible to their parents by 3;0 (Lynch et al., 1980) and to unfamiliar adults by their fourth birthday (Coplan & Gleason, 1988) even though intelligibility continues to increase after 4;0 (Hustad et al., 2020). School readiness may or may not coincide with **reading readiness**. The critical age hypothesis – for reading readiness – is that literacy acquisition is likely to be compromised if children are not intelligible by the age of 5;6, especially if they also have semantic and syntactic difficulties (Bishop & Adams, 1990). A conversational PCC below 50% when formal reading instruction starts (at about the age of 5;6) is associated with literacy acquisition difficulties, while persistent, mild speech production difficulties beyond the age of 6;9 are associated with literacy acquisition difficulties (Nathan et al., 2004).

Studies of diverse languages indicate that the consonant inventory is acquired early by monolingual children. For example, Malay-speaking children acquire all syllable-initial and syllable-final consonants by 4;6, except for syllable-final /s/, /h/ and /l/ (Phoon et al., 2014). Children acquiring Standard American English learn to produce all consonants except /θ/, with a mean age of acquisition below 6;0. (Crowe & McLeod, 2020; and see McLeod & Crowe, this volume). In Cantonese, Turkish, Putonghua, German, and Sesotho PCC measures at 6;0 exceed 98% (Zajdó, 2013). Taken together, these results suggest the early acquisition of consonants in general.

On the other hand, normative data from children acquiring Jordanian Arabic show PCCs of 90% between 6;0 and 6;10 (Amayreh & Dyson, 1998). Data from Icelandic show that /s/, /r/, /r̥/ and /ŋ/ in initial position, and /s/ in final position, are not yet acquired at 5;11 (Másdóttir et al., 2021). Spanish-speaking children acquire the labial fricative /β/ at a mean age of 6;0 to 6;11 (McLeod & Crowe, 2018). Further, some consonants are still erred at 8;6 in Turkish and Hungarian (McLeod & Crowe, 2018). Thus, a clinician might expect somewhat lower PCCs from multilinguals who speak Jordanian Arabic, Icelandic, Spanish, Turkish or Hungarian. *The acquisition of accurate consonant production is language-specific rather than universal, with some consonants typically on the later side.*

Myth 5: Consonants are Acquired at the Same Age Crosslinguistically

The belief that consonants across are acquired at roughly by the same age by children from diverse language backgrounds (Sander, 1972) is unfounded. There was a paucity of multilingual/crosslinguistic research in the 1970s and it was taken for granted that the estimates were valid for all typically developing children. Crosslinguistic research has since shown that, for example, the voiced palatal approximant /j/, which occurs in many of the world's languages has language-specific ages of acquisition in monolinguals. In Cantonese, /j/ is acquired between 1;3 and 2;1 (A. C. Y. Tse, 1991; Cheung, 1990; S. M. Tse, 1982; So & Dodd, 1995), and in Thai between 2;1 and 2;6 (Boonyathitisuk, 1982) or between 3;1 and 3;6 (Dardaranada, 1993). Icelandic children acquire /j/ between 2;6 and 2;11 (Másdóttir et al., 2021) while German-speaking children learn it by 3;0 to 3;5 (Fox & Dodd, 1999). Hungarian-speaking youngsters acquire /j/ between 3;0 and 4;0 (Nagy, 1980); and Japanese-speaking children, between 2;10–3;0 (Takagi & Yasuda, 1967) to 4;0–4;5 (Nakanishi et al., 1972). In contrast, /j/ is acquired late in Jordanian Arabic, between 6;0 and 6;6 (Amayreh, 2003; Amayreh & Dyson, 1998). Thus, the *age of acquisition for /j/ is language specific, with a range of four years across the languages that have been studied to date.*

Myth 6: Acquisition Order of Consonant Clusters Is Uniform Crosslinguistically

In similar vein to Myth 5 and the overgeneralization of Sander's (1972) conclusions, it must not be assumed that cluster acquisition occurs at similar ages crosslinguistically. Yavaş (2013) suggests that children acquiring different languages vary in correctly producing word-initial /#sC/ clusters in a picture-naming task. Children learning Germanic languages (such as Afrikaans, English, Dutch and Norwegian) are more successful with producing accurate consonant clusters where the second element is a continuant vs. a non-continuant (e.g., /sw/ and /sl/ are 'easier' than /sn/ and /st/). Conversely, children acquiring non-Germanic languages (such as Hebrew, Croatian, and Polish) show no such dichotomy. This is an example of a language-group pattern in acquisition. *This specific pattern for children learning Germanic languages must be considered by SLPs/SLTs when evaluating cluster accuracy in multilingual children with one or more Germanic languages.*

Myth 7: Speech Sounds in the Same Syllable Position Behave Uniformally Crosslinguistically

Research into monolingual children's learning of phonotactics began in the early 1990s (Zamuner & Kharlamov, 2016), with Friederici and Wessels (1993). Crosslinguistic investigations came later, perhaps partly accounting for a small knowledgebase for phonotactics and phonotactic development across languages. SLPs/SLTs with access to accurate age-of-acquisition differences in phonotactics in monolingual vs. multilingual children may find it beneficial. Over two decades ago, studies of Spanish-

German bilinguals demonstrated a higher rate of coda productions in Spanish bilinguals compared with monolinguals. Kehoe et al. (2001) and Lleó et al. (2003) argued that the source of the difference is that fewer constraints for coda consonants exist in Spanish. Here, we see an example of an acceleration process. That is, *an interlanguage effect that allows the acquisition of coda consonants earlier in bilinguals than in monolinguals.*

Myth 8: Certain Phonetic Features Do Not Change When a Language Learner Becomes a Multilingual

The phonetic inventories of multilinguals remain an under researched area with very little coverage in key textbooks (e.g., Ball, 2021; Shriberg et al., 2019; Williams et al., 2021) that include minimal to no sections on the developmental aspects of the phonetics of multilinguals. SLPs'/SLTs' clinical repertoires might be enhanced with better availability of information on *'interlanguage'* effects (Dickerson, 1975) such as segmental transfer phenomena (Fabiano-Smith & Goldstein, 2010). Sometimes, segments specific to one language 'transfer' to another language spoken by multilinguals, and at times, this can decrease their articulatory accuracy. Research on the development of VOT in multilinguals compared with monolinguals shows that multilingual children's stop systems display interlanguage effects in their categorical organization (Kehoe & Kannathasan, 2021; Lee & Iverson, 2012). Along with perceptual measures, *the importance of detailed phonetic analysis in the assessment and treatment of multilinguals cannot be overemphasized.*

Research Need

Further studies of diverse languages will help SLP/SLT clinicians and researchers understand and develop evidence-based procedures for the assessment and treatment of SSD in children speaking one or more non-English languages. Optimistically, the increased availability and widespread distribution of accurate, evidence-based information will help extinguish the myths discussed here.

Intercountry Adoption

Years before the 2008 Hague Convention on Protection of Children and Co-operation in Respect of Intercountry Adoption (the Convention) came into force, two of my nieces were adopted from mainland China, as infants. One, who was born in 1974 was raised in Taiwan, Scotland, and Australia, and the other, born in 1990 grew up in Canada. In those days, intercountry (or international) adoption of newborns and young babies was relatively usual in the industrialized world. The Convention is a multilateral treaty between Australia, Canada, China, Ireland, New Zealand, South Africa, the UK, the US, Vietnam and about 70 other countries. It provides safeguards for children and families involved in adoptions between participating countries and works to prevent the abduction, sale, or trafficking of children.

Nowadays, as Karen Pollock explains in A44, children adopted internationally (CAI) are generally *children* rather than babies. While some have typical developmental trajectories, many of them have identified special needs, health, or behaviour concerns; and/or have experienced psychological and emotional deprivation, poverty, malnutrition, and physical abuse; and/or have parental histories of mental illness; and/or were born through incest; and/or have had significant exposure Hepatitis C or D, and HIV/Aids. In general, they have only had exposure to a language of their birth country, or the language(s) of their carer(s), and either speak it, or are learning to, before they are exposed, unprepared, to the home country language. Because of the sudden language switch and poor or infrequent stimulation in orphanages, all children adopted internationally are potentially 'at risk' for speech-language delays.

Children Adopted Internationally (CAI) Who are Learning a Second First Language

Readers were introduced to **Dr. Karen Pollock** from the University of Alberta in Chapter 4 in the introduction to A20, Vowels and Vowel Disorders. Although her primary area of teaching and research is speech sound development and disorders, Karen

became interested in children who were adopted internationally as a new clinician in the early 1980s when she encountered a preschool client adopted from Korea with a profound SSD that was highly resistant to intervention. This interest was re-ignited in 1999 when she became the parent of a child adopted from China and participated in support groups for adoptive parents. She found that many parents had questions about speech-language expectations for their children, but at the time there was very little research available. What began as a personal interest quickly evolved into a line of research spanning more than 20 years and including children adopted from China, Haiti, and Ethiopia.

Q44.   Karen Pollock

What do we now know about the about the nature and course of speech-language acquisition in children adopted internationally (CAI)? When should we encourage parents to seek professional services, such as speech-language therapy or early intervention, and how can they be supported in the process? The current International Adoption landscape is marked by substantial changes. These changes include an overall drop in numbers of children adopted internationally; with a dramatic reduction in healthy infants finding new families overseas; and growth in the incidence of older children and children with special needs, especially from the People's Republic of China (PRC). What preparation, in terms of professional consultation, might parents undertake when planning to adopt a child from overseas with a known cognitive or communication disability, or loosely specified as so called additional needs?

A44.   Karen E. Pollock: The Continually Shifting Landscape of International Adoption

Parents have welcomed children from other countries into their homes through adoption for decades. Most children have come from Asia,

Eastern Europe, Africa, and South America, in response to dramatic situations including war, political upheaval, extreme poverty, social stigmatization, or strict population control policies. But the international adoption landscape is continually changing (Selman, 2009). Adoptions from South Korea started in 1953 and dominated through the 1970s and 1980s in North America but began to drop rapidly in 1989 when South Korea implemented a plan to gradually limit the program. From 1989 to 1991, thousands of children were adopted, throughout the industrialized world, from Romania following the collapse of the Ceausescu regime; the Romanian adoption program continued at a reduced level before closing in 2004. International adoptions from Russia and China started in the early 1990s and dominated for the next 20 years, both rising to a peak in 2004–05 before starting a steady decline. As adoptions from China and Russia decreased, those from other countries (e.g., Ethiopia, Guatemala, Haiti) increased.

Most research on speech-language development in Children Adopted Internationally (CAI) included children who were adopted between the mid-1990s and mid-2010s, when adoptions from Russia and China predominated. Since then, the Russian international adoption program has closed, and although adoptions from China are still possible, the number and type of adoptions have changed (U.S. Department of State, 2022). In 1999, children adopted from China were primarily infants (98% girls, 94% under 2 years of age, 49% under 1 year), 'left to be found' because of China's one-child policy and the high value placed on boys in Chinese culture historically. Most were reported to be in generally good health, although many arrived with growth and developmental delays or medical problems such as anaemia, Hepatitis B, or elevated lead levels. These were typically resolved with adequate nutrition and medical care post-adoption. In 2000, China implemented laws to allow older children and those with special needs to be adopted internationally and prospective adoptive families who already had biological children were required to be open to accepting children with special

needs (e.g., cleft lip and palate, heart defects, and other visible disabilities). Adoptions from China continued to rise through 2004–05, but subsequently there was a sharp decline in the overall number of children adopted from the PRC, presumably related to the relaxation of the one-child policy, which ended in 2016 under General Secretary Xi Jinping's leadership. At the same time, adoptions of boys, older children, and children with special needs increased. From 2005 to 2009, special needs adoptions rose from 14 to 66% in the US and from 6 to 34% in France (Miller et al., 2016). Today, nearly all CAI from China are older children or have special needs. In 2019, roughly half were boys, none were under 1 year, 31% were under 2 years, 35% were 3–4 years of age, and 34% were 5–13 years of age. In addition, many had pre-identified special needs such as cleft lip and palate, congenital heart disease, spina bifida, missing or malformed digits or limbs, and impaired vision or hearing, and others were found to have 'unexpected special needs' following placement, often involving behavioural or emotional problems (Miller et al., 2016). To date, there has been little research on language development in CAI adopted at older ages and even less on those with special needs.

Language Development in CAI – What do we Know?

No matter the circumstances, children adopted internationally (CAI) experience a unique pattern of linguistic exposure. They hear only the language of their birth country prior to adoption, and then, because most adoptive parents do not speak the child's birth language, they hear only the language of their adoptive family after adoption. Consequently, children lose their birth language abilities rapidly, within weeks according to some estimates. In essence, they become monolingual speakers of the adoption language shortly after adoption but have had insufficient time to acquire age-appropriate skills in the new language. Because language acquisition in CAI differs from that of other bilingual or second language learners, the term 'second first language' learners has been adopted (e.g., Roberts et al., 2005). Lacking the scaffold that ongoing first language capabilities provides, the reality for these children is that they are 'starting over' with learning the new language (Genesee & Delcenserie, 2016).

Early researchers of second first language acquisition anticipated delays based on two assumptions. First, they believed the second first language learning situation was bound to impact development detrimentally. Second, they expected early environmental deprivation related to orphanage care to evoke significant delays in cognition and language. Indeed, studies of children adopted from Romania during the early 1990s supported these hypotheses, with the prevalence of language delays shortly after arrival extending from 60 to 94% (e.g., Rutter & English and Romanian Adoptees (ERA) Study Team, 1998).

Findings from subsequent studies in the late 1990s through to the early 2000s, however, suggested that the extreme neglect/deprivation suffered by Romanian orphans and their struggles post-adoption were not typical of CAI generally. In fact, most CAI from Russia and China arriving under 2;0 demonstrate remarkable resilience following placement in an enriched environment. Although significant variation is observed during the first 12 months post-adoption (e.g., Pollock, 2005), most children adopted under 2;0 'catch up' to (or even exceed) norms for non-adopted monolingual peers following only a year or two of exposure to English (Roberts et al., 2005). Despite promising group trends, however, most studies have also reported that some (from 5 to 22%) CAI continue to struggle with the acquisition of English beyond two years post-adoption (Glennen & Bright, 2005) and additional exposure to the adoption language is not always sufficient to close the gap (Delcenserie et al., 2013; Roberts et al., 2005). SLPs/SLTs and researchers have also questioned whether CAI with average or better skills during the preschool years might encounter challenges with more complex and abstract language as they reach the school-age years, where language is critical for academic performance and literacy acquisition.

School-age language and literacy outcomes are mixed for children adopted under 2;0. Studies of children in early elementary grades, including those adopted from China, Russia, Haiti, and other countries, find that most perform at or above average compared to norming samples (e.g., Dalen & Theie, 2019; Delcenserie et al., 2013; Glennen, 2015, 2021; Glennen & Bright, 2005; Pollock, 2020; K. Scott et al., 2008). However, some have ongoing difficulties with morphosyntax, short-term memory, or social or pragmatic language skills. Interestingly, despite reported weaknesses in morphosyntax and short-term memory, Scott and colleagues found that phonological processing, reading comprehension and decoding skills of CAI were like those of non-adopted peers (K. A. Scott et al., 2013; K. Scott et al., 2008).

Overall, across multiple studies of children adopted under 2;0, it appears that vocabulary and reading are areas of strength during the early elementary years, presumably due to the enriched and stimulating environment post-adoption. Relative weaknesses in short-term memory, pragmatic and social skills, and expressive syntax may be linked to delayed onset of exposure to the adoption language and/or lingering effects of suboptimal pre-adoption care. Many parents report seeking additional educational support, including SLP/SLT provision, reading instruction, and general academic tutoring (Dalen & Theie, 2019; Glennen & Bright, 2005; K. Scott et al., 2008).

Less research has been completed with children adopted over 2;0. Older children have more fully developed birth language abilities and greater cognitive maturity, which may aid their transition to a new language, but they also may have spent more time in institutional settings. In addition, the older at adoption, the more language there is to learn to match age expectations. Glennen (2009) described this 'perfect storm' of issues surrounding children and the increasing challenges faced by children adopted at or nearing school-age. She found that children adopted from Eastern Europe between 2 and 5 years of age showed rapid growth in vocabulary and receptive language. However, one year later 40% still had below average expressive language skills and their utterances contained grammatical errors reflecting transfer or interference from Russian (e.g., incorrect use of articles, pronoun case errors, naming and word-finding errors), something not observed in children adopted under 2;0. A longitudinal study of children in Norway who were adopted between 4 and 15 years of age (from China, Russia,

Ethiopia, Haiti, Ghana, Columbia, and Ukraine) found a higher than expected percentage of children scoring below cut-offs for clinically significant impairments at 1, 2, and 3 years post-adoption (receptive language – 68%, 38%, 42%; expressive language – 68%, 57%, 32%; reading – 44%, 29%, 21%; Helder et al., 2016). Significant improvements from Year 1 to Year 3 were seen for receptive language and reading, but not for expressive language. At Year 3, the percentage of children with scores associated with clinical concerns was still higher than that seen for children adopted at younger ages.

CAI with pre-identified special needs have typically been excluded from research on speech-language development to avoid confounding factors. Interestingly, Tan et al. (2007) found no difference between CAI with and without special needs in parent reports of behavioural problems or developmental delays at adoption; however, they did not include specific measures of language development. One subgroup of special needs adoptions that has received some attention in the literature is children with cleft palate, who are likely to undergo surgery later or require secondary surgery post-adoption. Although most reports focus on medical care and surgical treatment, Morgan, et al. (2017) examined language development in two groups of children with cleft palate, one adopted from China and the other nonadopted. Both groups demonstrated mild delays in language development, but those who had been adopted tended to perform more poorly, especially those who were adopted at older ages. While language development appears to be only mildly impacted, a retrospective review of CAI with cleft lip and/or palate (Kaye et al., 2019) found that the CAI were more likely to have moderate to severe articulation disorders (79%) and many had persistent articulation issues years after adoption.

Speech Sound Development in CAI – What do we Know?

There has been surprisingly little research specifically on speech acquisition in second first language learners (Pollock, 2007 for a detailed summary of the available studies). In two longitudinal small-N studies (Pollock et al., 2003; Price et al., 2006) of children adopted from China as infants/toddlers, the researchers found considerable individual variation in early phonological measures, such as canonical babbling ratio, phonetic inventory size and diversity, and proportion of monosyllables. However, the majority (7 out of 8) of participants performed within normal limits on a standardized articulation test at 3;0 and/or had normal range PCCs and none of the early speech measures taken at 6 months post-adoption predicted performance at 3;0.

Small group studies of infants/toddlers adopted from Russia and China (Glennen, 2007; Roberts et al., 2005) found that only 7–11% had below average articulation scores when compared to test norms 1–2 years post-adoption. More detailed analyses, including PCC-Revised, PMLU, and phonological processes were reported by Pollock (2007, 2020) for children adopted from China and Haiti. Mostly, they produced developmental errors comparable to those of non-adopted peers, such as cluster reduction, stopping, and gliding.

Importantly, no studies have reported evidence of cross-linguistic interference from the birth language in the speech of children adopted under 2;0. In contrast, anecdotal reports of children adopted at older ages frequently include examples of birth language interference, like those seen in child second language learners. For Glennen (2014, 2016) reported that children adopted from Russia at 4 years of age fronted English /dʒ/ and /tʃ/ to their Russian affricate equivalents /dz/ ad /ts/ and those adopted at 5 years had vowel and syllable stress errors; however, these interference errors decreased over the first year and scores on single word articulation tests matched age expectations 12–15 months post-adoption.

Implications for Assessment and Intervention with CAI – When and How to Seek Help

Assessing the second first language abilities of CAI presents challenges for SLPs/SLTs, particularly during the first year post-adoption. While the birth language is undergoing rapid attrition and the transition to the emerging adopted language is proceeding, it is difficult (if not impossible) to determine whether apparent delays relate to this natural transition or are evidence of developmental communication delays that predated adoption.

It is essential to gather as much information as possible on the child's development in the birth language; this is especially true for children adopted at older ages. Glennen (2009) shared a list of pre-adoption questions specifically for children adopted at older ages, including questions about literacy and academic abilities for children old enough to have attend school in the birth country. Signs of delayed development in the birth language should be considered true delays or disorders and warrant SLP/SLT services upon arrival; delaying services while the child transitions to the adoption language will likely not resolve underlying disorders that existed pre-adoption.

In newly adopted younger children (under 2 years), assessments should focus more on universal (non-language-specific) measures such as joint attention, gestures, symbolic play, quantity and quality of vocalizations, and number of different consonants produced (Glennen, 2007; Pollock, 2005). Language-specific measures, such as vocabulary and utterance length, may also be used to determine the rate of acquisition of the adoption language over the first one- or two-years post-adoption but should be compared to reference data (or local norms) for other CAI adopted from Eastern Europe and China at similar ages (Glennen, 2014, 2016; Pollock, 2005, 2020). Children who are progressing at a slower pace than their CAI peers should be referred for early intervention.

Children adopted as pre-schoolers (2–5 years of age) should begin speaking in the adoption language soon after adoption. The older they are, the more quickly they learn new words. For example, Glennen (2016) reported that within 3 months post-adoption, children adopted at 2 years produced 64 words on average, but those adopted at 3 or 4 years produced over 160 words and were beginning to combine words. CAI not demonstrating rapid growth in vocabulary in the new language should be referred for a thorough assessment that includes hearing and non-verbal cognition as well as speech sound production, receptive and expressive language, and utterance length. Standardized tests may be used to gather information and to identify strengths and weaknesses, but scores should not be used to make clinical decisions. Although limited local norms are available for children adopted over 2;0, they are useful in determining appropriate expectations for CAI (Glennen, 2016). Spontaneous language sample analysis and dynamic assessment methods are also important in obtaining a more complete picture of the child's communication abilities and potential.

Following a reasonable transition period, standardized tests normed on monolingual speakers of the adoption language may be used with CAI. Glennen (2016) suggests the following guidelines for transition time: 12–17 months at adoption – 9 months; 18–35 months at adoption – 15 months; 3–4 years at adoption – 3 years. However, she also notes that receptive language and speech sound production abilities may require less time, while expressive language (especially MLU) may take longer. An estimated transition time for children adopted over 5 years is not available. Because attrition is so rapid in CAI, direct assessments in the birth language are valid only if completed within a few months of arrival. Standardized tests in the adoption language should be interpreted with caution and alternative evidence from language sample analysis or dynamic assessment used to supplement test scores.

Any child adopted internationally is potentially 'at risk' for speech-language delays, by virtue of the abrupt language switch and inadequate stimulation in orphanages. This necessitates parents being watchful regarding development during the first year at home, and, if concerns emerge, seeking an SLP/SLT opinion. As a rule of thumb for families, if vocabulary, utterance length, and intelligibility gains are sluggish, a comprehensive speech-language evaluation is indicated, and intervention may be necessary. For older children and those with pre-identified special needs, the situation is more complicated, as they face additional medical considerations. In such cases, a coordinated multidisciplinary assessment and intervention plan is essential.

Miller et al. (2016) provide an excellent overview of how changing trends in international adoption impact the amount and type of pre-adoption preparation and post-adoption support that parents need. Consultation with a paediatric adoption medicine specialist is recommended both before and after adoption. Prior to adoption, they can provide an overview of the scope of pre-identified and unexpected special needs typically encountered and counsel the family as they consider which diagnosis (or diagnoses) they are willing/able to accept. Once a referral is received, the adoption specialist can assist in reviewing the documentation provided, identify uncertainties (e.g., red flags for additional syndromes), educate the parents about specific conditions and treatments/outcomes, and if necessary, seek additional feedback from other specialists (e.g., cardiologists, surgeons). Upon arrival, they can complete a full examination, manage medical conditions, and coordinate referrals for sub-specialty care. In addition to the paediatrician, Miller et al. stress the importance of psychological/psychiatric support and counselling, as well as supports available through other adoption professionals (e.g., social workers) and parent support groups. The importance of support from 'experienced adoption-sensitive' individuals cannot be overstated and is critical to establishing realistic expectations and facilitating positive outcomes.

The same is true for speech-language professionals; not every SLP/SLT is experienced in working with CAI and familiar with the growing research base and evidence-based guidelines. Newly adopted toddlers are frequently assessed by early intervention teams and provided speech-language intervention, even though they are *already* functioning at the top of their peer group according to local norms. At the other extreme, stories of older internationally adopted children being denied services are even more concerning, with schools insisting that children be placed in ESL classrooms rather than receive SLP/SLT services. ESL programs are not designed to meet the needs of second first language learners or children with language delays/impairments. Parents and SLPs/SLTs must familiarize themselves with current research and be prepared to advocate for appropriate services and educate other professionals and administrators about the unique circumstances of children adopted internationally and the nature of second first language acquisition.

Protracted Phonological Development

So, what do we mean by protracted phonological development? We mean simply that phonological, or speech development happens over an extended or protracted period. The term 'speech sound disorders' is currently more in vogue and common but focuses its attention on speech sounds rather than all the parts of speech and its structure and contains the negative term 'disorders'. We prefer a term that has a positive connotation – we don't know if the person will develop the speech that is typical of their target area, but we'd like to give them the hope that they could.

Bernhardt et al., 2014

The words above are from a video tutorial (https://phonodevelopment.sites.olt.ubc.ca) in which readers can discover more about the work of the authors of Q45, Drs. Barbara May Bernhardt, Daniel Bérubé, and Glenda Mason in the international crosslinguistic research project on children's phonological acquisition.

Dr. Barbara May Bernhardt is a Professor Emerita, School of Audiology and Speech Sciences, University of British Columbia, Registered Speech-Language Pathologist (Inactive). Barbara May Bernhardt was on faculty at the University of British Columbia from 1990 to 2017 and has been a speech-language pathologist since 1972. Her primary focus is phonological development, assessment, and intervention across languages. In collaboration with co-investigator Dr. Joseph Paul Stemberger of the University of British Columbia and colleagues in over 15 countries, she has been conducting an international crosslinguistic project in children's phonological acquisition (phonodevelopment.sites.olt.ubc.ca) since 2004. Other areas of expertise include the utilization of ultrasound in speech therapy, language development, assessment and intervention, and approaches to service delivery for Indigenous people in Canada. The 'magic' of language keeps her engaged in voluntary work post-retirement, but she is finding more time for singing, dancing, cycling, cross-country skiing, hiking and most importantly, family and friends.

Dr. Daniel Bérubé is a speech-language pathologist and a faculty member of the speech-language pathology program at the University of Ottawa. He teaches courses pertaining to speech sound disorders and language disorders in school-aged children. Since 2013, he has collaborated on an international cross-linguistic project in phonological development. Other ongoing research include a Health Canada project assessing the oral language and pre-literacy skills of bilingual French-English children as well as a Consortium National de Formation en Santé project to standardize a screening tool to evaluate speech intelligibility in bilingual French-English speaking children. He is a father of two children who have grown up bilingual. His advice to living a healthy lifestyle is to spend time in mountains and to ignore things that cannot be controlled.

Dr. Glenda Mason is a Lecturer and Research Associate, Registered Speech-Language Pathologist, School of Audiology and Speech Sciences, University of British Columbia, Vancouver, Canada. Glenda Mason has over 30 years of clinical experience, mostly school based. Her major clinical research interest, phonological development in multisyllabic words, was motivated by observations of ongoing phonological and literacy difficulties for school-aged children with 'normalized' speech in short words. Glenda's focus has been on quantifying whole-word accuracy in multisyllabic words through application of an interactive nonlinear phonological framework. On that basis, she has developed a metric that has been integrated into Phon (Hedlund & Rose, 2020). Glenda's goal is to use the metric to acquire Canadian normative data, and to investigate speech production variability for both face-to-face and virtual assessment environments. Glenda also teaches graduate courses in developmental phonological and language/literacy disorders.

Q45.   Barbara May Bernhardt, Daniel Bérubé and Glenda Mason: Constraint-based Non-linear Phonology across Languages

Could you please update readers on developments in applications of constraint-based non-linear phonology for the analysis of developmental data, particularly as they concern findings from your international crosslinguistic research, since 2013. What are the implications of your findings for clinical practice?

A45.   Barbara May Bernhardt, Daniel Bérubé and Glenda Mason: Constraints-based Nonlinear Phonology – Updates in the Crosslinguistic Context

Researchers have been studying phonological development in a variety of languages within the framework of constraints-based nonlinear phonology since the 1990s. In this update, we review the framework and outline key findings since 2013 from a crosslinguistic project, exemplifying the investigatory process with one language, French, and looking to the future.

Constraints-based Nonlinear Phonology

Nonlinear ('multilinear') theories (as theorized in linguistics) describe hierarchically organized levels ('tiers') of autonomous phonological form: the phrase, word, foot, syllable, onset/rime, timing unit, segment, feature (manner, laryngeal place). Speech production (output) is the result of competition (ranking) between various positive (survival/faithfulness) and negative (prohibition/markedness) constraints. For example, if a negative constraint prohibiting consonants in syllable-final position (codas) is stronger (higher-ranked) than constraints promoting survival of certain consonants or features, no codas will appear in output. If survival of codas is more important than their actual content, a default consonant may appear in coda to preserve structure (e.g., [ʔ]). Phonological development entails 'shifts' in the relative importance of the various constraints across the hierarchy. In our crosslinguistic project we set out to compare phonological development among languages for children with typical (TD) and protracted phonological development (PPD).

The Crosslinguistic Project: From 2013

Following a research program initiated by Bernhardt (1990), an international crosslinguistic project in phonological development started in 2003 with Angela Ullrich of Germany and was later funded by a Canadian federal funding agency (SSHRC 410–2009–0348, 611–2012–0164). For each language, investigators: (1) create phonological assessment tools based on the same (nonlinear) principles; (2) conduct and report on studies of various aspects of the phonological hierarchy; (3) educate clinicians regarding practice; and (4) where possible, share data on Phonbank located at www.phon.ca. The project has given rise to many publications, some of which are displayed in Table A45.10.1, and a discussion of key outcomes follows.

Table A45.1 Crosslinguistic project: Selected publications since 2013

Language[a]	Group Data	Domain(s)	Case-based: Analysis [An], Treatment [Tx]
Akan	Amoako et al. (2020)	**All**	
Bulgarian	Bernhardt et al. (2019)	**Consonants**	
English	Mason (2018a)	**Multisyllabic words**	Feehan et al. (2015): **PPD Tx**
French (Canada)	Bérubé et al. (2020)	**Interaction: Structure, consonants**	Bérubé et al. (2015a), **PPD An.**
German	Bernhardt et al. (2014) Romonath and Bernhardt (2017)	**Word-initial fricatives** **Word structure**	
Greek			Babatsouli (2019), **TD An.**
Kuwaiti Arabic	Ayyad et al. (2016)	**Consonants**	
Spanish	Bernhardt et al. (2015)	**Word structure**	
Swedish			Lundeborg Hammarström and Stembergerss (2022), Tx.
Tagalog	Chen et al., 2016		
Multiple	Stemberger and Bernhardt (2018)	Word-initial clusters with tap/trill, singleton /ɾ/, /r/ /l/ Whole Word Match	

Additional assessment tools are available for Anishinaabemowin (Ojibwe), Brazilian Portuguese, Farsi, Polish, Punjabi, Tagalog and French of France at phonodevelopment.sites.olt.ubc.ca.

Key Outcomes

1. Whole Word Match (WWM)

WWM indicates match of the *whole word* with the target: consonants, vowels, stress, segment length. SLPs/SLTs/researchers can set criterion-based cut-offs in WWM to distinguish PPD/TD. Across languages, Bérubé et al. (2020) found preliminary cut-off levels of 40–45% WWM for 3-year-olds, 50–60% for 4-year-olds, and 60–75% for 5-year-olds. As more data are collected, this measure will increase in specificity/sensitivity but already has potential for identification of PPD in multilingual assessment. The SLP/SLT can observe whether a child's whole-word productions match the target transcriptions without transcribing the child's productions. In comparing the child's WWM across the child's languages, the SLP/SLT can then consider whether a child's presumed PPD in the SLP's/SLT's language is a result of additional language learning or represents a more pervasive difficulty in phonological development. If the latter, phonetic transcription, and phonological analysis would ensue. Early results in an SLP/SLT listener study suggest that SLPs/SLTs can judge WWM relatively well even in unfamiliar languages, indicating clinical promise for this measure.

2. Structure-segment Interactions

Studies continue to demonstrate the vital importance of examining word structure influences on segment (consonant and vowel) production, e.g., a special issue of *Clinical Linguistics & Phonetics*, 2018 on clusters with tap/trill, *32*(5–6), e.g., Stemberger and Bernhardt (2018); Mason (2018b); Bernhardt et al. (2019); Bérubé et al. (2020).

3. Word Structure in Intervention

Treatment studies continue to show the value of targeting word structure for accelerating developmental progress in children with constraints in both word structure and segments (Feehan et al., 2015, English; Lundeborg et al., 2019, Swedish).

4. Feature Combination Effects

Children's segments (consonants/vowels) may show production of many phonological features of a language but a lack of feature combinations that make up the full segmental inventory. A combinatorial view of segments (e.g., Bernhardt et al., 2014, German/English) provides therapeutic strategies aimed at drawing links between related phoneme classes (Feehan et al., 2015, English).

5. Inventory Differences Create Different Opportunities in Multilingual Intervention

Segments of a language's inventory are more likely to appear as substitutions in that language than in a language without those targets (Bernhardt et al., 2014, for German/English). Further, if a feature is part of many different segments in a language, it is more likely to appear in substitutions than in a language where it is less frequent, e.g., [+spread glottis] in Icelandic is present in /h/, voiceless fricatives, voiceless sonorants, pre-/post-aspirated stops, and substitutions often contain that feature (Bernhardt, Hanson et al., 2015: Icelandic versus English). Treatment strategies can exploit these differences in a multilingual context, taking content from one language to support change in another.

A Canadian French Example

We turn now to Daniel Bérubé who briefly recounts his involvement for Canadian French in the crosslinguistic project and applications to multilingual research.

Initially, research into Canadian French phonology was guided by linear phonological frameworks (e.g., MacLeod et al., 2011). The crosslinguistic project, based on nonlinear phonology, posited that principles of phonology required going beyond single consonants to consider consonant-vowel interactions, syllables, and properties of whole words. In addition, nonlinear theories were supported by clinical observations that children may appear to have similar phonologies but differ in the complexity of the words that are attempted and produced (Bérubé & McLeod, 2022). The crosslinguistic project has guided research and clinical outcomes about phonology for monolingual and multilingual children who speak Canadian French. Outcomes include: (1) two assessment tools: (a) a screening tool: *Test de phonologie du rançais canadien – dépistage* (Bérubé et al., 2015a, [Test of French Canadian phonology – Screening]) and a similar but expanded full assessment measure, i.e., *Test de phonologie du français canadien* (Bérubé et al., 2013; [Test of Canadian French phonology]); (2) a study showing the influence of word structure constraints on segment production (Bérubé et al., 2020); (3) educating clinicians on how to implement nonlinear analysis for assessment (Bérubé et al., 2020) and goal setting (Bérubé et al., 2015a, 2015b) and educating students through coursework; and (4) data sharing of Phon analyses (Hedlund & Rose, 2020) to facilitate knowledge mobilization (Bérubé et al., 2020), with future sharing through Phonbank planned. From its monolingual beginnings, the Canadian French section of the project has considered Canada's multilingual context as an officially bilingual French-English country with over 60 indigenous languages and many immigrant languages. In upcoming studies, we will: a) examine how environmental factors and language structure influence phonological development and vocabulary in bilingual children (English/Arabic, English/French, English/Spanish and more); and b) collect normative data for bilingual children's phonology and vocabulary skills in their spoken languages and examine how these abilities are associated with reading acquisition.

Quo Vadimus?

The crosslinguistic study has focused on preschool children, aged 3 to 5 years. As school-aged children develop their phonology, some may need continued support for resolution of residual rhotic or sibilant mismatches and/or multisyllabic word (MSW) production. Strengthening phonological knowledge and production skills also provides a stronger foundation for literacy development. Mason (2018a, 2018b) has addressed later phonological acquisition for English, particularly MSW development.

Mason (2018b) evaluated a metric for evaluating nonlinear phonological components of MSWs. The phonological aspects of the metric were incorporated into Phon (Hedlund & Rose, 2020) as the *Multisyllabic Nonlinear Analysis* (MNLA) and streamlines computation at all levels of phonology: the whole word, word structure and segments/features, individual components. Mason (2018a) also designed a flipbook test to elicit productions in English: *Comprehensive Assessment of Multisyllabic Words; CAMSWə*. The *CAMSWə* includes 42 mono- and di-syllables with relatively simple word structure, and 44 two- to five–syllable MSWs with a subset of 15 more challenging MSWs to evaluate variability/consistency. This word list was adapted from word lists in the *Computerized Articulation and Phonology Evaluation System* (Masterson & Bernhardt, 2001). Normative data collection for *CAMSWə* is currently underway for monolingual and bilingual speakers in Canada (of the largest language groups: Cantonese, Mandarin, Punjabi, Tagalog). Procedures have been adapted for virtual administration, a foundation for future virtual clinical application.

Further to future planning, the study in WWM perception is a foundation for new training tools for SLPs/SLTS in multilingual assessment. We will also continue to build criterion referenced measures for clinical applications from our databases for the various languages and add to our project website as tools and measures become available.

Recommended Resources

The project website, https://phonodevelopment.sites.olt.ubc.ca (Bernhardt & Stemberger, 2015, updated 2021), provides tutorials on transcription and nonlinear analysis, many free test materials and resources, and treatment activity videos in several languages (plus secret bonus footage)!

Acknowledgments

The authors thank the many collaborators and research assistants for the project, and in particular, Dr. Joseph P. Stemberger, linguist and lead co-investigator at the University of British Columbia.

The Topic of Change

The authors in Chapter 10 all address the topic of change. Michelle Pascoe (A39) was impelled to change the status quo when her students, who were first-language speakers of the indigenous South African languages: Setswana, SiSwati, and isiXhosa, asked where they could find information on speech and language acquisition in languages other than English, only to find very little that was helpful. Pascoe and her colleagues, some of whom were students, were bent on rectifying the situation. The changes that followed included preliminary normative data and assessment tools for, isiXhosa, isiZulu, Setswana, and adaptations of *The Intelligibility in Context Scale* into South Africa's 11 official languages (Pascoe & McLeod, 2016). This important endeavour is ongoing.

The change agenda for Benjamin Munson and Alayo Tripp (A40) revolves around language variation and change through a sociophonetics lens. They call for SLPs/SLTs who haven't already done so, to move beyond *only* considering cognitive, linguistic, perceptual, and motor factors to explain an individual's SSD, and become cognisant of the potential roles of sociolinguistic knowledge and social preferences in children's learning, and embrace the inclusivity that comes with that.

Brian Goldstein (A41) also suggests that SLPs/SLTs may need to change, particularly in terms of changing set when approaching increasing caseloads of multilingual children with SSD. This might involve dispelling persistent myths about crosslinguistic acquisition (examined by Zajdó, A43), upgrading cultural competence (and possibly abandoning some misperceptions), and studying the extensive current research literature on multilingualism and the role of the parents of multilingual children in assessment and intervention (Jensen de López et al., 2021).

The contribution by Sharynne McLeod and Kathryn Crowe (A42) embodies two examples of change. First, the incredible changes that occur cross-linguistically, over a comparatively short time, in typically developing children's speech acquisition and intelligibility. Second, their analysis of consonant acquisition by children growing up speaking English in the US stimulated what seemed like a seismic shift in the normative reference data available to SLPs, changing their expectations for typical consonant acquisition, particularly for /ɹ/ (Harold, 2018; updated 2019, 2020).

In A43, Krisztina Zajdó, who is on a mission to change unhelpful beliefs about multilingual children learning two or more languages, challenges eight unhelpful myths. Karen Pollock (A44) explains the changes that have occurred in international adoption, describing it as a constantly shifting landscape, and the changes that children (as opposed to babies) adopted internationally usually experience, emotionally, environmentally, culturally, linguistically, and socially. Barbara May Bernhardt, Daniel Bérubé and Glenda Mason (A48) describe the changes – in the form of impressive progress – that have occurred in the international crosslinguistic research project since 2013.

The change theme continues in Chapter 11, where changes in technology, and developments in professional communication are addressed, while Chapter 12 contains a discussion of practice-change.

References

Amayreh, M. M. (2003). Completion of the consonant inventory of Arabic. *Journal of Speech, Language, and Hearing Research*, 46(3), 517–529. https://doi.org/10.1044/1092-4388(2003/042)

Amayreh, M. M., & Dyson, A. T. (1998). The acquisition of Arabic consonants. *Journal of Speech, Language, and Hearing Research*, 41(3), 642–653. https://doi.org/10.1044/jslhr.4103.642

American Speech-Language-Hearing Association. (n.d.). *Learning two languages.* https://www.asha.org/public/speech/development/learning-two-languages

Amoako, W. K., Stemberger, J. P., Bernhardt, B. M., & Tessier, A.-M. (2020). Acquisition of consonants among typically developing Akan-speaking children: A preliminary report. *International Journal of Speech-Language Pathology*, *22*(6), 626–636. https://doi.org/10.1080/17549507.2020.1825804

Ayyad, H. S., Bernhardt, B. M., & Stemberger, J. P. (2016). Kuwaiti Arabic. Acquisition of singleton consonants. *International Journal of Language & Communication Disorders*, *51*(5), 531–545. https://doi.org/10.1111/1460-6984.12229

Babatsouli, E. (2019). A phonological assessment test for child Greek. *Clinical Linguistics & Phonetics*, *33*(7), 601–627. https://doi.org/10.1080/02699206.2019.1569164

Ball, M. (Ed.). (2021). *Manual of clinical phonetics.* Routledge.

Bauman-Waengler, J. (2020). *Articulation and phonology in speech sound disorders: A clinical focus* (6th ed.). Pearson.

Bernhardt, B. (1990). *The application of nonlinear phonological theory to intervention with six phonologically disordered children.* Unpublished doctoral dissertation, University of British Columbia.

Bernhardt, B. M., Hanson, R., Perez, D., Ávila, C., Lleó, C., Stemberger, J. P., Carballo, G., Mendoza, E., Fresneda, D., & Chávez-Peón, M. (2015). Word structures of Granada Spanish-speaking preschoolers with typical versus protracted phonological development. *International Journal of Language & Communication Disorders*, *50*(3), 298–311. https://doi.org/10.1111/1460-6984.12133

Bernhardt, B. M., Ignatova, D., Amoako, W., Aspinall, N., Marinova-Todd, S., Stemberger, J. P., & Yokota, K. (2019). Bulgarian consonant acquisition in preschoolers with typical versus protracted phonological development. *Journal of Monolingual and Bilingual Speech*, *1*(2), 143–181. https://doi.org/10.1558/jmbs.v1i2.11801

Bernhardt, B. M., Romonath, R., & Stemberger, J. P. (2014). A comparison of fricative acquisition in German and Canadian English-speaking children with protracted phonological development. In M. Yavas (Ed.), *Unusual productions in phonology: Universals and language-specific considerations* (pp. 102–127). Psychology Press.

Bernhardt, B. M., & Stemberger, J. P. (2015, updated 2021). https://phonodevelopment.sites.olt.ubc.ca

Bérubé, D., Bernhardt, B. M., & Stemberger, J. (2013). Un test de phonologie du français: Construction et utilisation. *Canadian Journal of Speech-Language-Pathology and Audiology*, *37*(1), 26–40.

Bérubé, D., Bernhardt, B. M., & Stemberger, J. P. (2015a). A test of Canadian French phonology: Construction and use. *Canadian Journal of Speech-Language Pathology and Audiology*, *39*(1), 61–100. https://cjslpa.ca/files/2015_CJSLPA_Vol_39/No_01/CJSLPA_Spring_2015_Vol_39_No_1_Berube_et_al.pdf

Bérubé, D., Bernhardt, B. M., Stemberger, J. P., & Bertrand, A. (2015b). Analyse phonologique en français manitobain: étude de cas selon la phonologie non linéaire [Phonological analysis in Manitoba French: Case study in nonlinear phonology]. *Rééducation orthophonique*, *253*, 105–148.

Bérubé, D., Bernhardt, B. M., Stemberger, J. P., & Ciocca, V. (2020). Development of singleton consonants in French-speaking children with typical versus protracted phonological development: The influence of word length, word shape and stress. *International Journal of Speech-Language Pathology*, *22*(6), 637–647. https://doi.org/10.1080/17549507.2020.1829706

Bérubé, D., & McLeod, A. A. M. (2022). A comparison of two phonological screening tools for French-speaking children. *International Journal of Speech-Language Pathology*, *24*(1), 22–32. https://doi.org/10.1080/17549507.2021.1936174

Bishop, D. V. M., & Adams, C. (1990). A prospective study of the relationship between specific language impairment, phonological disorders and reading retardation. *The Journal of Child Psychology and Psychiatry*, *31*(7), 1027–1050. https://doi.org/10.1111/j.1469-7610.1990.tb00844.x

Blackburn, J. F. (2012). The effect of dialect instruction on student knowledge of and attitudes toward African American English. *Communication Disorders Quarterly*, *34*(4), 220–229. https://doi.org/10.1177%2F1525740111430524

Bleile, K. M. (2020). *Speech sound disorders for class and clinic* (4th ed.). Plural.

Bleses, D., Basbøll, H., & Vach, W. (2011). Is Danish difficult to acquire? Evidence from Nordic past-tense studies. *Language and Cognitive Processes*, *26*(8), 1193–1231. https://doi.org/10.1080/0169096 5.2010.515107

Boonyathitisuk, P. (1982). *Articulatory characteristics of kindergarten children aged three to four years eleven months in Bangkok*. [Unpublished Master's thesis]. Mahidol University.

Chambers, J. K. (2007). *Sociolinguistics*. The Blackwell encyclopedia of sociology.

Chen, R.K., Bernhardt, B.M., & Stemberger, J.P. (2016). Phonological assessment and analysis tools for Tagalog: Preliminary development. *Clinical Linguistics & Phonetics*, *30*(8), 599–627. https://doi.org/10.3109/02699206.2016.1157208

Cheung, P. (1990). *The acquisition of Cantonese phonology in Hong Kong: A cross-sectional study*. [Unpublished B.Sc. project]. University College London.

Clark, E. V. (2016). *First language acquisition* (3rd ed.). Cambridge University Press.

Clausen, M. C., & Fox-Boyer, A. (2017). Phonological development in Danish-speaking children: A normative cross-sectional study. *Clinical Linguistics & Phonetics*, *31*(6), 440–458. https://doi.org/10.1080/02699206.2017.1308014

Coplan, J., & Gleason, J. R. (1988). Unclear speech: Recognition and significance of unintelligible speech in preschool children. *Pediatrics*, *82*(3), 447–452. PMID: 3405680

Crowe, K., & McLeod, S. (2020). Children's English consonant acquisition in the United States: A review. *American Journal of Speech-Language Pathology*, *29*(4), 2155–2169. https://doi.org/10.1044/2020_AJSLP-19-00168

Dalen, M., & Theie, S. (2019). Academic achievement among adopted and nonadopted children in early school years. *Adoption Quarterly*, *22*(3), 199–218. https://doi.org/10.1080/10926755.2019.1627448

Dardarananda, R. (1993). *The life and work of professor Dardarananda: Collection of articles from Ramathibodi hospital*. Division of Communicative Disorders, Mahidol University.

Davis, B. L. (2007). Applications of typical acquisition information to understanding of speech impairment. In S. McLeod (Ed.), *The international guide to speech acquisition* (pp. 50–54). Thomson Delmar Learning.

Delcenserie, A., Genesee, F., & Gautier, K. (2013). Language abilities of internationally adopted children from China during the early school years: Evidence for early age effects? *Applied Psycholinguistics*, *34*(3), 541–568. https://doi.org/10.1017/S0142716411000865

Dickerson, L. J. (1975). The learner's interlanguage as a system of variable rules. *TESOL Quarterly*, *9*(4), 401–407. https://doi.org/10.2307/3585624

Dodd, B. (2005). *Differential diagnosis and treatment of children with speech disorder* (2nd ed.). Whurr Publishers.

Dodd, B., Holm, D., & Li, W. (1997). Speech dis- order in preschool children exposed to Cantonese and English. *Clinical Linguistics and Phonetics*, *11*, 229–243. https://doi.org/10.3109/02699209708985193

Donegan, P. J. (2013). Normal vowel acquisition. In M. J. Ball & F. E. Gibbon (Eds.), *Handbook of vowels and vowel disorders* (pp. 24–60). Taylor & Francis.

Eckert, P. (2008). Variation and the indexical field 1. *Journal of Sociolinguistics*, *12*(4), 453–476. https://doi.org/10.1111/j.1467-9841.2008.00374.x

Fabiano-Smith, L., & Barlow, J. A. (2010). Interaction in bilingual phonological acquisition: Evidence from phonetic inventories. *International Journal of Bilingual Education and Bilingualism*, *13*(1), 81–97. https://doi.org/10.1080/13670050902783528

Fabiano-Smith, L., & Goldstein, B. A. (2010). Phonological acquisition in bilingual Spanish-English speaking children. *Journal of Speech, Language, and Hearing Research*, *53*(1), 160–178. https://doi.org/10.1044/1092-4388(2009/07-0064)

Feehan, A., Francis, C., Bernhardt, B. M., & Colozzo, P. (2015). Outcomes of phonological and morphosyntactic intervention for twin boys with protracted speech and language development. *Child Language Teaching and Therapy*, *31*, 53–69. http://dx.doi.org/10.1177/0265659014536205

Fey, M. E. (1986). *Language intervention in young children*. College Hill Press.

Fogle, P. T. (2020). *Essentials of communication sciences and disorders* (2nd ed.). Jones & Bartlett Learning.

Foulkes, P., Docherty, G. J., & Watt, D. (2005). Phonological variation in child-directed speech. *Language*, *81*(1), 177–206. https://doi.org/10.1353/lan.2005.0018

Fox, A. V., & Dodd, B. J. (1999). Der Erwerb des phonologischen Systems in der deutschen Sprache. *Sprache-Stimme-Gehör*, *23*, 183–191. https://doi.org/10.1055/s-2004-835864

Friederici, A. D., & Wessels, J. M. (1993). Phonotactic knowledge and its use in infant speech perception. *Perception & Psychophysics*, *54*(3), 287–295. https://doi.org/10.3758/bf03205263

Fung, P., Schertz, J., & Johnson, E. K. (2021). The development of gendered speech in children: Insights from adult L1 and L2 perceptions. *JASA Express Letters*, *1*(1), 014407. https://doi.org/10.1121/10.0003322

Genesee, F., & Delcenserie, A. (2016). *Starting over – The language development in internationally-adopted children*. John Benjamins. https://doi.org/10.1075/tilar.18

Gildersleeve-Neumann, C., Kester, E., Davis, B., & Peña, E. (2008). English speech sound development in preschool-aged children from bilingual English-Spanish backgrounds. *Language, Speech, and Hearing Services in Schools*, *39*(3), 314–328. https://doi.org/10.1044/0161-1461(2008/030)

Glennen, S. (2007). Predicting language outcomes for internationally adopted children. *Journal of Speech, Language, and Hearing Research*, *50*(2), 529–548. https://doi.org/10.1044/1092-4388(2007/036)

Glennen, S. (2009). Speech and language guidelines for children adopted from abroad at older ages. *Topics in Language Disorders*, *29*(1), 50–64. http://dx.doi.org/10.1097/TLD.0b013e3181976df4

Glennen, S. (2014). A longitudinal study of language and speech in children who were internationally adopted at different ages: Outcomes and assessment guidelines. *Language, Speech, and Hearing Services in Schools*, *45*(3), 185–203. https://doi.org/10.1044/2014_lshss-13-0035

Glennen, S. (2015). Internationally adopted children in the early school years: Relative strengths and weaknesses in language abilities. *Language, Speech, and Hearing Services in Schools*, *46*(1), 1–13. https://doi.org/10.1044/2014_LSHSS-13-0042

Glennen, S. (2016). Speech and language clinical issues in internationally adopted children. In F. Genesee & A. Delcenserie (Eds.), *Starting over: The language development in internationally adopted children* (pp. 147–177). John Benjamins.

Glennen, S. (2021). Oral and written language abilities of school-age internationally adopted children from Eastern Europe. *Journal of Communication Disorders*, *93*, 106127. https://doi.org/10.1016/j.jcomdis.2021.106127

Glennen, S., & Bright, B. (2005). Five years later: Language in school-age internationally adopted children. *Seminars in Speech and Language*, *26*(1), 86–101. https://doi.org/10.1055/s-2005-864219

Goldstein, B. (2006). Clinical implications of research on language development and disorders in bilingual children. *Topics in Language Disorders*, *26*(4), 318–334.

Goldstein, B., & Bunta, F. (2012). Positive and negative transfer in the phonological systems of bilingual speakers. *International Journal of Bilingualism*, *16*(4), 388–401. https://doi.org/10.1177/1367006911425817

Goldstein, B., Bunta, F., Lange, J., Rodriguez, J., & Burrows, L. (2010). The effects of measures of language experience and language ability on segmental accuracy in bilingual children. *American Journal of Speech-Language Pathology*, *19*(3), 238–247. https://doi.org/10.1044/1058-0360(2010/08-0086)

Goldstein, B., Fabiano, L., & Washington, P. (2005). Phonological skills in predominantly English, predominantly Spanish, and Spanish-English bilingual children. *Language, Speech, and Hearing Services in Schools*, *36*(3), 201–218. https://doi.org/10.1044/0161-1461(2005/021)

Goldstein, B., & Iglesias, A. (2001). The effect of dialect on phonological analysis: Evidence from Spanish-speaking children. *American Journal of Speech-Language Pathology*, *10*(4), 394–406. https://doi.org/10.1044/1058-0360(2001/034)

Goldstein, B., & McLeod, S. (2012). Typical and atypical multilingual speech acquisition. In S. McLeod & B. Goldstein (Eds.), *Multilingual aspects of speech sound disorders in children* (pp. 84–100). Multilingual Matters.

Goldstein, B. A., & Fabiano, L. (2007, February 13). Assessment and intervention for bilingual children with phonological disorders. *The ASHA Leader*, *12*(2), 6–7, 26–27, 31. https://doi.org/10.1044/leader.FTR2.12022007.6

Grech, H., & Dodd, B. (2008). Phonological acquisition in Malta: A bilingual learning context. *International Journal of Bilingualism*, *12*, 155–171. https://doi.org/10.1177%2F1367006908098564

Guiberson, M., & Atkins, J. (2012). Speech-language pathologists' preparation, practices, and perspectives on serving culturally and linguistically diverse children. *Communication Disorders Quarterly*, *33*(3), 169–180. https://doi.org/10.1177/1525740110384132

Harold, M. P. (2018 December; Updated 2019, August 2020). *That one time a journal article on speech sounds broke the SLP Internet*. [Blog Post]. https://www.theinformedslp.com/how-to/that-one-time-a-journal-article-on-speech-sound-norms-broke-the-slp-internet

Harte, J., Oliveira, A., Frizelle, P., & Gibbon, F. (2016). Children's comprehension of an unfamiliar speaker accent: A review. *International Journal of Language & Communication Disorders*, *51*(3), 221–235. https://doi.org/10.1111/1460-6984.12211

Hedlund, G., & Rose, Y. (2020). *Phon 3.1* [Computer Software]. https://phon.ca

Helder, E., Mulder, E., & Gunnoe, M. (2016). A longitudinal investigation of children internationally adopted at school age. *Child Neuropsychology*, *22*(1), 39–64. https://doi.org/10.1080/09297049.2014.967669

Holm, A., & Dodd, B. (1999a). A longitudinal study of the phonological development of two Cantonese-English bilingual children. *Applied Psycholinguistics*, *20*, 349–376. https://doi.org/10.1017/S0142716499003021

Holm, A., & Dodd, B. (1999b). An intervention case study of a bilingual child with a phonological disorder. *Child Language Teaching & Therapy*, *15*, 139–158. https://doi.org/10.1177/026565909901500203

Holm, A., & Dodd, B. (2006). Phonological development and disorder of bilingual children acquiring Cantonese and English. In H. Zhu & B. Dodd (Eds.), *Phonological development and disorders in children: A multilingual perspective* (pp. 286–325). Multilingual Matters.

Holm, A., Dodd, B., & Ozanne, A. (1997). Efficacy of intervention for a bilingual child making articulation and phonological errors. *International Journal of Bilingualism*, *1*(1), 55–69. https://doi.org/10.1177%2F136700699700100105

Holm, A., Dodd, B., Stow, C., & Pert, S. (1998). Speech disorder in bilingual children: Four case studies. *Osmania Papers in Linguistics*, *22-23*, 46–64. http://ajslp.pubs.asha.org/article.aspx?articleid=2629126. http://arts.osmania.ac.in/Journals/Linguistics/Volume%2022-23.pdf

Hua, Z. (2002). *Phonological development in specific contexts*. Multilingual Matters.

Hua, Z., & Dodd, B. (2000). The phonological acquisition of Putonghua (Modern Standard Chinese). *Journal of Child Language*, *27*(1), 3–42. https://doi.org/10.1017/s030500099900402x

Hua, Z., & Dodd, B. (2006). *Phonological development and disorders in children: A multilingual perspective*. Multilingual Matters.

Hustad, K. C., Mahr, T., Natzke, P. E. M., & Rathouz, P. J. (2020). Development of speech intelligibility between 30 and 47 months in typically developing children: A cross-sectional study of growth. *Journal of Speech, Language & Hearing Research*, *63*(6), 1675–1687. https://doi.org/10.1044/2020_jslhr-20-00008

Ingram, D. (2002). The measurement of whole-word productions. *Journal of Child Language*, *29*, 713–733. https://doi.org/10.1017/S0305000902005275

International Expert Panel on Multilingual Children's Speech. (2012). *Multilingual children with speech sound disorders: Position paper*. Research Institute for Professional Practice, Learning and Education (RIPPLE). Charles Sturt University. http://www.csu.edu.au/research/multilingual-speech/position-paper

Ireland, M., McLeod, S., Farquharson, K., & Crowe, K. (2020). Evaluating children in U.S. public schools with speech sound disorders: Considering federal and state laws, guidance, and research. *Topics in Language Disorders*. https://doi.org/10.1097/TLD.000000000000022

Jakielski, K. J., & Gildersleeve-Neumann, C. E. (2018). *Phonetic science for clinical practice*. Plural.

Jakobson, R. (1941/1968). *Kindersprache, Aphasie und allgemeine Lautgesetzte [Child language, aphasia and phonological universals]*. Mouton.

Jensen de López, K. M., Lyons, R., Novogrodsky, R., Baena, S., Feilberg, J., Harding, S., Kelić, M., Klatte, I. S., Mantel, T. C., Tomazin, M. O., Ulfsdottir, T. S., Zajdó, K., & Rodriguez-Ortiz, I. R. (2021). Exploring parental perspectives of childhood speech and language disorders across 10 countries: A pilot qualitative study. *Journal of Speech, Language, and Hearing Research*, *64*(5), 1739–1747. https://doi.org/10.1044/2020_JSLHR-20-00415

Johnston, W. R. (2017). *Historical international adoption statistics*, United States and World. Johnston Archive. http://www.johnstonsarchive.net/policy/adoptionstatsintl.html

Julien, H. M., & Munson, B. (2012). Modifying speech to children based on their perceived phonetic accuracy. *Journal of Speech, Language and Hearing Research*, *55*(6), 1836–1849. https://doi.org/10.1044/1092-4388(2012/11-0131)

Kamhi, A. G., & Pollock, K. E. (2005). *Phonological disorders in children: Clinical decision making in assessment and intervention*. Paul H. Brookes.

Kaye, A., Che, C., Chew, W., Stueve, E., & Jiang, S. (2019). Cleft care of internationally adopted children from China. *The Cleft Palate-Craniofacial Journal*, *56*(1), 46–55. https://doi.org/10.1177/1055665618771423

Kehoe, M., & Kannathasan, K. (2021). Development of voice onset time in monolingual and bilingual French-speaking children. *Lingua*, *252*, 102937. https://doi.org/10.1016/j.lingua.2020.102937

Kehoe, M., Trujillo, C., & Lleó, C. (2001). Bilingual phonological acquisition: An analysis of syllable structure and VOT. In K. F. Cantone & M. O. Hinzelin (Eds.), *Proceedings of the colloquium on structure, acquisition and change of grammars: Phonological and syntactic aspects* (pp. 38–54). Universität Hamburg, Arbeiten zur Mehrsprachigkeit.

Kgoleng, K. (May 23, 2022). *Black writers and publishers are South Africa's 'linguistic orphans'*. Mail & Guardian. https://mg.co.za/opinion/2022-05-23-opinion-black-writers-and-publishers-are-south-africas-linguistic-orphans

Khoza-Shangase, K., & Mophosho, M. (2021). Language and culture in speech-language and hearing professions in South Africa: Re-imagining practice. *The South African Journal of Communication Disorders, 68*(1), e1–e9. https://doi.org/10.4102/sajcd.v68i1.793

Kim, M., & Pae, S. (2007). Korean speech acquisition. In S. McLeod (Ed.), *The international guide to speech acquisition* (pp. 472-482). Thomson Delmar Learning.

Koenig, M. A., & Harris, P. L. (2005). Preschoolers mistrust ignorant and inaccurate speakers. *Child Development, 76*(6), 1261–1277. https://doi.org/10.1111/j.1467-8624.2005.00849.x

Kohnert, K. (2008). *Language disorders in bilingual children and adults*. Plural Publishing.

Kohnert, K., & Derr, A. (2012). Language intervention with Bilingual children. In B. Goldstein (Ed.), *Bilingual language development and disorders in Spanish-English speakers* (2nd ed., pp. 337–356). Paul H. Brookes Publishing Co.

Kohnert, K., Ebert, K. D., & Pham, G. (2020). *Language disorders in bilingual children and adults* (3rd ed.). Plural Publishing.

Kohnert, K., Yim, D., Nett, K., Kan, P. F., & Duran, L. (2005). Intervention with linguistically diverse preschool children: A focus on developing home language(s). *Language, Speech, and Hearing Services in Schools, 36*(3), 251–26. https://doi.org/10.1044/0161-1461(2005/025)

Labov, W., Ash, S., & Boberg, C. (2008). *The Atlas of North American English: Phonetics, phonology and sound change*. Walter de Gruyter.

Langdon, H. W., & Saenz, T. (2015). *Working with interpreters and translators: A guide for speech-language pathologists and audiologists*. Plural Publishing.

Lee, S. A. S., & Iverson, G. K. (2012). Stop consonant productions of Korean-English bilingual children. *Bilingualism: Language and Cognition, 15*(2), 275–287. https://doi.org/10.1017/S1366728911000083

Lleó, C., Kuchenbrandt, I., Kehoe, M., & Trujillo, C. (2003). Syllable final consonants in Spanish and German monolingual and bilingual acquisition. In N. Müller (Ed.), *Vulnerable domains in multilingualism* (pp. 191–220). John Benjamins.

Lundeborg Hammarström, I., & Stemberger, J. P. (2022). Consonants lost: A Swedish girl with protracted phonological development. *Clinical Linguistics & Phonetics, 36*(9), 820–831. https://doi.org/10.1080/02699206.2021.1988147

Lynch, J. I., Brookshire, B. L., & Fox, D. R. (1980). *A parent - child cleft palate curriculum: Developing speech and language*. CC Publications.

MacLeod, A. A. N., Sutton, A., Trudeau, N., & Thordardottir, E. (2011). Phonological Development in Québécois French: A cross-sectional study of preschool aged children. *International Journal of Speech Language Pathology, 13*(2), 93–109. https://doi.org/10.3109/17549507.2011.487543

Mahura, O., & Pascoe, M. (2016). The acquisition of Setswana segmental phonology in children aged 3;0–6;0 years: A cross-sectional study. *International Journal of Speech-Language Pathology*. http://dx.doi.org/10.3109/17549507.2015.1126639

Maphalala, Z., Pascoe, M., & Smouse, M. (2014). Phonological development of first language isiXhosa-speaking children aged 3;0–6;0 years: A descriptive cross-sectional study. *Clinical Linguistics & Phonetics, 28*(3), 176–194. https://doi.org/10.3109/02699206.2013.840860

Másdóttir, T., McLeod, S., & Crowe, K. (2021). Icelandic children's acquisition of consonants and consonant clusters. *Journal of Speech, Language, and Hearing Research, 64*(5), 1490–1502. https://doi.org/10.1044/2021_JSLHR-20-00463

Mason, G. (2018a). *Comprehensive Assessment of Multisyllabic Words; CAMSWə*. Unpublished test protocol, University of British Columbia.

Mason, G. (2018). School-aged children's phonological accuracy in multisyllabic words on a whole-word metric. *Journal of Speech, Language, and Hearing Research, 61*(12), 2869–2883. https://doi.org/10.1044/2018_JSLHR-S-17-0137

Masteson, J., & Bernhardt, B. M. (2001). *Computerized Articulation and Phonology Evaluation System (CAPES)*. Pearson.

McLeod, S. (Ed.). (2007). *The international guide to speech acquisition*. Thomson Delmar Learning.

McLeod, S. (2020). Intelligibility in context scale: Cross-linguistic use, validity, and reliability. *Speech, Language and Hearing, 23*(1), 9–16. https://doi.org/10.1080/2050571X.2020.1718837

McLeod, S., & Baker, E. (2017). *Children's speech: An evidence-based approach to assessment and intervention*. Pearson.

McLeod, S., & Crowe, K. (2018). Children's consonant acquisition in 27 languages: A cross-linguistic review. *American Journal of Speech-Language Pathology, 27*(4), 1546–1571. https://doi.org/10.1044/2018_AJSLP-17-0100

McLeod, S., & Goldstein, B. (Eds.). (2012). *Multilingual aspects of speech sound disorders in children*. Multilingual Matters.

McLeod, S., Harrison, L. J., & McCormack, J. (2012). Intelligibility in Context Scale: Validity and reliability of a subjective rating measure. *Journal of Speech, Language, and Hearing Research*, *55*(2), 648–656. https://doi.org/10.1044/1092-4388(2011/10-0130)

McLeod, S., Verdon, S., & International Expert Panel on Multilingual Children's Speech. (2017). Tutorial: Speech assessment for multilingual children who do not speak the same language(s) as the speech-language pathologist. *American Journal of Speech-Language Pathology*, *26*(3), 691–7008. https://doi.org/10.1044/2017_ajslp-15-0161

McLeod, S., Verdon, S., Baker, E., Ball, M. J., Ballard, E., David, A. B., Bernhardt, B. M., Bérubé, D., Blumenthal, M., Bowen, C., Brosseau-Lapré, F., Bunta, F., Crowe, K., Cruz-Ferreira, M., Davis, B., Fox-Boyer, A., Gildersleeve-Neumann, C., Grech, H., Goldstein, B., & International Expert Panel on Multilingual Children's Speech. (2017). Tutorial: Speech assessment for multilingual children who do not speak the same language(s) as the speech-language pathologist. *American Journal of Speech-Language Pathology*, *26*(3), 691–708. https://doi.org/10.1044/2017_ajslp-15-0161

McLeod, S., Verdon, S., Bowen, C., & the International Expert Panel on Multilingual Children's Speech. (2013). International aspirations for speech-language pathologists' practice with multilingual children with speech sound disorders: Development of a position paper. *Journal of Communication Disorders*, *46*(4), 375–387. https://doi.org/10.1016/j.jcomdis.2013.04.003

Mdlalo, T., Flack, P. S., & Joubert, R. W. (2019). The cat on a hot tin roof? Critical considerations in multilingual language assessments. *The South African Journal of Communication Disorders*, *66*(1), e1–e7. https://doi.org/10.4102/sajcd.v66i1.610

Miller, L., Pérouse de Montclos, P., & Sorge, F. (2016). Special needs adoption in France and USA 2016: How can we best prepare and support families? *Neuropsychiatrie de l'Enfance et de l'Adolesence*, *64*(5), 308–316. https://doi.org/10.1016/j.neurenf.2016.05.003

Morgan, A., Bellucci, C., Coppersmith, J., Linde, S., Curtis, A., Albert, M., O'Gara, M., & Kapp-Simon, K. (2017). Language development in children with cleft palate with or without cleft lip adopted from non-English-speaking countries. *American Journal of Speech-Language Pathology*, *26*(2), 342–354. https://doi.org/10.1044/2016_AJSLP-16-0030

Mukong, A. K., Van Walbeek, C., & Ross, H. (2017). Lifestyle and income-related inequality in health in South Africa. *International Journal for Equity in Health*, *16*(1), 1–14. https://doi.org/10.1186/s12939-017-0598-7

Munson, B., & Babel, M. (2019). The phonetics of sex and gender. In W. F. Katz & P. F. Assmann (Eds.), *The Routledge handbook of phonetics* (pp. 499–525). Routledge.

Munson, B., Lackas, N., & Koeppe, K. (2019). The longitudinal development of gendered speech production in children: Patterns and predictors. Oral Presentation at the Boston University Conference on Language Development, Boston, MA: Boston University.

Nagy, J. (1980). *Öt-hat éves gyermekeink iskolakészültsége [Preparedness for school of our five-six years old children]*. Akadémiai Kiadó.

Nakanishi, Y., Owada, K., & Fujita, N. (1972). K_onkensa to sono kekka ni kansuru k_satsu. *Tokyo Gakugei Daigaku Tokushu Kyoiku Shisetsu Hokoku*, *1*, 1–19.

Nathan, L., Stackhouse, J., Goulandris, N., & Snowling, M. J. (2004). The development of early literacy skills among children with speech difficulties: A test of the "critical age hypothesis". *Journal of Speech, Language and Hearing Research*, *47*(2), 377–391. https://doi.org/10.1044/1092-4388(2004/031)

National Academies of Sciences, Engineering, and Medicine NASEM. (2016). *Parenting matters: Supporting parents of children ages 0-8*. The National Academies Press.

Owens, R. E., & Farinella, K. A. (2019). *Introduction to communication disorders: A lifespan evidence-based perspective* (6th ed.). Pearson.

Paradis, J. (2001). Do bilingual two-year-olds have separate phonological systems? *The International Journal of Bilingualism*, *5*(1), 19–38. https://doi.org/10.1177%2F13670069010050010201

Pascoe, M., & Jeggo, Z. (2019). Speech acquisition in monolingual children acquiring isiZulu in rural KwaZulu-Natal, South Africa. *Journal of Monolingual and Bilingual Speech*, *1*, 94–117. https://doi.org/10.1558/jmbs.11082

Pascoe, M., Mahura, O., & Le Roux, J. (2018). South African English speech development: Preliminary data from typically developing pre-school children in Cape Town. *Clinical Linguistics & Phonetics*, *32*(12), 1145–1161. https://doi.org/10.1080/02699206.2018.1510985

Pascoe, M., Mahura, O., Le Roux, J., Danvers, E., de Jager, A., Esterhuizen, N., Naidoo, C., Reynders, J., Senior, S., & van der Merwe, A. (2018). Speech development in three-year-old children acquiring isiXhosa and English in South Africa. In E. Babatsouli, D. Ingram, & N. Müller (Eds.), *Crosslinguistic encounters in language acquisition: Typical and atypical development*. Multilingual Matters.

Pascoe, M., Mahura, O., & Rossouw, K. (2020). Transcribing and transforming: Towards inclusive, multilingual child speech training for South African speech-language therapy students. *Folia Phoniatrica et Logopaedica*, Special Issue on Transcription of Children's Speech, *72*(2), 108–111. https://doi.org/10.1159/000499427

Pascoe, M., & McLeod, S. (2016). Cross-cultural adaptation of the intelligibility in context scale for South Africa. *Child Language Teaching & Therapy*, *32*(3), 327–343. https://doi.org/10.1177/0265659016638395

Pascoe, M., Rossouw, K., Fish, L., Jansen, C., Manley, N., Powell, M., & Rosen, L. (2016). Speech processing and production in two-year-old children acquiring isiXhosa: A tale of two children. *South African Journal of Communication Disorders. Special Edition: Language Acquisition and Impairment in the African Languages, 63*(2), 1–16. http://dx.doi.org/10.4102/sajcd.v63i2.134

Pascoe, M., Rossouw, K., & Mahura, O. (2018). Core vocabulary intervention for an isiXhosa-English speaking child with speech sound difficulties. *Southern African Linguistics and Applied Language Studies*, *36*(4), 313–328. https://doi.org/10.2989/16073614.2018.1548292

Pascoe, M., & Smouse, M. (2012). *Masithethe*: Speech and language development and difficulties in isiXhosa. *South African Medical Journal*, *102*(6), 469–471. https://doi.org/10.7196/SAMJ.5554

Perry, T. L., Ohde, R. N., & Ashmead, D. H. (2001). The acoustic bases for gender identification from children's voices. *The Journal of the Acoustical Society of America*, *109*(6), 2988–2998. https://doi.org/10.1121/1.1370525

Phạm, B., & McLeod, S. (2019). Vietnamese-Speaking Children's Acquisition of Consonants, Semivowels, Vowels, and Tones in Northern Viet Nam. *Journal of Speech, Language, and Hearing Research, 62*(8), 2645–2670. https://doi.org/10.1044/2019_JSLHR-S-17-0405

Phoon, H. S., Abdullah, A. C., Lee, L. W., & Murugaiah, P. (2014). Consonant acquisition in the Malay language: A cross-sectional study of preschool aged Malay children. *Clinical Linguistics & Phonetics, 28*(5), 329–345. https://doi.org/10.3109/02699206.2013.868517

Pollock, K. E. (2005). Early language growth in children adopted from China: Preliminary normative data. *Seminars in Speech and Language*, *26*(1), 22–32. https://doi.org/10.1055/s-2005-864213

Pollock, K. E. (2007). Speech acquisition in second first language learners (children who were adopted internationally). In S. McLeod (Ed.), *International guide to speech acquisition* (pp. 137–145). Thomson Delmar Learning.

Pollock, K. E. (2020). Second first language acquisition following international adoption. In F. Li, K. E. Pollock, & R. Gibb (Eds.), *Child bilingualism and second language learning* (pp. 189–219). John Benjamins.

Pollock, K. E., Price, J. R., & Fulmer, K. C. (2003). Speech-language acquisition in children adopted from China: A longitudinal investigation of two children. *Journal of Multilingual Communication Disorders, 1*(3), 184–193. https://doi.org/10.1080/14769670310001603853

Price, J. R., Pollock, K. E., & Oller, D. K. (2006). Speech and language development in six infants adopted from China. *Journal of Multilingual Communication Disorders*, *1;4*(2), 108–127. https://doi.org/10.1080/14769670601092622

Ray, J. (2002). Treating phonological disorders in a multilingual child: A case study. *American Journal of Speech-Language Pathology*, *11*(3), 305–315. https://doi.org/10.1044/1058-0360(2002/035)

Roberts, J., Pollock, K., Krakow, R., Price, J., Fulmer, K., & Wang, P. (2005). Language development in preschool-aged children adopted from China. *Journal of Speech, Language, and Hearing Research*, *48*(1), 93–107. https://doi.org/10.1044/1092-4388(2005/008)

Romonath, R., & Bernhardt, B. M. (2017). Erwerb prosodischer Wortstrukturen bei Vorschulkindern mit und ohne phonologische Störungen [Prosodic word structure acquisition in preschool children with and without phonological disorders]. *Forschung Sprache, 1*, 91–107. https://forschung-sprache.eu/fileadmin/user_upload/Dateien/Heftausgaben/2017-1/5-70-2017-01-06.pdf

Rossouw, K., & Pascoe, M. (2018). Intervention for bilingual speech sound disorders: Description of an isiXhosa-English speaking child. *South African Journal of Communication Disorders*, *65*(1), a566. https://doi.org/10.4102/sajcd.v65i1.566

Rutter, M., & English and Romanian Adoptees (ERA) Study Team. (1998). Developmental catch-up, and deficit, following adoption after severe global early privation. *Journal of Child Psychology and Psychiatry, and Allied Disciplines*, *39*(4), 465–476. PMID: 9599775

Sander, E. K. (1972). When are speech sounds learned? *Journal of Speech and Hearing Disorders*, *37*(1), 55–63. https://doi.org/10.1044/jshd.3701.55

Scott, K., Roberts, J., & Krakow, R. (2008). Oral and written language development of children adopted from China. *American Journal of Speech-Language Pathology*, *17*(2), 150–160. https://doi.org/10.1044/1058-0360(2008/015)

Scott, K. A., Pollock, K. E., Roberts, J. A., & Krakow, R. (2013). Phonological processing skills of children adopted internationally. *American Journal of Speech-Language Pathology*, *22*(4), 673–683. https://doi.org/10.1044/1058-0360(2013/12-0133)

Selman, P. (2009). The rise and fall of intercountry adoption in the 21st century. *International Social Work*, *52*(5), 575–594. https://doi.org/10.1177%2F0020872809337681

Shriberg, L. D., Kent, R. D., McAllister Byun, T., & Preston, J. L. (2019). *Clinical phonetics* (5th ed.). Pearson.

Smit, A. B., Hand, L., Freilinger, J. J., Bernthal, J. E., & Bird, A. (1990). The Iowa articulation norms project and its Nebraska replication. *Journal of Speech and Hearing Disorders*, *55*(4), 779–798. https://doi.org/10.1044/jshd.5504.779

Smith, N. V. (1973). *The acquisition of phonology*. Cambridge University Press.

So, L. K. H., & Dodd, B. (1995). The acquisition of phonology by Cantonese-speaking children. *Journal of Child Language*, *22*(3), 473–495. https://doi.org/10.1017/S0305000900009922

Southwood, F., & van Dulm, O. (2015). The challenge of linguistic and cultural diversity: Does length of experience affect South African speech-language therapists' management of children with language impairment? *South African Journal of Communication Disorders*, *62*(1), E1–E14. https://doi.org/10.4102/sajcd.v62i1.71

Southwood, F., White, M. J., Brookes, H., Pascoe, M., Ndhambi, M., Yalala, S., Mahura, O., Mössmer, M., Oosthuizen, H., Brink, N., & Alcock, K. (2021). Sociocultural factors affecting vocabulary development in Young South African children. *Frontiers in Psychology*, *12*, 642315. https://doi.org/10.3389/fpsyg.2021.642315

Stackhouse, J., & Wells, B. (2002). *Children's speech and literacy difficulties II: Identification and intervention*. Whurr Publishers.

Stemberger, J. P., & Bernhardt, B. M. (2018). Tap and trill clusters in typical and protracted phonological development: Challenging segments in complex phonological environments. Introduction to the special issue. *Clinical Linguistics & Phonetics*, *32*(5–6), 563–575. https://doi.org/10.1080/02699206.2017.1370019

Strand, S., & Lindsay, G. (2009). Evidence of ethnic disproportionality in special education in an English population. *The Journal of Special Education*, *43*(3), 174–190. https://doi.org/10.1177%2F0022466908320461

Stuart-Smith, J. (2007). Empirical evidence for gendered speech production: /s/ in Glaswegian. In J. Cole & J. I. Hualde (Eds.), *Laboratory phonology 9*. Mouton de Gruyter.

Takagi, S., & Yasuda, A. (1967). Seij_y_ji no k_onn_ryoku. *Sh_ni Hoken Igaku*, *25*, 23–28.

Tan, T.X., Marfo, K., & Dedrick, R.F. (2007). Special needs adoption from China: Exploring child-level indicators, adoptive family characteristics, and correlates of behavioral adjustment. *Children and Youth Services Review*, *29*(10), 1269–1285. https://doi.org/10.1016/j.childyouth.2007.05.001

Templin, M. C. (1957). *Certain language skills in children: Their development and interrelationships*. Institute of Child Welfare, Monograph 26. University of Minnesota Press.

Thomas, E. R., & Bailey, G. (2015). Segmental phonology of African American English. *The Oxford Handbook of African American Language*, 403–419. https://doi.org/10.1093/oxfordhb/9780199795390.013.13

Trecca, F., Bleses, D., Højen, A., Madsen, T. O., & Christiansen, M. H. (2020). When too many vowels impede language processing: An eye-tracking study of Danish-learning children. *Language and Speech*, *63*(4), 898–918. https://journals.sagepub.com/doi/full/10.1177/0023830919893390

Tripp, A., Feldman, N. H., & Idsardi, W. J. (2021). Social inference may guide early lexical learning. *Frontiers in Psychology*, *12*(645247), 1–19. https://doi.org/10.3389/fpsyg.2021.645247

Tse, A. C. Y. (1991). *The acquisition process of Cantonese phonology: A case study*. [Unpublished M. Phil. Thesis]. University of Hong Kong.

Tse, S. M. (1982). *The acquisition of Cantonese phonology*. [Unpublished PhD thesis]. University of British Columbia.

U.S. Department of State. (2022). *Intercountry adoptions – Adoption statistics.* https://travel.state.gov/content/travel/en/Intercountry-Adoption/adopt_ref/adoption-statistics-esri.html

UNICEF. (2012). *School readiness: A conceptual framework.* UN Children's Fund. www.unicef.org/earlychildhood/files/Child2Child_Conceptual Framework_FINAL(1).pdf

van Haaften, L., Diepeveen, S., van den Engel-hoek, L., de Swart, B., & Maassen, B. (2020). Speech sound development in typically developing 2–7-year-old Dutch-speaking children: A normative cross-sectional study. *International Journal of Language & Communication Disorders, 55*(6), 971–987. https://doi.org/10.1111/1460-6984.12575

Weismer, G., & Brown, D. K. (2021). *Introduction to communication sciences and disorders: The scientific basis of clinical practice.* Plural.

Williams, A. L., McLeod, S., & McCauley, R. J. (2021). *Interventions for speech sound disorders in children* (2nd ed.). Paul H. Brookes.

Williams, C. J., & McLeod, S. (2012). Speech-language pathologists' assessment and intervention practices with multilingual children. *International Journal of Speech-Language Pathology, 14*(3), 292–305. https://doi.org/10.3109/17549507.2011.636071

Williamson, G. (2008–2021). *SLTinfo.* https://www.sltinfo.com

Williamson, G. (2015, May 26). *Age of acquisition of speech sounds.* https://www.sltinfo.com/ess101age-of-acquisition-of-speech-sounds

World Health Organization (WHO). (2007). WHO Workgroup for development of version of ICF for Children. International classification of functioning, disability and health - Version for children and youth: 2013-CY. World Health Organization.

Yavaş, M. (2013). Acquisition of #sC clusters: Universal grammar vs. language-specific grammar. *Letras de Hoje, 48*(3), 355–361. https://revistaseletronicas.pucrs.br/ojs/index.php/fale/article/view/14996/9915

Yavaş, M. (2020). *Applied English phonology* (4th ed.). Wiley.

Yavaş, M., & Goldstein, B. (1998). Phonological assessment and treatment of bilingual speakers. *American Journal of Speech-Language Pathology, 7*(2), 49–60. https://doi.org/10.1044/1058-0360.0702.49

Zajdó, K. (2002). *The acquisition of vowels in Hungarian-speaking children aged two to four years: A cross-sectional study.* [Unpublished doctoral dissertation]. University of Washington.

Zajdó, K. (2013). Cross-linguistic trends in the acquisition of speech sounds. In B. Peter & A. A. N. MacLeod (Eds.), *Comprehensive perspectives on speech sound development and disorders* (pp. 249–274). Nova.

Zamuner, T. S., & Kharlamov, V. (2016). Phonotactics and syllable structure in infant speech perception. In J. L. Lidz, W. Snyder, & J. Pater (Eds.), *Oxford Handbook of developmental linguistics* (pp. 27–42). Oxford University Press.

Zarifian, T., & Fotuhi, M. (2020). Phonological development in Persian-speaking children: A cross-sectional study. *International Journal of Speech-Language Pathology, 22*(6), 614–625. https://doi.org/10.1080/17549507.2020.1758209

Chapter 11
Technology, Communication, and SSD

The topic areas in Chapter 11 relate to technology and communication in one form or another. The first topic area is information and communication technology (ICT) as it relates to SLPs/SLTs and children's speech sound disorders. The emphasis is on protecting users' privacy – as far as possible – and staying safe online, while using social media platforms and other ICT for professional purposes.

The second topic area is in two parts: telepractice, and technology assisted SLP/SLT such as Apps. Telepractice (or telehealth) delivery of clinical services to clients, clinical education to students, and continuing professional development (CPD) content to SLPs/SLTs is explored by Williams, Thomas, & Caballero in A46.

The third topic area comprises two Articulatory Visual Biofeedback technologies for assessing and treating SSD: electropalatography (EPG) and ultrasound tongue imaging (Cleland & Scobbie, A47). Both originated as pioneering phonetics lab work in measuring tongue gestures and constrictions in typical speakers, later proving applicable to SLPs'/SLTs' practice with children and young people with protracted or 'residual' speech impairment.

Then follow four discussions of aspects of our work that sometimes have prominent ICT components, and which are firmly to do with intra- and inter-professional communication. They cover communities of practice (CoPs) in communication sciences and disorders (McComas, A48); collaborations between teachers and SLPs/SLTs, around children with speech and reading difficulties (Neilson, A49; A50); and heartening, and often transdisciplinary, advances in communication and clinical research alliances between academic researchers, university teachers, and hands-on practitioners (Froud & Randazzo, A51) in the service of our clients.

ICT and Online Safety

ICT includes products and software applications (Apps) that enable users to store, retrieve, manipulate, transmit or receive information electronically in a digital form. Increasingly, SLPs/SLTs must be technologically savvy enough to operate the ICT that we use professionally and personally. A 'tech savvy' individual has the appropriate skills and intuitive knowledge to use relevant devices effectively and an understanding of technical concepts that allows their application in different contexts. For example, by using their general knowledge of software in combination with the manual, the individual can work out how to run a new computer or mobile application. Most tech-savvy people can operate basic hardware and software tools, such as an operating system and web browser. That said, even a technically competent ICT user can succumb to some of the pitfalls, limitations, and risks of life online. These include privacy breaches, cyberbullying ('trolling') in social media, internet fraud, data loss, security violations, and more. All users are potentially susceptible, even with strong and unique passwords; active avoidance of abuse, scams, phishing, and unwanted tracking; downloading files and Apps only from trusted sources; *regular* file backups, software updates, password changes, and reviews of browser security settings; using anti tracking software or, if it is legal in their country, using a Virtual Private Network (VPN), and reading the fine print before entering 'agree'. An understanding of higher risk ICT environments helps to minimise these vulnerabilities.

Social Media

Social media depend on web-based ICT that supports interactive online platforms. To function, social media rely on connections between people who produce and/or co-produce, disseminate and share information, news, commentary and ideas in virtual communities or networks, hence *online communities*, and *social networks*. The platforms include blogs, hosted on 'free' blogging sites, or microblogging sites such as Twitter, which was an SLP/SLT stronghold until it changed hands in late 2022, or Mastodon on the 'Fediverse' which may or may not become the platform of choice.

Customers and Products

If an online service comes at no monetary cost, the user is often – unwittingly or knowingly – the merchandise, and not the simply the consumer. This may sound familiar, as the maxim, 'If you're not paying for it, you're not the customer, you're the product'

with variations, has circulated the internet since about 2010. Users, or 'customers' of social media, generate content, by blogging or microblogging, posting to Facebook Groups; reviewing on eBay, Goodreads, TripAdvisor, Rotten Tomatoes or YouTube sites; providing details in Academia, Linkedin, or ORCiD; allowing 'personalised preferences' on Foxtel or Netflix; using SlideShare; 'allowing' Apps, bookmarking, messaging, liking, listing, tweeting, and retweeting in Twitter, or boosting, favouriting, and posting in Mastodon. Of course, users also consume valuable content; for example, on journal sites by downloading and self-archiving open access or subscription articles, reference managing (e.g., in EndNote, Mendeley, Scopus, or Web of Science).

Ostensibly free products can come with potential hidden – or not so hidden – costs in the forms of privacy violations, intrusive phone calls, phishing attempts, push notification advertising, junk email, ad hominem attack, threats, trolling, bullying and harassment, or internet fraud endeavours that range from bumbling, obvious and absurd through to shrewd and convincing. Free services include browsers (Google Chrome, Firefox, Opera, Safari, etc.), e-Bay (e-Bay Plus attracts a modest annual fee), Facebook, Flickr, Google Scholar, Gmail, Hotmail, Instagram, ORCiD, Pinterest, and ResearchGate and the free versions of Academia and LinkedIn, Also free are search engines (e.g., Google with more than 91% of the market share, Microsoft Bing with about 3.1%, Yahoo, DuckDuckGo, and the Internet Archive), WhatsApp, and YouTube and the free versions of free versions of Skype, Twitter, and Zoom. Those that come at minimal cost include at Microsoft Office 365, for cents per day.

Third Party Tracking

Whether or not they 'accept cookies', users visit, engage in, talk about services, and are tracked by a third party – the ever-present customer intelligence hunters and gatherers who 'share' (sell) customers' details, purposefully, as desirable commodities. Noting that both third party trackers and advertising ('clickbait') can be blocked or minimised, customer intelligence is the process of collecting and analysing information about customers' personal and social profiles, preferences, and purchasing patterns.

Using third party cookies and other means, the types of intelligence gathered may include the music and books you like, movies you've watched and/or rated, your preferred mass media outlets (e.g., TV channels and newspapers), default browser and frequent searches. Information is also amassed about your activities (e.g., your hobbies, sport, and travel), interests, banking, and shopping patterns (e.g., bank sites, department stores, e-Bay categories, pharmacies, and supermarkets you frequent).

Among the identifying and demographic details collected and analysed will be your affiliations (e.g., religious, organizational, and political), age, campaigns (e.g., petitions signed, and causes supported), education (degrees and alma mater), games and puzzles (e.g., Wordle), family (e.g., children, and their ages), gender, health, fitness and well-being, income, location including the value of your owned or rented property, marital status, occupation, real name and pseudonyms, professional affiliations (e.g., association memberships), subscriptions (e.g., journals), your banking institution, the types of credit cards you use, and more. The third party's aim is to 'profile' you, building (for them) deeper, more effective customer relationships, improving (their) strategic decision-making, and strengthening (their) targeted marketing, tailored advertising, and curated offers.

Intelligence gathering can be around a customer's behaviour: in-store, in call centre and help-desk conversations, telephone surveys, and in browser-and-click contexts. It includes the person's buying patterns, in areas as diverse as, Amazon, the App Store, eBay, pharmacies, and supermarkets; conference registrations and accommodation and holiday bookings, insurance, and travel; the financial institutions, credit, debit, store and loyalty cards used for purchases, subscriptions and donations; and Afterpay and PayPal activity.

Customer intelligence also includes explicit and implicit feedback a person gives online such as likes, emojis, re-tweets, reactions, lists, and customer reviews and ratings (e.g., assigning an eBay seller stars, or rating hospitality venues in TripAdvisor); their alignment with activity and diet trackers (e. g., Apple Watch, Fitbit, MyFitnessPal), budget tracking and financial planning Apps, political and social justice issues (e.g., signing, commenting, and 'sharing' online

petitions. and supporting individuals, and causes (e.g., in Avaaz, Change, GetUP! and SumOfUs).

Blogging and micro-blogging sites often occupy more than one category, for example, Linkedin is mostly seen as a networking and jobhunting site, but it also offers a blogging option with easy-to-use tools, and it offers pre-existing professional audiences in Linkedin Groups. Other blogging sites are Blogger, Blogspot (e.g., Sharynne McLeod's https://speakingmylanguages.blogspot.com which focuses on typical and atypical speech development in mono- and multilingual children, and human rights, and Pamela Snow's blog on language, literacy, vulnerable young people, and social justice: http://pamelasnow.blogspot.com, Joomla (e.g., my https://www.speech-language-therapy.com) Medium, Tumblr, Weebly, and WordPress (e.g., Susan Rvachew's blog that has a section on child phonology and other SLP/SLT topics, and another that complements Rvachew and Brosseau-Lapré (2018). https://developmentalphonologicaldisorders.wordpress.com).

Other platforms support collaborative projects (e.g., Wikipedia®); content communities such as SlideShare, and YouTube (e.g., Edythe Strand's CAS videos: http://tiny.cc/kvcruz); content curation tools (e.g., LiveBinders, and Mendeley); Facebook groups (e.g., www.facebook.com/groups/clinicalresearchslps, www.facebook.com/groups/EBPSLPs, www.facebook.com/groups/E3BPforSSD, and one dedicated to ReST: https://www.facebook.com/groups/1765072333528566), Instagram, LinkedIn, and Twitter; news networking sites (e.g., Digg); virtual game-worlds (e.g., Minecraft, and SocioTown); and virtual social worlds (e.g., IMVU, Kaneva, and Second Life).

Participation in Twitter, and Mastodon in the Fediverse

Established in 2006, Twitter proved a helpful resource, pre- and post-pandemic, for a range of communication disorders' topics, until it changed ownership in late October 2022. The most prominent topics that related primarily to children and young people and SLP/SLT were Alternative and Augmentative Communication (AAC), Autism, Developmental Language Disorder (DLD), and Speech Sound Disorder (SSD).

Following the sale of Twitter, and consequent plummeting standards, many professionals have joined the Mastodon Fediverse, to use instead of, or as well as Twitter, and at the time of writing the future of Twitter was questionable. The word 'Fediverse' is a portmanteau of federation and universe. It is an ensemble of 'federated' (interconnected) servers (called 'instances') used for web publishing and file hosting. While independently hosted, the instances can communicate with each other, so it does not necessarily matter which you join. On the numerous instances, all of which are advertisement-free and published using open source (free) software, people can create one or more so-called identities (accounts). The identities can communicate over the instances' boundaries.

Social media generally, and Mastodon and Twitter specifically, are not for everyone, but it is worth signing up for a Mastodon account to test the water, and see if it is helpful to you, professionally. Introductory information is available here https://fedi.tips/mastodon-and-the-fediverse-beginners-start-here and here https://blog.joinmastodon.org/2018/08/mastodon-quick-start-guide

One step forward in clinician-researcher relations is attributable to an increase in the number of 'open access' publications in our field, and these are often signposted and shared in social media. As mentioned in Chapter 6, there are apparent increases in SLPs'/SLTs' reading of research articles (or at least downloading and intending to read them), engagement with theoretical frameworks, and knowledge-brokering (Douglas et al., 2022). To an extent, this increased activity is attributable to health professionals, their professional associations, and their major publishers accessing social media more frequently and strategically.

Erskine and Hendricks (2021) identified four Twitter strategies medical journals use promotionally: tweeting links to articles, infographics, and podcasts, and hosting monthly internet-based journal clubs. They recommended that journals and researchers should combine these strategies to maximize research impact and capture audiences with a variety of learning methods.

In SLP/SLT, Twitter subscribers include, or have included, individual academics, students, practitioners, and researchers, private (independent) and government funded practices, SLP/SLT university departments,

professional associations (e.g., @ASHAweb, @IASLT, @NZSTAComms, @RCSLT, @SAC_OAC, and @SpeechPathAus), journals (e.g., @AmerCleftPalate, @ASHAjournals, @CLTTjournal, @IJLCD, @IJSLP, @SIGPerspectives, and @SpeechLangHear), advocacy groups, charities, and not for profit organizations. All have increased their Twitter engagement, participating more actively by augmenting clinical research impact (Davidson et al., 2022; Finn, 2019), initiating topics, adding to discussion, sharing information and resources, promoting relevant hashtags.

Lurkers – not as Ominous as They Sound

As well as contributory subscribers, all kinds of social media have non-contributory (but not necessarily *passive*) participants, called lurkers. References to lurking as an (innocuous) online behaviour have been around since 2003 when IRC chat groups, and message boards began. Lurkers, or those who lurk, are members of or subscribers to an interactive online community such as a mailing list, group chat, or forum who only contribute by being there and reading, observing, or listening. As a behaviour, lurking is variable within and across individuals and not an all-or-none behaviour. A person might post regularly to a professional interest Facebook group, SIG (Special Interest Group), or mailing list while hanging back in other social media discussions and chats in contexts such as Linkedin, ResearchGate, and Twitter.

When I asked three seasoned SLP participants in, and researchers of social media about their lurking behaviour, one said, '*I can be a lurker and a poster all in one hour at times. It depends on my mood, the social media platform, the community, the topic or topics of interest, my opinions on said topics*'. Then came this from another, '*It's not binary, not passive lurker versus active contributor. The purpose of logging in to a social media site varies from moment and you find you're just reading and thinking, or reading and expressing your thoughts and sharing content, or engaging with others in the co-production aspects of expressing, as well*'. And from a third, '*Sometimes I'm there to read, learn, and lurk, particularly on Linguistics and Education mailing lists. Generally, the participants there are more knowledgeable than me, taking me out of my comfort zone, so I stay in the shadows. That doesn't mean I'm passive, just that I rarely post. If a topic, question, or issue I'm "across" comes up, I may chime in'.*

Most internet users lurk sometimes. For example, when new to a forum, an SLP/SLT might decide that it would be sensible to browse or view other people's input to judge the quality, mood, and relevance to them, of participation before (1) unsubscribing, (2) contributing when they are ready, or when a pertinent topic arises, (3) or asking a burning question, or (4) continuing to lurk. By convention, if a lurker switches to posting, messaging, or tweeting they may introduce themselves as a 'long-time lurker, first-time poster' but not necessarily in those words, often with a request for the larger group to forgive any newbie (novice) blunders. Then again, some individuals frequent social media often but lurk because they enjoy reading ('content consumption') rather than posting, or they feel uncomfortable posting perhaps perceiving the community as hostile or unsafe, or like one where they had a bad experience, or they think they have little to contribute, or are intimidated by some community members because of their high profile or air of authority.

A Survey of Twitter Lurkers (Infrequent Tweeters)

Using the terms *lurker* and *infrequent tweeter* synonymously, Odabaş (2022) defined lurkers as subscribers who never tweet, or tweet infrequently at a rate of fewer than five per month. Interested to provide insight into their behaviour on the platform and their reasons for being there, Odabaş reported her well-designed survey of Twitter lurkers. She found that about 21% of lurkers and 55% of more active tweeters visit Twitter daily. A further 38% of infrequent tweeters go there weekly, if not daily, and the remaining 41% go a few times a month or less frequently. Lurkers mainly reply to others' tweets rather than initiating topics (e.g., by asking a question), contributing content and information (e.g., by tweeting links to journal articles, copying the journal's Twitter handle into the tweet, and authors' handles if available), giving collegial support (e.g.,

mentoring new participants in a topic area of mutual interest, or encouraging students who tweet relevant content), promoting relevant hashtags (e.g., the tag for a national conference or campaign such as Better Hearing and Speech Month: #BHSM), commenting, retweeting, quote-tweeting, or liking. Odabaş found that 76% of lurkers said they used Twitter to see other viewpoints and to see what others were saying with only 6% expressing their own opinions. When she asked their main reason for visiting the site *most* frequent tweeters and *most* lurkers nominated entertainment, but interestingly, 13% of the lurkers and 5% of more frequent tweeters specified seeing different viewpoints as their top motivation.

Odabaş (2022), which is freely available online, may give readers the impression that Twitter subscribers fall into two camps: those who lurk and those who do not; but as explained above, it is more nuanced than that.

Realizing the Benefits of Social Media

*There are many barriers that prevent **medical professionals** from participating on social media. These include lack of time and technology skills and unfavorable perceptions of risk and profit. Healthcare professionals may feel they are unable to make a real difference or are not needed because others participate. However, with awareness and planning, these barriers can be overcome quite easily. And those who overcome them will discover many returns on their invested time, including increased empathy for patient concerns, improved communication and clinical skills, early notification of research findings, **lifelong medical education** and making new connections with colleagues around the world.*

(Patrick, 2019, p. 164)

These words from Michael D. Patrick Jr., MD introduce a chapter called *Myths that Prevent Medical Professionals from Engaging*, in a book that he co-edited on the topic of social media for medical professionals. If 'speech-language professionals' replaced 'medical professionals' and 'lifelong SLP/SLT education or CPD' replaced 'lifelong medical education', the sentiments would be perfectly apt for us. Patrick explores 12 myths that deter doctors from participating in social media, all of which apply to SLP/SLT. Addressing Myth 11, *'I don't get anything in return'* he commented, *'As professionals, we have a social responsibility that extends beyond our income- generating patients. The health and wellness of communities, states and countries depend, in part, on our involvement in matters of public health and health literacy. Social media represents tremendous opportunity to impact these elements on a national (and international) scale, and the result of our collective effort serves to improve the quality of life we all enjoy.'* Then, he listed tangible impacts and benefits of social media investment (pp. 162–163).

1. Making a positive impact on health literacy and public health.
2. Keeping up with changing evidence.
3. Achieving heightened patient empathy and sharpening clinical skills.
4. Connecting with distant colleagues.
5. Raising awareness of our work.

The Yahoo! Groups' Shutdown

Yahoo Groups (2001–2020) was one of the world's largest troves of online message boards, with an optional email or email digest component, with 113 million users, and nine million Groups using 22 languages. The then owner, Verizon Media, terminated the Groups in 2020 due to unfettered sharing of child pornography, and wrongheaded advice focusing on child trafficking, unlawful international adoptions, 'private re-homing' of unwanted international adoptees, and other illegalities (e.g., Twohey, 2013). This left a gap, and one of the casualties was the EBP-focused speech-language pathology discussion group, phonologicaltherapy (Bowen, 2001). As list owner, I observed that the once vibrant participation in phonologicaltherapy discussions dwindled from 2015 as Facebook, with its superior functionality, found its stride, and group members

turned to less research-oriented, and less theoretically sound content. However, phonologicaltherapy continued to attract SLPs/SLTs and students seeking 'therapy tips and ideas' in the message, links, and files archives.

Around the same time, clinicians and academics worldwide increased and promoted their professional (lab) and personal (SLP/SLT-topic specific) websites and blogs as never before. They also furthered their active engagement in Facebook, Instagram, Linkedin, ResearchGate, Twitter, and YouTube. Membership of Facebook groups like Clinical Research for SLPs, E^{3}BP for SSD, ReST – Rapid Syllable Transition Training, SLPs for Evidence Based Practice, and The Write Stuff: A ComDis Writing Group, ballooned and maintained research focus.

COVID-19, a Digital Surge, and Telepractice

The Yahoo! Groups' closure coincided with the start of the COVID-19 pandemic. A 'digital surge' (De' et al., 2020) followed, due to lockdowns, physical distancing, and the need to adapt and continue providing services as best we could. Privileged SLPs/SLTs in industrialised countries, and their clients with access, became familiar, adept, and innovative with videoconferencing and telehealth.

Zoom- and MS Teams-fatigue notwithstanding, primary, secondary and all forms of postsecondary education were delivered online in unprecedented volumes, as were CPD and SIG events, research forums, conferences, and web meetings, and an unforeseen boom occurred in the digital and e-commerce sectors. Developers seized opportunities to improve new platforms such as the secure and private telepractice software, Coviu released in 2015 (Sutherland et al., 2017), with a new version with improvements released fortnightly (Silvia Pfeiffer, Coviu https://www.coviu.com Founder and CEO, personal correspondence April 2022).

In 2020, Coviu took second place on Deloitte's list of fastest growing companies with 11,553% growth. That year, the number of telehealth consultations on the Coviu platform across health professions rose from 400 daily, peaking at 25,000 per day, before settling down to around 16-to-20,000 per day, amounting to over 7 million consultations, and counting to September 2022. Some 10-to-15 percent of consultations are conducted by SLPs/SLTs in Australia (where it began), the UK, and the US, and telepractice, via Coviu and other platforms, flourished.

Three Telepractitioners

Readers met **Dr. Pam Williams** at the top of Q33 in Chapter 8 and will recall that she has expertise in motor speech disorders and in delivering training courses. Pam had already run in-person training courses for SLPs/SLTs on CAS/DVD and NDP3 for over 30 years, but in June 2020, she was challenged to deliver such training virtually via Zoom, in collaboration with Reeves Consultancy and Training Ltd. trading as Course Beetle. With no previous experience of videoconferencing, she has presented numerous sets of online modules with more planned, to audiences including delegates from the UK, Ireland, Australia, New Zealand, Singapore, Canada, and the USA.

Dr. Donna Thomas is a speech pathologist, lecturer and clinical educator at The University of Sydney, Australia. Her research focusses on assessment and treatment for children with moderate-severe speech sound disorders, clinical education, and telepractice. In 2020–2021, Donna was a member of the Speech Pathology Australia (SPA) telepractice working party, which reviewed the evidence for telepractice assessment and treatment, and developed resources to support speech pathologists seeking to use telepractice.

Nicole Caballero is a certified speech-language pathologist at the Gebbie Speech-Language-Hearing Clinic and Speech Production Laboratory at Syracuse University. In her clinical work, she conducts assessments and provides treatment to preschoolers and school-age children with speech sound disorders. Nicole participates in research on the diagnosis and treatment of speech sound disorders, including treatment delivered using telepractice.

Q46. Pam Williams, Donna Thomas, and Nicole Caballero: SSD Services and Professional Education via Telepractice

Increasingly, SLPs/SLTs engage with their clients and their families, undergraduate and graduate students, and CPD/CEU/PD/PRO-D/training participants via telepractice. To date, there is a sparse but largely helpful literature to guide them, whether they are working with children and young people with speech sound disorder (SSD), providing clinical education or delivering professional development events on SSD in general, or motor speech disorder (MSD) in particular. What advice would you give newcomers to telepractice in terms of the technical skills required, mastering the technology, communicating with peers, students, parents, or caregivers, performing assessment, and delivering intervention? What ethical and legal issues must be considered when working across state or national boundaries, and when negotiating contracts with online professional development providers?

A46. Pam Williams, Donna Thomas, and Nicole Caballero: Telepractice in SSD: Application for Assessment, Treatment, Training, and Clinical Education

Heading our 'what to advise novice teletherapists or educators' checklist are to:

- approach telepractice optimistically and not anticipate (or dread) undue resistance from **clients** or **CPD participants**.
- turn to *your own* national **professional association** for information and guidance.
- identify **ethical** and **legal** requirements specific to your jurisdiction, being sure to check your association's 3-Rs: resources, rules, and regulations.
- survey the relevant, recent, peer reviewed **literature** on telepractice.

- seek **technical advice** and guard against being intimidated by the technology.
- be aware that many helpful, **practical resources** are available.

In the following sections, we cover these areas, in the order that they appear on our checklist. Then follow sections on student education and CPD/CEU/PD/PRO-D/training delivered online. Professional development (PD) is usually called continuing professional development (CPD) in Australia, Ireland, New Zealand, South Africa, and the UK, CEUs in the States, and PRO-D in Canada. CPD is often simply called 'training' in the UK and Ireland. For brevity, we call it CPD here.

Approach Telepractice Optimistically

Prior to the COVID-19 pandemic, few SLPs/SLTs routinely delivered services via telepractice. When they did, it was mostly for clients living in rural and remote areas. More widespread telepractice delivery was hampered by clients' access to technology and reliable internet, as well as the clinician's perceptions of, and attitudes to telepractice. In 2020 however, when in-person services were not possible due to COVID-19 public health measures, telepractice acceptance and uptake ballooned internationally (Aggarwal et al., 2020; Campbell & Goldstein, 2021; Fong et al., 2021). For example, a survey study of American paediatric SLPs showed the percentage of clinicians employing telepractice rose from 18% prior to the pandemic to 90% in March–October 2020 (Campbell & Goldstein, 2021). This enabled a new generation of SLPs to have hands-on telepractice experience, and in doing so, to increase their confidence and proficiency. Most of these clinicians saw a role for telepractice in their ongoing clinical work, beyond the pandemic period (Campbell & Goldstein, 2021; Kollia & Tsiamtsiouris, 2021). Pleasingly, Campbell & Goldstein's 2021 survey study revealed that neither the number of years working in the SLP profession, nor their workplace settings made a difference to telepractice adoption during the pandemic or willingness to continue with tele-

practice in the future. Their findings indicated that learning how to conduct telepractice and feeling comfortable with the technology is not beyond any of us.

While some clients may be initially hesitant, once they've experienced telepractice, most find it convenient and acceptable, and in many cases, prefer it to in-person sessions (Filbay et al., 2021). The same can be true for student education and CPD experiences. The rapid adoption of telepractice during COVID-19 gave clinicians, clients and CPD participants reason to be optimistic about its ongoing role in SLP practice.

Your Professional Association as a Telepractice Resource

Up-to-date information and guidance may be available on professional associations websites. Most of the six Mutual Recognition Agreement (MRA) associations (ASHA in the US, IASLT in Ireland, NZSTA in New Zealand, the RCSLT in the UK, SAC-OAC in Canada, and SPA in Australia) have web-based information regarding telepractice. For example, ASHA, IASLT, RCSLT and SPA each have a telepractice position statement, technical report, summary of telepractice evidence, and information about local licensure, ethical considerations, and reimbursement. ASHA's resources, which are available to members and international affiliates, include a Telepractice Practice Portal, Evidence Map and Special Interest Group (SIG18), as well as the ASHA Learning Pass to access Continuing Education Units (CEUs). Drawing on and acknowledging the RCSLT and SPA guidelines, IASLT has developed and posted, in a private members' area, a statement on telepractice which they kindly shared with us. It comprises a short evidence brief, a suite of recorded webinars, and links to external resources. The RCSLT updated their telepractice and communications technology guidelines in 2020, and SPA updated the telepractice policy, position statement, and evidence summary across a range of practice areas in 2021. Reassuringly, the associations' revisions, updates, and developments of new telepractice materials are ongoing, in response to both fluid situations nationally and internationally, and to their members' needs and feedback.

Legal and Ethical Requirements

SLPs/SLTs must ensure they meet national and local legal and ethical requirements. For example, ASHA states that telepractice sessions must be equivalent in quality to in-person services (as does IASLT), and that the SLP and/or Audiologist must be licensed in both the state they are located and the state the client is located at the time of service. Additional licensure and telepractice policies, reimbursement guidelines, and security requirements vary by state, and it is clinicians' responsibility to verify this information with state licensure boards and regulating departments. New clinicians completing their clinical fellowships should obtain guidance from the Council for Clinical Certification in Audiology and Speech-Language Pathology (CFCC) on telepractice as a supervision mechanism and/or as a mechanism to accumulate hours. The Audiology and Speech-Language Pathology Interstate Compact (ASLP-IC) was activated in 2021, allowing licensed clinicians in member states to apply for a privilege to practice across all ASLP-IC states.

In the UK, SLTs must adhere to professional standards set by the Health Professions and Care Council (HCPC), and to UK legislation, on matters such as information governance and data protection regulation (GDPR). Informed consent (verbal or written) from service-users to participate in telepractice is required. Practitioners should obtain specific consent before audio or video recording sessions and ensure they comply with local and national guidance, including privacy laws, regarding storage of such recordings.

SPA members should familiarise themselves with Government, AHPRA, and professional association resources that are pertinent to telepractice in all settings. If they have transitioned from practising in an institutional setting including private practice 'rooms' to working from home, they should confirm they have Professional Indemnity and Public Liability cover, remembering that they have a Duty of Care to themselves and others. The Telepractice Resources page contains a FAQ document about international standards to observe when members source or provide services internationally.

Peer-Reviewed Literature

Practitioners are advised to check recent peer-reviewed literature for evidence concerning the application of telepractice, summaries of which are available on the ASHA, IASLT, RCSLT and SPA websites. In terms of equivalency of telepractice for SSD assessment, the evidence is mixed (Taylor et al., 2014). Telepractice assessments reveal similar findings to in-person assessments when screening for the presence or absence of an SSD (Ciccia et al., 2011), rating connected speech intelligibility (Waite et al., 2006) and oral musculature assessments (OMA) (Waite et al., 2012). Without access to ideal camera positioning and good lighting, however, some aspects of OMA have fair to poor reliability (Waite et al., 2006, 2012). When conducting single-word assessments, the results are generally similar in telepractice and in-person contexts, with a few noteworthy caveats (Eriks-Brophy et al., 2008; Jessiman, 2003; Waite et al., 2006).

Although assessments conducted via telepractice reliably indicate whether a sound is in error, telepractice assessors don't always perceive the same error as an in-person assessor. The sounds that are most difficult to identify via telepractice are fricatives, affricates, voiceless consonants, s-clusters, and those without visible articulation (e.g., /tʃ/ and /l/; Eriks-Brophy et al., 2008; Jessiman, 2003; Waite et al., 2006). Additionally, abnormal nasal resonance is difficult to identify via telepractice (Hill et al., 2006). Most of the challenges with telepractice speech assessment are overcome when the child wears a lapel microphone (Jessiman, 2003), the clinician wears good quality headphones, the examiner can review recordings of the child's productions and a facilitator at the child's site assists with camera angle and lighting (Waite et al., 2012).

In well-controlled research, Campbell and Goldstein (2022) investigated the reliability of speech assessment with the GFTA-3 (Goldman & Fristoe, 2015) in three listening conditions: 1. live in-person, 2. synchronous telepractice with a consumer-grade microphone, and 3. synchronous telepractice without a microphone. In previous SSD-related telepractice studies, researchers have used equipment with higher specifications than is available to most clients. Indeed, many clients choose to engage in telepractice without a microphone and if one is worn, it will likely be inexpensive. Campbell & Goldstein reported no significant difference between SLPs' judgements on the GFTA-3 via any of the listening conditions. The authors noted, however, that despite no significant differences between conditions on scoring reliability, SLP participants reported they continued to prefer in-person over a telehealth speech sound assessment.

In terms of SSD treatment, outcomes are mostly equivalent when delivered in-person and via telepractice (Wales et al., 2017). Grogan-Johnson et al. (2011); Grogan-Johnson et al. (2013) found that school-age children who received traditional SSD treatment, which included discrimination training, and acquisition and generalization of a target speech sound through several substages from syllables to structured conversation, via telepractice and children who received the same therapy in-person made similar and significant gains. Additionally, a retrospective study comparing in-person and telepractice intervention found no difference in functional outcomes between the two groups (Coufal et al., 2018). Preliminary evidence supports the use of telepractice to implement ReST treatment (see McCabe, A32) for five children with CAS (Thomas et al., 2016; and see, Bahar et al., 2022) and the multiple opposition approach for two children with severe phonological disorders (Lee, 2018).

Technical Skills for Clinical Services

The selection of appropriate technology is vital to maximize therapeutic benefits. Both the clinician and the client must have consistent and reliable internet connection and a computer or a 10-inch or greater tablet with a webcam. Smaller devices such as smartphones limit viewing the clinician's face and of the materials being shown. Although not required, some clinicians prefer two monitors, with one displaying a full-size image of the videoconferencing platform and the second displaying materials. A minimum internet speed of 3MB is recommended to ensure video and audio quality (ASHA, n.d.). Free internet speed test websites, such as speedtest. net, are available to monitor bandwidth. Ideally, both the SLP/SLT and the client wear headsets to ensure audio quality and reduce background noise. If a parent or facilitator is actively involved in the session, a 3.5 mm splitter can be used to connect multiple headphones, with the child's microphone connected to the computer via a USB port or wirelessly.

Teletherapists in the US must (and those elsewhere are advised to) select a HIPAA compliant videoconferencing platform to host sessions, choosing between a general video platform (i.e., HIPAA-compliant versions of Zoom or Google Meet) or a therapy specific platform (i.e., Blink Session, Coviu). Helpful features for SSD therapy include screen-sharing, annotation features, a digital whiteboard, chat function, screen-recording, and remote mouse access. A trial period ('try before you buy') to test platform functionality and compatibility may be available on request.

The RCSLT website includes a comparison of available digital platforms. SLPs/SLTs adopting telepractice should be aware that individual employers may restrict the choice of digital platform; for example, SLTs employed by the National Health Service (NHS) are restricted to using either AccuRx or Attend Anywhere digital platforms.

Practical Advice

- Prior to the first session, conduct a 10-minute 'telepractice familiarization session' to troubleshoot technology issues, trial features (i.e., screen sharing), and answer any questions. Ideally, this session is free or not counted towards the service limit.
- Consider providing the family with a written document outlining instructions for using the technology and expectations (see, Werfel et al., 2021 for examples).

- Discuss expectations regarding the caregiver's role (e.g., be present for the session, facilitate the child's engagement, ensure the client's face is on the screen, troubleshoot technological issues).
- Consider whether you can schedule more-frequent sessions than were permissible with in-person sessions, as the family will avoid travel time and costs, and the client may benefit from increased session frequency (Allen, 2013).
- Seek digital versions of published tests. Pearson Assessment's Q-global platform has digital versions of the DEAP (Dodd et al., 2006) and the GFTA-3 (Goldman & Fristoe, 2015).
- If the speech sound assessment you prefer is unavailable for use on a digital platform, use unpublished tests and/or create your own stimuli designed for your client.
- The knowledge and skills you utilize when selecting an intervention approach, determining treatment goals, and preparing session activities for in-person therapy will extend to telepractice. Consider how you would implement in-person therapy and make appropriate adaptations.
- Check whether the session materials can be scanned legitimately, noting that copyright materials must not be scanned. Scanned paper materials can be shared via screen share and made interactive with features such as annotation and providing the child with mouse control.
- Free digital materials and activities of varying quality are widely available from, for example, Pinterest, Facebook Groups dedicated to telepractice speech therapy, and SLP/SLT blogs. Low-cost digital resources are available via TeachersPayTeachers (TPT) and Boom Cards.
- As with in-person therapy, reinforcers should motivate the child and incorporate their interests. Game breaks may include online games, a short YouTube video, or drawing on a virtual whiteboard. Reinforcers can also include materials from the child's environment (i.e., a favorite toy) and movement breaks (i.e., star jumps).

- Conversational speech can be practised with games and activities from websites such as PBSKids, ABCya, Poki, and Funbrain.
- Review online material prior to the session to check for inappropriate content, advertisements, or pop-ups.

Student Education

Telepractice provides opportunities for SLP/SLT students to conduct clinical sessions and/or receive clinical education ('telesupervision') when the educator, client and/or student are geographically distant (Martin et al., 2017). This enables the conduct of clinical placements in geographically remote sites, and for the placements to continue when in-person sessions are on hold, as in a pandemic. Telesupervision is acceptable to educators and meets the learning needs of students (Nagarajan et al., 2016). Although student use of telepractice is feasible, it adds a layer of complexity compared with in-person sessions (Overby & Baft-Neff, 2017). One main benefit of telesupervision is that the educator can provide real-time 'silent' feedback the clients' awareness, via the private chat function of the telepractice portal (Beiting & Nicolet, 2020). Silent feedback (also known as BITEye) increases student autonomy, circumvents session interruptions, and is most efficient when the educator limits messages to 10 words or fewer (Beiting & Nicolet, 2020).

CPD/CEU/PD/PRO-D/Training

CPD, by any synonymous name, is a *requirement* for most SLPs/SLTs. In-person short training courses on specific clinical topics have traditionally been a popular form of CPD, but the physical presence of participants and presenters at such courses ranged from difficult to impossible during the COVID-19 pandemic. Training providers and hosts of SIGs or Clinical Excellence Networks (CENs) adapted swiftly, offering CPD events online.

With no literature to guide practice, presenters and hosts had to be flexible, adapting their resources for online delivery, knowing that they needed adequate technological skills to perform professionally and effectively. Equally, CPD participants have required essential 'tech savvy', equipment and again, flexibility to gain from these novel virtual experiences. Participants report, in post-training evaluations, certain advantages associated with online training, such as no travel requirements, reduced costs and controlled time commitments (personal communication (04.12.2020) Dot Reeves, Director Training & Consultancy Ltd, trading as Course Beetle). Furthermore, online training can closely mirror in-person experiences when tools such as Breakout rooms are used for small group work and discussions and questions are invited verbally or via a Chat facility.

Just as a written contract for service provision is drawn up between an SLP/SLT and a client, there should be a written contract between a training provider and speaker, specifying terms and conditions and considering contractual and legal requirements. Speakers should negotiate such terms and conditions, ensuring they are satisfied with the security and protection put in place for online delivery. Agreement should be reached on how the:

- **participants** will access handouts and other course resources to protect the speaker's intellectual property (e.g., distributed as pdfs via email; or made available as view only, print or download options through an encrypted portal, using software, such as Vitrium).
- **provider** plans to restrict participants from sharing resources without permission (e.g., through a written document asking participants not to share; or watermarking downloadable content to a registered participant).
- **speaker** regards their sessions being recorded. If, after careful thought, they are willing for this to happen, they must be clear on how such recordings might be used. If recordings are made, additional protection may be required for some aspects, such as removing, editing, and/or pixilating video clips to protect clients' identity.

Summary

Telepractice was already well established for some SLPs/SLTs, however the COVID-19 pandemic pushed many others to use it to deliver clinical services, student education and CPD activities. In future, it is likely to continue as a routine part of clinical practice, alongside in-person services. Newcomers to telepractice do not need to be concerned; there is a wealth of advice, guidance, and resources available to support them.

Technology Assisted SLP/SLT (TASLP/SLT)

Survey responses from 80 British SLTs on the use of TASLT in assessing, treating, and motivating children with phonological delay, reported by Kuschmann et al. (2021) showed that 25% of respondents did not use TASLT for telepractice (telehealth) assessment or treatment. The 75% that did used a desktop or laptop computer (35%), a landline (27%), a tablet/iPad (34%), and a smartphone (10%), with 12% of SLTs having access to a single device (either a landline telephone, computer, or tablet). The research team noted a clear trend towards using devices to support face-to-face assessment (47%) and treatment (82%) rather than replacing it or performing evaluations and intervention remotely using devices. The SLTs used apps and computer software for articulation, minimal pairs, and phonological awareness intervention (see Joffe A23 for an insightful response), voice recording and phonetic transcription. Reportedly, the SLTs' use of technology was aimed at increasing client motivation (82%), facilitating home practice (63%), and speech analysis (48%).

Kuschmann et al. listed the SLTs' 'major barriers' to TASLT, notably unavailability of devices in clinics, followed by practitioners' lack of awareness of suitable apps, the absence of permission to instal apps on NHS devices, and a general scarcity of appropriate software.

As it stands, the use of technology in speech-language pathology provision in the UK appears to be largely determined by each individual clinician's knowledge and willingness to engage with technology, combined with determination to overcome institutional and client barriers at various stages of treatment. Joint efforts at individual, local, national as well as international levels will be required to tackle these challenges and effect the change needed to equip speech-language pathology services with the technological resources and skills that can benefit clients' communication.

Kuschmann et al., 2021, p. 152

Apps

In the Kuschmann et al. British study, Just 55% of the 80 participants used apps, compared to 77% of 69 school based SLPs in the US (Olszewski et al., 2022).

Regrettably, the popularity and demand for TASLP/SLT interventions for SSD are not associated with a comparable volume of evidence 'for' or 'against' their use and efficacy (Peterson et al., 2022). Indeed, Furlong et al. (2018) searched systematically for publicly available apps finding 132 that were intended for SSD treatment. Only 19/132 apps (14%) were deemed to have probable value in treating children with SSD. This pointed to a mismatch between software development and the scrupulous requirements of evidence-based clinical practice. There is, therefore, a pressing need for more research on apps designed for SSD intervention to allow SLPs/SLTs to make confident, evidence-based decisions about which to adopt (Furlong et al., 2018; Olszewski et al., 2022; Peterson et al., 2022). For years there have been promising signs that the general lack of rigorous research into apps might change (e.g., *Say Bananas:*, Ahmed et al., 2022; the free *SAILS App* for iPad: Rvachew A18; and *SCIP-2:*, Williams, 2016) but much more must be done.

Generalist SLPS/SLTS and Biofeedback Instrumentation

SLP/SLT clinicians working with children and young people with unclear speech encounter clients with atypical articulatory gestures who do not meet the criteria for a diagnosis of developmental dysarthria or CAS, but who, to a skilled observer, have a subtle motoric difficulty that is neurologically based, structurally based or both. In private conversation, therapists may refer to their speech presentation as dysarthria-like, apraxia-like, or even dysarthric-y or dyspraxic-y.

The diagnostic landscape shifted somewhat when Shriberg et al. (2010, 2011) developed extensions to the Speech Disorders Classification system (SDCS), coining the term Motor Speech Disorders–Not Otherwise Specified (MSD-NOS), later re-labelled as Speech Motor Delay (SMD; Shriberg et al., 2019) as a better fit for this 'in between' population (see Chapter 2). Some two decades later, little has changed regarding treatment options for SLPs/SLTs without easy access to biofeedback instrumentation.

They might correctly diagnose SMD, but then intervene with 1) an articulation therapy following a sound-by-sound methodology in a traditional 'van Riper therapy' sensorimotor paradigm (Bauman-Waengler, 2020, pp. 271–281), or 2) a phonological therapy focusing on perception and production of minimal pairs in a linguistically motivated approach (Baker, 2021), 3) some combination of the previous two, or 4) deliver therapy based on the Principles of Motor Learning (PML) such as the Speech Systems Approach which focuses on increasing intelligibility in developmental dysarthria (Pennington, A30), or an intervention designed for children with CAS, like DTTC (Strand, A31), ReST (McCabe, A32), and NDP3 (Williams, A33).

Articulation therapy, phonological therapy and PML-based therapy combine *auditory* perception (listening) and *visual* attention to the therapist (watching) as active ingredients, expected to promote immediate and longer-term intelligibility gains. In treatment, clients are urged constantly to 'listen to me and watch my face'. But the *auditory-visual* combination of ear training and face-watching may not be sufficiently powerful to modify hard-to-observe erred articulatory gestures in the SMD population.

This is particularly so for older children and young people with entrenched lingual errors, who may have had years of intervention that was a poor fit for their needs, and who are likely disenchanted and bored with the whole thing. Might Visual Biofeedback (VBF) interventions, such as electropalatography (EPG) and ultrasound, that provide real-time articulatory feedback in the form of *visual* displays of largely out-of-sight articulatory placement capture their interest and stimulate renewed cooperation in these therapy veterans? Who better to ask about articulatory visual biofeedback

(VBF) instrumentation than Joanne Cleland and James Scobbie?

Dr. Joanne Cleland is a Reader in Speech and Language Therapy at the University of Strathclyde in Glasgow, Scotland. Her research focuses on instrumental techniques, particularly ultrasound tongue imaging, for the assessment and treatment of children with Speech Sound Disorders. She uses instrumental articulatory techniques to measure tongue-shape and movement during speech to answer theoretical questions about the underlying nature of speech disorder in children with persistent SSDs. This is coupled with ongoing collaborative work with clinical colleagues measuring the effectiveness of ultrasound visual biofeedback as an intervention for children with persistent SSDs, including in cleft lip and palate.

Dr. Jim Scobbie is professor of speech sciences at Queen Margaret University, Edinburgh. After an undergraduate degree in Linguistics with Artificial Intelligence, his doctoral research concentrated on formalism in theoretical and computational phonology. Since coming to QMU to work on a project on covert contrast in disordered speech with Fiona Gibbon and Bill Hardcastle in 1993, he has worked on the phonetics/phonology interface in sociolinguistics, laboratory phonology, child speech development and in clinical contexts. His particular focus is on the use of ultrasound and articulatory phonetics in research. As director of the CASL Research Centre, he has also contributed to his colleagues' projects that use ultrasound in swallowing research and phonetics teaching (the SeeingSpeech resource).

Q47. Joanne Cleland and James M. Scobbie: Visual Biofeedback Interventions

What is in the current range of articulatory visual biofeedback (VBF) instrumentation for SLPs/SLTs in specialist settings to use in a speech motor-learning paradigm for children and youth with erred, apparently intractable lingual articulations? What factors should a generalist SLP/SLT be thinking about when referring their clients for assessment of VBF suitability? What can the young clients and their parents expect of the assessment process, and intervention if it transpires? What evi-

dence is currently available to support the application of VBF? Cleland et al. (2019) report the variability of generalization in a case series of fifteen 6-to-15-year-old children with heterogeneous SSDs who received VBF. Remarkably, ten went from non-stimulable status at initial assessment to achieving their targeted articulation within one or two 1-hour treatment sessions. What evidence based and affordable VBF devices or applications are currently on the market, in development or on the horizon for generalist clinicians with modest budgets and what would you like to see in future research and development?

A47. Joanne Cleland and James M. Scobbie: Practical Options for Articulatory Feedback in the Speech Clinic

Articulatory Visual Biofeedback for treating SSDs currently comprises two main techniques: electropalatography (EPG) and ultrasound tongue imaging. Both techniques were pioneered in the phonetics laboratory for measuring lingual gestures and constrictions in typical speakers but have been applied in the speech therapy clinic with children with persistent SSDs. Each technique can show tongue movement (ultrasound) or tongue-palate contact (EPG) in real time, providing the client with a novel type of feedback about their own articulations. This 'knowledge of performance' (KP) about the movements of the tongue augments 'knowledge of results'(KR) about the perceptual correctness of an articulation (Maas et al., 2008), and can enable speakers with intractable SSDs to achieve new articulations (Sugden et al., 2019). Each of these techniques fits well with a motor learning paradigm, particularly with the pre-practice phase of intervention (Cleland & Preston, 2020; McCabe, A32). In this phase, the SLP/SLT essentially teaches the client how to make an appropriate articulatory gesture relevant to the speech sound in error, and to suppress inappropriate ones. Authors of some case studies report that using biofeedback leads to quick acquisition of new articulatory gestures, even after previous unsuccessful intervention (e.g., Gibbon et al., 1993; Modha et al., 2008). Typically, errors are either residual distortions of consonants like /r/ or /s/; persistent developmental neutralizations such as velar fronting; or compensatory articulations associated with cleft lip and palate such as backing. Once the client can achieve an acceptable new articulation in at least a single syllable, the practice phase of intervention reinforces these new articulations so that they are learnt, retained, and generalised with decreasing conscious effort and increasing automaticity. Typically, practice involves increasingly complex contexts, building from single syllables to short words, phrases, and conversational speech.

Since VBF uses a motor learning paradigm, suitable clients for these interventions share characteristics with suitable clients for other motor speech or articulation interventions. A major pre-requisite for motor-based intervention is clients' motivation and adequate attention to cope with drill-based practice (Dugan et al., 2019). Thus, clients are usually over seven years old, although some research studies with younger children have taken place (Heng et al., 2016). Typically, clients have one or two lingual speech sounds in error that may have been resistant to other intervention approaches (Preston et al., 2020). VBF has also been useful in therapy with clients with cleft lip and palate (Roxburgh et al., 2021), Down syndrome (Wood et al., 2019), hearing impairment (Bernhardt et al., 2003), persistent SSD (Cleland et al., 2019) and Childhood Apraxia of Speech (Preston et al., 2013).

Rather than being adopted because it is suitable for a specific client group, clients are typically referred for biofeedback because they have a particular difficulty achieving a specific lingual speech sound and this has not been remediated by non-instrumental approaches such as articulation or phonological intervention. Biofeedback is therefore suitable for various SSD subtypes, particularly articulation disorder, Speech Motor Delay, or other motor speech disorders.

Where to refer clients to is an ongoing problem. Access to articulatory VBF has most often been via funded research studies with strict protocols. This picture is changing, however, with some specialist schools and some community clinics in the United Kingdom and the Republic of Ireland having access to instrumentation, particularly to ultrasound. Although EPG and ultrasound may in theory be suited to different clients, in practice the clinician will be constrained by which instrumentation is available.

For the most part, clinics (including most university clinics) do not have a choice of different instruments available to suit each individual client's needs. This is especially the case with EPG which requires expensive individualised hardware in the form of a custom-made pseudo-palate with embedded electrodes. This EPG palate allows the client to see their own tongue-palate contact patterns in real time and has the advantage that it shows not only front/back contact of the tongue, but also lateral bracing, which is particularly relevant for sibilant production, especially lateral lisps (Dagenais et al., 1994). The major drawback of EPG is that each palate costs in the region of $200USD to $600USD, depending on the system used. Moreover, because the pseudo-palate needs to fit snugly against the roof of the mouth, clients must have stable secondary dentition in place to support it, and that is usually established by, or soon after the seventh birthday. A dentist can advise on whether a client's dentition is suitable for EPG.

In contrast, ultrasound does not require individualised equipment, however, there are still initial outlay costs. Even clinicians working in a hospital environment may find that ultrasound machines available locally are not suitable for speech intervention as only some probes and set ups are suitable for imaging the tongue (Cleland, 2021). Moreover, if the clinician wants to record ultrasound to support assessment, as is recommended, the machine must operate at a high enough frame rate to capture speech events without distortion or blurring, as well as being synchronised accurately with the audio signal (Wrench & Scobbie, 2006).

The Assessment and Intervention Process

Children and young people referred for biofeedback can expect that both assessment and intervention involve the instrumentation. For EPG, a suitability evaluation will normally take place first, followed by at least one visit to a dentist for an impression to be taken of the upper teeth and palate. In the case of ultrasound, assessment with the technique can begin right away. Assessment normally consists of a thorough investigation of phonology, articulation, oromotor skills, and stimulability in CV, VC and CVC. Probe lists, focussing on the client's consonant or vowel errors should be utilised. The consonant or vowel in error should be elicited in a variety of word positions and vowel/consonant environments. Minimal pairs should be elicited where relevant. Single words, including multisyllabic words, and connected speech should also be sampled. The speech sample is normally collected as a simultaneous EPG/ultrasound and audio recording.

This process allows the clinician to identify whether the client can accurately produce the sounds in error in any context and to determine whether the error sounds show any specific articulatory patterns. In particular, the clinician will look for evidence of covert contrast where a putative merger of two or more phonemes is signalled by productions with subtly different articulatory configurations (Gibbon & Lee, 2017). The clinician will also look for other articulatory errors such as undifferentiated lingual gestures or reduced complexity of tongue shape (Kabakoff et al., 2021). All these error types suggest motor control immaturity, underlining the appropriateness of a motor-based intervention rather than a phonological intervention.

Following assessment, the clinician will choose one or two consonants or vowels to target in intervention. Target selection is often straightforward as, typically, clients with residual speech sound disorders have only one or two speech sounds in error. In more complex cases, the clinician should focus on errors which are amenable to treatment with the instrumentation available (i.e., involve either tongue shape for ultrasound or tongue-palate-contact for EPG) and which evidence the largest number of errors on assessment (Cleland et al., 2019). In line with the motor learning paradigm, intervention is often drill based, with a high number of trials (at least 100) per session. The client can expect to sit at a computer and guided by the clinician, use the visual information on the screen to try to change incorrect articulatory

gestures. A video, illustrating ultrasound biofeedback intervention for two clients aged 17 and 5 years that accompanies the Cleland and Preston (2020) chapter is available to registered users via the book's Download Hub (https://downloads.brookespublishing.com).

The clinician will use canonical EPG patterns or ultrasound tongue shapes to show the client static targets for the correct articulation. Short dynamic visual models in which the canonical targets are readily identified are also useful. These can be provided via live demonstration of the correct articulation by the clinician or by using pre-recorded videos of typical speakers. This pre-practice phase, where the client attempts to modify the erroneous articulation, is arguably the most demanding part of the intervention for the client. Some clients may spend several sessions in this pre-practice phase of intervention or never achieve the target intervention despite multiple sessions (Preston et al., 2016), while others may acquire their new speech sound in as little as one to two sessions (Cleland et al., 2019). The characteristics of children and young people who are likely to respond to the intervention and in what time frame is not yet fully understood, however it is possible that distortions of later acquired speech sounds such as /r/ may be more resistant to treatment and that auditory perceptual acuity might affect treatment progress (Cialdella et al., 2021). Intervention is usually delivered once or twice a week in sessions of around an hour for about 14 weeks (Sugden et al., 2019), although this varies considerably.

Evidence for the effectiveness of biofeedback is variable. Most published intervention studies are single case reports or case series, with only a few small group studies, although there are at least two ongoing randomised control trials of ultrasound biofeedback currently underway (McAllister et al., 2020, Cleland et al., 2021). A systematic review of ultrasound biofeedback (Sugden et al., 2019) showed that that most studies show good evidence for the effectiveness of ultrasound, but larger scale well-controlled studies are needed. For EPG, there are many small n studies, but few group studies: a 2009 Cochrane review of EPG for clients with cleft lip and palate (Lee et al., 2009) found only one RCT met inclusion criteria. It therefore remains difficult to give clients clear information on the likely success of biofeedback interventions. This is problematic when other types of interventions might be suitable because it should be noted that many studies, particularly EPG studies, have tended to enrol only children and young people for whom previous intervention had failed. After the biofeedback intervention, it is likely that clients will need further intervention, perhaps using a motor-learning paradigm (without the instrumentation) to generalise their new articulations.

The Future of Biofeedback

EPG and ultrasound are unlikely to become available in every community clinic. Rather, they are more likely to be specialist techniques available at regional centres. The techniques are expensive, potentially involving specialist training and ongoing practice for clinicians to confidently interpret the EPG patterns or ultrasound tongue shapes.

Biofeedback devices which use acoustic information only and are compatible with smartphones or home computers are a potential future goal. Much progress has already been made in using acoustic biofeedback for treating /r/ distortions (McAllister Byun, et al., 2017) including the freely available 'staRt app' (https://wp.nyu.edu/byunlab/projects/start/download-start). However, the app is targeted towards treating distortions of /r/, with a particular emphasis on speakers of standard American English, which may limit its generalisability. Moreover, each class of segmental or structural phonetic error requires a different acoustic basis for analysis and perhaps a different approach to feedback. The same goes for prosodic and voice problems. However, acoustic analysis has two enormous advantages over articulatory analysis: namely the accessibility of modern speech technologies and the limited hardware they require (microphone and computer).

The recent explosion in Automatic Speech Recognition (ASR) – for example, Alexa and Google Assistant, and Siri – exploits technologies which will likely be applied to create acoustics-driven biofeedback tools which show children their speech errors in near-real time. Similar technologies have been applied to pronunciation training for adults learning a second language (O'Brien et al., 2018). Although these systems detect mispronunciations accurately there remains a need for better software which can combine accurate ASR with teaching instruction. Accuracy of ASR for children's voices remains problematic, and of disordered children and young people's voices even more so. Basic technical challenges are compounded by the need to provide reliable real-time visualizations of mergers or errors that are useful in a therapeutic context. Nevertheless, some commercially available apps show promise (for example, Hair et al., 2019) for disordered speech. Acoustic feedback is not, however, directly informative of speech production. There is no easy one-to-one mapping of acoustic parameters to articulatory gestures: acoustically similar productions can be created from a variety of articulatory configurations. EPG and ultrasound, however, show important individual articulatory parameters directly. They also reveal problematic speech production behaviour, which is silent or covert, for example, groping of the articulators. It is not surprising therefore that current acoustic-based biofeedback devices cannot tell a client whether an error is present or not, for a wide variety of consonants and vowels, nor to provide both client and clinician with reliable real-time information about how the articulators are moving. The future of biofeedback therefore needs to include both acoustic and articulatory solutions.

Communities of Practice (CoPs)

Communities of practice (CoPs) are a collaborative knowledge transfer strategy that can be used for evidence-based practice implementation.
Alary Gauvreau et al., 2019

Although the term Communities of Practice (Wegner et al., 2002; Wegner & Snyder, 2000; Wenger, 1998) was coined before the turn of the century (Lave &

Wenger, 1991), little research had been conducted into their effect on EBP implementation. Available reports include Barwick et al. (2009), Buysse et al. (2003), Terry et al. (2020), and Thomson et al. (2013), with signs that more is to come (e.g., Elbrink et al., 2021). The SLP/SLT research in this area is sparse, but with outstanding exceptions, e.g., Alary Gauvreau et al. (2019) evaluating an Aphasia CoP. They concluded that 'SLPs can include more participation-based approaches in their aphasia rehabilitation practice within a CoP intentionally designed to support learning, reflection, interaction and collaboration among peers.'

Wenger (1998) said that to be identified as such, a community of practice should have three distinct characteristics: 1) *Domain*: a shared interest; 2) *Practice*: a shared body of knowledge, experiences, and techniques; and 3) *Community*: a self-selected group of people who care enough about the topic to participate in regular interactions. Karen McComas has been a CoP advocate and participant for many years, contributing information about them to the 2009 and 2015 editions of this book.

Dr. Karen McComas is a Professor of Communication Disorders and the Executive Director for the Center for Teaching and Learning (CTL) at Marshall University in Huntington, West Virginia, USA. She holds the ASHA Certificate of Clinical Competence in Speech-Language Pathology and Audiology. McComas is a founding member of a community of research practice (CoRP) and was the principal investigator for a narrative, collaborative ethnographic research study exploring the faculty and student community. Additional research interests include narrative studies about identity development in women researchers (McComas, 2014), the experiences and lives of caregivers and persons with disabilities in Appalachia, and Appalachian discourse. In the CTL, McComas develops and delivers programming for faculty to enhance their knowledge and skill sets for teaching, research, and community engagement. To that end, McComas has initiated a new digital humanities project involving the collection of oral histories and life stories, using a team of undergraduate researchers, as part of a community revitalization project.

Q48. Karen Mccomas

Usually, Communities of Practice (CoP) are small groups who meet over several sessions, and whose discussions are facilitated by an experienced leader in the field. A CoP can be clinical or non-clinically based with a focus on mutual interests and support, group-based learning, sharing of information and resources, and problem solving. In the second edition of this book, you answered the question: How can the socialisation experience of being a member of a disciplinary community help the transformation from student to ethical practitioner?' Can you please elaborate the same question considering more recent developments, challenges, and publications?

A48. Karen McComas: Communities of Practice in CSD: Sources of Support and Transformation

When Dr. Bowen invited me to contribute to the newest edition of *Children's Speech Sound Disorders*, I readily agreed and planned to take a different path from my contributions to earlier editions of the text. I added this to my task list with plans to complete the work well before the deadline. Not long after, however, COVID-19 stopped the world and I, like many of you, shifted into crisis mode – where I have remained for well over a year now.

Even though I have been a practising SLP and a faculty member in a CSD program for over 44 years, I now spend most of my time providing professional development for faculty members, promoting, and fostering the development of innovative approaches to teaching and learning, and doing what persons employed in higher education refer to as 'other duties as assigned'. Still, throughout the COVID-19 pandemic, I had a daily window into the worlds of my first – and primary – professional community of speech pathologists. In that window, I saw my daughter continue her work as a Speech Language Pathologist at a university hospital; enthusiastically leaving her house each morning and putting her smile back on before she returned at the end of the day. She repeatedly assured me (and perhaps herself) that she was the safest member of our family, but I saw the stress, worry, sadness, and loneliness etched on her face.

Meanwhile, my 4-year-old grandson, at home with his little brother and his dad (who had never worked from home and never had a four-year-old and one-year-old as 'co-workers'), started speech therapy via Telehealth. It was challenging for many reasons, but Miss Alice, his SLP, set aside her preferences for in-person treatment and learned what she needed to do to engage her patients virtually. Throughout his stay-at-home period, she met with him weekly. During that time, he 'won' several prizes – a testament to his progress but mostly to her efforts.

Looking through both windows, I could see two women and a man–each one strong, brave, and resilient in their individual ways – adapting to a once-in-a-lifetime (we hope) circumstance and doing so with equal measures of grace and guts. All three were impressive, but I marvelled at how much the SLPs accomplished and wondered how they were able to be so successful in such unfamiliar and frightening times. I doubt that many practising clinicians completed coursework on how to ethically provide services during a global pandemic. Yet, the achievements and successes of these two women were frequent enough throughout that time to know they were not accidental. Perhaps, I theorised, their successes evolved because they were standing shoulder to shoulder with other members of an incredibly large and strong community of practice with which they identified and to which they belonged.

I think about these two ideas, professional identities, and communities of practice, often and these were the topics of my contributions to earlier editions of this text. In the first edition, I described the importance of facilitating the development of disciplinary, or professional, identities in students. Further, I described the salient characteristics of a discipline and how those characteristics shape disciplinary

identities. Disciplines are recognised and distinguished from one another by the issues a discipline deems worthy of investigating; the inquiry approaches a discipline gives credence to; the literature the discipline identifies as authoritative; and the language (including foundational ideas and concepts), that expresses the discipline's ethical, evidentiary, and pragmatic approaches to practice.

For the second edition of the text, I shifted my theoretical description of disciplinary, or professional, identities to make a practical suggestion about how to foster identity development. In other words, I suggested that we invite students to become active members in our professional communities of practice. I went on to describe a community of practice to which I once belonged. Participants were both students and faculty and it was a transformative experience for many of the participants, me included. More specifically, the scholarly activity of the faculty drastically increased, and student participants reported gains in their own abilities to ask questions and read the primary literature and textbooks (preferring the former readings over the latter). In addition, they reported an increase in their confidence as scholars and researchers.

Communities of Practice and Support

Often loosely organised, communities of practice are tightly knit learning organizations. They reflect ways of being, prioritise what must be known and when it must be known, and present real opportunities to use knowledge in contextually appropriate ways. Every community of practice has members with varying degrees and types of experience and varying levels of participation. Members who are most actively engaged with the community stand to learn the most, but even those who participate along the periphery can also learn. All members of the community share the responsibility for the quality, the significance, and the longevity of the community.

Communities of practice are generally defined by a domain, or a shared interest; the community, or the people who share that interest; and the practice, or the things community members do. The practice is what distinguishes communities of practice from other kinds of learning organizations, such as professional learning communities. Members of a community of practice acquire new knowledge about the shared area of interest in the service of developing and refining new skills (practice). The close and supportive relationships that develop among community members spurs their growth and development.

Communities of practice sustain us during the regular course of our work. And, when we find ourselves facing new and global forces, like a pandemic, communities of practice can lift us up and encourage us, ensuring continuity of care for our patients. The concept of communities of practice is not new to SLPs/SLTs. We are used to meeting one another to talk about professional issues and we have numerous models of communities of practice, including our national organizations, regional and local organizations, and special interest groups. We 'meet' by email, telephone, and video call; at professional conferences, in the staff lunchroom, and while exiting the building at the end of the day. These interactions with our colleagues provide us with the support we require to keep on, especially when times are hard and a little bit scary. Our colleagues provide professional and emotional support; and when we are weary, as many have been during COVID-19 and its aftermath, they let us rest our heads on their shoulders.

High Impact Practices and Transformation

In addition to being supportive, communities of practice can be transformative. They offer opportunities for participants to create professional coherence by integrating theory (knowledge) and practice (skills) to accomplish certain tasks. Because communities of practice are learning organizations, the educational literature on high-impact practices (HIPs) in teaching and learning can help

us better understand the transformative nature of communities of practice. HIPs have repeatedly been shown to have a positive impact on students from many backgrounds and to increase rates of student retention and engagement. Some of the commonly used high-impact practices ask students to participate in some of the following: first year experiences, common intellectual experiences, learning communities, writing intensive courses, collaborative assignments and projects, undergraduate research, global learning courses and experiences, community-based learning, internships, or capstone experiences (called final-year projects in the UK; Kuh, 2008).

Communities of practice are inherently conducive to supporting numerous HIPs. As learning organizations, communities of practice provide participants with a common intellectual experience in a learning community. Many communities of practice set their sights beyond learning and seek to put their learning into practice by completing collaborative projects, research, or some type of community-based learning and engagement. Even so, the literature suggests that to achieve transformation, HIPs must be done well (consistently, intentionally, and innovatively) and must give learners opportunities to (Kuh, 2008):

1. exert great effort
2. build substantive relationships
3. engage across differences
4. receive rich feedback
5. apply and test what they are learning in new situations
6. reflect on the people they are becoming

Most communities of practice meet several, if not all, of those benchmarks. Members are expected to exert effort to learn; build relationships to achieve their aims; and remain open to different ideas, perspectives, experiences, and cultures. Communities of practice sustain us during the regular course of our work. And, when we find ourselves faced with new and global forces, like a pandemic, communities of practice can lift us up and encourage us, ensuring continuity of care for our patients.

Idea to Implementation

This all leads into the next, and final, question: How can educational programs provide enough opportunities so that all students might participate in a community of practice? Two sources of inspiration that can provide more than enough ideas for communities of practice immediately come to mind.

The first source of inspiration is the Scope of Practice upheld by our professional organizations. A quick glance at ASHA's Scope of Practice (American Speech-Language-Hearing Association, 2016) reveals five professional practice domains (advocacy and outreach, supervision, education, administration/leadership, and research) along with numerous service delivery domains (collaboration; counselling; prevention and wellness; screening; assessment; treatment; modalities, technology, and instrumentation; and population and systems). Each of these domains could serve as the focus, or shared interest, for a community of practice; combining domains expands the possibilities even more (e.g., advocacy and outreach coupled with prevention and wellness). While not all domains are appropriate for all students (e.g., those relating to intervention and assessment practices), there are enough areas that could engage students at all levels.

A second source of inspiration is to look outside of our own academic departments for communities of practice students might join or for potential partners to join in starting a new community of practice. Areas to consider include education, political science and public policy, healthcare management, particularly to related fields in education, public policy and political science, healthcare management, public health, and sociology.

The relationship between participating in a community of practice and developing disciplinary identities is a symbiotic one. The community shapes identity which, in turn, shapes the community. Participating in a community of practice is a powerful way to develop and build a professional identity – to become an ethical practitioner. Given the importance of communities of practice in supporting and sustaining our discipline, as evidenced most recently during the COVID-19 pandemic, integrating future SLPs/SLTs into communities of practice from the beginning of their academic careers is a sound investment in their futures and the future of the discipline.

Collaboration with Educators: Meeting Halfway

The COVID-19 pandemic was well into its second year when an SLP/SLT CoP met via video chat to discuss collaboration with educators. As explained above, CoPs are small groups who meet over several sessions, and whose discussions are facilitated by an experienced leader in the field. Whether an SLP/SLT CoP is clinically or non-clinically based, the focus is on group-based learning, sharing and problem solving. This CoP included participant from all the Mutual Recognition nations: Australia, Canada, Ireland, New Zealand, the UK and the US, and several other countries. They were experienced SLPs/SLTs, accustomed to working face-to-face, in classrooms, with children with speech, language and literacy difficulties.

They began by discussing the ups and downs of remote (online) assessment and treatment, but the conversation soon became bogged down as they shared tales of problems communicating with their clients' teachers. *'They don't "get it" when we talk about language; their terminology seems different from ours', 'They're quite ready to blame parents when students are slow with their reading', 'They make no connections between speech, language and literacy', 'They are locked into using non-evidence-based approaches to reading instruction like Whole Language, Reading Recovery, multi-cueing', 'They can't see the relevance of SLP/SLT for slow- and low-progress readers. I often feel like an intruder, poaching their skillset', 'They don't mention the Science of Reading or accountability; I mean, what are they taught at university?', 'If I mention the interplay of phonics, vocabulary, comprehension, fluency, syntax, and discourse—they kind of glaze over'.* The downhearted mood was interrupted when the facilitator interjected cheerfully, *'They, they, they! Enough with the teacher-bashing! Do you want to hear a good news story?'*

The members listened attentively as their colleague told of numerous successful classroom collaborations with a teacher who was well-informed about all aspects of spoken and written language – and skilled and confident in delivering explicit instruction. '*I wish...*,' one of them said. Another spoke up, '*I think we come across as "superior" or all-knowing because of our commitment to EBP. For a "communication professional", I'm not terribly good at explaining the science or why it's important to me. And, while teachers might tend to blame parents, I'm too inclined to go along with those who blame teachers. I need to lift my game*'.

The facilitator guided reflection on these points, gently suggesting they meet teachers halfway, recognizing their expertise and experience. '*I found it easier to communicate teachers about individual students when I realised that their Initial Teacher Education (ITE) equipped so many of them with a restricted view of both language and reading, an unsatisfactory reliance on ineffective reading programs, practices and routines, an inadequate range of materials, and a culture devoid of encouragement to understand and stay abreast of relevant research*'.

The facilitator, whom I was mentoring, debriefed in a Zoom call, and as I listened, several questions for Roslyn Neilson began to form. The results are Q49 and Q50. **Dr. Roslyn Neilson** is a speech-language pathologist in private practice who has worked for many years in supporting literacy development, both in schools and in a private clinic. She has researched and published several phonological awareness assessments.

Q49. Roslyn Neilson: The Science of Reading

There are obvious tensions between instruction provided explicitly by teachers who are well versed in the science of reading, as well as the inextricable connections between language and literacy (Snow, 2016). If you were invited to step in and advise the CoP on supporting teachers at each stage of their professional development, what would you emphasize? How would you counsel university personnel who are tasked with their ITE? What safeguards might be put in place to ensure the delivery of

evidence-based reading instruction, and could it be accomplished within a generation?

A49. Roslyn Neilson: Putting Teachers and SLPs/SLTs on the Same Page: Phonemic Awareness and Responding to Students' Errors

From the point of view of a speech-language pathologist who has worked collaboratively with teachers of early literacy and supported students with reading difficulties for many years, I would like to offer two suggestions in response to the questions posed here. Suggestion 1. involves advising universities to include a compulsory Introduction to Phonetics module in the (admittedly crowded) ITE undergraduate years. Suggestion 2. is to ensure that classrooms are conducive to teachers controlling the ways they can respond when students practising their early literacy skills make errors.

1. Enhancing Practice through Linguistic Knowledge

Some foundational experience in phonetics would enrich the practice of almost all teachers across the school years, not only those involved in early literacy education. The potential benefits of a course like this go beyond providing important and interesting linguistic knowledge as part of a rounded education. I suggest that for teachers, the essential value of studying phonetics involves what I refer to as 'sharpening' of phonemic awareness, or the awareness of the phonemes in spoken words (Scarborough et al., 1998).

When you study Phonetics 101 and learn how to do phonetic transcription, you are taught how to take what is, for literate people, an 'unnatural' step in listening for the sounds in words: you are taught how to focus on the sounds undistracted by the letters used to spell the words. It is surprisingly difficult. Why would teachers benefit from their phonemic awareness being 'sharpened' in a phonetics course? Teachers, like most literate adults, are generally able to read and spell nonwords accurately, which suggests that they can work with sound-letter relationships quite competently – so it is not immediately obvious why there might be an issue with their phonemic awareness. The problem is that, like most literate adults, teachers tend to show weaknesses on phonemic awareness tasks where the spelling of the words involved gets in the way of the analysis of the sounds. This is a problem that crops up all the time in early literacy lessons. Some teachers, for example, might treat it as an error if a child says that the last *sound* in the word box is /s/, expecting the correct answer to be 'x'. Similarly, some teachers who are teaching beginning readers segmentation and blending skills might expect them to blend the phonemes /æ/ and /s/ into the word *as* (where letter 's' is pronounced /z/) rather than realizing that a child who is really listening carefully will come up with the word *ass*.

Incorrect assumptions like these made by teachers are often labelled as evidence of their poor phonemic awareness – which is not only disheartening for teachers but also misguided. As Scarborough et al. (1998) put it, phonemic awareness becomes 'dulled' as our ability to read builds. Ehri (2014) explains this phenomenon in a model of the development of our lexical representations – our knowledge about words – as we learn to read. The phonological information (how the word sounds) and the orthographic information (how the word is spelled) become, as Ehri (2014) describes it 'bonded'. As the lexicon becomes more fully specified in terms orthographic knowledge, the letters tend to dominate and, as it were, push the sounds into the background. It is much easier to think of letters, which are concrete and easy to visualise, than to think about sounds, which are transient.

If, therefore, teachers could use the experience of a Phonetics 101 course to learn – or recapture – the art of focussing on sounds and ignoring letters, they would be in a better position to give accurate explanations of the oddities of the English alphabetic code to their students, and to understand and troubleshoot the difficulties their students might encounter.

The benefits of 'sharpened' phonemic awareness for teachers are likely to be relevant beyond the early primary years, too. Teachers in higher grades will be better able to help students to learn to spell complex words that crop up in all the discipline areas if they can ensure that their students understand the spelling of the words, rather than trying to use rote memorization. This enriched approach to spelling involves students understanding where the words came from (their etymology), e.g., bouquet is spelled that way because it came from French; how the letters correspond to (and don't correspond to) the phonemes in words; as well as how important words parts, or morphemes, are represented. Spelling practice can be a useful part of learning and understanding new vocabulary (Ehri, 2014).

It is common practice for SLPs/SLTs to offer short in-services to practising teachers that involve basic phonetics, and while this is a welcome band-aid, it would be ideal if this kind of catch-up were never needed.

2. Teachers Responding (In Class) to Children's Errors

My second suggestion encompasses goals that are less tangible. It involves ensuring that classroom arrangements are in place that allow teachers to be in control of how they can respond when students make errors while practising their early literacy skills. Dehaene (2020) points out that feedback following errors is one of the pillars of teaching and learning. Making an error, Dehaene argues, is an indication of learners having made an incorrect prediction as they extend their knowledge and stretch their skills. When such errors occur, immediate, supportive, and accurate feedback about the students' predictions is an ideal way to support their learning. If errors are not corrected, however, the incorrect predictions are not adjusted, and the errors themselves morph into bad habits.

While it is not difficult for SLPs/SLTs working with individual clients or small groups in a clinic setting to provide immediate, accurate and supportive feedback for errors, it is a challenge for classroom teachers with over 20 students in a class. And yet every time students who have not yet mastered as skill are sent off unsupervised to practice that skill on a phonics worksheet, or to read a difficult text to themselves, or to practise their letter formation, or even to learn their spelling homework, they are put at risk of learning bad habits rather than progressing their literacy skills.

Those early literacy classrooms that place a priority on discovery learning and small group self-teaching run a particularly serious risk of errors being practised – including guessing habits becoming entrenched as a word recognition strategy, and transcription errors involved in 'invented spelling' story writing. Teachers have debated at length the problem of over-correcting students' independent writing attempts, raising the obvious issue of overwhelming students with red marks on the page. But it could be argued that requiring students to write something that is so far beyond their mastery level that all those corrective red marks are needed, sets them up for failure in terms of efficient learning.

The easiest way for a teacher to minimise the practising of errors, I suggest, is as follows. Run at least a core portion of literacy instruction as an explicit, systematic, teacher-directed whole-class activity where the engagement and accuracy of all student responses can be monitored using tools such as mini white-boards. This teaching strategy allows teachers to notice when students have indeed practised a new skill to mastery, and to note when they have not mastered a skill and should therefore not be left to flounder as they practise their errors.

For those teachers who instinctively reject an explicit, direct instruction strategy on the grounds that is too rigid for them, a conversation with an SLP/SLT about the nature of errors and the importance of accurate feedback following errors might be a good place to start. The SLP/SLT would have to be as supportive as possible about respecting the practical difficulties of classroom teaching. It is likely that there are many teachers who

are already sensitive to the challenge of providing feedback for errors, and who have developed their own strategies; they might have much to offer SLPs/SLTs who may themselves not have enough classroom experience to be able to support other teachers to rise to the challenge.

How Long Might Practice-Change Take?

Could my suggestions be accomplished within a generation of teachers? Including basic phonetics in ITE could certainly be accomplished if the decision were made; it might have to be imposed from above. There is some evidence that the improvement in teachers' skill with analysing the phonological level of language would be reflected in more effective teaching (Stainthorp, 2020), but more research is needed. My second suggestion about the role of errors involves a larger cultural change. Advocates of direct instruction are, however, becoming increasingly creative in finding ways to support schools as they more towards a more consistent understanding of the role of errors in student learning (e.g., Brooks et al., 2021), and I see no reason why those cultural changes could not eventually occur.

Learning to Read and Reading to Learn

Readers met **Dr. Roslyn Neilson** in the preamble to A49 and will recall that she is an SLP with a strong clinical practice background in supporting children's literacy development, and a research background that has focused particularly on phonological awareness assessment. She was the Speech Pathology Australia (SPA) 2012 National Tour speaker on the topics 'Learning to read' and 'Reading to learn' and has presented numerous, invited pre- and in-service lectures and workshops for teachers. She was transferred to Life Membership of SPA in 2018.

Q50. Roslyn Neilson: Co-Occurring Speech, Language, Reading, and Writing Difficulties

What are the inter-related speech and language weaknesses that place children in an at-risk category for literacy difficulties? What can be done to help, and what are the implications for the collaborative classroom?

A50. Roslyn Neilson: Early Literacy Difficulties: Speech Language Professionals as Collaborators

In the decades since I started working in literacy development, SLPs/SLTs have increasingly included in their caseloads children who are experiencing reading and writing difficulties. This extension of our traditional practice brings with it the extra challenge of collaborating constructively with teachers and school systems as well as with clients and their families. There is a complex interface between oral language difficulties and literacy problems (Snow, 2016), and it takes careful negotiation to establish why and how support for children with literacy difficulties is the business of SLPs/SLTs as well as belonging in the domain of teachers. It is also very important – and at times difficult – to ensure that SLP/SLT intervention is in harmony with what the children are being taught at school.

The oft-cited 'Simple View of Reading' (see, Hoover & Tunmer, 2020) makes the point that reading is rather complicated. Successful reading involves two dimensions of skills: (a) recognizing written words efficiently and (b) understanding what is read. Children with reading difficulties fall into three groups along these two dimensions (Nation, 2019): those who do not recognise words efficiently; those who have difficulty understanding what they read; and those who struggle with both sets of skills. In practice the groups of children with literacy problems often overlap, and this means that it is important that SLPs/SLTs are aware of the all the strands of component skills that combine to enable successful reading (Scarborough, 2001).

Although SLP/SLT skills are relevant to both dimensions of the Simple View of Reading, I will not focus on language comprehension here. Instead, I will discuss contributions SLPs/SLTs can make to the acquisition of word recognition, since this ability tends to be seen as the more salient aspect of learning to read in the early years of school.

Many children who struggle with reading have an early history of oral speech and language difficulties (Catts et al., 2002) or have a familial history of dyslexia (Snowling et al., 2003), or have spent their pre-school years in an environment that was not conducive to the development of foundational literacy skills (Smith et al., 2021). SLPs/SLTs may therefore often be able to offer some advance warning of the risk of reading difficulties at the point that an at-risk child enters school. This means that adaptations can be made if necessary, so that children are not left in a wait-to-fail situation once they start school.

What are the pre-school speech and language problems that can act as warning signals? The strongest factor seems to be language delay (Catts et al., 2002), although speech sound disorders do make a modest contribution to the risk, especially if they are associated with language disorder and/or if the speech difficulties persist into the school years (Hayiou-Thomas et al., 2017; Nathan et al., 2004). Leitão and Fletcher (2004) report that early, unusual, non-developmental processes (e.g., Initial Consonant Deletion, in English) are more likely than common developmental errors (such as interdental or dentalised substitutions for /s/ and /z/) to be associated with literacy problems. Among Leitão and Fletcher's participants, reading accuracy and spelling scores also showed similar trends. Rvachew (2007) reports that early speech perception difficulties are also related to risk of reading problems. Signs of weakness in speech production may be evident beyond errors on single sounds; Masso et al. (2017) report observing difficulty with producing polysyllabic words in preschool children at risk of reading difficulties. Teachers can usefully be alerted to notice when this problem persists into the school years and school age children struggle to pronounce phonologically complex words (e.g., *computer, congratulations, Aboriginal*).

Many early speech and language difficulties may seem to have resolved by school age, with children's conversation sounding 'normal to the naked ear' (Paul & Norbury, 2012, p. 394). The role of SLPs/SLTs in making the link between oral and written language difficulties nevertheless remains important well after children have entered school; Overby et al. (2007) report that half of a group of teachers listening to recordings of moderately intelligible second graders judged that the children were not at risk for literacy difficulties. This finding suggests that large numbers of teachers may not be alert to the associated learning implications of expressive phonological difficulties, even though they may recognise the social repercussions.

There are several other aspects of phonological processing that are related to reading progress, all involving difficulties that may not be obvious in conversation. Word recognition problems are often attributed to an umbrella concept referred to as 'core phonological deficit' (Kilpatrick, 2015), with a cluster of weaknesses potentially identified (Mundy & Hannant, 2020). SLPs/SLTs are well positioned to carry out fine-grained assessments that can help to identify students who may need extra support, and they may be able to suggest appropriate adaptations in the classroom.

The most widely recognised phonological weakness associated with reading difficulty is in phonemic awareness, or the ability to identify and manipulate the sounds in spoken words. Based on a meta-analysis of relevant research into reading instruction, phonemic awareness was identified as one of five cornerstones of literacy development (National Reading Panel, 2000), and the concept has been the subject of vast amounts of research over the past decades (see, e.g., Kilpatrick, 2015). Difficulty with manipulating sounds means that children may be slow or inefficient at retrieving and blending phonemes as they try to read words. When children with weak phonemic awareness are learning to remember words, they tend to develop rather imprecise mappings between sounds and letters (Ehri, 2014). SLPs/SLTs may contribute by not only providing ongo-

ing phonemic awareness assessments but also explaining to teachers the implications of the information obtained and suggesting ways that students might be supported.

When there are early concerns about slow (or no) reading progress, it may be useful for SLPs/SLTs to assess Rapid Automatized Naming (RAN), a task that requires children to name known items in a visual array as quickly as they can. RAN scores are reported to be strongly correlated with reading ability, and it has been suggested that the RAN task presents a microcosm of the skills required in reading (Norton & Wolf, 2012). While RAN performance itself is not a target for intervention, the presence of difficulties is a strong indication that children may need continued extra support in learning to read.

Phonological working memory is a problem for many children with reading difficulties (Gathercole & Alloway, 2008). If SLPs/SLTs provide assessments of working memory and nonword repetition (Gathercole, et al. 2006), they can point out to teachers how children may struggle to hold unfamiliar sequences of sounds in their minds as they try to read.

SLPs/SLTs can make several positive contributions to ongoing teaching support for children with word recognition difficulties. While debates in the educational context about how phonics should be taught have not yet been settled, many schools do include systematic phonics teaching in their early literacy programs, providing explicit and sequenced instruction about sound-letter relationships. This is particularly useful for children with weak phonological skills because the alternative instructional approach – that is, using meaning as the prime means of guessing the identity of words – invites children with phonological difficulties to bypass phonology and rely on contextual cues to identify unfamiliar words, rather than attempting to decode them precisely. This is a strategy that leaves them vulnerable to an inability to read new words independently (Nicholson, 1993).

Even when children do have the substantive benefit of explicit phonics instruction in the classroom, SLPs/SLTs still have a key role to play in supporting children with weak phonological processing. Most systematic synthetic phonics programs tend to assume that learners have normal underlying phonological skills. Teachers assume that children know what is meant when they are asked to 'sound out' words, that they can easily retrieve the letter-sound associations they have been taught, and that they are able hold sounds in working memory. When children do not learn easily, it can be difficult for teachers to pinpoint the exact problem, let alone work out ways to scaffold the children's attempts. It can be useful for SLPs/SLTs to work with teachers to develop well-planned adaptations to their teaching routines, supporting strategies such as making phonemic awareness explicit, practising letter-sound connections, and blending skills to mastery, and reducing cognitive load to free up working memory resources.

Some school systems are not in favour of systematic phonics teaching, instead preferring an instructional approach that prioritizes meaning during early reading instruction. In this situation I have found it useful to work with both the teacher and the child on strategies for supporting the child's spelling, rather than focussing on reading. This change of focus can defuse a potentially harmful clash of opinions about reading instruction, and the word study skills involved in good spelling instruction can allow much of the necessary explicit teaching to be provided. This focus also allows parents to be involved constructively in homework activities.

Finally, when children experience ongoing difficulties with learning to recognise words despite reasonable instruction and support, SLPs/SLTs may be ideally placed to act as advocates for the children and families who are likely to be navigating – and possibly floundering – through the social, clinical, and educational minefield that involves the diagnosis of 'dyslexia' (Bowen & Snow, 2017). It is perhaps at this point that it is most crucial to work towards a collaborative SLP/SLT approach that involves consideration of the educational context and the research evidence as well as the client, to provide children with reading difficulties the best possible chance to participate successfully in a literate society.

Theoreticians and Interventionists: A Matter of Trust

If critical advances in health behavior theory depend on an iterative process by which theoreticians and interventionists cooperate in the testing and evaluation of theoretical principles, individuals in both camps need to not only recognize the goals and values of each group, but also trust each other's ability to advance our understanding of both theory and practice.

Rothman, 2004

The final contribution to this chapter, and to this book (Froud & Randazzo, A51) is an exploration of the encouraging rise in clinical research alliances that is becoming increasingly apparent in our learned journals and scholarly meetings. Often cross disciplinary, transdisciplinary, or multidisciplinary, improved communication between academe and hands-on practitioners produce collaborative research partnerships in which all parties – theoreticians, researchers, and other university faculty, and interventionists – make invaluable contributions.

Dr. Karen Froud is the director of the Neurocognition of Language Lab, and Associate Professor of Neuroscience and Education in the Department of Biobehavioral Sciences at Teachers College, Columbia University, in New York. Trained as a Speech and Language Therapist in the UK, she holds a PhD in Linguistics from University College London, and her research is concerned with the neurophysiological underpinnings of linguistic processing and representation in normal and disordered language. She teaches graduate research methods courses and maintains a wide range of collaborative research projects in linguistics and neuroscience, including work on the neural correlates of child speech disorders.

Dr. Melissa Randazzo is Assistant Professor in the Department of Communication Sciences and Disorders at Adelphi University, where she directs the Neurocognition of Communication Disorders Lab. She holds a PhD in Communication Sciences and Disorders from Columbia University. Her research examines the neural correlates of multisensory integration in communication disorders, as well as clinical and research self-efficacy in CSD students and faculty. She is a speech-language pathologist, recognized for advanced training and expertise in Childhood Apraxia of Speech (CAS) by the Childhood Apraxia of Speech Associations of North America (CASANA, or Apraxia Kids). She teaches graduate-level courses in paediatric speech sound disorders and research methods.

Q51. Karen Froud and Melissa Randazzo: Theoretical Models and Frameworks

It is noticeable in the SLP/SLT literature and from interactions with academics, students, and practitioners, that there is a narrowing of the research-to-practice divide between clinical practice and training since you addressed this topic in the previous editions of this book. Since the gap has shifted,

1. are we now more effectively convincing clinicians that we need theoretical models and frameworks, and
2. that it is both ethical and possible to stay abreast of the literature in general and theoretical advances in particular?
3. How can we maintain the momentum, and continue to advance?

A51. Karen Froud and Melissa Randazzo: Minding the Gap: The Narrowing Theory-to-Practice Divide in SLP/SLT Training and Practice

Relationships between mental representations and speech signals are quite opaque, yet our profession works exactly at this interface: between speech and language, receptive and expressive modalities, perception and production, sensorimotor and cognitive processes. A productive way to yield greater understanding of the interfaces between sensory and cognitive phenomena has been to identify the processes involved in relating them to real world referents. Models of such processes have potential to simplify and guide remediation approaches

for greater generalization of therapeutic gains (e.g., Lee, 2018; Lundeborg Hammarström et al., 2019; Bernhardt et al., 2010), but applying these theoretical frameworks to diagnosis, treatment planning, and intervention requires consistent and systematic engagement with research. Since previous editions of this book, there has been increasing recognition in the classroom and field that engagement with theoretical frameworks and associated research enhances our understanding and remediation of speech and language disorders – indeed, mandates for evidence-based practice (EBP) in SLP/SLT are established in many countries. However, barriers to EBP implementation remain, with three main kinds of obstacles making it more difficult for clinicians to tackle the research literature: Pedagogical, investigational, and practical.

Pedagogical Barriers

When training future clinical professionals, we provide instruction in theoretical frameworks associated with areas of practice; but how successfully do we direct this theoretical grounding towards the practicalities of clinical work? Greater exposure to EBP principles and research during graduate training (and clinical fellowships where they are required) results in greater reported use of EBP by practicing clinicians, and a more positive perspective on its applicability (Zipoli & Kennedy, 2005). Nevertheless, clinicians still report a lack of confidence in their ability to critically evaluate research findings, especially statistical analyses (Greenwell & Walsh, 2021). Indeed, Crais and Savage (2020) reported that doctoral students in SLP/SLT identified limited skills in statistics and research design as primary barriers to PhD completion.

Directed training in EBP seems to have positive effects (Thome et al., 2020), but relationships between such directed training and engagement with research in professional practice appear to be mediated by various factors, especially perceptions of self-efficacy. For example, Spek et al. (2013) evaluated a curriculum addressing EBP implementation skills, finding that student clinicians feel uncertain about the nature and applicability of EBP despite increasing EBP knowledge and skills over time. They note that feelings of competence and self-efficacy stimulate intrinsic motivation, hence affecting willingness to use EBP. Therefore, to engage clinicians with research, we must first ensure that students are *empowered* to tackle relevant literature and apply it to clinical decision-making. To be effective in promoting clinician engagement with the research literature, training in research must emphasize self-efficacy and student perceptions of research utility – not the methods and theories alone (McCurtin & Roddam, 2012; Pasupathy & Bogschutz, 2013).

Investigational Barriers

Determining best practices in SLP/SLT rests on the existence of relevant high-quality research, which can be lacking. For example, Roberts et al. (2020) showed that only 25% of articles in ASHA journals between 2008-18 reported on clinical research, with fewer than 1% reporting on implementation. Even when relevant research does exist, translating findings to inform clinical decision-making remains challenging (Furlong et al., 2018, T. Hoffman et al., 2017; Leitão, this volume), and clinicians report lacking confidence to reproduce research methods and outcomes within clinical practice (e.g., Lancaster et al., 2010). Clinical decision-making in SLP/SLT is affected by multiple variables, including service-related, family, and client factors (Furlong et al., 2018); such multi-pronged, eclectic approaches are typically not reflected in the controlled conditions under which research is conducted.

To investigate intervention practices in real-life contexts, more qualitative and mixed methods research is needed. However, these methodologies are minimally represented in the SLP/SLT literature (Damico & Simmons-Mackie, 2003; Wium & Louw, 2018). This situation is compounded by biases in research, such as the exclusion of some populations from clinical trials (e.g., Elman, 2006) and uneven representation of disorders in available clinical research (Roberts et al., 2020). For instance, Shriberg et al. (1997) describe both the low population prevalence of idiopathic Childhood Apraxia of Speech, and the lack of consensus regarding relevant pathognomonic signs; such factors hinder the sample size required for research that is higher on the evidence hierarchy (e.g., randomized controlled trials). These issues interact with well-documented publication biases that render null findings – especially relevant for evaluating which interventions are *not* effective – scarce in the literature (e.g., Chow, 2018).

Practical Barriers

Time is the most frequently reported, although not the only, barrier to research engagement for clinicians (e.g., Fulcher-Rood et al., 2020; L. M. Hoffman et al., 2013; Thome et al., 2020; Zipoli & Kennedy, 2005). L. M. Hoffman et al. (2013) found that only 9% of U.S. public school based SLPs surveyed (around 249 out of 2,762 respondents representing 28 states) had any scheduled time for research; of these, more than half reported research time limited from 1-30 minutes per week, and another quarter reported a weekly allocation of 31-60 minutes. Furlong et al. (2018) showed that caseload size, scheduling constraints, and a lack of access to resources constitute barriers to research engagement; while Greenwell and Walsh (2021) identified additional barriers including a lack of funds for resources such as journal articles at work and at home, a lack of confidence in expertise required to search and interpret the literature, and differences in workplace culture.

Implementation of research in clinical settings is also subject to practical constraints. The disconnect between controlled experimental conditions and the messy reality of clinical practice constitutes a 'mismatch in research agendas' (McCurtin & Roddam, 2012), whereby investigators conducting relevant work may lack clinical backgrounds and hence have little understanding of clinicians' research needs. In their call to increase implementation research in SLP/SLT, Olswang and Prelock (2015) describe how the current research pipeline of 'pushing information into practice' requires clinicians to independently determine how to adapt laboratory-controlled findings to real life settings. In contrast, implementation science investigates optimal ways to apply EBP (Dollaghan, 2007) to clinical practice. This is one barrier that can be partially overcome by changes in research approaches, considered further below.

Overcoming Barriers

All these obstacles exist in critical tension with the imperative to provide best, most efficacious practices for our clients. As a result, clinicians have reported negative self-judgements related to the standards of their clinical practice, alongside feelings of compromise and frustration (Furlong et al., 2018). Requiring EBP is one thing but making it a feasible and accessible part of daily practice comes with significant challenges. However, potential supports exist within each domain described above.

During training, research skills can be taught from problem-based or case-based perspectives, and specific skills needed to engage with research for EBP can be explicitly addressed and familiarized. By relating statistical and experimental methods directly to practice, students can be empowered to engage with research literature and interpret it for their own applications. Strategies such as the Critically Appraised Topic: CAT (White et al., 2017), or using a search framework such as PICO to bridge from clinical to research questions (Hutcheson, 2017), can be applied rapidly to both qualitative and quantitative research (Skeat & Roddam, 2019), supporting clinicians in critical evaluation of topics and methods where they may not have specific expertise. If such strategies are explicitly taught during graduate preparation, clinicians may feel more prepared to engage with research that they otherwise consider beyond their expertise. Research engagement can be rendered approachable when clinicians have

built sufficient self-efficacy – a mindset that should be directly addressed during training (Pasupathy & Bogschutz, 2013).

Relatedly, it is crucial for researchers to link findings explicitly to intervention approaches (Furlong et al., 2018), ensuring transparency in reporting while maintaining rigour. This might mean adopting qualitative approaches, instead of or in addition to experimental frameworks that can seem isolated from clinical practice (Damico & Simmons-Mackie, 2003); or it might mean explicitly acknowledging limitations of experimental approaches and offering concrete suggestions for interpreting findings within real-world clinical contexts. Damico and Simmons-Mackie (2003) call for more qualitative research in SLP/SLT, potentially an advantage for studying highly-context-dependent phenomena like the complex interactions between client and clinician. Crooke and Olswang (2015) describe the concept of practice-based research (PBR), that brings rigorous research methods to bear on practice-oriented issues. Such approaches illustrate how shifting away from the imperative for strictly experimental methods in clinically related research could help to contextualize the many factors that impact intervention efficacy.

Clarifying and standardizing descriptions of treatment approaches under investigation could also ameliorate the impact of mismatched investigator/clinician goals. For example, Turkstra et al. (2016) proposed a 'rehabilitation treatment taxonomy' whereby researchers conducting clinically oriented studies can clearly specify aspects of an intervention. Based on this, Baker et al. (2018) developed the Phonological Intervention Taxonomy, a hierarchical framework for understanding similarities and distinctions between intervention approaches. This taxonomy highlights commonalities between approaches while identifying the less common features that might require more explicit instruction for application. This promotes implementation in clinical settings by identifying the inherent flexibility of different approaches and which factors facilitate treatment effects, reflecting clinicians' characteristically eclectic approaches to intervention (Lancaster et al., 2010).

All investigators should be working to publish in open-source outlets to ensure accessibility and visibility. Journals behind paywalls are becoming ever more limited in their relevance and application – including journals maintained by our regulatory bodies and/or professional associations, who promote evidence-based practice and research engagement while maintaining some of the barriers affecting such practices. Researchers can also share their own work more widely, for example, by posting online summaries, materials, and practical suggestions that can be made freely available – for example, as seen in the '2 languages 2 worlds' blog (Goldstein et al., 2008 and onwards). Dunst (2017) exemplifies another approach, whereby in-depth syntheses of research are implemented to develop tools for clinical contexts – and then those tools are also shared. Storkel's (2018) tutorial on the complexity approach for phonological disorders, written for a clinical audience, is another example. The tutorial outlined the theoretical underpinnings of the approach, with concrete examples, acknowledgment of barriers to implementation, and scaffolded instructions. The 'Multilingual Children's Speech' online initiative (McLeod, 2012) is another dynamic web-based resource where McLeod and her collaborators collate information and resources about speech sound disorders in many languages. It provides supporting research, assessment instruments, and background information in linguistics, phonetics, language development, and speech sound disorders for audiences ranging from parents to professionals.

With respect to clinical practice, our regulators and professional associations must support efforts to make training and research part of the job by working with clinical settings to clarify practice standards. There are some notable ongoing research initiatives by regulatory bodies – such as the Royal College of Speech and Language Therapists (2015) Research Priorities project, or the establishment of clinician-academic research communities through the Irish Association of Speech and Language Therapists (McCurtin & O'Connor, 2020). Resource gaps can be addressed through research sharing and by managers building in time and access during the workday, rather than crowding schedules and caseloads. While recognizing the practical reasons behind heavy caseloads, denying methods known to increase efficiency in practice is a false economy. Acknowledging the axiomatic centrality of research will only support the work.

Finally, with an eye to supporting the self-efficacy of readers: by engaging with the work in this volume, *you are already* undertaking the effort to engage with research in support of practice. Clinicians and clinical educators *can* shift mindsets and practices; assimilate new theoretical developments and discuss these with colleagues; develop and implement strategies for assessment and intervention that have a firm theoretical grounding. Our professional regulatory bodies *can* explicitly acknowledge the reality that informed and ethical clinical practice is much more than 'knee-to-knee time' and do their part to remove barriers to accessing research. By adopting these approaches, not only do we provide better training and care, but we also contribute data and experience that can guide the development of more fine-grained theories of speech and language – hence opening the way forward for more effective and efficient interventions. The gap is closing; let's maintain the momentum.

References

ASHA. (n.d.). Telepractice. American Speech-Language-Hearing Association. https://www.asha.org/practice-portal/professional-issues/telepractice/

Aggarwal, K., Patel, R., & Ravi, R. (2020). Uptake of telepractice among speech-language therapists following COVID-19 pandemic in India. *Speech, Language and Hearing*, 228–234. https://doi.org/10.1080/2050571X.2020.1812034

Ahmed, B., Ballard, K. J., Kelly, G., & McLeod, S. (2022). *Say bananas! Equitable access to speech intervention for rural children*. Abstract from Speech Pathology Australia 2022 National Conference, Melbourne, Victoria, Australia. Speech Pathology Australia. https://web.archive.org/save/https://www.speechpathologyaustralia.org.au/SPAConf2022/Program/Conf_abstract_Oral.aspx?SubId=41

Alary Gauvreau, C., Le Dorze, G., Kairy, D., & Croteau, C. (2019). Evaluation of a community of practice for speech-language pathologists in aphasia rehabilitation: A logic analysis. *BMC Health Services Research*, *19*(1), 530. https://doi.org/10.1186/s12913-019-4338-0

Allen, M. M. (2013). Intervention efficacy and intensity for children with speech sound disorder. *Journal of Speech, Language and Hearing Research*, *56*(3), 865–877. https://doi.org/10.1044/1092-4388(2012/11-0076)

American Speech-Language-Hearing Association. (2016). *Scope of practice in speech-language pathology* [Scope of Practice]. Available from www.asha.org/policy

Bahar, N., Namasivayam, A. K., & van Lieshout, P. (2022). Telehealth intervention and childhood apraxia of speech: A scoping review. *Speech, Language and Hearing*, *25*(4), 450–462.

Baker, E. (2021). Minimal pairs intervention. In A. L. Williams, S. McLeod, & R. J. McCauley (Eds.), *Interventions for speech sound disorders in children* (2nd ed., pp. 33–60). Paul H. Brookes Publishing Co.

Baker, E., Williams, A. L., McLeod, S., & McCauley, R. (2018). Elements of phonological interventions for children with speech sound disorders: The development of a taxonomy. *American Journal of Speech-Language Pathology*, *27*(3), 906–935. https://doi.org/10.1044/2018_ajslp-17-0127

Barwick, M. A., Peters, J., & Boydell, K. (2009). Getting to uptake: Do communities of practice support the implementation of evidence-based practice? *Journal of the Canadian Academy of Child and Adolescent Psychiatry*, *18*(1), 16–29. http://www.ncbi.nlm.nih.gov/pmc/articles/pmc2651208

Bauman-Waengler, J. (2020). *Articulatory and phonological impairments: A clinical focus* (6th ed.). Pearson Education, Inc.

Beiting, M., & Nicolet, G. (2020). Screenless teletherapy and silent telesupervision: Leveraging technology for innovative service delivery and clinician training in speech-language pathology during the COVID-19 era. *CommonHealth*, *1*(3), 106–120. https://doi.org/10.15367/ch.v1i3.413

Bernhardt, B. M., Gick, B., Bacsfalvi, P., & Ashdown, J. (2003). Speech habilitation of hard of hearing adolescents using electropalatography and ultrasound as evaluated by trained listeners. *Clinical Linguistics & Phonetics*, *17*(3), 199–216. https://doi.org/10.1080/0269920031000071451

Bernhardt, B. M., Bopp, K. D., Daudlin, B., Edwards, S. M., & Wastie, S. E. (2010). Nonlinear phonological intervention. In A. L. Williams, S. McLeod, & R. J. McCauley (Eds.), *Interventions for speech sound disorders in children* (pp. 315–331). Brookes.

Bowen, C. (2001). *Children's speech sound disorders (phonologicaltherapy) discussion group*. http://groups.yahoo.com/neo/groups/phonologicaltherapy/info (2001-to-2019).

Bowen, C., & Snow, P. (2017). *Making sense of interventions for children with developmental disorders*. J&R Press Ltd.

Brooks, C., Burton, R., & Hattie, J. (2021). Feedback for learning. In K.-A. Allen, A. Reupert, & L. Oades (Eds.), *Building better schools with evidence-based policy* (pp. 65–70). Routledge. https://doi.org/10.4324/9781003025955

Buysse, V., Sparkman, K. L., & Wesley, P. W. (2003). Communities of practice: Connecting what we know with what we do. *Exceptional Children*, *69*(3), 263–277. http://dx.doi.org/10.1177/001440290306900301

Campbell, D. R., & Goldstein, H. (2021). Genesis of a new generation of telepractitioners: The COVID-19 pandemic and pediatric speech-language pathology services. *American Journal of Speech-Language Pathology*, *30*(5), 2143–2154. https://doi.org/10.1044/2021_AJSLP-21-00013

Campbell, D. R., & Goldstein, H. (2022). Reliability of scoring telehealth speech sound assessments administered in real-world scenarios. *American Journal of Speech-Language Pathology*, *31*(3), 1338–1353. https://doi.org/10.1044/2022_AJSLP-21-00219

Catts, H. W., Fey, M. E., Tomblin, J. B., & Zhang, X. (2002). A longitudinal investigation of reading outcomes in children with language impairments. *Journal of Speech, Language & Hearing Research*, *45*(6), 1142–1157. https://doi.org/10.1044/1092-4388(2002/093)

Chow, J. C. (2018). Prevalence of publication bias tests in speech, language, and hearing research. *Journal of Speech, Language, and Hearing Research*, *61*(12), 3055–3063. https://doi.org/10.1044/2018_jslhr-l-18-0098

Cialdella, L., Kabakoff, H., Preston, J., Dugan, S., Spencer, C., Boyce, S., Tiede, M., Whalen, D., & McAllister, T. (2021). Auditory-perceptual acuity in rhotic misarticulation: Baseline characteristics and treatment response. *Clinical Linguistics & Phonetics*, *35*(1), 19–42. https://doi.org/10.1080/02699206.2020.1739749

Ciccia, A. H., Whitford, B., Krumm, M., & McNeal, K. (2011). Improving the access of young urban children to speech, language, and hearing screening via telehealth. *Journal of Telemedicine and Telecare*, *17*(5), 240–244. https://doi.org/10.1258/jtt.2011.100810

Cleland, J. (2021). Ultrasound tongue imaging. In M. J. Ball (Ed.), *Manual of clinical phonetics* (1st ed.). Routledge. https://doi.org/10.4324/9780429320903. (2021).

Cleland, J., Crampin, L., & Campbell, L. (2021). Ultrasound visual biofeedback versus standard treatment for children with cleft lip and palate. *ISRCTN Registry*. https://doi.org/10.1186/ISRCTN17441953

Cleland, J., & Preston, J. (2020). Biofeedback interventions. In A. L. Williams, S. McLeod, & R. McCauley (Eds.), *Interventions for speech sound disorders in children* (2nd ed., pp. 573–599).

Cleland, J., Scobbie, J. M., Roxburgh, Z., Heyde, C., & Wrench, A. (2019). Enabling new articulatory gestures in children with persistent speech sound disorders using ultrasound visual biofeedback. *Journal of Speech, Language, and Hearing Research, 62*(2), 229–246. https://doi.org/10.1044/2018_JSLHR-S-17-0360

Coufal, K., Parham, D., Jakubowitz, M., Howell, C., & Reyes, J. (2018). Comparing traditional service delivery and telepractice for speech sound production using a functional outcome measure. *American Journal of Speech-Language Pathology, 27*(1), 82–90. https://doi.org/10.1044/2017_ajslp-16-0070

Crais, E.R., & Savage, M.H. (2020). Communication Sciences and Disorders PhD Graduates' Perceptions of their PhD Program. *Perspectives of the ASHA Special Interest Groups, 5*, 463–478. https://doi.org/10.1044/2020_persp-19-00107

Crooke, P. J., & Olswang, L. B. (2015). Practice-based research: Another pathway for closing the research–practice gap. *Journal of Speech, Language, and Hearing Research, 58*(6), S1871–S1882. https://doi.org/10.1044/2015_JSLHR-L-15-0243

Dagenais, P. A., Critz-Crosby, P., & Adams, J. B. (1994). Defining and remediating persistent lateral lisps in children using electropalatography. *American Journal of Speech-Language Pathology, 3*(3), 67–76. https://doi.org/10.1044/1058-0360.0303.67

Damico, J. S., & Simmons-Mackie, N. N. (2003). Qualitative research and speech-language pathology: A tutorial in the clinical realm. *American Journal of Speech-Language Pathology, 12*(2), 131–143. https://doi.org/10.1044/1058-0360(2003/060)

Davidson, M. M., Mahendra, N., & Nicholson, N. (2022). Creating clinical research impact through social media: Five easy steps to get started. *Perspectives of the ASHA Special Interest Groups, 7*(3), 669–678. https://doi.org/10.1044/2022_PERSP-21-00208

De', R., Pandey, N., & Pal, A. (2020). Impact of digital surge during Covid-19 pandemic: A viewpoint on research and practice. *International Journal of Information Management, 55*, 102171. https://doi.org/10.1016/j.ijinfomgt.2020.102171

Dehaene, S. (2020). *How we learn: The new science of education and the brain*. Penguin Books.

Dodd, B., Zhu, H., Crosbie, S., Holm, A., & Ozanne, A. (2006). *Diagnostic evaluation of articulation and phonology (DEAP)*. The Psychological Corporation.

Dollaghan, C. A. (2007). *The handbook for evidence-based practice in communication disorders*. Paul H. Brookes.

Douglas, N. F., Feuerstein, J. L., Oshita, J. Y., Schliep, M. E., & Danowski, M. L. (2022). Implementation science research in communication sciences and disorders: A scoping review. *American Journal of Speech-Language Pathology, 31*(3), 1054–1083. https://doi.org/10.1044/2021_AJSLP-21-00126

Dugan, S., Li, S. R., Masterson, J., Woeste, H., Mahalingam, N., Spencer, C., Mast, T. D., Riley, M. A., & Boyce, S. E. (2019). Tongue part movement trajectories for /r/ using ultrasound. *Perspectives of the ASHA Special Interest Groups, 4*(6), 1644–1652. https://doi.org/10.1044/2019_PERS-19-00064

Dunst, C. J. (2017). Research foundations for evidence-informed early childhood intervention performance checklists. *Education Science, 7*(4), 78. https://doi.org/10.3390/educsci7040078

Ehri, L. C. (2014). Orthographic mapping in the acquisition of sight word reading, spelling memory, and vocabulary learning. *Scientific Studies of Reading, 18*(1), 5–21. https://doi.org/10.1080/10888438.2013.819356

Elbrink, S. H., Elmer, S. L., & Osborne, R. H. (2021). Are communities of practice a way to support health literacy: A study protocol for a realist review. *BMJ open, 11*(8), e048352. http://dx.doi.org/10.1136/bmjopen-2020-048352

Elman, R. J. (2006). Evidence-based practice: What evidence is missing? *Aphasiology, 20*(02–04), 103–109. https://doi.org/10.1080/02687030500472256

Eriks-Brophy, A., Quittenbaum, J., Anderson, D., & Nelson, T. (2008). Part of the problem or part of the solution? Communication assessments of Aboriginal children residing in remote communities using videoconferencing. *Clinical Linguistics and Phonetics, 22*(8), 589–609. https://doi.org/10.1080/02699200802221737

Erskine, N., & Hendricks, S. (2021). The use of Twitter by medical journals: Systematic review of the literature. *Journal of Medical Internet Research*, *23*(7), e26378. https://doi.org/10.2196/26378

Filbay, S., Hinman, R., Lawford, B., Fry, R., & Bennell, K. (2021, April). *Telehealth by allied health practitioners during the COVID-19 pandemic; An Australian wide survey of clinicians and clients*. The University of Melbourne. https://healthsciences.unimelb.edu.au/departments/physiotherapy/chesm/research-overview/allied-health-telehealth

Finn, P. (2019). The impact of social media on communication sciences and disorders: A need for examination and research. *Perspectives of the ASHA Special Interest Groups*, *4*(2), 224–227. https://doi.org/10.1044/2019_PERS-ST-2019-0001

Fong, R., Tsai, C. F., & Yiu, O. Y. (2021). The implementation of telepractice in speech language pathology in Hong Kong during the COVID-19 pandemic. *Telemedicine Journal and e-Health: The Official Journal of the American Telemedicine Association*, *27*(1), 30–38. https://doi.org/10.1089/tmj.2020.0223

Fulcher-Rood, K., Castilla-Earls, A., & Higginbotham, J. (2020). What does evidence-based practice mean to you? A follow-up study examining school-based speech-language pathologists' perspectives on evidence-based practice. *American Journal of Speech-Language Pathology*, *29*(2), 688–704. https://doi.org/10.1044/2019_ajslp-19-00171

Furlong, L., Serry, T., Erickson, S., & Morris, M. E. (2018). Processes and challenges in clinical decision-making for children with speech-sound disorders. *International Journal of Language & Communication Disorders*, *53*(6), 1124–1138. https://doi.org/10.1111/1460-6984.12426

Gathercole, S. E., & Alloway, T. P. (2008). *Working memory and learning: A practical guide for teachers*. Sage.

Gathercole, S. E., Alloway, T. P., Willis, C., & Adams, A. M. (2006). Working memory in children with reading disabilities. *Journal of Experimental Child Psychology*, *93*(3), 265–281. https://doi.org/10.1016/j.jecp.2005.08.003

Gibbon, F., Dent, H., & Hardcastle, W. (1993). Diagnosis and therapy of abnormal alveolar stops in a speech-disordered child using electropalatography. *Clinical Linguistics & Phonetics*, *7*(4), 247–267. https://doi.org/10.1080/02699209308985565

Gibbon, F. E., & Lee, A. (2017). Electropalatographic (EPG) evidence of covert contrasts in disordered speech. *Clinical Linguistics & Phonetics*, *31*(1), 4–20. https://doi.org/10.1080/02699206.2016.1174739

Goldman, R., & Fristoe, M. (2015). *Goldman-Fristoe test of articulation* (3rd ed.). Pearson Clinical Assessment.

Goldstein, B., Peña, E., Kiran, S., Mahendra, N., & Simon-Cereijido, G. (2008 and onwards). *2 languages 2 worlds*. https://2languages2worlds.wordpress.com

Greenwell, T., & Walsh, B. (2021). Evidence-based practice in speech-language pathology: Where are we now? *American Journal of Speech-Language Pathology*, *30*(1), 186–198. https://doi.org/10.1044/2020_ajslp-20-00194

Grogan-Johnson, S., Gabel, R., Taylor, J., Rowan, L., Alvares, R., & Schenker, J. (2011). A pilot investigation of speech sound disorder intervention delivered by telehealth to school-age children. *International Journal of Telerehabilitation*, *3*(1), 31–41. https://doi.org/10.5195/ijt.2011.6064

Grogan-Johnson, S., Schmidt, A. M., Schenker, J., Alvares, R., Rowan, L. E., & Taylor, J. (2013). A comparison of speech sound intervention delivered by telepractice and side-by-side service delivery models. *Communication Disorders Quarterly*, *34*(4), 210–220. https://doi.org/10.1177/1525740113484965

Hair, A., Ballard, K. J., Ahmed, B., & Gutierrez-Osuna, R. (2019). *Evaluating automatic speech recognition for child speech therapy applications*. The 21st International Conference on Computers and Accessibility, Pittsburgh, PA, USA. Journal ACM Transactions on Accessible Computing. https://doi.org/10.1145/3308561.3354606

Hayiou-Thomas, M. E., Carroll, J. M., Leavett, R., Hulme, C., & Snowling, M. J. (2017). When does speech sound disorder matter for literacy? The role of disordered speech errors, co-occurring language impairment and family risk of dyslexia. *Journal of Child Psychology and Psychiatry, and Allied Disciplines*, *58*(2), 197–205. https://doi.org/10.1111/jcpp.12648

Heng, Q., McCabe, P., Clarke, J., & Preston, J. L. (2016). Using ultrasound visual feedback to remediate velar fronting in preschool children: A pilot study. *Clinical Linguistics & Phonetics*, *30*(3–5), 382–397. https://doi.org/10.3109/02699206.2015.1120345

Hill, A. J., Russell, T. G., Cahill, L. M., Ward, E. C., & Clark, K. M. (2006). An internet-based telerehabilitation system for the assessment of motor speech disorders: A pilot study. *American*

Journal of Speech-Language Pathology, 15(1), 45–56. https://doi.org/10.1044/1058-0360(2006/006)

Hoffman, L. M., Ireland, M., Hall-Mills, S., & Flynn, P. (2013). Evidence-based speech-language pathology practices in schools: Findings from a national survey. *Language, Speech, and Hearing Services in Schools, 44*(3), 266–280. https://doi.org/10.1044/0161-1461(2013/12-0041)

Hoffman, T., Bennett, S., & Del Mar, C. (2017). *Evidence-based practice across the health professions.* Elsevier.

Hoover, W. A., & Tunmer, W. E. (2020). *The cognitive foundations of reading and its acquisition: A framework with applications connecting teaching and learning.* Springer.

Hutcheson, K. A. (2017). Developing a clinical question into a research question: The "use it or lose it" example. *Perspectives of the ASHA Special Interest Groups, 2*(13), 147–154. https://doi.org/10.1044/persp2.SIG13.147

Jessiman, S. M. (2003). Speech and language services using telehealth technology in remote and underserviced areas. *Journal of Speech-Language Pathology and Audiology, 27*(1), 45–51. https://www.cjslpa.ca/files/2003_JSLPA_Vol_27/No_01_1-92/Jessiman_JSLPA_2003.pdf

Kabakoff, H., Harel, D., Tiede, M., Whalen, D. H., & McAllister, T. (2021). Extending ultrasound tongue shape complexity measures to speech development and disorders. *Journal of Speech, Language, and Hearing Research, 64*(7), 2557–2574. https://doi.org/10.1044/2021_JSLHR-20-00537

Kilpatrick, D. (2015). *Essentials of assessing, preventing, and overcoming reading difficulties.* John Wiley & Sons., Inc.

Kollia, B., & Tsiamtsiouris, J. (2021). Influence of the COVID-19 pandemic on telepractice in speech-language pathology. *Journal of Prevention & Intervention in the Community, 49*(2), 152–162. https://doi.org/10.1080/10852352.2021.1908210

Kuh, G. D. (2008). *High-impact educational practices: What they are, who has access to them, and why they matter.* Association of American Colleges and Universities.

Kuschmann, A., Nayar, R., Lowit, A., & Dunlop, M. (2021). The use of technology in the management of children with phonological delay and adults with acquired dysarthria: A UK survey of current speech-language pathology practice. *International Journal*

of Speech-Language Pathology, 23(2), 145–154. https://doi.org/10.1080/17549507.2020.1750700

Lancaster, G., Keusch, S., Levin, A., Pring, T., & Martin, S. (2010). Treating children with phonological problems: Does an eclectic approach to therapy work? *International Journal of Language & Communication Disorders, 45*(2), 174–181. https://doi.org/10.1080/13682820902818888

Lave, J., & Wenger, E. (1991). *Situated learning: Legitimate peripheral participation.* Cambridge University Press.

Lee, A. S. Y., Law, J., & Gibbon, F. E. (2009). Electropalatography for articulation disorders associated with cleft palate. *Cochrane Database of Systematic Reviews,* (3). https://doi.org/10.1002/14651858.CD006854.pub2

Lee, S. A. (2018). The treatment efficacy of multiple opposition phonological approach via telepractice for two children with severe phonological disorders in rural areas of West Texas in the USA. *Child Language Teaching and Therapy, 34*(1), 63–78. https://doi.org/10.1177/0265659018755527

Leitão, S., & Fletcher, J. (2004). Literacy outcomes for students with speech disorders: Longterm follow-up. *International Journal of Language & Communication Disorders, 39*(2), 245–256. https://doi.org/10.1080/13682820310001619478

Lundeborg Hammarström, I., Svensson, R. M., & Myrberg, K. (2019). A shift of treatment approach in speech language pathology services for children with speech sound disorders–a single case study of an intense intervention based on non-linear phonology and motor-learning principles. *Clinical Linguistics & Phonetics, 33*(6), 518–531. https://doi.org/10.1080/02699206.2018.1552990

Maas, E., Robin, D. A., Hula, S. N. A., Freedman, S. E., Wulf, G., Ballard, K. J., & Schmidt, R. A. (2008). Principles of motor learning in treatment of motor speech disorders. *American Journal of Speech-Language Pathology, 17*(3), 277–298. https://doi.org/10.1044/1058-0360(2008/025)

Martin, P., Lizarondo, L., & Kumar, S. (2017). A systematic review of the factors that influence the quality and effectiveness of telesupervision for health professionals. *Journal of Telemedicine and Telecare, 24*(4), 271–281. https://doi.org/10.1177/1357633×17698868

Masso, S., Baker, E., McLeod, S., & Wang, C. (2017). Polysyllable speech accuracy and predictors of later literacy development in preschool children with speech sound disorders. *Journal of Speech, Language & Hearing Research, 60*(7), 1887–1890. https://doi.org/10.1044/2017_JSLHR-S-16-0171

McAllister Byun, T., Campbell, H., Carey, H., Liang, W., Park, T. H., & Svirsky, M. (2017). Enhancing intervention for residual rhotic errors via app-delivered biofeedback: A case study. *Journal of Speech, Language, and Hearing Research, 60*(6S), 1810–1817. https://doi.org/10.1044/2017_JSLHR-S-16-0248

McAllister Byun, T. M. (2017). Efficacy of visual–Acoustic biofeedback intervention for residual rhotic errors: A single-subject randomization study. *Journal of Speech, Language, and Hearing Research, 60*(5), 1175–1193. https://doi.org/10.1044/2016_JSLHR-S-16-0038

McAllister, T., Preston, J. L., Hitchcock, E. R., & Hill, J. (2020). Protocol for correcting residual errors with spectral, ultrasound, traditional speech therapy randomized controlled trial (C-RESULTS RCT). *BMC Pediatrics, 20*(1), 66. https://doi.org/10.1186/s12887-020-1941-5

McComas, K. L. (2014). Dig your heels in and fight! How women become researchers in communication sciences and disorders. J & R Press.

McCurtin, A., & O'Connor, A. (2020). Building a collaborative research community of practice and supporting research engagement in speech-language pathology: Identification of stakeholder priorities. *JBI Evidence Implementation, 18*(4), 368–375. https://doi.org/10.1097/xeb.0000000000000229

McCurtin, A., & Roddam, H. (2012). Evidence-based practice: SLTs under siege or opportunity for growth? The use and nature of research evidence in the profession. *International Journal of Language and Communication Disorders, 47*(1), 11–26. https://doi.org/10.1111/j.1460-6984.2011.00074.x

McLeod, S. (2012). *Multilingual children's speech.* Charles Sturt University. http://www.csu.edu.au/research/multilingual-speech

Modha, G., Bernhardt, B. M., Church, R., & Bacsfalvi, P. (2008). Case study using ultrasound to treat /ɹ. *International Journal of Language & Communication Disorders, 43*(3), 323–329. https://doi.org/10.1080/13682820701449943

Mundy, I. R., & Hannant, P. (2020). Exploring the phonological profiles of children with reading difficulties: A multiple case study. *Dyslexia, 26*(4), 441–426. https://doi.org/10.1002/dys.1667

Nagarajan, S., McAllister, L., McFarlane, L., Hall, M., Schmitz, C., Roots, R., Drynan, D., Avery, L., Murphy, S., & Lam, M. (2016). Telesupervision benefits for placements: Allied health students' and supervisors' perceptions. *International Journal of Practice-Based Learning in Health and Social Care, 4*(1), 16–27. https://doi.org/10.18552/ijpblhsc.v4i1.326

Nathan, L., Stackhouse, J., Goulandris, N., & Snowling, M. J. (2004). The development of early literacy skills among children with speech difficulties: A test of the "critical age hypothesis". *Journal of Speech, Language & Hearing Research, 47*(2), 377–391. https://doi.org/10.1044/1092-4388(2004/031)

Nation, K. (2019). Children's reading difficulties, language, and reflections on the simple view of reading. *Australian Journal of Learning Difficulties, 24*(1), 47–73. https://doi.org/10.1080/19404158.2019.1609272

National Reading Panel. (2000). *Report of the National Reading Panel: Teaching children to read: An evidence-based assessment of the scientific research literature on reading and its implications for reading instruction.* National Institute of Child Health and Human Development.

Nicholson, T. (1993). The case against context. In G. B. Thompson, W. E. Tunmer, & T. Nicholson (Eds.), *Language and education library, 4. Reading acquisition processes* (pp. 91–104). Multilingual Matters.

Norton, E., & Wolf, M. (2012). Rapid automatized naming (RAN) and reading fluency: Implications for understanding and treatment of reading disabilities. *Annual Review of Psychology, 63,* 427–452. http://doi.org/10/1146/annurev-psych-120710-100431

O'Brien, M. G., Derwing, T. M., Cucchiarini, C., Hardison, D. M., Mixdorff, H., Thomson, R. I., Strik, H., Levis, J. M., Munro, M. J., Foote, J. A., & Levis, G. M. (2018). Directions for the future of technology in pronunciation research and teaching. *Journal of Second Language Pronunciation, 4*(2), 182–207. https://doi.org/10.1075/jslp.17001.obr

Odabaş, M. (2022). *5 facts about Twitter lurkers.* Pew Research Center. Pew Research. https://www.pewresearch.org/fact-tank/2022/03/16/5-facts-about-twitter-lurkers

Olswang, L. B., & Prelock, P. A. (2015). Bridging the gap between research and practice: Implementation science. *Journal of Speech, Language, and Hearing Research, 58*(6), S1818–S1826. https://doi.org/10.1044/2015_JSLHR-L-14-0305

Olszewski, A., Smith, E., & Franklin, A. D. (2022). Speech-language pathologists' feelings and practices regarding technological apps in school service delivery. *Language, Speech, and Hearing Services in Schools, 53*(4), 1051–1073. https://doi.org/10.1044/2022_LSHSS-21-00150

Overby, M., Carrell, T., & Bernthal, J. (2007). Teachers' perceptions of students with speech sound disorders. *Language, Speech & Hearing Services in Schools, 38*(4), 327–341. https://doi.org/10.1044/0161-1461(2007/035)

Overby, M. S., & Baft-Neff, A. (2017). Perceptions of telepractice pedagogy in speech-language pathology: A quantitative analysis. *Journal of Telemedicine and Telecare, 23*(5), 550–557. https://doi.org/10.1177/1357633x16655939

Pasupathy, R., & Bogschutz, R. J. (2013). An investigation of graduate speech-language pathology students' SLP clinical self-efficacy. *Contemporary Issues in Communication Science and Disorders, 40*, 151–159. https://doi.org/10.1044/cicsd_40_f_151

Patrick, M. D. (2019). Myths that prevent medical professionals from engaging. In D. R. Stukus, M. D. Patrick, & K. E. Nuss (Eds.), *Social media for medical professionals*. Springer, Cham. https://doi.org/10.1007/978-3-030-14439-5_3

Paul, R., & Norbury, C. F. (2012). *Language disorders form infancy to adolescence* (4th ed.). Elsevier.

Peterson, L., Savarese, C., Campbell, T., Ma, Z., Simpson, K. O., & McAllister, T. (2022). Telepractice treatment of residual rhotic errors using app-based biofeedback: A pilot study. *Language, Speech, and Hearing Services in Schools, 53*(2), 256–274. https://doi.org/10.1044/2021_LSHSS-21-00084

Preston, J. L., Brick, N., & Landi, N. (2013). Ultrasound Biofeedback Treatment for Persisting Childhood Apraxia of Speech. *American Journal of Speech-Language Pathology, 22*(4), 627–643. https://doi.org/10.1044/1058-0360(2013/12-0139)

Preston, J. L., Hitchcock, E. R., & Leece, M. C. (2020). Auditory perception and ultrasound biofeedback treatment outcomes for children with residual /ɹ/ distortions: A randomized controlled trial. *Journal of Speech, Language, and Hearing Research, 63*(2), 444–455. https://doi.org/10.1044/2019_JSLHR-19-00060

Preston, J. L., Maas, E., Whittle, J., Leece, M. C., & McCabe, P. (2016). Limited acquisition and generalisation of rhotics with ultrasound visual feedback in childhood apraxia. *Clinical Linguistics & Phonetics, 30*(3–5), 363–381. https://doi.org/10.3109/02699206.2015.1052563

Roberts, M. Y., Sone, B. J., Zanzinger, K. E., Bloem, M. E., Kulba, K., Schaff, A., Davis, K. C., Reisfeld, N., &

Goldstein, H. (2020). Trends in clinical practice research in ASHA journals: 2008–2018. *American Journal of Speech-Language Pathology, 29*(3), 1629–1639. https://doi.org/10.1044/2020_AJSLP-19-00011

Rothman, A. J. (2004). "Is there nothing more practical than a good theory?": Why innovations and advances in health behavior change will arise if interventions are used to test and refine theory. *The International Journal of Behavioral Nutrition and Physical Activity, 1*(1), 11. https://doi.org/10.1186/1479-5868-1-11

Roxburgh, Z., Cleland, J., Scobbie, J. M., & Wood, S. E. (2021). Quantifying changes in ultrasound tongue-shape pre- and post-intervention in speakers with submucous cleft palate: An illustrative case study. *Clinical Linguistics & Phonetics*, 1–19. https://doi.org/10.1080/02699206.2021.1973566

Royal College of Speech and Language Therapists (2015). *Research priorities*. https://www.rcslt.org/members/research/research-priorities

Rvachew, S. (2007). Phonological processing and reading in children with speech sound disorders. *American Journal of Speech-Language Pathology, 16*(3), 260–270. https://doi.org/1058-0360/07/1603-260

Rvachew, S., & Brosseau-Lapré, F. (2018). *Developmental phonological disorders: Foundations of clinical practice* (2nd ed.). Plural Publishing.

Scarborough, H. (2001). Connecting early language and literacy to later reading (dis)abilities: Evidence, theory, and practice. In S. Neuman & D. Dickinson (Eds.), *Handbook of early literacy research* (pp. 97-110). Guilford Press.

Scarborough, H., Ehri, L., Olson, R., & Fowler, A. (1998). The fate of phoneme awareness beyond the early school years. *Scientific Studies of Reading, 2*(2), 115–142. https://doi.org/10.1207/s1532799xssr0202_2

Shriberg, L. D., Aram, D. M., & Kwiatkowski, J. (1997). Developmental apraxia of speech: I. Descriptive and theoretical perspectives. *Journal of Speech, Language, and Hearing Research, 40*(2), 273–85. https://doi.org/10.1044/jslhr.4002.273

Shriberg, L. D., Campbell, T. F., Mabie, H. L., & McGlothlin, J. H. (2019). Initial studies of the phenotype and persistence of speech motor delay (SMD). *Clinical Linguistics & Phonetics, 8*(33), 737–756. https://doi.org/10.1080/02699206.2019.1595733

Shriberg, L. D., Fourakis, M., Hall, S., Karlsson, H. K., Lohmeier, H. L., McSweeny, J., Potter, N. L.,

Scheer-Cohen, A. R., Strand, E. A., Tilkens, C. M., & Wilson, D. L. (2010). Extensions to the speech disorders classification system (SDCS). *Clinical Linguistics & Phonetics, 24*(10), 795–824. https://doi.org/10.3109/02699206.2010.503006

Shriberg, L. D., Potter, N. L., & Strand, E. A. (2011). Prevalence and phenotype of childhood apraxia of speech in youth with galactosemia. *Journal of Speech, Language, and Hearing Research, 54*(2), 487–519. https://doi.org/10.1044/1092-4388(2010/10-0068)

Skeat, J., & Roddam, H. (2019). The qualCAT: Applying a rapid review approach to qualitative research to support clinical decision-making in speech language pathology practice. *Evidence-Based Communication Assessment and Intervention, 13*(12), 3–14. https://doi.org/10.1080/1748 9539.2019.1600292

Smith, J., Levicks, P., Neilson, R., Mensah, F., Goldfield, S., & Bryson, H. (2021). Prevalence of language and pre-literacy difficulties in an Australian cohort of 5-year-old children experiencing adversity. *International Journal of Language & Communication Disorders, 56*(2), 389–401. https://doi.org/10.1111/1460-6984.12611

Snow, P. C. (2016). Elizabeth Usher memorial lecture: Language is literacy is language – Positioning speech-language pathology in education policy, practice, paradigms, and polemics. *International Journal of Speech-Language Pathology, 18*(3), 216–228. https://doi.org/10.3109/17549507.2015.1 112837

Snowling, M. J., Gallagher, A., & Frith, U. (2003). Family risk of dyslexia is continuous: Individual differences in the precursors of reading skill. *Child Development, 74*(2), 358–373. https://doi.org/10. 1111/1467-8624.7402003

Spek, B., Wieringa-de Waard, M., Lucas, C., & Van Dijk, N. (2013). Teaching evidence-based practice (EBP) to speech–language therapy students: Are students competent and confident EBP users? *International Journal of Language & Communication Disorders, 48*(4), 444–452. https://doi.org/10.1111/1460-6984.12020

Stainthorp, R. (2020). A national intervention in teaching phonics: A case study from England. *The Educational and Developmental Psychologist, 37*(2), 114–122. https://doi.org/10.1017/edp.2020.14

Storkel, H. L. (2018). The complexity approach to phonological treatment: How to select treatment targets. *Language, Speech, and Hearing Services in Schools, 49*(3), 463–481. https://doi.org/10.1044/2017_lshss-17-0082

Sugden, E., Lloyd, S., Lam, J., & Cleland, J. (2019). Systematic review of ultrasound visual biofeedback in intervention for speech sound disorders. *International Journal of Language & Communication Disorders, 54*(5), 705–728. https://doi.org/10.1111/1460-6984.12478

Sutherland, R., Trembath, D., Hodge, A., Drevensek, S., Lee, S., Silove, N., & Roberts, J. (2017). Telehealth language assessments using consumer grade equipment in rural and urban settings: Feasible, reliable, and well tolerated. *Journal of Telemedicine and Telecare, 23*(1), 106–115. https://doi.org/10.1177/1357633×15623921

Taylor, O. D., Armfield, N. R., Dodrill, P., & Smith, A. C. (2014). A review of the efficacy and effectiveness of using telehealth for paediatric speech and language assessment. *Journal of Telemedicine and Telecare, 20*(7), 405–412. https://doi.org/10.1177/1357633×14552388

Terry, D. R., Nguyen, H., Peck, B., Smith, A., & Phan, H. (2020). Communities of practice: A systematic review and meta-synthesis of what it means and how it really works among nursing students and novices. *Journal of Clinical Nursing, 29*(3–4), 370–380. https://doi.org/10.1111/jocn.15100

Thomas, D. C., McCabe, P., Ballard, K. J., & Lincoln, M. (2016). Telehealth delivery of rapid syllable transitions (ReST) treatment for childhood apraxia of speech. *International Journal of Language & Communication Disorders, 51*(6), 654–671. https://doi.org/10.1111/1460-6984.12238

Thome, E. K., Loveall, S. J., & Henderson, D. E. (2020). A survey of speech-language pathologists' understanding and reported use of evidence-based practice. *Perspectives of the ASHA Special Interest Groups, 5*(4), 984–999. https://doi.org/10.1044/2020_persp-20-00008

Thomson, L., Schneider, J., & Wright, N. (2013). Developing communities of practice to support the implementation of research into clinical practice. *Leadership in Health Services, 26*(1), 20–33. https://doi.org/10.1108/17511871311291705

Turkstra, L. S., Norman, R., Whyte, J., Dijkers, M. P., & Hart, T. (2016). Knowing what we're doing: Why specification of treatment methods is critical for evidence-based practice in speech-language pathology. *American Journal of Speech-Language Pathology, 25*(2), 164–171. https://doi.org/10.1044/2015_ajslp-15-0060

Twohey, M. (2013). *The Child Exchange: Inside America's underground market for adopted children.* Reuters. https://www.reuters.com/investigates/adoption/#

article/part1 and https://www.reuters.com/investigates/adoption/#article/part2

Waite, M. C., Cahill, L. M., Theodoros, D. G., Busuttin, S., & Russell, T. G. (2006). A pilot study of online assessment of childhood speech disorders. *Journal of Telemedicine and Telecare, 12*(Suppl. 3), 92–94. https://doi.org/10.1258/135763306779380048

Waite, M. C., Theodoros, D. G., Russell, T. G., & Cahill, L. M. (2012). Assessing children's speech intelligibility and oral structures, and functions via an Internet-based telehealth system. *Journal of Telemedicine and Telecare, 18*(4), 198–203. https://doi.org/10.1258/jtt.2012.111116

Wales, D., Skinner, L., & Hayman, M. (2017). The efficacy of telehealth-delivered speech and language intervention for primary school-age children: A systematic review. *International Journal of Telerehabilitation, 9*(1), 55–70. https://doi.org/10.5195/ijt.2017.6219

Wegner, E., McDermott, R., & Snyder, W. (2002). *Cultivating communities of practice: A guide to managing knowledge.* Harvard Business School Press. 2002.

Wegner, E., & Snyder, W. (2000, January-February). Communities of practice: The organizational frontier. *Harvard Business Review*, 139–145. https://hbr.org/2000/01/communities-of-practice-the-organizational-frontier

Wenger, E. (1998). *Communities of practice: Learning, meaning, and identity.* Cambridge University Press.

Werfel, K. L., Grey, B., Johnson, M., Brooks, M., Cooper, E., Reynolds, G., ... Lund, E. A. (2021). Transitioning speech-language assessment to a virtual environment: Lessons learned from the ELLA study. *Language, Speech, and Hearing Services in Schools, 52*(3), 769–775. https://doi.org/10.1044/2021_LSHSS-20-00149

White, S., Raghavendra, P., & McAllister, S. (2017). Letting the CAT out of the bag: Contribution of critically appraised topics to evidence-based practice. *Evidence-Based Communication Assessment and Intervention, 11*(1–2), 27–37. https://doi.org/10.1080/17489539.2017.1333683

Williams, A. L. (2016). *SCIP 2: Sound contrasts in phonology 2 (1.0)* [mobile application Software]. App Store. https://itunes.apple.com

Wium, A.-M., & Louw, B. (2018). Mixed-methods research: A tutorial for speech-language therapists and audiologists in South Africa. *South African Journal of Communication Disorders, 65*(1). https://doi.org/10.4102/sajcd.v65i1.573

Wood, S. E., Timmins, C., Wishart, J., Hardcastle, W. J., & Cleland, J. (2019). Use of electropalatography in the treatment of speech disorders in children with Down syndrome: A randomized controlled trial. *International Journal of Language & Communication Disorders, 54*(2), 234–248. https://doi.org/10.1111/1460-6984.12407

Wrench, A. & Scobbie, J. (2006). *Spatio-temporal inaccuracies of video-based ultrasound images of the tongue.* Proceedings of the 7th International Seminar on Speech Production, 451–458. CASL, Queen Margaret University. https://eresearch.qmu.ac.uk/bitstream/handle/20.500.12289/2151/wrench_ISSP2006.pdf?sequence=1&isAllowed=y

Zipoli, R. P., Jr., & Kennedy, M. (2005). Evidence-based practice among speech-language pathologists: Attitudes, utilization, and barriers. *American Journal of Speech-Language Pathology, 14*(3), 208–220. https://doi.org/10.1044/1058-0360(2005/021)

Chapter 12
Change

This book contains a distillation of international research into typical and atypical speech development, and clinical practice in 'child speech', from the profession's inception until late 2022, with a few references with a 2023 or 2024 publication date. It spans aspects of acquisition, assessment, analysis, classification, and diagnosis of SSD; its co-occurring conditions, its consequences; and SSD-related service delivery, research dissemination and implementation science.

The work stems largely from three convictions. First, that competent, committed SLP/SLT students and clinicians want, need, and value clearly stated theory, well-grounded evidence, realistic implications for practice, and guidance for implementation in busy, real-world settings. Second – and this is more a hope than a conviction – that they like seeing these things in their historical context. And third, that clinical researchers and teaching faculty want the outcomes of their labours, built on prior scholarship, to be appreciated and used by those at the clinical coalface.

It is also grounded in personal clinical experience and an understanding that the threefold basis of good clinical thinking and decision-making is solid theory, robust evidence, and unambiguous principles of practice, with the client centre-stage. This achievable trifecta works best when individualized service provision focuses, at any given moment, on each unique client-and-family combination. To this end, respectful, holistic, explicitly principled ethical practice takes account of the impact of SSD on children's and their families' lives, emotions, and participation in society.

From Foundational Knowledge to Innovative Practices

The book incorporates foundational knowledge and research evidence from our own, and allied disciplines, alongside well-supported theoretical perspectives, and established principles of practice. These are coupled with practical approaches, procedures, techniques, and activities that SLPs/SLTs can apply flexibly as scientific clinicians, working with children with SSD and their caregivers. There is also information about nascent, emerging, and evolving areas of practice, and newer approaches to service delivery – particularly telepractice – necessitated by the COVID-19 pandemic among other catalysts.

Children's Speech Sound Disorders, Third Edition. Caroline Bowen.
© 2023 John Wiley & Sons Ltd. Published 2023 by John Wiley & Sons Ltd.

Innovation was the name of the game when everyone involved with SSD navigated the 'new normal' (Caffery et al., 2022) of COVID-times, stretching from December 2019. Everybody faced change whether they were children, families (Rodríguez-García & de la Mano-rodero, 2022), clinicians (Overby, 2023), or faculty and SLP/SLT students (Ng, 2023).

> *The profound effects of COVID-19 may change how future speech-language pathology students are educated. COVID-19 appeared to be a catalyst for technological advancement in university teaching and learning, as well as telepractice and simulation in clinical education. The transition of clinical teaching and learning accelerated by COVID-19, though seemingly intimidating, gave the global community of speech-language pathology educators an opportunity to go through a steep learning curve by trial and error. This has had benefits and drawbacks. Telepractice may improve access to and cost-effectiveness of healthcare. Yet technological infrastructure issues and personal data protection concerns should be adequately addressed for sustainable development of this service delivery mode.*
>
> Janet Ho-yee Ng, 2023, p. 236

Behind These Pages

When *Children's Speech Sound Disorders 3e* was commissioned in early 2020, everyone swung into gear: publisher, author, and the invited contributors. SARS-CoV-2 already loomed large in the news, but no one foresaw that the writing, editing, and production process, and our work practices, homelives, relationships, and selves would be impacted so broadly by the so-called interesting times.

In the collaborative writing and editing process, my appreciation grew for the steady handed editorial and production teams, and the contributors who displayed a combination of professionalism, resilience, and dedication, despite vying with the pandemic. Drawing on these qualities, the contributors tackled their topics deftly, conveying information straightforwardly, without oversimplifying or reducing academic rigour.

Evidence-based Guidelines and High-quality Care

Writing the contributions was a noteworthy achievement, as it is difficult for anyone – no matter their interest and expertise – to detail the essence of a large research agenda, or a significant body of work in 2,000 or so words, with the aim of providing readable, detailed-enough information for time-poor clinicians (Greenwell & Walsh, 2021) with full workloads, for whom reading the literature may be a rare or rationed luxury.

A common aspect of the contributions was that their authors cited evidence. When researchers publish work that is associated with robust, clinically applicable evidence, the concepts of research dissemination and implementation science are rarely far from their thoughts.

> *Implementation Science is the scientific study of methods to promote knowledge translation/the uptake of research and evidence-based guidelines into practice. The primary aim of Implementation Science is to improve the quality of clinical practice, and this often includes the study of healthcare professionals and organization behaviour/attitude, economic feasibility, and sustainability as well as clinical practice itself. Implementation Science has become increasingly popular in recent years with its focus on effective clinical changes in our economically challenged workplaces. All clinical researchers should be considering knowledge translation in their research programme designs to ensure that their research findings can be implemented as quickly and effectively as possible.*
>
> Miles, 2020, p. 1

Aside from a subset of academic entrepreneurs (Wurth et al., 2015), most researchers probably hope that once their work has been disseminated, and practitioners have read and understood its clinical implications, it will become common practice, so augmenting high-quality care. Unfortunately, research disseminationt can founder, and uptake by practitioners may be slow or non-existent. This means that common practice – some of it unproven, and pointless – can remain fixed in clinicians' repertoires. This does nothing to enhance client care.

When SLPs/SLTs say their work is fulfilling, or that they constantly learn from their clients, it probably means that they are delivering high quality care, driven by strong theory, evidence, and principles of practice. Moreover, those who are fortunate enough to work closely with other SLPs/SLTs and/or with a team of colleagues in other disciplines – medicine, for example – likely experience constant learning opportunities too, particularly around implementation science.

Don't Just do Something, Stand There

Examples of common practice, such as SLPs/SLTs using articulation intervention for phonological disorder (Joffe, A23) or perhaps less commonly now, NSOME to improve intelligibility (Lof, A24), attract pejorative descriptors within medicine. There, they are referred to as *entrenched practice* and *ineffective and untested practice* (Prasad & Ioannidis, 2014), *low value practices* (Farmer et al., 2022), *'things we do for no reason'* (Feldman, 2015), and *low-value care* (Keijzers et al., 2018, with the unexpected title 'don't just do something, stand there!'.

Verkerk et al. (2018) made an obvious link between the components of EBP versus low-value care, defining it as *'care that is unlikely to benefit the patient given the harms, cost, available alternatives, or preferences of the patient'* (p. 737). Accordingly, they devised a 3-way typology which is highly applicable to SLP/SLT practice, with the low-value care types corresponding with their reason for being of low-value:

- **Ineffectiveness** e.g., in terms of inappropriate treatment, uneconomic distribution of resources, or over-servicing.
- **Inefficiency** e.g., too low intensity and/or too low frequency to 'work'.
- **Unwantedness** i.e., effective, but remote from the client's preferences.

The authors explain the last category as follows:

...unwanted care...is of low value from the patients' perspective. Like 'inefficient care' it is in essence effective for the targeted condition

but becomes low value because it does not solve the individual patient's problem or does not fit the individual patient's preferences. Examples are vaccines and blood transfusions for patients with certain religious beliefs, chemotherapy for a patient that prefers palliative care, or surgery while the patient prefers conservative treatment. This category is probably the least well-known and least well-studied type of low-value care because it can only be identified and measured by assessing the patient's values.

Verkerk et al., 2018, p. 728

Seeing low-value care as a mounting phenomenon in western countries, Verkerk and colleagues' objective was to stimulate debate and encourage efforts to de-implement (stop delivering) inappropriate, ineffective, unproven, overused, harmful, and/or low-value health services and practices. They were strong advocates for de-implementation because they pictured it easing patient harm, refining processes of care, and lessening healthcare costs (cf., Norton et al., 2017).

Verkerk et al. (2018) also posited that different types of low-value care might require different, explicitly principled de-implementation strategies.

Abandoning ineffective medical practices and mitigating the risks of untested practices are important for improving patient health and containing healthcare costs. Historically, this process has relied on the evidence base, societal values, cultural tensions, and political sway, but not necessarily in that order. We propose a conceptual framework to guide and prioritize this process, shifting emphasis toward the principles of evidence-based medicine, acknowledging that evidence may still be misinterpreted or distorted by recalcitrant proponents of entrenched practices and other biases.

Prasad and Ioannidis, 2014, p. 1

De-implementation, and change away from entrenched practices, is a demanding process (Nicoll et al., 2021) that has been scrutinized through various lenses. For example, Montini and Graham (2015) unpacked historical, economic, professional, and social resistance to de-implementation of established practices.

De-implementing Customary SSD Practice in Scotland

In Scotland, Nicoll et al. (2021) conducted a retrospective case-based qualitative study of how treatment for SSD (called 'child speech' in the report) had changed across three National Health Service (NHS) SLT agencies (represented by 39 interviewees) and private practice (a further three interviewees). They focused on newer, evidence-based treatment approaches, dubbed 'non-traditional interventions' that had featured for decades in SLP/SLT research literature but that were not routinely practised, concluding that for clinicians:

> *Achieving coherence with these interventions was intellectually demanding because they challenged the traditional linguistic assumptions underpinning routine practice. Implementation was also logistically demanding, and therapists felt they had little agency to vary what was locally conventional for their service. In addition, achieving coherence took considerable relational work. Non-traditional interventions were often difficult to explain to children and parents, involved culturally uncomfortable repetitive drills and required therapists to do more tailoring of intervention for individual children.*
>
> Nicoll et al., 2021, p. 1

The Positives and Negatives of Business as Usual in SLP/SLT

On the positive side, in SLP/SLT, the terms 'common practice', 'everyday practice', and 'business as usual' apply to something that is typically or routinely done, because:

- The SLP/SLT is honouring the EBP principles of objective, balanced, responsible use of current research and the best available internal and external evidence, while respecting client preferences, to guide policy and practice decisions, such that consumer outcomes are improved. In simple terms, because there is evidence to show that it *does* work (Clark, 2003; Leitão, A1).
- Despite a limited evidence-base, its use can be justified ethically, based on its solid theoretical grounds, or because it *should* work (Clark, 2003; Leitão, A1).

By contrast, the disparaging terms – *entrenched*, *ineffective*, and *untested practice*, 'things we do for no reason', and *low-value care* – apply to SLP/SLT assessment and intervention practices, and caseload management approaches, that are implemented:

- As a habit or appeal to tradition, and/or
- To match workplace policy, or to meet cultural, societal, or political expectations, and/or
- Because practitioners do not know about, or do not acknowledge alternatives that are associated with more robust theory and/or stronger evidence, and/or
- Because an individual or organization is disinclined to relinquish it, and/or
- Because an individual practitioner 'just knows' it works (but cannot identify evidentiary support) or 'believes in it' (Gruber et al., 2003), and/or
- Because the necessary materials and equipment are readily to hand, and/or...
- ...in SLT child speech practice specifically, due to the perceived difficulty of the work involved in 'practice change' (Furlong et al., 2018; Nicoll, 2017).

Implementation Science: An Iterative Process

> *...the clinical researcher establishes the efficacy and then effectiveness of an innovation, and then hands it off to the implementation scientist to test ways of getting people to use it. This process as stated is overly simplistic because it suggests a unidimensional flow of tasks. [Really], the process is much more iterative as implementation experience may suggest changes in the clinical innovation to increase its external validity (while also taking steps to ensure fidelity to its core components, supporting internal validity).*
>
> Bauer and Kirchner, 2020

Establishing the effectiveness of a new methodology or treatment element is no guarantee of their routine adoption because contextual barriers can prevent it. Conversely, contextual facilitators can make it happen. Implementation science identifies and tackles such barriers and facilitators to enhance innovation uptake, or as Bauer and Kirchner say, 'to get people to use it'.

Researchers Would Likely Be Dismayed

Most researchers would likely be dismayed to learn that even after 20 years of research demonstrating good effectiveness for a given treatment, that treatment will remain unused by most clinicians, even when appropriate for the client at hand (Greenhalgh et al., 2004). Indeed, **the evidence on dissemination could not be clearer: Traditional methods** *such as conferences, clinical guidelines, and published journal articles repeatedly* **fall short** *as conduits for changing the behaviors of health care professionals (Beidas et al., 2012; Glasgow et al., 2012; Velligan et al., 2013). Practitioners require more than a published article to use an evidence-based practice (EBP).*

Douglas et al., 2015, p. S1827

Douglas and co-workers were dismayed, but not despairing. They identified facilitators that could increase the likelihood of an SLP/SLT choosing to implement evidence-based practices. Some of the strategies they found were informal knowledge sharing between the SLP/SLT and others, worksite coaching and mentoring, consistent access, for the SLP/SLT, to data relevant to implementation and feedback about their performance, open communication among workplace employees at every level, positive reinforcement, and organizational support. Such support could come from other SLPs/SLTs, workplace administrators, educational institutions and research centres, and professional organizations.

Asserting that these inputs were essential in advancing EBP use, Douglas et al. concluded that implementation science is not just a buzzword. Rather, they said is a gamechanger: '*a new field of study that can make a substantive contribution in communication sciences and disorders by informing research agendas, reducing health and education disparities, improving accountability and quality control, increasing clinician satisfaction and competence, and improving client outcomes.*' Furthermore, they declared that '*Exactly what factors enable a treatment to be used, how those factors should be addressed or managed, and the best practices for facilitating the use of an evidence-based treatment constitute the research agenda for implementation science.*'

Clinical SLPs/SLTs bear some responsibility for disappointing research dissemination and implementation, if they do not keep abreast of the evidence base, or learn to implement new interventions, for example. But the responsibility is not theirs alone. Resonating with Douglas et al. (2015): '*the evidence on dissemination could not be clearer: Traditional methods…fall short*', Feuerstein et al. (2022, p. 2) asked:

Why do we rely on what historically has been done, diffusion of evidence, rather than pursuing a more active approach to identifying the most salient and relevant content to share with audiences via their preferred mode of learning? The answers to these questions are complex and influenced by the systems in which researchers often conduct their work.

Practice Change

In their study, Nicoll et al. (2021) focused on practice change, as opposed to learning how to implement a new intervention. They found that when their SLT participants endeavoured to shift away from customary ('traditional') practice to adopting newer ('non-traditional') approaches to SSD they did so by

1. employing new approaches,
2. providing therapy more frequently for certain children, over a pre-set period,
3. trialling new approaches with certain children,
4. personalizing, or tailoring therapy to better meet individual children's needs,
5. training parents to implement the therapy, and
6. constantly tweaking the therapy to improve or revitalise it.

There were echoes, in the Nicoll and colleagues' results of Bauer and Kirchner (2020) who found that:

○ Practitioners' service setting or workplace – or context – was a powerful determinant of whether (or not) practice changes could happen.
○ Changing customary practice is hard work that requires careful planning.
○ Even if only one new intervention approach is under consideration, hearing or knowing about it is insufficient for implementation. To use it, the SLP/SLT must study and think about the

intervention itself, **candidacy**, **caseload**, and the **service**.

o First, considering the **intervention** includes knowing what is involved, learning necessary skills, planning how it can be organized, deciding whether it requires adaptation, and determining how it fits with everything else that occurs in the wider service context.

o In considering **candidacy** decisions must be made about who receives therapy and when.

o The **caseload** (how the SLP/SLT organizes their work) must be contemplated.

o Finally, thought must go into how the **service** might be impacted, e.g.,

• The costs of change to the service, and their likely duration – in weeks, months, or years.

• Modifications to treatment rooms to allow additional people to participate in sessions.

• Purchase of assessment and intervention materials and equipment.

• Fees for professional development or staff training.

• Time costs associated with capacity building.

Turning Typical Practice into Optimal Practice

In sum, SLPs'/SLTs' efforts to de-implement clinical practices supported by negligible evidence, in favour of practices with stronger efficiency, effects, efficacy, and effectiveness may be more successful and sustainable if **intervention**, **candidacy**, **caseload**, and **service** are well-thought-out at each step. Often, the process of refining what we do, practice change, and maintaining a personal best-practice attitude is probably easier within a mentor-mentee collaboration. In such two-way professional relationships, both parties stand to gain.

Of course, in the practice change process, across the board, for a client group, or for a single client, we are justly mindful of the client in their family and wider communicative milieu. When considering changing practice relative to a specific client, particularly if their progress is suboptimal, it is helpful to start with the four clinical questions about progress monitoring in children that were posed by Olswang and Bain (1994, p. 56) in a highly recommended article. The questions are repeated in boldface below, with my suggestions for supplementary questions:

• **Is the client responding to the treatment program?**
Are the targets I have chosen optimal for this client?
Would a treatment with a stronger evidence-base promote a stronger response?

• **Is significant, important change occurring?**
Have I gathered relevant data, or am I relying on clinical judgement?
Have I taken objective measurements that demonstrate any changes?
What have I measured?

• **Is treatment responsible for the change?**
Are threats to validity present: is treatment, or something else, evoking change?
Have treatment changes generalized to other untreated targets?
What is the nature of the generalization?

• **How long should a therapy target be treated?**
How much evidence of generalization is enough for *this* client?
What probes should I use?
Is the client's communicative milieu conducive to encouraging generalization?

The Last Words

In their thoughtful article about SLP/SLT practitioners adopting EBP, Greenwell and Walsh (2021) asked, 'where are we now?'. Predictably, they identified insufficient time for research (i.e., for reading and incorporating it into practice) and heavy workloads/caseloads as the most crushing barriers to EBP implementation. In an encouraging twist however, they also determined that participants who had experienced substantial EBP career training as students were less likely to perceive time as a barrier, and were more likely to apply, consistently, the components of EPB in their clinical practice.

These positive findings are potentially inspirational to the academics and clinical educators charged with the demanding task of preparing future SLPs/SLTs – the so-called SLP2b and SLT2b participants in social media – for the satisfactions, expectations and challenges of the workplace. It also fuels the profession's confidence in an optimistic future for SLP/SLT practice in general, and in practice with children with speech sound disorders specifically.

As evidenced here, SSD research and practice thrive, are rich in human and practical resources and goodwill, and exciting advances are ongoing. That is why the last words are *to be continued...*

References

Bauer, M. S., & Kirchner, J. (2020). Implementation science: What is it and why should I care? *Psychiatry Research*, *283*, 112376. https://doi.org/10.1016/j.psychres.2019.04.025

Beidas, R. S., Edmunds, J. M., Marcus, S. C., & Kendall, P. C. (2012). Training and consultation to promote implementation of an empirically supported treatment: A randomized trial. *Psychiatric Services (Washington, D.C.)*, *63*(7), 660–665. https://doi.org/10.1176/appi.ps.201100401

Caffery, L. A., Muurlink, O. T., & Taylor-Robinson, A. W. (2022). Survival of rural telehealth services post-pandemic in Australia: A call to retain the gains in the 'new normal'. *The Australian Journal of Rural Health*, *30*(4), 544–549. https://doi.org/10.1111/ajr.12877

Clark, H. M. (2003). Neuromuscular treatments for speech and swallowing: A tutorial. *American Journal of Speech-Language Pathology*, *12*(4), 400–415. https://doi.org/10.1044/1058-0360(2003/086)

Douglas, N. F., Campbell, W. N., & Hinckley, J. J. (2015). Implementation science: Buzzword or game changer? *Journal of Speech, Language, and Hearing Research*, *58*(6), S1827–S1836. https://doi.org/10.1044/2015_JSLHR-L-15-0302

Farmer, R., Zaheer, I., & Schulte, M. (2022). Disentangling low-value practices from pseudoscience in health service psychology. *Philosophical Psychology*. Advance online publication Advance onlineA. https://doi.org/10.1080/09515089.2022.2144193

Feldman, L. S. (2015). Choosing Wisely®: Things we do for no reason. *Journal of Hospital Medicine*, *10*(10), 696. https://doi.org/10.1002/jhm.2425

Feuerstein, J. L., Douglas, N. F., & Olswang, L. B. (2022). Dissemination research in communication sciences and disorders: A tutorial. *Journal of Speech, Language, and Hearing Research*, *65*(11), 4172–4180. https://doi.org/10.1044/2022_JSLHR-22-00421

Furlong, L., Serry, T., Erickson, S., & Morris, M. E. (2018). Processes and challenges in clinical decision-making for children with speech-sound disorders. *International Journal of Language & Communication Disorders*, *53*(6), 1124–1138. https://doi.org/10.1111/1460-6984.12426

Glasgow, R. E., Vinson, C., Chambers, D., Khoury, M. J., Kaplan, R. M., & Hunter, C. (2012). National institutes of health approaches to dissemination and implementation science: Current and future directions. *American Journal of Public Health*, *102*(7), 1274–1281. https://doi.org/10.2105/AJPH.2012.300755

Greenhalgh, T., Robert, G., Macfarlane, F., Bate, P., & Kyriakidou, O. (2004). Diffusion of innovations in service organizations: Systematic review and recommendations. *The Milbank Quarterly*, *82*(4), 581–629. https://doi.org/10.1111/j.0887-378x.2004.00325.x

Greenwell, T., & Walsh, B. (2021). Evidence-based practice in speech-language pathology: Where are we now? *American Journal of Speech-Language Pathology*, *30*(1), 186–198. https://doi.org/10.1044/2020_AJSLP-20-00194

Gruber, F. A., Lowery, S. D., Seung, H.-K., & Deal, R. (2003). Approaches to speech/language intervention and the true believer. *Journal of Medical Speech-Language Pathology*, *11*(2), 95–104. https://speech-language-therapy.com/pdf/truebelieverEBP.pdf

Keijzers, G., Cullen, L., Egerton-Warburton, D., & Fatovich, D. M. (2018). Don't just do something, stand there! The value and art of deliberate clinical inertia. *Emergency Medicine Australasia*, *EMA*, *30*(2), 273–278. https://doi.org/10.1111/1742-6723.12922

Miles, A. (2020). Tutorials in improving practice through implementation science. *Speech, Language and Hearing*, *23*(1), 1. https://doi.org/10.1080/2050571X.2020.1718328

Montini, T., & Graham, I. D. (2015). "Entrenched practices and other biases": Unpacking the historical, economic, professional, and social resistance to de-implementation. *Implementation Science*, *10*, 24. https://doi.org/10.1186/s13012-015-0211-7

Ng, J. H.-Y. (2023). COVID-19 impact on education and training. In L. Cummings (Ed.), *COVID-19 and speech-language pathology*. Routledge.

Nicoll, A. (2017). *Speech and language therapy in practice: A critical realist account of how and why speech and language therapists in community settings in Scotland have changed their intervention for children with speech sound disorders*. [Unpublished doctoral dissertation]. University of Stirling. https://dspace.stir.ac.uk/handle/1893/27257

Nicoll, A., Maxwell, M., & Williams, B. (2021). Achieving 'coherence' in routine practice: A qualitative case-based study to describe speech and language therapy interventions with implementation in mind. *Implementation Science Communications*, 2(1), 56. https://doi.org/10.1186/s43058-021-00159-0

Norton, W. E., Kennedy, A. E., & Chambers, D. A. (2017). Studying de-implementation in health: An analysis of funded research grants. *Implementation Science*, 12(1), 144. https://doi.org/10.1186/s13012-017-0655-z

Olswang, L. B., & Bain, B. (1994). Data collection: Monitoring children's treatment progress. *American Journal of Speech-Language Pathology*, 3(3), 55–65. https://doi.org/10.1044/1058-0360.0303.55

Overby, M. S. (2023). Telepractice in child speech-language pathology during COVID-19. In L. Cummings (Ed.), *COVID-19 and speech-language pathology*. Routledge.

Prasad, V., & Ioannidis, J. P. (2014). Evidence-based de-implementation for contradicted, unproven, and aspiring healthcare practices. *Implementation Science*, 9, 1. https://doi.org/10.1186/1748-5908-9-1

Rodríguez-García, L., & de la Mano-rodero, P. (2022). What we learn from listening to families in early childhood tele-intervention during the pandemic. *Perspectives of the ASHA Special Interest Groups*, 7(5), 1551–1566. https://doi.org/10.1044/2022_PERSP-22-00021

Velligan, D., Mintz, J., Maples, N., Xueying, L., Gajewski, S., Carr, H., & Sierra, C. (2013). A randomized trial comparing in person and electronic interventions for improving adherence to oral medications in schizophrenia. *Schizophrenia Bulletin*, 39(5), 999–1007. https://doi.org/10.1093/schbul/sbs116

Verkerk, E. W., Tanke, M. A. C., Kool, R. B., van Dulmen, S. A., & Westert, G. P. (2018). Limit, lean or listen? A typology of low-value care that gives direction in de-implementation. *International Journal for Quality in Health Care*, 30(9), 736–739. https://doi.org/10.1093/intqhc/mzy100

Wurth, B., Howick, S., & MacKenzie, N. (2015). *Research for research's sake? A critical reflection on the unintended consequences of academic entrepreneurship*. Paper presented at the University-Industry Interaction Conference, Berlin, Germany. Unpublished. https://tinyurl.com/muhd6zuj

Contributor Index

Subject Index

Children's Speech Sound Disorders, Third Edition. Caroline Bowen.
© 2023 John Wiley & Sons Ltd. Published 2023 by John Wiley & Sons Ltd.